Biomarkers of Tumor Metastasis and Invasiveness

Biomarkers of Tumor Metastasis and Invasiveness

Editors

Daniel L. Pouliquen
Cristina Núñez González

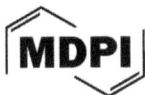

Basel • Beijing • Wuhan • Barcelona • Belgrade • Novi Sad • Cluj • Manchester

Editors
Daniel L. Pouliquen
Inserm U1307
CNRS UMR 6075, CRCI2NA
University of Angers
Angers
France

Cristina Núñez González
Facultade de Quimica
Universidade de Santiago
de Compostela
Santiago de Compostela
Spain

Editorial Office
MDPI
St. Alban-Anlage 66
4052 Basel, Switzerland

This is a reprint of articles from the Special Issue published online in the open access journal *Cancers* (ISSN 2072-6694) (available at: www.mdpi.com/journal/cancers/special_issues/metastasis_invasiveness).

For citation purposes, cite each article independently as indicated on the article page online and as indicated below:

Lastname, A.A.; Lastname, B.B. Article Title. *Journal Name* **Year**, *Volume Number*, Page Range.

ISBN 978-3-03928-590-7 (Hbk)
ISBN 978-3-0365-9999-1 (PDF)
doi.org/10.3390/books978-3-0365-9999-1

© 2024 by the authors. Articles in this book are Open Access and distributed under the Creative Commons Attribution (CC BY) license. The book as a whole is distributed by MDPI under the terms and conditions of the Creative Commons Attribution-NonCommercial-NoDerivs (CC BY-NC-ND) license.

Contents

About the Editors vii

Preface ix

Daniel L. Pouliquen and Cristina Núñez González
Biomarkers of Tumor Metastasis and Invasiveness
Reprinted from: *Cancers* 2023, 15, 5000, doi:10.3390/cancers15205000 1

Estefania Carrasco-Garcia, Lidia Lopez, Veronica Moncho-Amor, Fernando Carazo, Paula Aldaz and Manuel Collado et al.
SOX9 Triggers Different Epithelial to Mesenchymal Transition States to Promote Pancreatic Cancer Progression
Reprinted from: *Cancers* 2022, 14, 916, doi:10.3390/cancers14040916 5

Takehiro Tozuka, Rintaro Noro, Masahiro Seike and Kazufumi Honda
Benefits from Adjuvant Chemotherapy in Patients with Resected Non-Small Cell Lung Cancer: Possibility of Stratification by Gene Amplification of *ACTN4* According to Evaluation of Metastatic Ability
Reprinted from: *Cancers* 2022, 14, 4363, doi:10.3390/cancers14184363 25

Ishani H. Rao, Edmund K. Waller, Rohan K. Dhamsania and Sanjay Chandrasekaran
Gene Expression Analysis Links Autocrine Vasoactive Intestinal Peptide and ZEB1 in Gastrointestinal Cancers
Reprinted from: *Cancers* 2023, 15, 3284, doi:10.3390/cancers15133284 38

Qiwei Wu, Hsiang-i Tsai, Haitao Zhu and Dongqing Wang
The Entanglement between Mitochondrial DNA and Tumor Metastasis
Reprinted from: *Cancers* 2022, 14, 1862, doi:10.3390/cancers14081862 51

Daniel L. Pouliquen, Giacomo Ortone, Letizia Rumiano, Alice Boissard, Cécile Henry and Stéphanie Blandin et al.
Long-Chain Acyl Coenzyme A Dehydrogenase, a Key Player in Metabolic Rewiring/Invasiveness in Experimental Tumors and Human Mesothelioma Cell Lines
Reprinted from: *Cancers* 2023, 15, 3044, doi:10.3390/cancers15113044 69

Mitsunobu Oba, Yoshitsugu Nakanishi, Tomoko Mitsuhashi, Katsunori Sasaki, Kanako C. Hatanaka and Masako Sasaki et al.
CCR7 Mediates Cell Invasion and Migration in Extrahepatic Cholangiocarcinoma by Inducing Epithelial– Mesenchymal Transition
Reprinted from: *Cancers* 2023, 15, 1878, doi:10.3390/cancers15061878 86

Liangkun Huang, Fei Sun, Zilin Liu, Wenyi Jin, Yubiao Zhang and Junwen Chen et al.
Probing the Potential of Defense Response-Associated Genes for Predicting the Progression, Prognosis, and Immune Microenvironment of Osteosarcoma
Reprinted from: *Cancers* 2023, 15, 2405, doi:10.3390/cancers15082405 102

Hao Sun, Huibo Wang, Hongming Pan, Yanjiao Zuo, Ruihu Zhao and Rong Huang et al.
CD19 (+) B Cell Combined with Prognostic Nutritional Index Predicts the Clinical Outcomes of Patients with Gastric Cancer Who Underwent Surgery
Reprinted from: *Cancers* 2023, 15, 2531, doi:10.3390/cancers15092531 129

Mark Marsland, Amiee Dowdell, Sam Faulkner, Craig Gedye, James Lynam and Cassandra P. Griffin et al.
The Membrane Protein Sortilin Is a Potential Biomarker and Target for Glioblastoma
Reprinted from: *Cancers* 2023, *15*, 2514, doi:10.3390/cancers15092514 148

Chunyang Jiang, Mengyao Zhao, Shaohui Hou, Xiaoli Hu, Jinchao Huang and Hongci Wang et al.
The Indicative Value of Serum Tumor Markers for Metastasis and Stage of Non-Small Cell Lung Cancer
Reprinted from: *Cancers* 2022, *14*, 5064, doi:10.3390/cancers14205064 163

Katie Dunphy, Despina Bazou, Michael Henry, Paula Meleady, Juho J. Miettinen and Caroline A. Heckman et al.
Proteomic and Metabolomic Analysis of Bone Marrow and Plasma from Patients with Extramedullary Multiple Myeloma Identifies Distinct Protein and Metabolite Signatures
Reprinted from: *Cancers* 2023, *15*, 3764, doi:10.3390/cancers15153764 175

Li-Mei Chen and Karl X. Chai
Exosome-Mediated Activation of the Prostasin-Matriptase Serine Protease Cascade in B Lymphoma Cells
Reprinted from: *Cancers* 2023, *15*, 3848, doi:10.3390/cancers15153848 200

Marta Łukaszewicz-Zajac, Sara Paczek and Barbara Mroczko
A Disintegrin and Metalloproteinase (ADAM) Family—Novel Biomarkers of Selected Gastrointestinal (GI) Malignancies?
Reprinted from: *Cancers* 2022, *14*, 2307, doi:10.3390/cancers14092307 222

Marike S. Lombaers, Karlijn M. C. Cornel, Nicole C. M. Visser, Johan Bulten, Heidi V. N. Küsters-Vandevelde and Frédéric Amant et al.
Preoperative CA125 Significantly Improves Risk Stratification in High-Grade Endometrial Cancer
Reprinted from: *Cancers* 2023, *15*, 2605, doi:10.3390/cancers15092605 238

Fei-Yuan Yu, Qian Xu, Xiao-Yun Zhao, Hai-Ying Mo, Qiu-Hua Zhong and Li Luo et al.
The Atypical MAP Kinase MAPK15 Is Required for Lung Adenocarcinoma Metastasis via Its Interaction with NF-B p50 Subunit and Transcriptional Regulation of Prostaglandin E2 Receptor EP3 Subtype
Reprinted from: *Cancers* 2023, *15*, 1398, doi:10.3390/cancers15051398 250

Maurice Klein, Merle Wefers, Christian Hallermann, Henrike J. Fischer, Frank Hölzle and Kai Wermker
IMP3 Expression as a Potential Tumour Marker in High-Risk Localisations of Cutaneous Squamous Cell Carcinoma: IMP3 in Metastatic cSCC
Reprinted from: *Cancers* 2023, *15*, 4087, doi:10.3390/cancers15164087 265

Giovanna Casili, Sarah Adriana Scuderi, Marika Lanza, Alessia Filippone, Deborah Mannino and Raffaella Giuffrida et al.
Therapeutic Potential of BAY-117082, a Selective NLRP3 Inflammasome Inhibitor, on Metastatic Evolution in Human Oral Squamous Cell Carcinoma (OSCC)
Reprinted from: *Cancers* 2023, *15*, 2796, doi:10.3390/cancers15102796 280

About the Editors

Daniel L. Pouliquen

Daniel L. Pouliquen, PharmD, PhD, initially developed the characterization and applications of new NMR contrast agents for proton MRI. After a PostDoc (Dept. Radiology Massachusetts General Hospital, Boston, USA), as staff researcher (French National Institute of Health - Inserm), he designed superparamagnetic iron oxide nanoparticles (SPIO) for MRI applications. In 1995, he extended NMR relaxometry to the study of water states and dynamic properties in normal and tumor tissues, organisms under development (seeds, fish eggs, and embryos), and biological fluids. This led to demonstrate changes in the biophysics of water in tissues during carcinogenesis. He then explored the quantitative and qualitative changes in the different water phases in mitochondria and investigated the effects of phytochemicals in the prevention of cancers in mice and rats (myeloma, glioblastoma, 2001–2008). From 2008 to 2018, he established a biocollection of preneoplastic and neoplastic cell lines and experimental models of malignant mesothelioma (MM) for basic research on the biology of this aggressive cancer and the evaluation of new strategies of treatment (Inserm UMR 892 and UMR 1232 (team 4, CRCINA, Nantes)). Since 2019, he has worked on the identification of new biomarkers of cancer invasiveness by mass spectrometry using cell lines, experimental MM tumors, and formalin-fixed, paraffin-embedded sections of tumors from patients (CRCI2NA, ICO Cancer Center, Angers). To promote the exchange of ideas between researchers from different parts of the world working on common topics, he has edited two books on rat models of cancer (2012) and the use of curcumin for health implications (2014), an eBook on malignant mesothelioma, and two Special Issues dedicated to Curcuminoids in cancer research as well as biomarkers of cancer invasiveness and metastasis.

Cristina Núñez González

Dra. Nunez completed a PhD degree in chemistry from the University of Santiago de Compostela (Spain) in 2009. In 2010, she obtained a Post-Doctoral grant from the FCT-MEC-Portugal to work in the design of novel molecular sensors (2010-2013). She obtained a research contract (I2C) of the Xunta de Galicia and worked in the Dept of Geographical and Life Sciences of the Canterbury Christ Church University in UK (08/2013 to 04/2014). During this time, she obtained novel skills in Genomics and Biotechnology and then pursued her investigations on novel multifunctional nanomaterials with potential antitumor activity in the Chemistry Dept, Faculty of Science and Technology, at the University NOVA of Lisbon (Portugal). At 34 years of age, she had published 50 papers (41 after obtaining her PhD degree) in international peer review journals with an accumulated impact factor of 149, 341 citations, an h-index of 12, 31 of the 46 papers being published within the 25% higher impact factor in its knowledge area, including 1 published in the multidisciplinary scientific journal Chem. Soc. Rev. 2010 (39) 2948-76 (IP: 26.585). Additionally, 3 of these papers were published independently from her PhD supervisor and 17 were published with her as a senior (corresponding) author. The papers were published in different scientific areas, such as inorganic/organic materials (33), analytical chemistry (3), microscopy (2), nanotechnology (2), multidisciplinary science and general chemistry (5), and biological journals (4). Furthermore, she also participated as the co-author of book chapters and books. She was also a regular referee of 12 international journals, was co-author of 98 communications in national and international congresses, and participated in 27 national and international seminars, specialized courses, and congresses. She was also a member of 11 projects financed by national and international funding agencies.

Preface

The molecular characterization of tumors, investigated particularly through proteogenomic analyses, has led to a revolution in cancer research. Over the last decade, the development of quantitative proteomics, together with other major technological breakthroughs, have identified candidate biomarkers for diagnosis, prognosis, and drug efficacy/resistance follow-up. These improvements have allowed researchers to explore the capability of cancer cells to invade, metastasize, and finally, destroy normal tissues and organs. In parallel, new hypotheses have been formulated, and the means cancer cells use to exploit their surrounding environment have begun to be deciphered, leading to new therapeutic approaches. This Special Issue covers all these aspects, revealing new, recent insights on the molecular networks controlling the tumor invasiveness process; dynamic interactions between cancer cells; and the host stroma, stemness, and epithelial-to-mesenchymal transition, as well as the links between inflammation and tumor metastasis. The scope is extended to studies on all cancer histological types (original research articles and reviews) conducted on experimental tumor models, tumor samples, and/or biofluids from patients with cancer.

Daniel L. Pouliquen and Cristina Núñez González
Editors

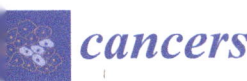

Editorial

Biomarkers of Tumor Metastasis and Invasiveness

Daniel L. Pouliquen [1,*] and Cristina Núñez González [2,*]

1. Inserm, CRCI²NA, CNRS, Université d'Angers, Nantes Université, F-49000 Angers, France
2. Research Unit, Lucus Augusti University Hospital (HULA), Servizo Galego de Saude (SERGAS), 27002 Lugo, Spain
* Correspondence: daniel.pouliquen@inserm.fr (D.L.P.); cristina.nunez.gonzalez@sergas.es (C.N.G.); Tel.: +33-241-352-854 (D.L.P.)

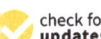

Citation: Pouliquen, D.L.; Núñez González, C. Biomarkers of Tumor Metastasis and Invasiveness. *Cancers* 2023, 15, 5000. https://doi.org/10.3390/cancers15205000

Received: 20 September 2023
Revised: 3 October 2023
Accepted: 11 October 2023
Published: 16 October 2023

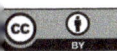

Copyright: © 2023 by the authors. Licensee MDPI, Basel, Switzerland. This article is an open access article distributed under the terms and conditions of the Creative Commons Attribution (CC BY) license (https://creativecommons.org/licenses/by/4.0/).

The identification of proteins as new cancer diagnostic and prognostic biomarkers continues to attract considerable attention in the oncology literature, especially in the context of invasion and metastasis activation process [1]. In this field, the most recent developments include, but are not restricted to, proteins linked to the epithelial-to-mesenchymal transition (EMT), extracellular vesicles [2], co-receptors for growth factors [3], cell surface receptor adaptor proteins [4], transcription factors [5], or scaffolding proteins [6]. In this Special Issue, 169 authors representing 98 affiliations from 18 countries over 4 continents have made 17 contributions, and it is a great honor and pleasure for the Editors to introduce this collective work which summarizes important insights in this field of research.

In link with previous findings on EMT [2], Carrasco-Garcia et al. reported that a member of the SOX transcription factors (encoded by *SRY*-related HMG-box genes) that bind to the minor groove in DNA, SOX9, and linked to stem cell activity exhibited an increased expression in both pancreatic ductal adenocarcinoma cell lines and human biopsies. This observation was associated with metastasis, poor prognosis, and resistance to therapy [7]. Subsequently, previously reported biomarkers of effective adjuvant chemotherapy of non-small-cell lung cancer were reviewed by Tozuka and colleagues. They showed that cytoskeletal protein actinin-4, (ACTN4), previously reported to induce EMT through upregulation of a transcriptional repressor of E-cadherin, Snail, represented a possible biomarker for identifying patients at high risk of postoperative recurrence [8]. An in silico gene expression analysis, conducted by Rao et al., also established that, among 760 genes examined from the PANCAN Cancer Genome Atlas, a novel association was observed between the expression of vasoactive intestinal peptide (VIP) in gastrointestinal cancers and ZEB1-mediated EMT [9].

EMT has also been associated with mitochondrial dysfunction, which regulates the tumor microenvironment, leading to more aggressive tumors. Wu and colleagues reviewed the recent progress in the regulation of cancer metastasis by mitochondrial DNA, showing its impact on different aspects, including resistance to anoikis, promotion of angiogenesis, cancer cell survival in the circulatory system, and colonization [10]. Moreover, mitochondrial dysfunction leads to metabolic reprogramming and proteome rewiring. In their cross-species investigation of mitochondrial metabolic differences between invasive and non-invasive mesothelioma of four experimental rat tumor models and ten patient-derived cell lines, Pouliquen et al. showed that the most impressive expression increase concerned one enzyme of the fatty acid oxidation, the long-chain acyl coenzyme A dehydrogenase (ACADL) [11].

Other components of the tumor microenvironments also influence EMT. In extrahepatic cholangiosarcoma, another type of aggressive tumor, Oba et al. found an association between one chemokine receptor, CCR7, which is primarily expressed in various immune cells, and EMT in human cell lines. Interestingly, their clinicopathological examination also revealed that high-grade CCR7 expression was one of the most adverse postoperative prognostic factors in patients undergoing surgical resections of this tumor and was associated with more tumor buds and mesenchymal status [12]. The involvement of immune tumor microenvironment in clinical management was also documented in osteosarcoma by Huang and colleagues. They highlighted the role and mechanism of three proteins associated with the immune infiltration and progression of this cancer type, BCL2 interacting protein 3, prostaglandin I2 synthase, and the adhesion plaque protein Zyxin [13], all of which having been previously individually classified as unfavorable prognosis biomarkers (https://www.proteinatlas.org/, accessed on 29 August 2023). Among immune cells, the role played by the infiltration of gastric cancer by lymphocyte subsets, combined with the Prognostic Nutritional Index, was also emphasized by Sun and colleagues. Their study revealed the peculiar role of CD19+ B cells to identify patients with a high risk of metastasis and recurrence after surgery [14].

For some aggressive types of cancers such as glioblastoma multiforme (GBM), since 2021, the grading includes molecular features of the tumor. To improve its characterization, the search for new diagnosis biomarkers has led to investigation of the protein cargo of extravesicles in the blood and cerebrospinal fluid, highlighting some potential candidates [15]. However, further work is required to translate the basic research into clinical practice. To date, a few molecular biomarkers have shown potential to predict the survival outcomes and treatment response in patients, with some limitations [16]. As other biomarkers need to be investigated, in this Special Issue, Marshland et al. revealed the clinical relevance of sortilin, a membrane receptor involved in the sorting and transporting of intracellular proteins, which represents a potential biomarker and therapeutic target for GBM [17].

Like sortilin, other proteins circulating in the blood of patients with invasive cancers were recently investigated. In a large study conducted on 3272 patients with non-small-cell lung cancer (NSCLC), Jiang and colleagues explored the roles of seven proteins to predict tumor metastasis and stage. They found that patients exhibiting combined increased levels of three serum tumor markers, carcinoembryonic antigen, cytokeratin-19 fragment, and carbohydrate antigen 199 tended to have higher tumor stages, while the two latter were indicative of lymphatic and distant metastasis [18]. In their combined analysis of blood plasma and bone marrow mononuclear cells proteomes from patients with multiple myeloma, Dunphy et al. also revealed that an aggressive, extramedullary form of this disease was associated with a significant differential abundance of three promising biomarkers, vascular cell adhesion molecule 1, pigment epithelium-derived factor, and hepatocyte growth factor activator [19].

Another field of investigation is represented by enzymes secreted into the extracellular spaces. One example was provided by the work of Chen and Chai on prostasin and matriptase, two membrane serine proteases showing opposite effects in solid epithelial tumors, that reciprocally activate each other. In B lymphoma cells, they explored the utility of prostasin exosomes in matriptase activation to initiate a prostasin–matriptase activation cascade and analyzed its impact on the invasive properties of different cell lines [20]. As remodeling of the extracellular matrix plays an important role in tumor progression, among zinc-dependent proteases, a growing interest concerns the A disintegrin and metalloproteinases family (ADAM), their involvement in gastrointestinal tumor progression being reviewed by Lukaszewicz-Zajac et al. They highlighted the promising significance of seven members of this family as potential prognostic biomarkers and therapeutics targets for these cancers [21].

Distant metastasis represents a major problem for invasive cancers, which frequently concerns lymph nodes. In this field, attempts to identify biomarkers of lymph node invasion are continuously produced, which have led, for example, to recently highlighting the role played by CD47 in the progression of colorectal cancer [22]. In the case of high-grade endometrial cancer, Lombaers et al. reported that the increased risk of lymph node metastasis observed in patients with stage III–IV disease was associated with elevated levels of cancer antigen 125 (CA125) and reduced overall survival, confirming its predictive value [23]. In patients with lung adenocarcinoma, Yu and colleagues revealed that the expression of one member of the mitogen-activated protein kinase family, MAPK15, was positively correlated with lymph node metastasis. Moreover, mechanistically, MAPK15 was shown to interact with p50 to promote the expression of the prostaglandin E2 receptor EP3 subtype at the transcriptional level, thereby enhancing cancer cell migration and metastasis [24]. In patients with squamous cell carcinoma (SCC) of the skin, Klein et al. reported that the high expression of the insulin-like growth factor 2 mRNA-binding protein 3 (IMP3) observed in 122 cases with high-risk localizations (lip, ear) was correlated with aggressiveness features, including lymph node metastases [25]. Finally, for another primary tumor site of this cancer, in the tongue tissue, Casili and colleagues used an in vivo orthotopic model of oral SCC to demonstrate the therapeutic potential of an inhibitor of one member of the nucleotide-binding domain leucine-rich repeat-containing receptors (NLRs), playing essential roles in immunity and inflammation. This protein, NOD-like receptor protein 3 (NLRP3), for which the activation of induces the assembly of multiprotein complexes known as inflammasomes, represents a potential prognostic biomarker for different cancer types [26,27]. They showed that treatment with this molecule modulated EMT in the tongue tissue as well as in metastatic organs such as lymph nodes [28].

In conclusion, we hope that this Special Issue will attract readers interested in this crucial topic in basic cancer research, which could help generate important future biomedical applications for the benefits of patients.

Author Contributions: Writing-original draft preparation, D.L.P. Writing-review and editing, D.L.P. and C.N.G. All authors have read and agreed to the published version of the manuscript.

Acknowledgments: This Special Issue is dedicated to the memory of my father, Henri Pouliquen (1928–2023), and to all the patients with invasive cancers who, in another world, could have beneficiated from this research for a better end of life.

Conflicts of Interest: The author declares no conflict of interest.

References

1. Veuger, J.; Kuipers, N.C.; Willems, S.M.; Halmos, G.B. Tumor markers and their prognostic value in sinonasal ITAC/Non-ITAC. *Cancers* **2023**, *15*, 3201. [CrossRef]
2. Giusti, I.; Poppa, G.; Di Fazio, G.; D'Ascenzo, S.; Dolo, V. Metastatic dissemination: Role of tumor-derived extracellular vesicles and their use as clinical biomarkers. *Int. J. Mol. Sci.* **2023**, *24*, 9590. [CrossRef]
3. Fernández-Palanca, P.; Payo-Serafín, T.; Méndez-Blanco, C.; San-Miguel, B.; Tuñon, M.J.; González-Gallego, J.; Mauriz, J.L. Neuropilins as potential biomarkers in hepatocellular carcinoma: A systematic review of basic and clinical applications. *Clin. Mol. Hepatol.* **2023**, *29*, 293–319. [CrossRef]
4. Lin, Y.; Cai, H. Biological functions and therapeutic potential of SHCBP1 in human cancer. *Biomed. Pharmacother.* **2023**, *160*, 114362. [CrossRef]
5. Liu, S.; Liu, X.; Lin, X.; Chen, H. Zinc finger proteins in the war on gastric cancer: Molecular mechanism and clinical potential. *Cells* **2023**, *12*, 1314. [PubMed]
6. Pintor-Romero, V.G.; Hurtado-Ortega, E.; Nicolás-Morales, M.L.; Gutiérrez-Torres, M.; Vences-Velázquez, A.; Ortuño-Pineda, C.; Espinoza-Rojo, M.; Navarro-Tito, N.; Cortés-Sarabia, K. Biological role and aberrant overexpression of syntenin-1 in cancer: Potential role as a biomarker and therapeutic target. *Biomedicines* **2023**, *11*, 1034.
7. Carrasco-Garcia, E.; Lopez, L.; Moncho-Amor, V.; Carazo, F.; Aldaz, P.; Collado, M.; Bell, D.; Gaafar, A.; Karamitopoulou, E.; Tzankov, A.; et al. SOX9 triggers different epithelial to mesenchymal transition states to promote pancreatic cancer progression. *Cancers* **2022**, *14*, 916. [CrossRef] [PubMed]
8. Tozuka, T.; Noro, R.; Seike, M.; Honda, K. Benefits from adjuvant chemotherapy in patients with resected non-small cell lung cancer: Possibility of stratification by gene amplification of ACTN4 according to evaluation of metastatic ability. *Cancers* **2022**, *14*, 4363. [CrossRef]
9. Rao, I.H.; Waller, E.K.; Dhamsania, R.K.; Chandrasekaran, S. Gene expression analysis links autocrine vasoactive intestinal peptide and ZEB1 in gastrointestinal cancers. *Cancers* **2023**, *15*, 3284. [CrossRef] [PubMed]
10. Wu, Q.; Tsai, H.-I.; Zhu, H.; Wang, D. The entanglement between mitochondrial DNA and tumor metastasis. *Cancers* **2022**, *14*, 1862. [CrossRef]
11. Pouliquen, D.L.; Ortone, G.; Rumiano, L.; Boissard, A.; Henry, C.; Blandin, S.; Guette, C.; Riganti, C.; Kopecka, J. Long-chain acyl coenzyme A dehydrogenase, a key player in metabolic rewiring/invasiveness in experimental tumors and human mesothelioma cell lines. *Cancers* **2023**, *15*, 3044. [CrossRef] [PubMed]

12. Oba, M.; Nakanishi, Y.; Mitsuhashi, T.; Sasaki, K.; Hatanaka, K.C.; Sasaki, M.; Nange, A.; Okumura, A.; Hayashi, M.; Yoshida, Y.; et al. CCR7 mediates cell invasion and migration in extrahepatic cholangiocarcinoma by inducing epithelial-mesenchymal transition. *Cancers* **2023**, *15*, 1878. [CrossRef] [PubMed]
13. Huang, L.; Sun, F.; Liu, Z.; Jin, W.; Zhang, Y.; Chen, J.; Zhong, C.; Liang, W.; Peng, H. Probing the potential of defense response-associated genes for predicting the progression, prognosis, and immune microenvironment of osteosarcoma. *Cancers* **2023**, *15*, 2405. [CrossRef] [PubMed]
14. Sun, H.; Wang, H.; Pan, H.; Zuo, Y.; Zhao, R.; Huang, R.; Xue, Y.; Song, H. CD19 (+) B cell combined with prognostic nutritional index predicts the clinical outcomes of patients with gastric cancer who underwent surgery. *Cancers* **2023**, *15*, 2531. [CrossRef]
15. Rackles, E.; Hernández Lopez, P.; Falcon-Perez, J.M. Extracellular vesicles as source for the identification of minimally invasive molecular signatures in glioblastoma. *Semin. Cancer Biol.* **2022**, *87*, 148–159. [CrossRef] [PubMed]
16. Sareen, H.; Ma, Y.; Becker, T.M.; Roberts, T.L.; de Souza, P.; Powter, B. Molecular biomarkers in glioblastoma: A systematic review and meta-analysis. *Int. J. Mol. Sci.* **2022**, *23*, 8835. [CrossRef]
17. Marshland, M.; Dowdell, A.; Faulkner, S.; Gedye, C.; Lynam, J.; Griffin, C.P.; Marshland, J.; Jiang, C.C.; Hondermarck, H. The membrane protein sortilin is a potential biomarker and target for glioblastoma. *Cancers* **2023**, *15*, 2514. [CrossRef] [PubMed]
18. Jiang, C.; Zhao, M.; Hou, S.; Hu, X.; Huang, J.; Wang, H.; Ren, C.; Pan, X.; Zhang, T.; Wu, S.; et al. The indicative value of serum tumor markers for metastasis and stage of non-small cell lung cancer. *Cancers* **2022**, *14*, 5064. [CrossRef] [PubMed]
19. Dunphy, K.; Bazou, D.; Henry, M.; Meleady, P.; Miettinen, J.J.; Heckman, C.A.; Dowling, P.; O'Gorman, P. Proteomic and metabolomic analysis of bone marrow and plasma from patients with extramedullary multiple myeloma identifies distinct protein and metabolite signatures. *Cancers* **2023**, *15*, 3764. [CrossRef]
20. Chen, L.-M.; Chai, K.X. Exosome-mediated activation of the prostasin-matriptase serine protease cascade in B lymphoma cells. *Cancers* **2023**, *15*, 3848. [CrossRef] [PubMed]
21. Łukaszewicz-Zając, M.; Pączek, S.; Mroczko, B. A disintegrin and metalloproteinase (ADAM) family—Novel biomarkers of selected gastrointestinal (GI) malignancies? *Cancers* **2022**, *14*, 2307. [CrossRef] [PubMed]
22. Oh, H.-H.; Park, Y.-L.; Park, S.-Y.; Myung, E.; Im, C.-M.; Yu, H.-J.; Han, B.; Seo, Y.-J.; Kim, K.-H.; Myung, D.-S.; et al. CD47 mediates the progression of colorectal cancer by inducing tumor cell apoptosis and angiogenesis. *Pathol. Res. Pract.* **2022**, *240*, 154220. [CrossRef]
23. Lombaers, M.S.; Cornel, K.M.C.; Visser, N.C.M.; Bulten, J.; Küsters-Vandevelde, H.V.N.; Amant, F.; Boll, D.; Bronsert, P.; Colas, E.; Geomini, P.M.A.J.; et al. Preoperative CA125 significantly improves risk stratification in high-grade endometrial cancer. *Cancers* **2023**, *15*, 2605. [CrossRef] [PubMed]
24. Yu, F.-Y.; Xu, Q.; Zhao, X.-Y.; Mo, H.-Y.; Zhong, Q.-H.; Luo, L.; Lau, A.T.Y.; Xu, Y.-M. The atypical MAP kinase MAPK15 is required for lung adenocarcinoma metastasis via its interaction with NF-kB p50 subunit and transcriptional regulation of prostaglandin E2 receptor EP3 subtype. *Cancers* **2023**, *15*, 1398. [CrossRef]
25. Klein, M.; Wefers, M.; Hallermann, C.; Fischer, H.J.; Hölzle, F.; Wermker, K. IMP3 expression as a potential tumour marker in high-risk localisations of cutaneous squamous cell carcinoma: IMP3 in metastatic cSCC. *Cancers* **2023**, *15*, 4087. [CrossRef] [PubMed]
26. Shi, F.; Wei, B.; Lan, T.; Xiao, Y.; Quan, X.; Chen, J.; Zhao, C.; Gao, J. Low NLRP3 expression predicts a better prognosis of colorectal cancer. *Biosci. Rep.* **2021**, *41*, BSR20210280. [CrossRef] [PubMed]
27. Saponaro, C.; Scarpi, E.; Sonnessa, M.; Cioffi, A.; Buccino, F.; Giotta, F.; Pastena, M.I.; Zito, F.A.; Mangia, A. Prognostic value of NLRP3 inflammasome and TLR4 expression in breast cancer patients. *Front. Oncol.* **2021**, *11*, 705331. [CrossRef] [PubMed]
28. Casili, G.; Scuderi, S.A.; Lanza, M.; Filippone, A.; Mannino, D.; Giuffrida, R.; Colarossi, C.; Mare, M.; Capra, A.P.; De Gaetano, F.; et al. Therapeutic potential of BAY-117082, a selective NLRP3 inflammasome inhibitor, on metastatic evolution in human oral squamous cell carcinoma (OSCC). *Cancers* **2023**, *15*, 2796. [CrossRef]

Disclaimer/Publisher's Note: The statements, opinions and data contained in all publications are solely those of the individual author(s) and contributor(s) and not of MDPI and/or the editor(s). MDPI and/or the editor(s) disclaim responsibility for any injury to people or property resulting from any ideas, methods, instructions or products referred to in the content.

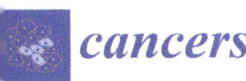

Article

SOX9 Triggers Different Epithelial to Mesenchymal Transition States to Promote Pancreatic Cancer Progression

Estefania Carrasco-Garcia [1,2,*], Lidia Lopez [1], Veronica Moncho-Amor [1,3], Fernando Carazo [4], Paula Aldaz [1], Manuel Collado [5], Donald Bell [3], Ayman Gaafar [6], Eva Karamitopoulou [7], Alexandar Tzankov [8], Manuel Hidalgo [9,10], Ángel Rubio [4], Manuel Serrano [11,12], Charles H. Lawrie [13,14], Robin Lovell-Badge [3] and Ander Matheu [1,2,14,*]

1. Cellular Oncology Group, Biodonostia Health Research Institute, 20014 San Sebastian, Spain; tslab.granada@hotmail.com (L.L.); veronica.moncho@biodonostia.org (V.M.-A.); paula.aldaz.donamaria@navarra.es (P.A.)
2. CIBER de Fragilidad y Envejecimiento Saludable (CIBERfes), 28029 Madrid, Spain
3. The Francis Crick Institute, London NW1 1AT, UK; donald.bell@crick.ac.uk (D.B.); robin.lovell-badge@crick.ac.uk (R.L.-B.)
4. School of Engineering, University of Navarra, 20009 San Sebastian, Spain; fcarazo@tecnun.es (F.C.); arubio@tecnun.es (Á.R.)
5. Health Research Institute of Santiago de Compostela (IDIS), Xerencia de Xestión Integrada de Santiago (XXIS/SERGAS), 15706 Santiago de Compostela, Spain; manuel.collado.rodriguez@sergas.es
6. Department of Pathology, Cruces University Hospital, 48903 Barakaldo, Spain; ayman.gaafareleraky@osakidetza.eus
7. Institute of Pathology, University of Bern, 3012 Bern, Switzerland; eva.diamantis@pathology.unibe.ch
8. Institute of Pathology, University Hospital Basel, 4056 Basel, Switzerland; alexandar.tzankov@usb.ch
9. Spanish National Cancer Research Centre (CNIO), 28029 Madrid, Spain; mah4006@med.cornell.edu
10. New York-Presbyterian Hospital/Weill Cornell Medical Center, New York, NY 10065, USA
11. Institute for Research in Biomedicine (IRB Barcelona), Barcelona Institute of Science and Technology (BIST), 08028 Barcelona, Spain; manuel.serrano@irbbarcelona.org
12. Catalan Institution for Research and Advanced Studies (ICREA), 08010 Barcelona, Spain
13. Molecular Oncology Group, Biodonostia Institute, 20014 San Sebastian, Spain; charles.lawrie@biodonostia.org
14. IKERBASQUE, Basque Foundation for Science, 48009 Bilbao, Spain
* Correspondence: estefania.carrasco@biodonostia.org (E.C.-G.); ander.matheu@biodonostia.org (A.M.); Tel.: +34-943-006073 (E.C.-G. & A.M.); Fax: +34-943-006250 (E.C.-G. & A.M.)

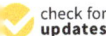

Simple Summary: Pancreatic cancers are lethal types of cancer. A majority of patients progress to an advanced and metastatic disease, which remains a major clinical problem. Therefore, it is crucial to identify critical regulators to help predict the disease progression and to develop more efficacious therapeutic approaches. In this work we found that an increased expression of the developmental factor SOX9 is associated with metastasis, a poor prognosis and resistance to therapy in pancreatic ductal adenocarcinoma patients and in cell cultures. We also found that this effect is at least in part due to the ability of SOX9 to regulate the activity of stem cell factors, such as BMI1, in addition to those involved in EMT and metastasis.

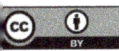

Abstract: Background: Pancreatic ductal adenocarcinoma (PDAC) is one of the most lethal cancers mainly due to spatial obstacles to complete resection, early metastasis and therapy resistance. The molecular events accompanying PDAC progression remain poorly understood. SOX9 is required for maintaining the pancreatic ductal identity and it is involved in the initiation of pancreatic cancer. In addition, SOX9 is a transcription factor linked to stem cell activity and is commonly overexpressed in solid cancers. It cooperates with Snail/Slug to induce epithelial-mesenchymal transition (EMT) during neural development and in diseases such as organ fibrosis or different types of cancer. Methods: We investigated the roles of SOX9 in pancreatic tumor cell plasticity, metastatic dissemination and chemoresistance using pancreatic cancer cell lines as well as mouse embryo fibroblasts. In addition, we characterized the clinical relevance of SOX9 in pancreatic cancer using human biopsies. Results: Gain- and loss-of-function of SOX9 in PDAC cells revealed that high levels of SOX9 increased migration and invasion, and promoted EMT and metastatic dissemination, whilst

SOX9 silencing resulted in metastasis inhibition, along with a phenotypic reversion to epithelial features and loss of stemness potential. In both contexts, EMT factors were not altered. Moreover, high levels of SOX9 promoted resistance to gemcitabine. In contrast, overexpression of SOX9 was sufficient to promote metastatic potential in *K-Ras* transformed MEFs, triggering EMT associated with Snail/Slug activity. In clinical samples, SOX9 expression was analyzed in 198 PDAC cases by immunohistochemistry and in 53 patient derived xenografts (PDXs). SOX9 was overexpressed in primary adenocarcinomas and particularly in metastases. Notably, SOX9 expression correlated with high vimentin and low E-cadherin expression. Conclusions: Our results indicate that SOX9 facilitates PDAC progression and metastasis by triggering stemness and EMT.

Keywords: SOX9; pancreatic cancer; plasticity; metastasis; EMT; chemoresistance

1. Introduction

Metastasis is a complex process by which cancer cells spread from the primary tumor and colonize distant tissues in the body. The process takes place through a sequence of steps including invasion across the surrounding extracellular matrix, intravasation and dissemination into the systemic circulation, and the extravasation and colonization of distant organs. The first steps of the process have been linked to the activation of the epithelial-mesenchymal transition (EMT), which confers to cancer cells mesenchymal characteristics that allow their dissemination from the primary tumor. In contrast, the "engraftment" of cancer cells in distant organs has been associated with the reverse process (i.e., mesenchymal-epithelial transition or MET) [1,2]. In EMT, the expression of epithelial cell adhesion molecules (E-cadherin, β-catenin and cytokeratins) is decreased, while the expression of mesenchymal proteins related to cell migration (vimentin, N-cadherin, etc.) is activated. Moreover, the participation of a network of transcription factors, including Snail, Slug, Twist and Zeb1, which repress the expression of cell adhesion molecules and trigger the manifestation of a mesenchymal phenotype, has been widely described [3,4]. It is noteworthy that EMT is not a binary process, since disseminated cancer cells can present intermediate phenotypes that are not completely epithelial or mesenchymal [3,5]. In addition, the EMT process may have other important implications for cancer cells such as the acquisition of stem cell-like properties [6–8], which are closely implicated in therapy resistance [9]. However, this is not always associated with EMT processes in the context of metastasis [1,10].

SOX9 is a member of the SOX family of developmental transcription factors, characterized by containing a high mobility group (HMG) DNA-binding protein domain. SOX9 plays a relevant role in development, governing cell fate specification and lineage commitment [11]. In the adult, SOX9 is involved in the regulation of homeostasis in several tissues including the pancreas, wherein it regulates stem cell maintenance and directs cell fate decisions in a dosage dependent manner [12,13]. Gain- and loss-of-function experiments have revealed that SOX9 activates EMT during embryonic development for neural crest delamination and cardiac valve formation [14,15], and also in different types of cancer [16–18]. Among them, it cooperates with members of the Snail/Slug family for metastatic progression in breast and lung cancers [8,19,20].

Pancreatic ductal adenocarcinoma (PDAC) is among the most lethal cancers, with a 5-year survival rate of less than 6% [21]. The poor prognosis of PDAC is mainly due to late diagnosis, spatial obstacles in resection, its high metastatic potential and its resistance to currently available chemotherapies [22–24]. The most effective therapeutic approach at present is surgical resection, yet most patients are diagnosed with an advanced stage disease and only a small proportion (around 15–20%) are eligible for surgery. Moreover, even in patients who receive surgical treatment, the majority of tumors will relapse [25]. Thus, unfortunately, pancreatic cancer still exhibits very close rates of incidence and mortality, with 458,918 new diagnoses and 432,242 deaths worldwide in 2018 [26], with metastasis being the leading cause of mortality.

Several studies have demonstrated the involvement of SOX9 in the initial steps of pancreatic carcinogenesis. Thus, SOX9 is required for the formation of acinar-ductal metaplasias (ADM) and their progression to pancreatic intraepithelial neoplasias (PanIN), through its activity downstream of oncogenic K-RAS or EGFR signaling [27–29]; however, its role in the advanced stages of pancreatic cancer is not well described. Some evidence indicates that high SOX9 may promote pancreatic cancer cell invasion and aggressiveness [30–32], as well as chemoresistance [33], while others have reported low levels of SOX9 expression [28,34]. In this study we wanted to address whether SOX9 promotes EMT along with other metastatic traits in pancreatic cancer.

2. Experimental Procedures

2.1. Human Samples

Human samples arranged in tissue microarrays (TMAs) were provided by the Molecular Pathology Division of the Institute of Pathology at the Basel University Hospital. Written informed consent was obtained from all patients prior to specimen collection.

2.2. Cell Culture

The pancreatic carcinoma cell lines Panc-1, RWP-1, IMIMPC-1, IMIMPC-2, BxPC-3, SKPC-1, SKPC-3, MiaPaca-2 and Hs766-T, were kindly provided by Dr. Real (CNIO) and Dr. Navarro (IMIM Medical Research Institute). All cell lines were mycoplasma free confirmed by the PCR-based detection of a conserved region of mycoplasma's 16S rRNA using a mycoplasma detection kit (Biotools). Cells were cultured as adherent monolayers at 37 °C and 5% CO_2 in a DMEM medium (Gibco) supplemented with 10% FBS (Gibco), 100 U/mL penicillin and 100 µg/mL streptomycin. Tumorspheres were cultured in DMEM/F12 medium (Sigma) supplemented with 20 ng/mL of EGF and bFGF (Sigma) growth factors, in the presence of N2 and B27. For the tumorsphere quantification studies, 1×10^3 cells/well were seeded in non-treated 12-wells flat bottom plates and fresh media was added every 3 days. After 10 days, the 1ry (primary) tumorspheres were counted. Then, the spheres were disaggregated with accutase, seeded for 2ry (secondary) tumorspheres and maintained for another 10 days in culture. MEFs with a gain of SOX9 function have been described previously [35].

2.3. Gene Silencing and Overexpression

For SOX9 silencing by shRNA, cell lines were lentivirally infected. The cells were infected with lentivirus harboring the shSOX9 plasmid #40644 (*sh1*) and the corresponding pLKO.1 puro control plasmid #8453 (*pLKO*) from Addgene, both gifts from Dr. Bob Weinberg. For the lentiviral SOX9 overexpression, the Addgene plasmid #36979, a gift from Bob Weinberg, was used. For BMI1 upregulation, the cells were infected with lentivirus harboring the plasmid pLenti CMV GFP Puro-Bmi1 (a gift from Jacqueline Lees). Lentiviral infections were performed as previously described [36]. All infections were performed at a MOI of 10 for 6 h.

2.4. mRNA Expression Analysis

Total RNA was extracted with Trizol (Life Technologies, Carlsbad, CA, USA). Reverse transcription was performed using the High-Capacity cDNA Reverse Transcription Kit (ThermoFisher, Waltham, MA, USA) according to the manufacturer's guidelines. Quantitative real-time PCR was performed in an ABI PRISM 7300 thermocycler (Applied Biosystems, Waltham, MA, USA) using a Power SYBR® Green Master Mix (ThermoFisher), 10 mmol/L of primers and 20 ng of cDNA. *GAPDH*, a housekeeping gene, was used as a positive control for quantification. The ΔΔCT method was used for relative quantification.

2.5. Western Blot and Immunofluorescence

Immunoblots and immunofluorescence were performed following standard procedures. Primary antibodies used were: SOX9 (AB5535, Millipore, Burlington, MA, USA), E-Cadherin (610181, BD Biosciences, San Jose, CA, USA), N-Cadherin (610920, BD Biosciences, San Jose, CA, USA), vimentin (M7020, Dako, Santa Clara, CA, USA), SNAIL (5243, AB clonal, Woburn, MA, USA), SLUG (bs-1382R, Bioss, Woburn, MA, USA) and β-actin (AC-15, Sigma, St. Louis, MO, USA).

2.6. In Vitro Assays for Migration and Invasion

For migration evaluation, wound healing (scratch) and transwell assays were performed. In the wound healing assays, the cells were seeded at a 90% confluency in 24-well flat bottom plates (triplicates) and 24 h later, a lineal artificial gap (scratch) was made with a sterile tip at the bottom of the wells. After removing the debris, the cells were serum-deprived for the duration of the experiment (48 h). Transwell migration was analyzed using Corning® Transwell® polycarbonate membrane inserts (#3422, Corning, NY, USA). Briefly, the cells were seeded into the insert compartment in medium without serum and the inserts were placed in wells of 24-well flat bottom plates containing medium with 10% of a fetal bovine serum as chemo-attractant. Then, 48 h later, the migrated cells were fixed and stained with 0.2% crystal violet in 5% formalin. To quantify the migration, the stain was dissolved and the absorbance was measured at 750 nm.

Invasion assays were performed using the QCM™ Collagen Cell Invasion Assay of Millipore (ECM551, Burlington, MA, USA). Invading cells were quantified 48 h after the seeding according to the manufacturer's staining protocol.

2.7. F-Actin Staining

For cytoskeletal visualization, F-Actin was labelled with phalloidin. Cells were grown onto 8 mm diameter coverslips and fixed in 3.7% formaldehyde at room temperature for 15 min. After washing with PBS, the cells were permeabilized with 0.2% Triton X-100 (Sigma, St. Louis, MO, USA) and blocked with a blocking solution (10% *v/v* donkey serum in PBS/0.1% *v/v* Triton X-100; PBST) for 1 h. Then, F-actin filaments were stained using Alexa 546-conjugated phalloidin (Molecular Probes, Eugene, OR, USA) for 20 min at room temperature and the coverslips were counterstained with 4′,6-diamidino-2-phenylindole (DAPI) and mounted. Images were acquired using a Leica SPE confocal microscope.

2.8. Colony Formation Assay

A total of 0.5×10^3 cells were seeded in 9.5 cm^2 wells (triplicates) in a DMEM medium. The medium was added every 3 days and after 10 days of culture the colonies formed were fixed with paraformaldehyde for 15 min at room temperature, stained with Giemsa and counted.

2.9. Soft Agar Foci

A total of 2.5×10^3 cells were seeded in 9.5 cm^2 wells (triplicates) in medium with 0.7% of agarose (top layer medium) on a bottom layer of medium with 1% of agar. The top layer medium was added every 3 days and after 15 days of culture the foci formed were counted.

2.10. In Vivo Carcinogenesis Assays

For subcutaneous injection, cells were harvested with trypsin/EDTA and resuspended in PBS, with 1×10^5 cells injected subcutaneously into both flanks of $Foxn1^{nu}/Foxn1^{nu}$ nude mice (8 weeks old). External calipers were used to measure the tumor size at the indicated time points from which tumor volume was estimated according to the formula: $\frac{1}{2}$ (length × width^2). For tumor initiation experiments, 1×10^4, 1×10^5 and 1×10^6 cells were injected into both flanks of $Foxn1^{nu}/Foxn1^{nu}$ mice and tumor appearance was monitored over time.

For metastasis assays, *wt* and *Z/Sox9tg* MEFs and RWP1 and Panc-1 *pLKO/sh1* cells were injected intravenously into the tail vein of $Foxn1^{nu}/Foxn1^{nu}$ mice. Metastatic *foci* were detected by in vivo imaging system and at endpoint mice were euthanized and *foci* were extirpated for pathologic and immunohistochemistry studies.

2.11. Immunohistochemistry

For immunohistochemistry, 4 micrometer-thick sections were incubated with primary antibodies: SOX9 (AB5535, Millipore, Burlington, MA, USA), BMI1 (05-637, Millipore, Burlington, MA, USA), Ki67 (ab15580, abcam, Cambridge, UK), Snail (ab85931, abcam, Cambridge, UK), E-Cadherin (610181, BD Biosciences, San Jose, CA, USA), vimentin (M7020, Dako, Santa Clara, CA, USA), β-Catenin (610154, BD Biosciences, San Jose, CA, USA), and cytokeratin 19 (TROMA-III, Max Plant Institute, Freiburg, Germany). The sections then were washed and incubated with a MACH 3 Rabbit Probe and MACH 3 Rabbit HRP-Polymer (M3R531, Biocare Medical, Pacheco, CA, USA). The color was developed with 3,3′ diaminobenzidine (DAB, SPR-DAB-060, Spring Bioscience, Pleasanton, CA, USA). Counterstaining with hematoxylin was performed to mark the cell nuclei.

2.12. Expression Microarrays

HuGene 2.0_st arrays from Affymetrix (Santa Clara, CA, USA) were used to analyze the expression changes in RWP-1 cells with SOX9 silencing. The microarray data preprocessing was performed using the TAC software provided by Affymetrix including batch effect removal and the annotation file that corresponds to chip hugene_2_0_st_v1. The design and contrast matrices simply compared the shSOX9 with the references. Functional enrichment analysis was performed using the Overrepresentation Enrichment Analysis provided by WebGestalt, using a hypergeometric distribution to test the GO categories overrepresented. The enrichment analysis was performed independently for up- and down-regulated genes. Genes are included in the list if the fold change was larger than 1.5 (or less than −1.5 for down-regulated genes) and the *p* value was below 0.05. The selected universe for the enrichment analysis were the genes included in the hugene_2_0_st_v1 array. The functional analysis considered only the non-redundant biological processes terms. The data discussed in this publication have been deposited in NCBI's Gene Expression Omnibus and are accessible in GSE193406.

2.13. Data Evaluation

Data are presented as mean values ± S.E.M. with the number of experiments (*n*) in parenthesis. Unless otherwise indicated, the statistical significance (*p*-values) was calculated using the Student's t-test. The correlation *p* values related to the correlation coefficient (calculated using the Spearman method) have been calculated using the correlation test. Asterisks (*, **, and ***) indicate statistical significance ($p < 0.05$, $p < 0.01$, and $p < 0.001$, respectively).

3. Results

3.1. SOX9 Overexpression Confers Metastatic Potential and Promotes EMT in K-Ras Transformed Cells

We examined whether SOX9 would facilitate the dissemination of cells to distant organs in vivo. For this, we used mouse embryo fibroblasts (MEFs), as they lack the ability to metastasize. *E1a/Ras* transformed MEFs that overexpress *Sox9* and *GFP* (*Z/Sox9tg*) and controls [35], were injected intravenously (tail vein) into nude mice. The progressive growth of these cells was traced in vivo and was detected in mice injected *with Z/Sox9tg* cells, but not in those injected with *wt* MEFs (Figure 1A). Consistent with these results, 100% of the *Z/Sox9tg* injected mice presented metastatic masses in the lungs or brain, whereas *wt* cells failed to establish metastases as judged by the absence of detectable tumors in these two organs or elsewhere (Figure 1B). The metastases found in the *Z/Sox9tg* injected mice were positive for SOX9 and GFP staining (Figure 1C), confirming that the tumors originated from *Z/Sox9tg* cells. Furthermore, along with the gain of metastatic potential, *Sox9* overexpression diminished the E-cadherin and increased Snail expression (Figure 1D).

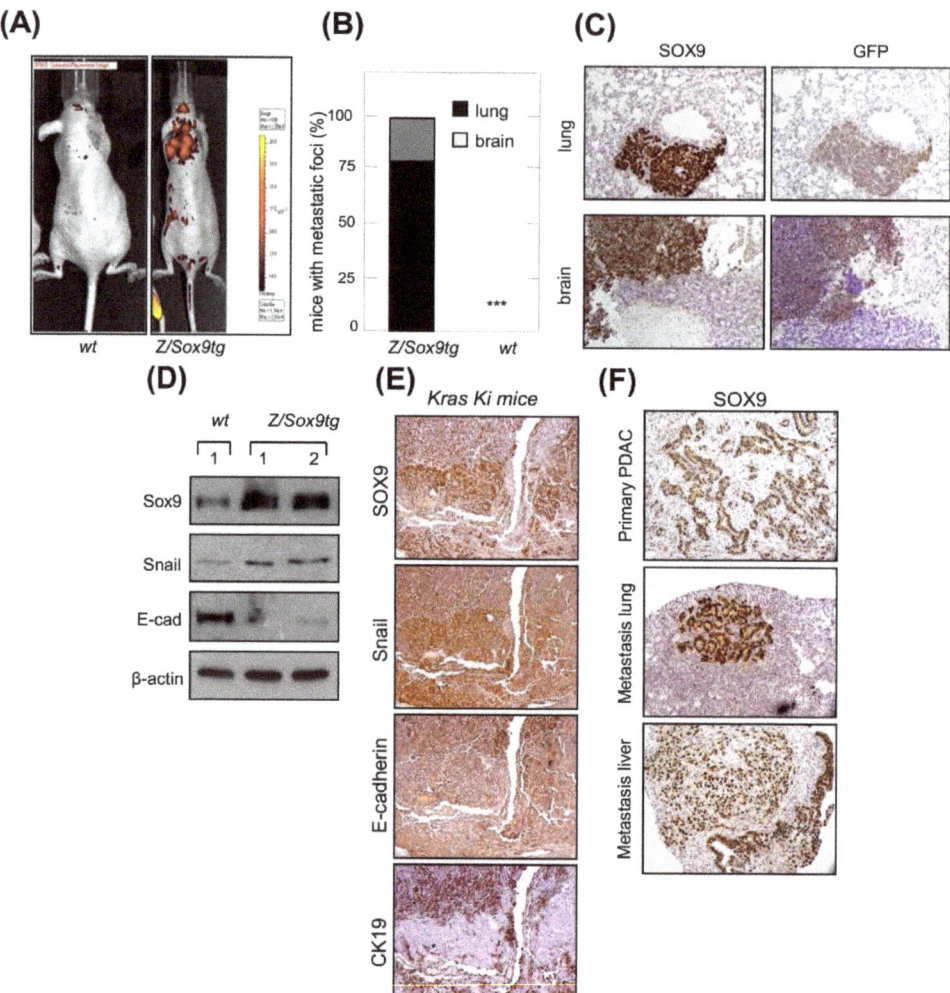

Figure 1. SOX9 overexpression promotes EMT and confers metastatic potential in *K-Ras* transformed cells. (**A**) Representative picture of metastatic tumors derived from intravenously injected *E1a/Ras* transformed MEFs with ectopic *Sox9* expression (*Z/Sox9tg*) (right, $n = 5$) or *wild type* MEFs (*wt*) (left, $n = 5$) in nude mice. Images obtained with an IVIS-200 in vivo imaging system. (**B**) Quantification of the percentage of nude mice that developed metastatic tumors derived from *Z/Sox9tg* ($n = 5$) and *wt* MEFs. (**C**) Sox9 and GFP expression analyzed by immunohistochemistry in lung and brain metastasis established by *E1a/Ras* transformed *Z/Sox9tg* MEFs. (**D**) Analysis by Western blot of Sox9, Snail and E-Cadherin levels in neoplastically transformed *wt* and *Z/Sox9tg* MEFs. (**E**) Serial sections of *K-Ras* G12V-induced lung adenocarcinomas stained with Sox9, Snail and the epithelial markers, E-cadherin and CK19. Representative image from at least three different mice. (**F**) Representative images of Sox9 expression analyzed by immunohistochemistry in sections from *K-Ras/p53$^{-/-}$* induced primary pancreatic tumors and metastatic tumors in lung and liver ($n = 5$). *** indicates statistical significance with $p < 0.001$.

The most intensely SOX9 staining cells in the *K-Ras G12V*-induced lung primary adenocarcinomas were also the areas of tumor growth at invasive sites [35]. In order to expand these observations, we analyzed these areas for different EMT markers. The cells most strongly expressing SOX9, displayed intense staining for the EMT transcription factor Snail and an absence or low levels of E-cadherin and CK19 epithelial markers (Figure 1E). To further study the association between SOX9 and metastasis, we checked its expression in pancreatic *K-Ras(G12V);p53*$^{-/-}$ mice, which develop pancreatic tumors with a highly metastatic activity affecting lung and liver [37]. In this context, the staining of SOX9 was very intense in primary PDAC and in both lung and liver metastatic nodes (Figure 1F).

3.2. SOX9 Overexpression Promotes EMT and Metastatic Traits in Pancreatic Cancer Cells

We tested whether high levels of SOX9 were sufficient to promote EMT in pancreatic cancer cells, which are classified as the tumor cell types with high SOX9 expression (Supplementary Figure S1A). To address this, we transduced primary epithelial BxPC-3 and IMIMPC-2 PDAC cell lines, which express endogenous low levels of SOX9 (Supplementary Figure S1B,C), with plasmids encoding *SOX9* or GFP. Immunoblotting revealed an overexpression of SOX9 in both cell lines (Figure 2A). In this context, SOX9 overexpression was associated with decreased E-cadherin along with higher vimentin and N-cadherin expression (Figure 2A,B), reflecting the activation of EMT. In agreement, SOX9 overexpressing cells presented a less cohesive organization when compared to control cells (Supplementary Figure S2A). Surprisingly, SOX9 overexpression did not alter the expression of SNAIL or other well-known EMT transcription factors such as SLUG or ZEB1 in BxPC-3 and IMIMPC-2 pancreatic cancer cells (Figure 2A; Supplementary Figure S2B); however, the expression of the BMI1 stem cell factor was elevated (Figure 2A).

As cancer cell motility and invasion into the basement membrane are associated with the induction of EMT and metastasis [6], we investigated these capabilities in pancreatic cancer cells overexpressing SOX9. For this, we performed scratch assays followed by live-cell microscopy, finding that PDAC cells with SOX9 overexpression displayed significantly enhanced migratory potential (Figure 2C; Supplementary Videos S1 and S2). Moreover, transwell assays also demonstrated that high levels of SOX9 boost invasion into collagen (Figure 2D). Successful colonization of distant organs requires active and highly proliferative cells to generate micrometastasis and macrometastasis [2,38]. We recently showed that ectopic SOX9 upregulation increased the proliferation of BxPC-3 and IMIMPC-2 cells [39]. This effect was paralleled by enhanced tumor growth over time in vivo (Figure 2E). Altogether, these observations establish that high levels of SOX9 in pancreatic cancer cells facilitate their acquisition of the cellular and molecular traits required for the metastatic dissemination and colonization.

3.3. Silencing of SOX9 Drives MET and Decreases Metastatic Potential

We then studied whether SOX9 knockdown could impair metastatic traits. For this, we silenced SOX9 in Panc-1 and RWP-1, two highly invasive and metastatic human pancreatic cancer cell lines, both with elevated endogenous levels of SOX9 (Supplementary Figure S1B). Western blotting confirmed the knockdown of SOX9 in both cell lines (Figure 3A). Phase contrast images and F-actin staining with phalloidin showed that cells with silenced SOX9 acquired an epithelial-like morphology (Figure 3B; Supplementary Figure S3A). According to this, SOX9 silencing increased the E-cadherin levels and reduced N-cadherin levels (Figure 3A,C), resembling the process of MET; however, the expression of *SNAIL*, *SLUG*, *ZEB1* or *PRRX1* was not altered in the SOX9-silenced cells, whereas BMI1 levels were reduced (Figure 3A; Supplementary Figure S3B). These results, together with the data presented above from the SOX9 overexpressing cells, suggest that EMT transcription factors are not linked to SOX9 functions in pancreatic cancer. Supporting this idea, their expression correlated negatively with SOX9 expression in human pancreatic cancer samples from the TCGA cohort (Supplementary Figure S3C).

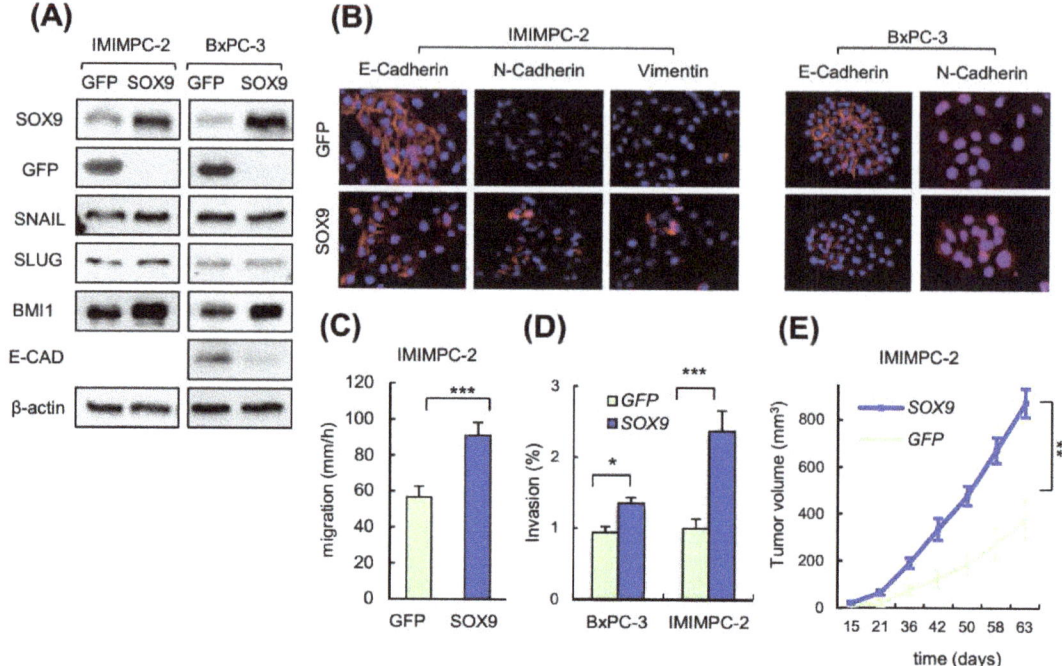

Figure 2. SOX9 overexpression promotes EMT and metastatic traits in pancreatic cancer cells. (**A**) Representative Western blot of GFP, SOX9, E-CAD, SNAIL, SLUG and BMI1 in IMIMPC-2 and BxPC-3 cell lines lentivirally transduced with plasmids harboring GFP or SOX9 coding sequences. (**B**) Representative images of epithelial (E-cadherin) and mesenchymal markers (N-cadherin and vimentin) expression detected by immunofluorescence in IMIMPC-2 and BxPC-3 cells transduced with GFP or SOX9 ($n = 3$). (**C**) Migration speed of IMIMPC-2 control and SOX9 cells calculated through live imaging studies ($n \geq 3$). (**D**) Relative invasion of BxPC-3 and IMIMPC-2 cell lines with ectopic SOX9 overexpression with respect to the invasion of cells transduced with GFP. Invasive cells analyzed using collagen transwell assays based in Boyden chamber ($n = 3$). (**E**) Tumor volume over time of subcutaneous tumors formed in nude mice by control and SOX9 transduced IMIMPC-2 cells ($n = 12$). Asterisks (*, **, and ***) indicate statistical significance ($p < 0.05$, $p < 0.01$, and $p < 0.001$, respectively).

We performed scratch assays with live-cell microscopy in pancreatic cancer cells with and without SOX9 silencing. Live-cell microscopy compositions from these assays revealed an impaired migration in SOX9 knockdown cells (Figure 3D; Supplementary Videos S2 and S3), which were able to form protrusive structures at the leading edge but seemed not to achieve the traction necessary to move efficiently forward. To give further insight into which cells are most efficient at wound healing in a competence context, we co-cultured IMIM-PC2 cells transduced with GFP and shSOX9 and we observed that the scratch was mainly closed by GFP transduced cells (Figure 3E, Supplementary Video S2). Accordingly, SOX9-silenced cells were found to invade the collagen matrix assays less efficiently than control cells (Figure 3F).

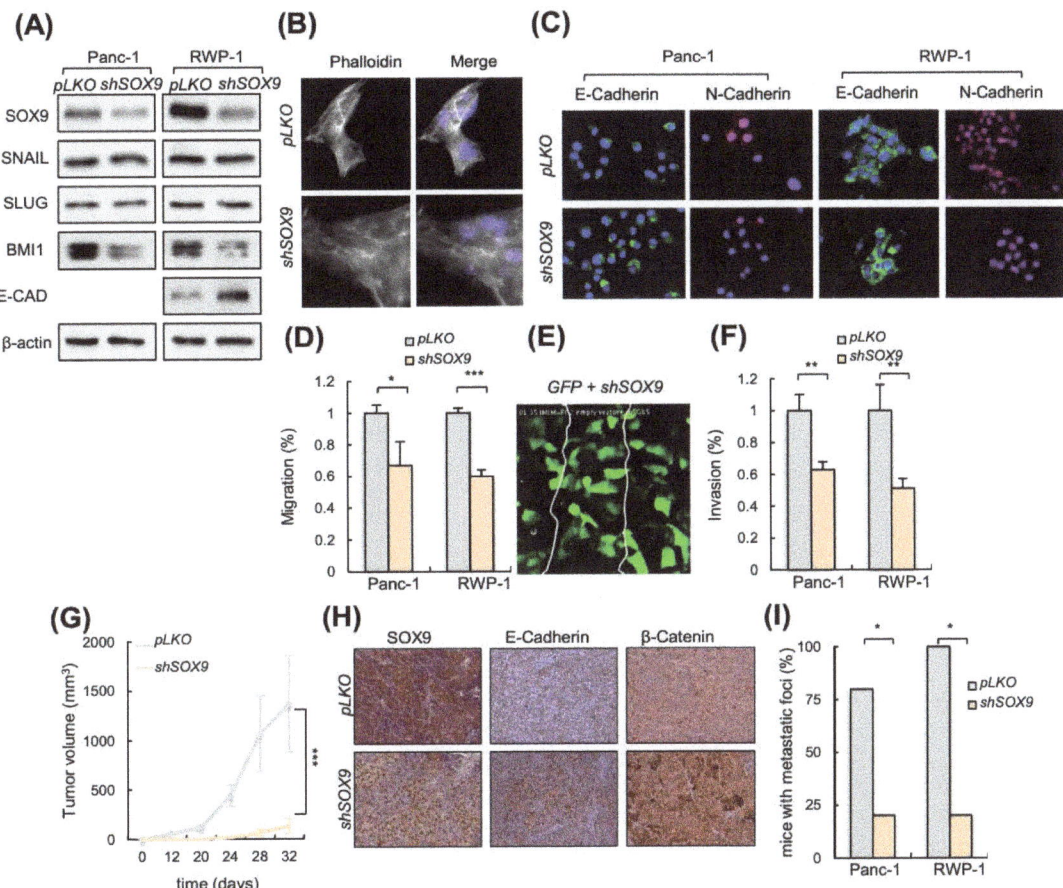

Figure 3. SOX9 knockdown drives MET and impairs metastasis. (**A**) Representative Western blot of SOX9, E-CAD, SNAIL, SLUG and BMI1 protein levels in Panc-1 and RWP-1 cell lines lentivirally infected with virus harboring a specific short hairpin RNA against SOX9 (*shSOX9*) or the corresponding empty vector (*pLKO*) ($n \geq 4$). (**B**) Images show filamentous actin (F-actin) labeled with phalloidin in RWP-1 *pLKO* and *shSOX9* cells. Nuclei were marked with DAPI, and the merged images are presented in right panel. (**C**) Representative images of E-Cadherin and N-Cadherin expression determined by immunofluorescence in Panc-1 and RWP-1 *pLKO* and *shSOX9* cells ($n = 3$). (**D**) Relative migration determined by transwell assays based in Boyden chamber ($n \geq 4$) in indicated cells and genotypes. (**E**) Frame at the time of wound closure (from Supplementary Video S2: down, middle panel) obtained in a scratch assay performed with a mix of IMIMPC-2 cells transduced with *GFP* or *shSOX9*. (**F**) Relative invasion of Panc-1 and RWP-1 cell lines with *shSOX9* with respect to *pLKO* cells. Invasive cells analyzed in vitro using collagen transwell assays based in Boyden chamber. (**G**) Tumor volume at the indicated time points of subcutaneous tumors formed by control *pLKO* and *shSOX9* RWP-1 cells ($n = 12$). (**H**) Representative images of SOX9, E-Cadherin and β-Catenin expression determined by immunohistochemistry in subcutaneous tumors represented in 3G. (**I**) Percentage of nude mice that developed metastatic *foci* derived from Panc-1 and RWP-1 *pLKO* and *shSOX9* cells in tail vein injection assays ($n = 5$). Asterisks (*, **, and ***) indicate statistical significance ($p < 0.05$, $p < 0.01$, and $p < 0.001$, respectively).

We performed in vivo studies in immunodeficient mice. When a subcutaneous inoculation route was used, tumors derived from *SOX9*-silenced cells exhibited a markedly reduced growth with respect to the tumors derived from control cells (Figure 3G). Of note, tumors derived from *SOX9*-silenced cells presented higher E-cadherin and β-catenin expression (Figure 3H), further supporting the link between SOX9 and the EMT process. Then, we compared the ability of control and *shSOX9* transduced cells to form metastatic *foci* in the lungs after intravenous injection in the tail vein. These experiments revealed a reduced metastatic potential in *SOX9*-silenced cells, with less than 20% of mice injected with *shSOX9* presenting *foci*, compared to almost 100% of the mice with controls that developed metastatic *foci* in their lungs (Figure 3I). These results altogether, support the notion that SOX9 activity is necessary for pancreatic cancer dissemination and colonization.

3.4. SOX9 Is Necessary for Pro-Metastatic Cancer Self-Renewal

We evaluated whether SOX9 might function in the maintenance of CSCs. We carried-out colony formation, soft agar and tumorsphere formation assays to examine the ability of cells to grow independently of attachment and their self-renewal potential in vitro. Silencing of SOX9 in the RWP-1 and Panc-1 cells resulted in a significant decline in the number of colonies and *foci* in soft agar (Figure 4A,B), and reduced the tumorsphere formation ability in stem-cell selective media (Figure 4C). To examine this further we analyzed the expression of the well-established pancreatic CSCs markers, *CD133*, *CD44*, *BMI1*, and *ALDH1* (39), which were significantly lower in *shSOX9* tumorspheres (Figure 4D). Consistent with these observations, SOX9 expression positively correlated with *CD44* and *BMI1* in the TCGA cohort samples (Supplementary Figure S3C). Moreover, the expression of *CD44* and *SOX9* increased according to tumor grade in the samples of patients (Figure 4E).

We determined the effect of *SOX9*-silencing on tumor initiation by performing subcutaneous injections upon limiting dilution transplantation in immunocompromised mice in vivo. We found that *SOX9*-silencing in both Panc-1 and RWP-1 cells resulted in a significant impairment of their tumorigenic ability (Figure 4F). The analysis using the ELDA software application revealed a diminished frequency of tumor-initiating/cancer stem cells in SOX9-silenced cells, with frequencies of 1/422,319 and 1/5,255,599 for the control and *shSOX9* cells, respectively (Figure 4G). Altogether, these results confirm that SOX9 sustains the self-renewal and tumor initiation activity in pancreatic cancer.

3.5. Transcriptomics Reveal Multiple Processes Differentially Expressed in SOX9-Silenced Cells

We performed expression microarrays in RWP-1 *pLKO* and *shSOX9* cells. An amount of 1091 genes were differentially expressed between conditions with p values below 0.05 and a fold change higher than 1.5 (or less than −1.5 for down-regulated genes). Functional enrichment analysis developed using the Overrepresentation Enrichment Analysis provided by WebGestalt and a hypergeometric distribution to test the GO categories overrepresented, revealed an alteration of different biological processes in agreement with the cellular features observed with SOX9 modulation. Thus, the establishment or maintenance of cell polarity, and the centriole assembly or regulation of microtubule-based processes, which are related to motility and migration, were downregulated in *SOX9*-silenced cells (Figure 5A). The two latter processes were also important in cytokinesis and cell division, which is concordant with the less proliferative phenotype exhibited by *SOX9*-silenced cells. Moreover, downregulation of neural tube development and post-embryonic development were detected in *SOX9*-silenced cells (Figure 5A). On the contrary, the stem cell differentiation processes were upregulated with *SOX9*-silencing (Figure 5B), which is in agreement with the SOX9 function in stem cell activity. Among the list of genes differentially expressed, genes involved in EMT and metastasis including *FGFR4*, *mTOR-RICTOR*, *PLK4*, and *PIK3CB* were found; however, EMT factors were not detected (Figure 5C). This result further supports that SOX9 controls different EMT states in pancreatic cancer cells.

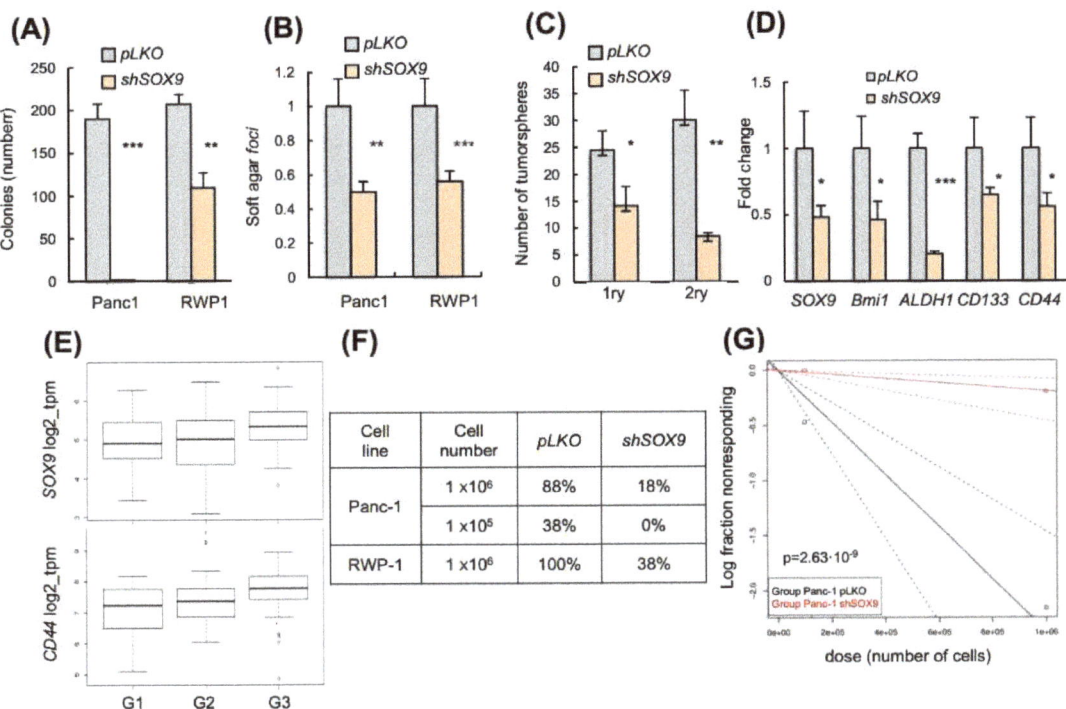

Figure 4. SOX9 is necessary for pro-metastatic cancer self-renewal. (**A**) Number of colonies formed by Panc-1 and RWP-1 *pLKO* and *sh1* ($n \geq 4$). (**B**) Relative number of soft agar foci formed by Panc-1 and RWP-1 *sh1* cells ($n = 4$). (**C**) Representative image and quantification of the number of primary (1ry) and secondary (2ry) tumorspheres formed by control and *sh1* RWP-1 cells ($n = 6$). (**D**) mRNA levels of cancer stem cell markers in 2ry tumorspheres ($n = 4$). (**E**) SOX9 and CD44 expression according to tumor grade in pancreatic cancer samples from the TCGA cohort (SOX9: $p = 0.0289$, $n = 147$; CD44: $p = 0.0038$, $n = 147$). (**F**) Tumor incidence in nude mice injected with Panc-1 and RWP-1 *pLKO* and *sh1* cells. (**G**) Plot representing the fraction of mice without tumors with respect to the dose of Panc1 cells subcutaneously injected. The slopes of the depicted solid lines correspond to the fraction of cells with tumor-initiating ability (black color: *pLKO* cells; red color: *sh1* cells. Chi square test for differences in stem cell frequencies: $p = 2.63 \times 10^{-9}$. Analysis performed using the ELDA software application (http://bioinf.wehi.edu.au/software/elda/). Accessed on 6 September 2021. Asterisks (*, **, and ***) indicate statistical significance ($p < 0.05$, $p < 0.01$, and $p < 0.001$, respectively).

3.6. BMI1 Stem Cell Factor Mediates SOX9 Activities

We have previously found that the transcriptional repressor BMI1, which is an important regulator of self-renewal, linked to EMT and metastasis in different cancers [40,41] including PDAC [42,43], is an effector of SOX9 activity [39]. We tested whether it could be involved in SOX9-mediated EMT and self-renewal activity. For this, we ectopically re-expressed *BMI1* in *SOX9*-silenced cells. Interestingly, ectopic *BMI1* restoration rescued the expression of N-cadherin and diminished the expression of E-cadherin (Figure 6A). In agreement with this, cells with *SOX9*-silencing and *BMI1* restoration exhibited a 3-fold increase in their invasive potential compared to cells with *SOX9*-silencing (Figure 6B). Moreover, the *BMI1* restoration increased in 3.4-fold the tumorsphere formation capacity of cells (Figure 6C). Accordingly, *BMI1* significantly fostered in vivo tumor growth (Figure 6D), as well as the number of Ki67 positive cells in vivo (Figure 6E). The link between SOX9 and

BMI1 was translated to clinical samples since their levels positively correlated in PDACs from the TCGA cohort (Figure 6F).

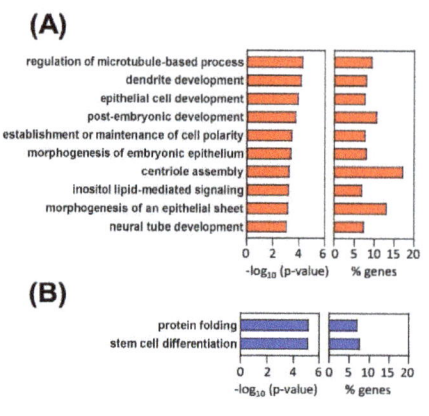

Figure 5. Multiple biological processes differentially expressed in *SOX9*-silenced cells. (**A**,**B**) Biological processes (BPs) altered in *shSOX9* RWP-1 cells. Gene ontology enrichment analysis from the differentially expressed genes were performed with WebGestalt (WEB-based Gene SeT AnaLysis Toolkit). Bar charts represent −log10 of the *p*-values and the percentage of genes belonging to the different BPs whose expression is altered. BPs (**A**) downregulated are represented in red and (**B**) upregulated in blue. (**C**) Differentially expressed genes in *SOX9*-silenced cells belonging to the identified BPs.

3.7. High Levels of SOX9 Confer Chemoresistance

Since our data indicated that SOX9 induces EMT and stemness, we reasoned that SOX9 might be involved in resistance to chemotherapy. Therefore, we exposed BxPC-3 cells to cytotoxic doses of gemcitabine in order to obtain drug-resistant cells (Figure 7A). These resistant cells were highly proliferative (Figure 7B), formed a higher number of tumorspheres (Figure 7C), and presented higher tumor initiation activity than the parental cells (Figure 7D). Gemcitabine-resistant cells exhibited a significantly elevated *SOX9* expression 5.2- and 6-fold in 1 µM and 10 µM concentrations, respectively, as well as increased levels of stem cell markers such as *CD133*, *BMI1*, *CD44* and *ESA* (Figure 7E). Moreover, the reduction in tumor volume exerted by the gemcitabine was significantly lower in tumors overexpressing SOX9 (Figure 7F). These results support the notion that SOX9 confers gemcitabine chemoresistance in pancreatic cancer.

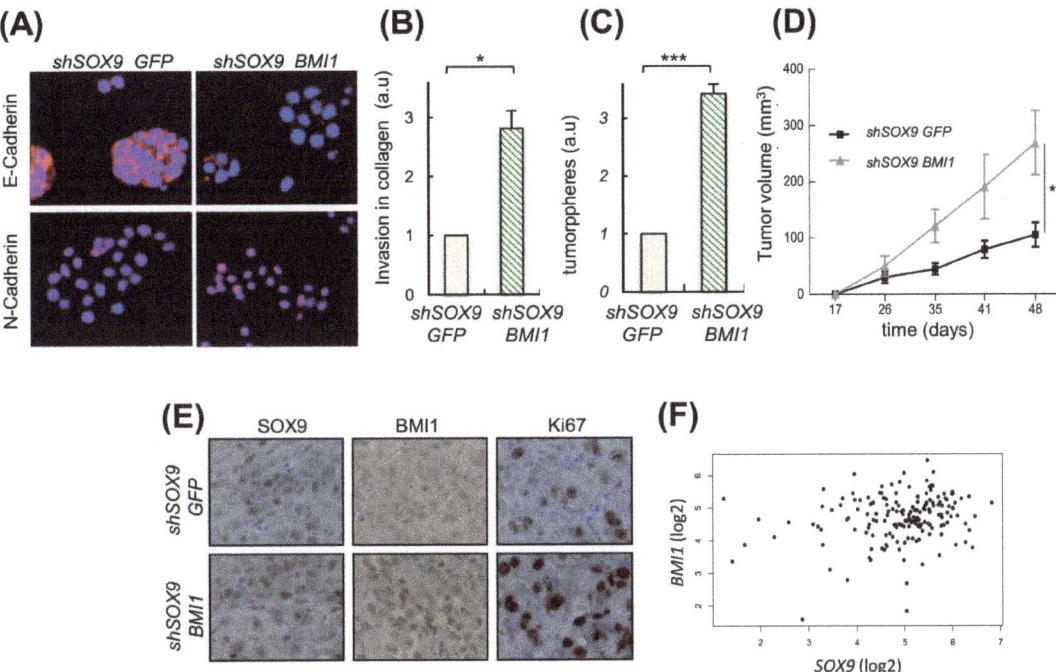

Figure 6. BMI1 is relevant in the metastatic potential induced by SOX9. (**A**) E-Cadherin and N-Cadherin expression analyzed by immunofluorescence in *SOX9*-silenced RWP-1 cells transduced with BMI1 (*shSOX9 BMI1*), and *SOX9*-silenced RWP-1 cells transduced with the corresponding empty plasmid (*shSOX9 GFP*). (**B**) Relative invasion determined by transwell assays for *shSOX9 BMI1* referred to *shSOX9GFP* (*n* = 4). (**C**) Relative number of tumorspheres (*n* = 3). (**D**) Average volume at the indicated time points of tumors derived from Panc-1 *shSOX9 BMI1* and *GFP* (10×10^4 cells/injection). (**E**) Representative images of SOX9, BMI1 and Ki67 expression determined by immunohistochemistry in subcutaneous tumors represented in 6D. (**F**) Correlation between the expression of SOX9 and BMI1 in pancreatic tumors of the TCGA cohort (cor = 0.19; *p* = 0.0137). * and *** indicate statistical significance with $p < 0.05$ and $p < 0.001$, respectively.

3.8. High Levels of SOX9 Are Associated with Reduced Survival and Correlate with EMT Markers

We investigated SOX9 expression in a large number of samples of healthy human pancreatic tissue, and in PanIN and PDAC by immunohistochemistry on a tissue microarray (TMA) [44]. SOX9 was expressed, although generally at low levels, in healthy pancreatic tissue, while its expression increased in PanIN lesions and was highest in PDAC (Figure 8A). Interestingly, metastatic samples (lymph nodes and distant organs) displayed very high SOX9 expression (+++) (Figure 8B). Consistent with this, the levels of SOX9 were higher in metastatic cell lines such as IMIMPC-1, RWP-1, Hs766T, and the highly pro-metastatic cell line Panc-1, than in the primary pancreatic cancer cell lines (Supplementary Figure S1B). Patient-derived xenografts (PDXs) represent to a certain extent the original human pancreatic tumors [45]. The distribution of SOX9 in a set of 53 engrafted tumors was reminiscent of patient data, with all of them displaying higher SOX9 mRNA expression (from 20- to 178-fold) compared to the average expression found in a group of 36 normal human pancreatic tissue samples (Figure 8C).

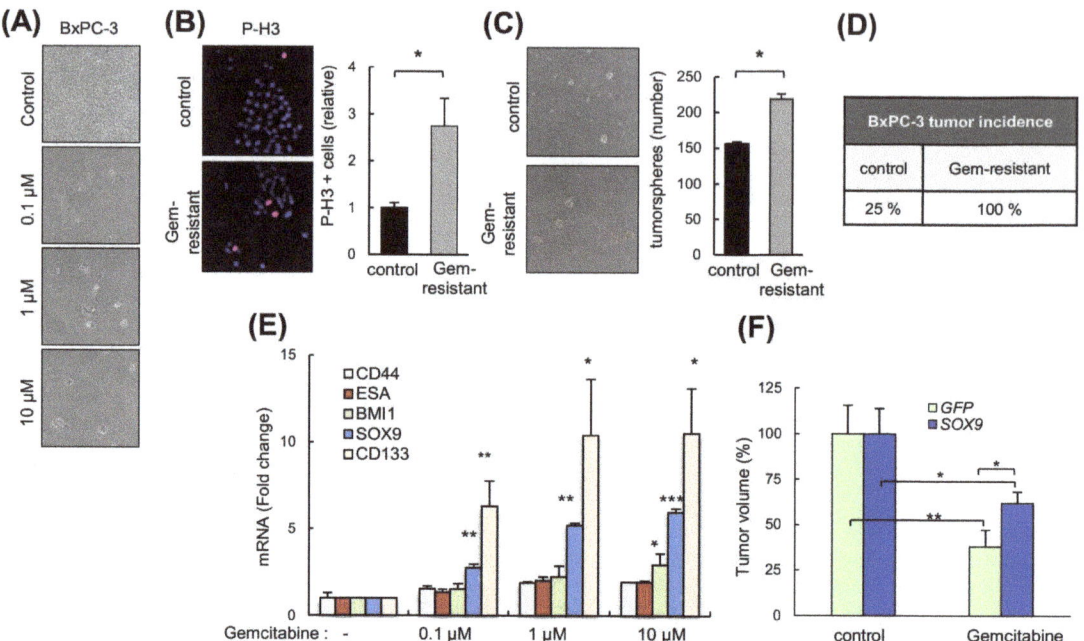

Figure 7. High levels of SOX9 confer chemoresistance. (**A**) Representative images of BxPC-3 cells untreated (parental) and gemcitabine-resistant cells after 120 h of treatment with different concentrations of gemcitabine (0.1, 1 and 10 µM). (**B**) Representative image and representation of the proportion of BxPC-3 and BxPC-3 gemcitabine-resistant cells (Gem-resistant) positive for the mitosis marker phospho-histone H3 (p-H3). (**C**) Representative image and quantification of the number of tumorspheres derived from BxPC-3 and BxPC-3 gemcitabine-resistant cells. (**D**) Percentage of subcutaneous tumors formed from BxPC-3 parental and gemcitabine-resistant cells (1×10^6 cells/injection). (**E**) *SOX9, CD133, BMI1, CD44* and *ESA* mRNA expression in BxPC-3 control and gemcitabine-resistant cells ($n = 4$). (**F**) Volume of tumors from IMIM-PC2 *GFP* and SOX9 cells in nude mice treated intraperitoneally once per week with vehicle or gemcitabine 5 mg/Kg ($n = 5$). Asterisks (*, **, and ***) indicate statistical significance ($p < 0.05$, $p < 0.01$, and $p < 0.001$, respectively).

Next, we investigated whether SOX9 expression was associated with EMT markers. For this, we analyzed the expression of E-cadherin (epithelial) and vimentin (mesenchymal) on the TMA. Consistent with previous studies [46,47], we observed high vimentin expression ($\geq$10% of cells) coupled with a total or partial loss of E-cadherin ($\leq$90% of cells) in PDAC (data not shown). Interestingly, the correlation analysis showed a positive association between SOX9 and vimentin expression (chi square, $p = 0.0006$) (Figure 8D). Alongside, there was an inverse correlation between SOX9 and E-cadherin expression (chi square, $p = 0.003$) (Figure 8D). Moreover, the analysis of the available information from The Cancer Genome Atlas (TCGA) project associated high SOX9 expression with reduced overall survival ($p = 0.011$) (Figure 8E), showing the relevance of SOX9 in the clinical progression of pancreatic cancer.

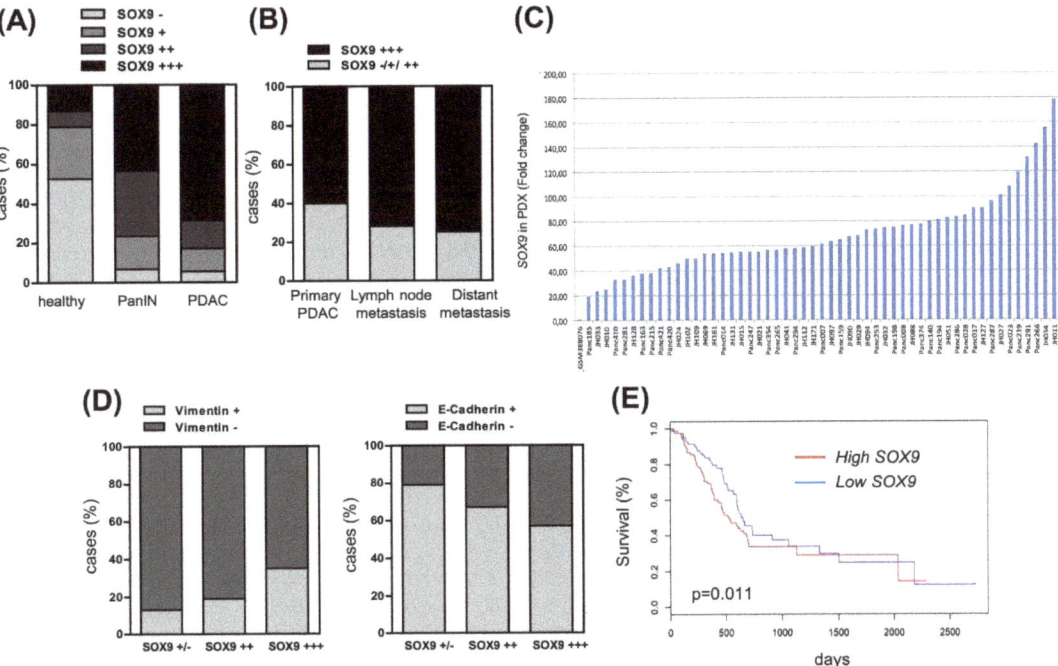

Figure 8. High levels of SOX9 are associated with PDAC progression and reduced survival. (**A**) SOX9 intensity analyzed by immunohistochemistry in a tissue microarray (TMA) composed by human samples of healthy pancreas ($n = 38$), PanIN ($n = 30$) and PDAC ($n = 198$). (−): 0–20 intensity grade; (+): 30–50 intensity grade; (++): 60–80 intensity grade; (+++): 90–100 intensity grade. (**B**) Distribution of SOX9 expression analyzed by immunochemistry in PDAC samples according to stage. Primary PDAC ($n = 58$), lymph node metastases ($n = 123$) and distant metastases ($n = 12$). (**C**) SOX9 mRNA expression in 53 pancreatic tumors from patient-derived xenografts (PDXs) relative to the average SOX9 expression level found in 36 samples of normal human pancreas. Expression in normal tissue is included as first line (GSM388076), whereas the remaining lines are the independent PDXs with the respective number in the bottom. (**D**) Negative association between SOX9 and vimentin protein expression (chi square, $p = 0.0006$) and positive association between SOX9 and E-Cadherin expression (chi square, $p = 0.003$) in human PDAC. Data obtained by immunohistochemistry in the TMA of 198 human PDAC samples. (**E**) Overall survival analysis of pancreatic cancer patients from the TCGA cohort according to SOX9 expression ($p = 0.011$, $n = 178$).

4. Discussion

Metastasis is the main cause of cancer deaths and remains the least understood process of cancer progression. This challenge is particularly important in pancreatic cancer, whereby the metastatic dissemination of cells occurs even at premalignant stages [48]. In this work, we demonstrate that SOX9 is necessary and sufficient for the activation and modulation of a tumorigenic EMT in pancreatic cancer, in a process that requires the activation of stemness pathways, but not critical EMT factors. Moreover, we ascertain that high levels of SOX9 are associated with poor patient survival and chemoresistance to gemcitabine.

We confirmed in clinical samples that SOX9 expression was particularly high in samples from metastases in both lymph nodes and distant organs. Importantly, through both gain- and loss-of-function approaches, we functionally demonstrated that SOX9 promotes the migration and invasion of pancreatic cancer cells and facilitates the metastatic dissemination and colonization of distant organs in vivo. Consistent with these observations, several studies have linked SOX9 activity to invasion and metastasis in pancreatic cancer [31,32,49] and additional types of cancer [20,50–53]. Our results are in agreement with the findings revealing that SOX9 activates context-dependent tumorigenic EMT programs [20,54–56]. Indeed, both gain- and loss-of-function approaches revealed that its activity is necessary for the induction of EMT and MET in K-Ras transformed cells and pancreatic tumor cells. Moreover, SOX9 correlated negatively with E-cadherin (epithelial marker) and positively with vimentin (mesenchymal marker) in human PDAC samples and pancreatic cells; however, the activation of EMT seems to be independent of SNAIL/SLUG or additional EMT transcription factors such as ZEB1 or PRRX1 in the advanced stages, because these transcription factors are not affected in pancreatic cancer cells with an altered expression of SOX9. Thus, our results show that SOX9 acts similarly to other EMT inducers including SNAIL, SLUG and ZEB1, which induce EMT along with stemness [6–8], and in contrast to PRRX1, which governs a pro-tumorigenic EMT not linked to stem cell properties [1,10].

Our results also support the notion that metastasis is in most cases dependent on EMT processes, which could be partial and are necessary for primary tumor cells to become motile and invasive [57]. Indeed, particularly in pancreatic cancer, a study using a mouse model with pancreas-specific alteration of pancreatic cancer driver genes, that harbored a lineage system to track the cells of epithelial origin, revealed that cancer circulating cells expressing mesenchymal markers were able to seed the liver [58]. In contrast, another study also using genetically engineered mouse models affirmed that EMT is dispensable for pancreatic cancer metastasis, but it is essential for therapy resistance [59], a phenomenon also observed in lung cancers [60]. This study showed that EMT specifically driven by Snail or Twist was not necessary for pancreatic cancer metastasis.

Our results also demonstrate that SOX9 confers resistance to chemotherapy in PDAC. In accordance with other studies, we observed an enrichment of the CSC compartment after gemcitabine exposure [61–64]. Importantly, SOX9 expression was elevated in gemcitabine resistant cells to a level only reached by CD133, one of the best-established stem cell markers in pancreatic cancer [62]. Additional studies also reported an increase of SOX9, although one of them of smaller magnitude, with lower concentrations of gemcitabine [30,33], suggesting a dose dependent effect of this agent. Taken together, these data link SOX9 to pancreatic CSCs and chemoresistance. In addition, our results further support the link between EMT and chemoresistance observed in pancreatic cancer [59,65]. Finally, we found that high levels of SOX9 correlated with poor patient survival. These results are in line with previous studies [33,66] and support the idea that SOX9 is a prognostic biomarker of pancreatic cancer.

5. Conclusions

In summary, we demonstrate that the developmental transcription factor, SOX9, confers cellular plasticity and promotes EMT in pancreatic cancer cells. This facilitates metastasis and promotes resistance to therapies, being both directly responsible for disease relapse and death. At the cellular level, SOX9 is a pleiotropic regulator of cancer cell activity governing additional functions to its well-known function regulating quiescence and self-renewal, such as EMT and metastasis. Mechanistically, we have identified stem cell factors rather than EMT factors as important mediators of the oncogenic activity of SOX9 in pancreatic cancer. Altogether, our findings highlight the relevance of SOX9 in pancreatic cancer outcomes due to its role in metastasis and to recurrence after therapy.

Supplementary Materials: The following supporting information can be downloaded at: https://www.mdpi.com/article/10.3390/cancers14040916/s1, Figure S1: High levels of SOX9 in pancreatic cancer cells, Figure S2: Characteristics of SOX9 overexpressing cells, Figure S3: Characteristics of SOX9 knock-down cells; Video S1: Frame composition showing motility and migration of IMIMPC-2 control (GFP) and SOX9 up-regulated (SOX9) cells in an in vitro scratch (wound healing) assay. Composition made from images acquired with a live cell imaging system over night, Video S2: Frame composition showing motility and migration performed by IMIMPC-2 cells with ectopic SOX9 overexpression or silencing in scratch (wound healing) assays. Up: Left panel: control cells (IMIM empty vector). Middle panel: IMIMPC-2 cells with ectopic SOX9 overexpression (IMIM OE SOX9). Right panel: SOX9-silencing cells (IMIM shSOX9). Down: Left panel: mix of IMIMPC-2 control cells harboring the empty vector with GFP (green cells) and IMIM-PC2 cells with ectopic SOX9 overexpression (IMIM empty vector+ IMIM OE SOX9). Middle panel: mix of IMIM-PC2 control cells harboring the empty vector with GFP (green cells) and IMIMPC-2 cells with SOX9-silencing (IMIM empty vector+ IMIM shSOX9), Video S3: Frame composition showing motility and migration performed by RWP-1 control (pLKO) and RWP-1 SOX9-silenced cells (sh1) in an in vitro scratch (wound healing) assay. Composition made from images acquired with a live cell imaging system over night.

Author Contributions: E.C.-G., L.L., V.M.-A. and P.A. performed the experiments in pancreatic cell lines; M.C. and M.S. provided reagents and performed experiments in K-Ras mice; D.B. performed in vivo imaging experiments; A.G., E.K., A.T. and C.H.L. collected clinical data and samples from the patients, evaluated the patients and completed the clinical experiments; M.H. assisted with PDX analysis; F.C., Á.R. and C.H.L. performed the transcriptomic analysis; R.L.-B. provided reagents, coordinated experiments and assisted in project design and writing; A.M. and E.C.-G. directed the project, contributed to data analysis and wrote the manuscript. All authors have read and agreed to the published version of the manuscript.

Funding: E.C.-G. was a recipient of a Stop Fuga de Cerebros postdoctoral fellowship and holds a Miguel Servet contract (CP19/00085) from the Instituto de Salud Carlos III (ISCIII). P.A. was a recipient of a predoctoral fellowship from the AECC foundation. V.M.-A., D.B. and R.L.-B. were supported by the Francis Crick Institute which receives its core funding from Cancer Research UK (FC001107), the UK Medical Research Council (FC001107), and the Wellcome Trust (FC001107). Work in the laboratory of M.S. was funded by the IRB, and by grants from Spanish Ministry of Economy co-funded by European Regional Development Fund (SAF2017-82613-R), European Research Council (ERC-2014-AdG/669622), Secretaria d'Universitats i Recerca del Departament d'Empresa i Coneixement of Catalonia (Grup de Recerca consolidat 2017 SGR 282) and "laCaixa" Foundation. Work in the laboratory of A.M. was supported by grants from ISCIII and FEDER Funds (CP16/00039, DTS16/00184, PI16/01580, DTS18/00181, PI18/01612, CP19/00085), Diputacion Foral Gipuzkoa (112/18), and Industry and Health Departments of the Basque Country.

Institutional Review Board Statement: The study was conducted according to the guidelines of the Declaration of Helsinki, and approved by the clinical research Ethics Committee of the Basque country (CEIC-E) code 02-2012 and Guipuzcoa Health Research Ethics Committee code 07-2013.

Informed Consent Statement: Informed consent was obtained from all subjects involved in the study.

Data Availability Statement: The data that support the findings of this study are included in the manuscript or in Supplementary Figures. Microarray data are openly available in GEO database with access number GSE193406.

Acknowledgments: The authors thank the Histology Platform of the Biodonostia Health Research Institute for their help.

Conflicts of Interest: The authors declare no conflict of interest.

References

1. Ocana, O.H.; Corcoles, R.; Fabra, A.; Moreno-Bueno, G.; Acloque, H.; Vega, S.; Barrallo-Gimeno, A.; Cano, A.; Nieto, M.A. Metastatic colonization requires the repression of the epithelial-mesenchymal transition inducer Prrx1. *Cancer Cell* **2012**, *22*, 709–724. [CrossRef]
2. Tsai, J.H.; Donaher, J.L.; Murphy, D.A.; Chau, S.; Yang, J. Spatiotemporal regulation of epithelial-mesenchymal transition is essential for squamous cell carcinoma metastasis. *Cancer Cell* **2012**, *22*, 725–736. [CrossRef]
3. Nieto, M.A.; Huang, R.Y.; Jackson, R.A.; Thiery, J.P. Emt: 2016. *Cell* **2016**, *166*, 21–45. [CrossRef]
4. Fazilaty, H.; Rago, L.; Kass Youssef, K.; Ocana, O.H.; Garcia-Asencio, F.; Arcas, A.; Galceran, J.; Nieto, M.A. A gene regulatory network to control EMT programs in development and disease. *Nat. Commun.* **2019**, *10*, 5115. [CrossRef]
5. Pastushenko, I.; Brisebarre, A.; Sifrim, A.; Fioramonti, M.; Revenco, T.; Boumahdi, S.; Van Keymeulen, A.; Brown, D.; Moers, V.; Lemaire, S.; et al. Identification of the tumour transition states occurring during EMT. *Nature* **2018**, *556*, 463–468. [CrossRef]
6. Mani, S.A.; Guo, W.; Liao, M.J.; Eaton, E.N.; Ayyanan, A.; Zhou, A.Y.; Brooks, M.; Reinhard, F.; Zhang, C.C.; Shipitsin, M.; et al. The epithelial-mesenchymal transition generates cells with properties of stem cells. *Cell* **2008**, *133*, 704–715. [CrossRef] [PubMed]

7. Wellner, U.; Schubert, J.; Burk, U.C.; Schmalhofer, O.; Zhu, F.; Sonntag, A.; Waldvogel, B.; Vannier, C.; Darling, D.; zur Hausen, A.; et al. The EMT-activator ZEB1 promotes tumorigenicity by repressing stemness-inhibiting microRNAs. *Nat. Cell Biol.* **2009**, *11*, 1487–1495. [CrossRef] [PubMed]
8. Ye, X.; Tam, W.L.; Shibue, T.; Kaygusuz, Y.; Reinhardt, F.; Ng Eaton, E.; Weinberg, R.A. Distinct EMT programs control normal mammary stem cells and tumour-initiating cells. *Nature* **2015**, *525*, 256–260. [CrossRef] [PubMed]
9. van Staalduinen, J.; Baker, D.; Ten Dijke, P.; van Dam, H. Epithelial-mesenchymal-transition-inducing transcription factors: New targets for tackling chemoresistance in cancer? *Oncogene* **2018**, *37*, 6195–6211. [CrossRef] [PubMed]
10. Beck, B.; Lapouge, G.; Rorive, S.; Drogat, B.; Desaedelaere, K.; Delafaille, S.; Dubois, C.; Salmon, I.; Willekens, K.; Marine, J.C.; et al. Different levels of Twist1 regulate skin tumor initiation, stemness, and progression. *Cell Stem Cell* **2015**, *16*, 67–79. [CrossRef] [PubMed]
11. Kamachi, Y.; Kondoh, H. Sox proteins: Regulators of cell fate specification and differentiation. *Development* **2013**, *140*, 4129–4144. [CrossRef] [PubMed]
12. Seymour, P.A.; Freude, K.K.; Dubois, C.L.; Shih, H.P.; Patel, N.A.; Sander, M. A dosage-dependent requirement for Sox9 in pancreatic endocrine cell formation. *Dev. Biol.* **2008**, *323*, 19–30. [CrossRef]
13. Furuyama, K.; Kawaguchi, Y.; Akiyama, H.; Horiguchi, M.; Kodama, S.; Kuhara, T.; Hosokawa, S.; Elbahrawy, A.; Soeda, T.; Koizumi, M.; et al. Continuous cell supply from a Sox9-expressing progenitor zone in adult liver, exocrine pancreas and intestine. *Nat. Genet.* **2011**, *43*, 34–41. [CrossRef] [PubMed]
14. Akiyama, H.; Chaboissier, M.C.; Behringer, R.R.; Rowitch, D.H.; Schedl, A.; Epstein, J.A.; de Crombrugghe, B. Essential role of Sox9 in the pathway that controls formation of cardiac valves and septa. *Proc. Natl. Acad. Sci. USA* **2004**, *101*, 6502–6507. [CrossRef]
15. Cheung, M.; Chaboissier, M.C.; Mynett, A.; Hirst, E.; Schedl, A.; Briscoe, J. The transcriptional control of trunk neural crest induction, survival, and delamination. *Dev. Cell* **2005**, *8*, 179–192. [CrossRef] [PubMed]
16. Panda, M.; Tripathi, S.K.; Biswal, B.K. SOX9: An emerging driving factor from cancer progression to drug resistance. *Biochim. Biophys. Acta Rev. Cancer* **2021**, *1875*, 188517. [CrossRef]
17. Carrasco-Garcia, E.; Lopez, L.; Aldaz, P.; Arevalo, S.; Aldaregia, J.; Egana, L.; Bujanda, L.; Cheung, M.; Sampron, N.; Garcia, I.; et al. SOX9-regulated cell plasticity in colorectal metastasis is attenuated by rapamycin. *Sci. Rep.* **2016**, *6*, 32350. [CrossRef]
18. Huang, J.Q.; Wei, F.K.; Xu, X.L.; Ye, S.X.; Song, J.W.; Ding, P.K.; Zhu, J.; Li, H.F.; Luo, X.P.; Gong, H.; et al. SOX9 drives the epithelial-mesenchymal transition in non-small-cell lung cancer through the Wnt/beta-catenin pathway. *J. Transl. Med.* **2019**, *17*, 143. [CrossRef] [PubMed]
19. Luanpitpong, S.; Li, J.; Manke, A.; Brundage, K.; Ellis, E.; McLaughlin, S.L.; Angsutararux, P.; Chanthra, N.; Voronkova, M.; Chen, Y.C.; et al. SLUG is required for SOX9 stabilization and functions to promote cancer stem cells and metastasis in human lung carcinoma. *Oncogene* **2016**, *35*, 2824–2833. [CrossRef]
20. Guo, W.; Keckesova, Z.; Donaher, J.L.; Shibue, T.; Tischler, V.; Reinhardt, F.; Itzkovitz, S.; Noske, A.; Zurrer-Hardi, U.; Bell, G.; et al. Slug and Sox9 cooperatively determine the mammary stem cell state. *Cell* **2012**, *148*, 1015–1028. [CrossRef]
21. Siegel, R.L.; Miller, K.D.; Jemal, A. Cancer statistics, 2019. *CA Cancer J. Clin.* **2019**, *69*, 7–34. [CrossRef] [PubMed]
22. Burris, H.A., 3rd; Moore, M.J.; Andersen, J.; Green, M.R.; Rothenberg, M.L.; Modiano, M.R.; Cripps, M.C.; Portenoy, R.K.; Storniolo, A.M.; Tarassoff, P.; et al. Improvements in survival and clinical benefit with gemcitabine as first-line therapy for patients with advanced pancreas cancer: A randomized trial. *J. Clin. Oncol.* **1997**, *15*, 2403–2413. [CrossRef] [PubMed]
23. Conroy, T.; Desseigne, F.; Ychou, M.; Bouche, O.; Guimbaud, R.; Becouarn, Y.; Adenis, A.; Raoul, J.L.; Gourgou-Bourgade, S.; de la Fouchardiere, C.; et al. FOLFIRINOX versus gemcitabine for metastatic pancreatic cancer. *N. Engl. J. Med.* **2011**, *364*, 1817–1825. [CrossRef]
24. Von Hoff, D.D.; Ervin, T.; Arena, F.P.; Chiorean, E.G.; Infante, J.; Moore, M.; Seay, T.; Tjulandin, S.A.; Ma, W.W.; Saleh, M.N.; et al. Increased survival in pancreatic cancer with nab-paclitaxel plus gemcitabine. *N. Engl. J. Med.* **2013**, *369*, 1691–1703. [CrossRef] [PubMed]
25. Ghaneh, P.; Kleeff, J.; Halloran, C.M.; Raraty, M.; Jackson, R.; Melling, J.; Jones, O.; Palmer, D.H.; Cox, T.F.; Smith, C.J.; et al. The Impact of Positive Resection Margins on Survival and Recurrence Following Resection and Adjuvant Chemotherapy for Pancreatic Ductal Adenocarcinoma. *Ann. Surg.* **2019**, *269*, 520–529. [CrossRef]
26. Bray, F.; Ferlay, J.; Soerjomataram, I.; Siegel, R.L.; Torre, L.A.; Jemal, A. Global cancer statistics 2018: GLOBOCAN estimates of incidence and mortality worldwide for 36 cancers in 185 countries. *CA Cancer J. Clin.* **2018**, *68*, 394–424. [CrossRef]
27. Prevot, P.P.; Simion, A.; Grimont, A.; Colletti, M.; Khalaileh, A.; Van den Steen, G.; Sempoux, C.; Xu, X.; Roelants, V.; Hald, J.; et al. Role of the ductal transcription factors HNF6 and Sox9 in pancreatic acinar-to-ductal metaplasia. *Gut* **2012**, *61*, 1723–1732. [CrossRef]
28. Kopp, J.L.; von Figura, G.; Mayes, E.; Liu, F.F.; Dubois, C.L.; Morris, J.P.t.; Pan, F.C.; Akiyama, H.; Wright, C.V.; Jensen, K.; et al. Identification of Sox9-dependent acinar-to-ductal reprogramming as the principal mechanism for initiation of pancreatic ductal adenocarcinoma. *Cancer Cell* **2012**, *22*, 737–750. [CrossRef]
29. Chen, N.M.; Singh, G.; Koenig, A.; Liou, G.Y.; Storz, P.; Zhang, J.S.; Regul, L.; Nagarajan, S.; Kuhnemuth, B.; Johnsen, S.A.; et al. NFATc1 Links EGFR Signaling to Induction of Sox9 Transcription and Acinar-Ductal Transdifferentiation in the Pancreas. *Gastroenterology* **2015**, *148*, 1024–1034.e1029. [CrossRef]

30. Sun, L.; Mathews, L.A.; Cabarcas, S.M.; Zhang, X.; Yang, A.; Zhang, Y.; Young, M.R.; Klarmann, K.D.; Keller, J.R.; Farrar, W.L. Epigenetic regulation of SOX9 by the NF-kappaB signaling pathway in pancreatic cancer stem cells. *Stem Cells* **2013**, *31*, 1454–1466. [CrossRef]
31. Camaj, P.; Jackel, C.; Krebs, S.; De Toni, E.N.; Blum, H.; Jauch, K.W.; Nelson, P.J.; Bruns, C.J. Hypoxia-independent gene expression mediated by SOX9 promotes aggressive pancreatic tumor biology. *Mol. Cancer Res.* **2014**, *12*, 421–432. [CrossRef]
32. Li, J.; Chen, X.; Zhu, L.; Lao, Z.; Zhou, T.; Zang, L.; Ge, W.; Jiang, M.; Xu, J.; Cao, Y.; et al. SOX9 is a critical regulator of TSPAN8-mediated metastasis in pancreatic cancer. *Oncogene* **2021**, *40*, 4884–4893. [CrossRef]
33. Higashihara, T.; Yoshitomi, H.; Nakata, Y.; Kagawa, S.; Takano, S.; Shimizu, H.; Kato, A.; Furukawa, K.; Ohtsuka, M.; Miyazaki, M. Sex Determining Region Y Box 9 Induces Chemoresistance in Pancreatic Cancer Cells by Induction of Putative Cancer Stem Cell Characteristics and Its High Expression Predicts Poor Prognosis. *Pancreas* **2017**, *46*, 1296–1304. [CrossRef]
34. Tanaka, T.; Kuroki, T.; Adachi, T.; Ono, S.; Hirabaru, M.; Soyama, A.; Kitasato, A.; Takatsuki, M.; Hayashi, T.; Eguchi, S. Evaluation of SOX9 expression in pancreatic ductal adenocarcinoma and intraductal papillary mucinous neoplasm. *Pancreas* **2013**, *42*, 488–493. [CrossRef]
35. Matheu, A.; Collado, M.; Wise, C.; Manterola, L.; Cekaite, L.; Tye, A.J.; Canamero, M.; Bujanda, L.; Schedl, A.; Cheah, K.S.; et al. Oncogenicity of the developmental transcription factor Sox9. *Cancer Res.* **2012**, *72*, 1301–1315. [CrossRef]
36. Santos, J.C.; Carrasco-Garcia, E.; Garcia-Puga, M.; Aldaz, P.; Montes, M.; Fernandez-Reyes, M.; de Oliveira, C.C.; Lawrie, C.H.; Arauzo-Bravo, M.J.; Ribeiro, M.L.; et al. SOX9 Elevation Acts with Canonical WNT Signaling to Drive Gastric Cancer Progression. *Cancer Res.* **2016**, *76*, 6735–6746. [CrossRef]
37. Guerra, C.; Schuhmacher, A.J.; Canamero, M.; Grippo, P.J.; Verdaguer, L.; Perez-Gallego, L.; Dubus, P.; Sandgren, E.P.; Barbacid, M. Chronic pancreatitis is essential for induction of pancreatic ductal adenocarcinoma by K-Ras oncogenes in adult mice. *Cancer Cell* **2007**, *11*, 291–302. [CrossRef]
38. Chaffer, C.L.; Weinberg, R.A. A perspective on cancer cell metastasis. *Science* **2011**, *331*, 1559–1564. [CrossRef] [PubMed]
39. Aldaz, P.; Otaegi-Ugartemendia, M.; Saenz-Antonanzas, A.; Garcia-Puga, M.; Moreno-Valladares, M.; Flores, J.M.; Gerovska, D.; Arauzo-Bravo, M.J.; Sampron, N.; Matheu, A.; et al. SOX9 promotes tumor progression through the axis BMI1-p21(CIP). *Sci. Rep.* **2020**, *10*, 357. [CrossRef] [PubMed]
40. Yang, M.H.; Hsu, D.S.; Wang, H.W.; Wang, H.J.; Lan, H.Y.; Yang, W.H.; Huang, C.H.; Kao, S.Y.; Tzeng, C.H.; Tai, S.K.; et al. Bmi1 is essential in Twist1-induced epithelial-mesenchymal transition. *Nat. Cell Biol.* **2010**, *12*, 982–992. [CrossRef] [PubMed]
41. Kreso, A.; van Galen, P.; Pedley, N.M.; Lima-Fernandes, E.; Frelin, C.; Davis, T.; Cao, L.; Baiazitov, R.; Du, W.; Sydorenko, N.; et al. Self-renewal as a therapeutic target in human colorectal cancer. *Nat. Med.* **2014**, *20*, 29–36. [CrossRef] [PubMed]
42. Song, W.; Tao, K.; Li, H.; Jin, C.; Song, Z.; Li, J.; Shi, H.; Li, X.; Dang, Z.; Dou, K. Bmi-1 is related to proliferation, survival and poor prognosis in pancreatic cancer. *Cancer Sci.* **2010**, *101*, 1754–1760. [CrossRef] [PubMed]
43. Proctor, E.; Waghray, M.; Lee, C.J.; Heidt, D.G.; Yalamanchili, M.; Li, C.; Bednar, F.; Simeone, D.M. Bmi1 enhances tumorigenicity and cancer stem cell function in pancreatic adenocarcinoma. *PLoS ONE* **2013**, *8*, e55820. [CrossRef] [PubMed]
44. Karamitopoulou, E.; Pallante, P.; Zlobec, I.; Tornillo, L.; Carafa, V.; Schaffner, T.; Borner, M.; Diamantis, I.; Esposito, F.; Brunner, T.; et al. Loss of the CBX7 protein expression correlates with a more aggressive phenotype in pancreatic cancer. *Eur. J. Cancer* **2010**, *46*, 1438–1444. [CrossRef]
45. Martinez-Garcia, R.; Juan, D.; Rausell, A.; Munoz, M.; Banos, N.; Menendez, C.; Lopez-Casas, P.P.; Rico, D.; Valencia, A.; Hidalgo, M. Transcriptional dissection of pancreatic tumors engrafted in mice. *Genome Med.* **2014**, *6*, 27. [CrossRef]
46. Hong, S.M.; Li, A.; Olino, K.; Wolfgang, C.L.; Herman, J.M.; Schulick, R.D.; Iacobuzio-Donahue, C.; Hruban, R.H.; Goggins, M. Loss of E-cadherin expression and outcome among patients with resectable pancreatic adenocarcinomas. *Mod. Pathol.* **2011**, *24*, 1237–1247. [CrossRef]
47. Handra-Luca, A.; Hong, S.M.; Walter, K.; Wolfgang, C.; Hruban, R.; Goggins, M. Tumour epithelial vimentin expression and outcome of pancreatic ductal adenocarcinomas. *Br. J. Cancer* **2011**, *104*, 1296–1302. [CrossRef]
48. Tuveson, D.A.; Neoptolemos, J.P. Understanding metastasis in pancreatic cancer: A call for new clinical approaches. *Cell* **2012**, *148*, 21–23. [CrossRef]
49. Kaushik, G.; Seshacharyulu, P.; Rauth, S.; Nallasamy, P.; Rachagani, S.; Nimmakayala, R.K.; Vengoji, R.; Mallya, K.; Chirravuri-Venkata, R.; Singh, A.B.; et al. Selective inhibition of stemness through EGFR/FOXA2/SOX9 axis reduces pancreatic cancer metastasis. *Oncogene* **2021**, *40*, 848–862. [CrossRef]
50. Wang, G.; Lunardi, A.; Zhang, J.; Chen, Z.; Ala, U.; Webster, K.A.; Tay, Y.; Gonzalez-Billalabeitia, E.; Egia, A.; Shaffer, D.R.; et al. Zbtb7a suppresses prostate cancer through repression of a Sox9-dependent pathway for cellular senescence bypass and tumor invasion. *Nat. Genet.* **2013**, *45*, 739–746. [CrossRef]
51. Cheng, P.F.; Shakhova, O.; Widmer, D.S.; Eichhoff, O.M.; Zingg, D.; Frommel, S.C.; Belloni, B.; Raaijmakers, M.I.; Goldinger, S.M.; Santoro, R.; et al. Methylation-dependent SOX9 expression mediates invasion in human melanoma cells and is a negative prognostic factor in advanced melanoma. *Genome Biol.* **2015**, *16*, 42. [CrossRef] [PubMed]
52. Larsimont, J.C.; Youssef, K.K.; Sanchez-Danes, A.; Sukumaran, V.; Defrance, M.; Delatte, B.; Liagre, M.; Baatsen, P.; Marine, J.C.; Lippens, S.; et al. Sox9 Controls Self-Renewal of Oncogene Targeted Cells and Links Tumor Initiation and Invasion. *Cell Stem Cell* **2015**, *17*, 60–73. [CrossRef] [PubMed]
53. Laughney, A.M.; Hu, J.; Campbell, N.R.; Bakhoum, S.F.; Setty, M.; Lavallee, V.P.; Xie, Y.; Masilionis, I.; Carr, A.J.; Kottapalli, S.; et al. Regenerative lineages and immune-mediated pruning in lung cancer metastasis. *Nat. Med.* **2020**, *26*, 259–269. [CrossRef] [PubMed]

54. Ma, Y.; Shepherd, J.; Zhao, D.; Bollu, L.R.; Tahaney, W.M.; Hill, J.; Zhang, Y.; Mazumdar, A.; Brown, P.H. SOX9 is Essential for Triple-Negative Breast Cancer Cell Survival and Metastasis. *Mol. Cancer Res.* **2020**, *18*, 1825–1838. [CrossRef] [PubMed]
55. Li, T.; Huang, H.; Shi, G.; Zhao, L.; Li, T.; Zhang, Z.; Liu, R.; Hu, Y.; Liu, H.; Yu, J.; et al. TGF-beta1-SOX9 axis-inducible COL10A1 promotes invasion and metastasis in gastric cancer via epithelial-to-mesenchymal transition. *Cell Death Dis.* **2018**, *9*, 849. [CrossRef] [PubMed]
56. Kawai, T.; Yasuchika, K.; Ishii, T.; Miyauchi, Y.; Kojima, H.; Yamaoka, R.; Katayama, H.; Yoshitoshi, E.Y.; Ogiso, S.; Kita, S.; et al. SOX9 is a novel cancer stem cell marker surrogated by osteopontin in human hepatocellular carcinoma. *Sci. Rep.* **2016**, *6*, 30489. [CrossRef] [PubMed]
57. Liao, T.T.; Yang, M.H. Hybrid Epithelial/Mesenchymal State in Cancer Metastasis: Clinical Significance and Regulatory Mechanisms. *Cells* **2020**, *9*, 623. [CrossRef]
58. Rhim, A.D.; Mirek, E.T.; Aiello, N.M.; Maitra, A.; Bailey, J.M.; McAllister, F.; Reichert, M.; Beatty, G.L.; Rustgi, A.K.; Vonderheide, R.H.; et al. EMT and dissemination precede pancreatic tumor formation. *Cell* **2012**, *148*, 349–361. [CrossRef] [PubMed]
59. Zheng, X.; Carstens, J.L.; Kim, J.; Scheible, M.; Kaye, J.; Sugimoto, H.; Wu, C.C.; LeBleu, V.S.; Kalluri, R. Epithelial-to-mesenchymal transition is dispensable for metastasis but induces chemoresistance in pancreatic cancer. *Nature* **2015**, *527*, 525–530. [CrossRef]
60. Fischer, K.R.; Durrans, A.; Lee, S.; Sheng, J.; Li, F.; Wong, S.T.; Choi, H.; El Rayes, T.; Ryu, S.; Troeger, J.; et al. Epithelial-to-mesenchymal transition is not required for lung metastasis but contributes to chemoresistance. *Nature* **2015**, *527*, 472–476. [CrossRef] [PubMed]
61. Quint, K.; Tonigold, M.; Di Fazio, P.; Montalbano, R.; Lingelbach, S.; Ruckert, F.; Alinger, B.; Ocker, M.; Neureiter, D. Pancreatic cancer cells surviving gemcitabine treatment express markers of stem cell differentiation and epithelial-mesenchymal transition. *Int. J. Oncol.* **2012**, *41*, 2093–2102. [CrossRef] [PubMed]
62. Hermann, P.C.; Huber, S.L.; Herrler, T.; Aicher, A.; Ellwart, J.W.; Guba, M.; Bruns, C.J.; Heeschen, C. Distinct populations of cancer stem cells determine tumor growth and metastatic activity in human pancreatic cancer. *Cell Stem Cell* **2007**, *1*, 313–323. [CrossRef]
63. Shah, A.N.; Summy, J.M.; Zhang, J.; Park, S.I.; Parikh, N.U.; Gallick, G.E. Development and characterization of gemcitabine-resistant pancreatic tumor cells. *Ann. Surg. Oncol.* **2007**, *14*, 3629–3637. [CrossRef] [PubMed]
64. Jimeno, A.; Feldmann, G.; Suarez-Gauthier, A.; Rasheed, Z.; Solomon, A.; Zou, G.M.; Rubio-Viqueira, B.; Garcia-Garcia, E.; Lopez-Rios, F.; Matsui, W.; et al. A direct pancreatic cancer xenograft model as a platform for cancer stem cell therapeutic development. *Mol. Cancer Ther.* **2009**, *8*, 310–314. [CrossRef]
65. Arumugam, T.; Ramachandran, V.; Fournier, K.F.; Wang, H.; Marquis, L.; Abbruzzese, J.L.; Gallick, G.E.; Logsdon, C.D.; McConkey, D.J.; Choi, W. Epithelial to mesenchymal transition contributes to drug resistance in pancreatic cancer. *Cancer Res.* **2009**, *69*, 5820–5828. [CrossRef] [PubMed]
66. Huang, L.; Holtzinger, A.; Jagan, I.; BeGora, M.; Lohse, I.; Ngai, N.; Nostro, C.; Wang, R.; Muthuswamy, L.B.; Crawford, H.C.; et al. Ductal pancreatic cancer modeling and drug screening using human pluripotent stem cell- and patient-derived tumor organoids. *Nat. Med.* **2015**, *21*, 1364–1371. [CrossRef]

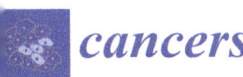

Review

Benefits from Adjuvant Chemotherapy in Patients with Resected Non-Small Cell Lung Cancer: Possibility of Stratification by Gene Amplification of *ACTN4* According to Evaluation of Metastatic Ability

Takehiro Tozuka [1], Rintaro Noro [1], Masahiro Seike [1] and Kazufumi Honda [2,3,*]

1. Department of Pulmonary Medicine and Oncology, Graduate School of Medicine, Nippon Medical School, Tokyo 113-8603, Japan
2. Department of Bioregulation, Graduate School of Medicine, Nippon Medical School, Tokyo 113-8602, Japan
3. Institution for Advanced Medical Science, Nippon Medical School, Tokyo 113-8602, Japan
* Correspondence: k-honda@nms.ac.jp

Simple Summary: The establishment of biomarkers that can identify individuals at high risk of early recurrence after surgery will be an important issue in decision-making for perioperative therapy. In this review, we describe potential biomarkers for predicting the likelihood of recurrence in patients who undergo surgery for stage I NSCLC. ACTN4 is a possible biomarker for identifying patients at high risk of postoperative recurrence, and patients with gene amplification of *ACTN4* might thus benefit the most from adjuvant chemotherapy.

Abstract: Surgical treatment is the best curative treatment option for patients with non-small cell lung cancer (NSCLC), but some patients have recurrence beyond the surgical margin even after receiving curative surgery. Therefore, therapies with anti-cancer agents also play an important role perioperatively. In this paper, we review the current status of adjuvant chemotherapy in NSCLC and describe promising perioperative therapies, including molecularly targeted therapies and immune checkpoint inhibitors. Previously reported biomarkers of adjuvant chemotherapy for NSCLC are discussed along with their limitations. Adjuvant chemotherapy after resective surgery was most effective in patients with metastatic lesions located just outside the surgical margin; in addition, these metastatic lesions were the most sensitive to adjuvant chemotherapy. Thus, the first step in predicting patients who have sensitivity to adjuvant therapies is to perform a qualified evaluation of metastatic ability using markers such as actinin-4 (ACTN4). In this review, we discuss the potential use of biomarkers in patient stratification for effective adjuvant chemotherapy and, in particular, the use of ACTN4 as a possible biomarker for NSCLC.

Keywords: non-small cell lung cancer; adjuvant chemotherapy; biomarker; actinin-4; metastatic ability

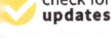

Citation: Tozuka, T.; Noro, R.; Seike, M.; Honda, K. Benefits from Adjuvant Chemotherapy in Patients with Resected Non-Small Cell Lung Cancer: Possibility of Stratification by Gene Amplification of *ACTN4* According to Evaluation of Metastatic Ability. *Cancers* **2022**, *14*, 4363. https://doi.org/10.3390/cancers14184363

Academic Editors: Daniel L. Pouliquen and Cristina Núñez González

Received: 19 July 2022
Accepted: 2 September 2022
Published: 7 September 2022

Publisher's Note: MDPI stays neutral with regard to jurisdictional claims in published maps and institutional affiliations.

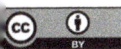

Copyright: © 2022 by the authors. Licensee MDPI, Basel, Switzerland. This article is an open access article distributed under the terms and conditions of the Creative Commons Attribution (CC BY) license (https://creativecommons.org/licenses/by/4.0/).

1. Introduction

Lung cancer is the leading cause of cancer death worldwide [1]. (NSCLC) non-small cell lung cancer (NSCLC) accounts for 85% of all lung cancers [2]. Almost 20% of patients have early-stage disease (stage I–II) and around 30% of patients have locally advanced disease (stage III) at the time of diagnosis of NSCLC [3]. Surgical resection is the best curative treatment option for patients with NSCLC. However, local or systemic relapse of the disease is common despite complete resection. Five-year overall survival (OS) rates are reported to be about 70%, 50–60%, and 35% for pathological stages IB, IIA–IIB, and IIIA NSCLC, respectively [4].

Adjuvant chemotherapy is performed to prevent recurrence in patients who undergo complete resection of NSCLC. Adjuvant cisplatin-based chemotherapy is the standard treatment for postoperative patients with stage IIA–IIIA NSCLC. Pooled analysis of several clinical trials has shown that adjuvant cisplatin-doublet chemotherapy improved the 5-year disease-free survival (DFS) rate by 5.8% and the 5-year OS rate by 5.4% [5] Moreover, the IMpower 010 trial demonstrated that atezolizumab after adjuvant platinum-based chemotherapy improved DFS in postoperative patients who were selected by programmed death-ligand 1 [PD-L1] expression [6]. The ADAURA trial demonstrated that osimertinib improved DFS in epidermal growth factor receptor (EGFR) mutation-positive stage IB–IIIA disease following complete resection [7]. However, a pooled analysis of several clinical trials showed that some patients without adjuvant chemotherapy achieved five-year DFS and that the rate of overall grade 3 to 4 toxicity was 66% in patients with adjuvant platinum-based chemotherapy [5]. As a result, some patients with lung cancer were cured by chest surgery alone, and adjuvant chemotherapy may be overtreatment for such patients [5]. An economic analysis of a randomized trial of adjuvant vinorelbine plus cisplatin suggested a high cost-effectiveness of this combined treatment compared with other standard healthcare interventions [8]. However, a pilot study revealed that patients undergoing cancer treatment may change their treatment to defray out-of-pocket costs because of financial burden [9]. In particular, molecularly targeted therapies and immune checkpoint inhibitors (ICIs) may increase economic toxicity for cancer patients due to the high prices of these drugs [10]. From the perspective of reducing adverse events and saving on the medical costs of adjuvant chemotherapy, biomarkers that can predict the likelihood of recurrence after surgery would be of great interest. In contrast, some patients with completely resected NSCLC may have minimal residual disease (MRD) that is undetectable radiographically due to the limits of imaging resolution. Therefore, it is important to establish biomarkers that can predict the risk of recurrence of lung cancer. To date, many studies have investigated specific gene expression, gene signature, and excision repair cross-complementation group 1 (ERCC1), which is related to cisplatin (CDDP) sensitivity, as candidate biomarkers for adjuvant chemotherapy in patients with NSCLC [11–25]. However, a robust biomarker has not yet been established and clinical application has been challenging because it is difficult to quantify the biomarkers and determine the cutoff values. It is generally considered that patients with MRD are the best candidates for adjuvant chemotherapy, as the presence of MRD beyond the surgical margin is known to be a strong indicator of the metastatic ability of the primary site. Thus, there is a need for biomarkers that can accurately evaluate the metastatic ability of the primary site and thus help decide the strategy for precision adjuvant chemotherapy.

Actinin-4 (ACTN4) is an anti-binding protein involved in cancer invasion and metastasis [23]. In various cancers, including lung cancer, increased protein expression of ACTN4 indicates malignancy and metastatic potential [26–28]. Gene amplification of *ACTN4* located on 19q13 is also significantly associated with metastatic potential in various types of cancer [29–31]. We have recently reported that increased protein expression and gene amplification of ACTN4 can be a promising biomarker for adjuvant chemotherapy in postoperative patients with NSCLC [32–34]. In this review, we discuss the role of ACTN4 in the process of tumor progression and the usefulness of ACTN4 as a potential biomarker for selecting patients most likely to benefit from adjuvant chemotherapy.

2. Adjuvant Chemotherapy in NSCLC

Previous clinical trials have demonstrated improvements in DFS and OS following adjuvant cisplatin-based chemotherapy for resected NSCLC [35–37]. A meta-analysis including five clinical trials also showed that cisplatin-based adjuvant chemotherapy prolonged OS compared with surgery alone (hazard ratio [HR], 0.89; 95% confidence interval [CI], 0.82–0.96). Adjuvant cisplatin-doublet chemotherapy achieved a 5.4% improvement in the 5-year OS rate [5]. However, some of these patients had severe adverse events (AEs). In the meta-analysis, the rates of grade 3 or 4 AEs and of grade 4 AEs were reported to be 66% and 32%, respectively. Although toxicity types differed according to the chemotherapeutic regimen, the most frequent AE was neutropenia. Treatment-related deaths were reported as 0.9%. Subset analysis by stage of cancer showed possible harm in stage IA (HR, 1.40; 95%CI, 0.95–2.06) [5]. The clinical benefits of adjuvant chemotherapy tend to be higher at more advanced stages [5]. In Japan, adjuvant therapy with tegafur/uracil (UFT) is recommended for patients with stage IA–IB NSCLC after complete resection [38]. A meta-analysis of adjuvant UFT in NSCLC demonstrated that surgery plus UFT prolonged OS compared with surgery alone (HR, 0.74; 95%CI, 0.61–0.88) [38,39].

Molecular targeted therapy has been a standard treatment for advanced NSCLC patients with driver mutations such as EGFR mutation or anaplastic lymphoma kinase (ALK) rearrangement. Clinical trials of adjuvant chemotherapy using tyrosine kinase inhibitors (TKIs) have been conducted perioperatively in patients with EGFR-mutant NSCLC. In the RADIANT randomized controlled trial, Erlotinib was compared to placebo in patients with completely resected stage IB–IIIA NSCLC [40]. In a subgroup analysis of the RADIANT trial, erlotinib prolonged DFS (HR, 0.61; 95%CI: 0.38–0.98) but not OS (HR, 1.09; 95%CI: 0.55–2.16) compared to placebo in patients with EGFR-mutant NSCLC. The ADJUVANT trial compared gefitinib (oral for two years) with cisplatin plus vinorelbine (four cycles) in stage II–IIIA NSCLC patients with common EGFR mutations (exon 19 deletion or exon 21 L858R mutation) after complete resection [41]. DFS was significantly longer in the gefitinib group (HR, 0.60; 95%CI, 0.42–0.87), but there was no significant difference in OS between the groups (HR, 0.92; 95%CI, 0.62–1.36). In the IMPACT trial, adjuvant gefitinib (oral for two years) did not prolong DFS and OS compared with cisplatin plus vinorelbine (four cycles) in patients with completely resected Stage II–IIIA NACLC with common EGFR mutations [42]. The ADAURA trial compared osimertinib (oral for three years) with placebo in stage IB–IIIA NSCLC patients with common EGFR mutations after complete resection. In that study, the physician decided whether patients received adjuvant platinum-based chemotherapy before administration of osimertinib or placebo. Adjuvant osimertinib significantly prolonged DFS compared with placebo (HR, 0.17; 99.06%CI, 0.11–0.26), although OS was immature [7]. These results suggest that adjuvant chemotherapy using EGFR-TKI may become a treatment option in the near future, but toxicity and medical cost should be considered. Therefore, it is necessary to identify biomarkers for detecting patients with a high risk of recurrence and those who would benefit from adjuvant EGFR-TKI.

ICIs including anti-programmed cell death 1 (PD-1) antibodies, anti-PD-L1 antibodies, and anti-cytotoxic T-lymphocyte-associated protein 4 (CTLA-4) antibodies have greatly improved prognosis in patients with metastatic NSCLC. ICIs have recently moved from the second-line to the first-line setting for metastatic NSCLC patients without driver mutations [43–47]. At present, ICIs play an important role in the treatment of locally advanced NSCLC. The PACIFIC trial revealed that durvalumab after chemoradiotherapy prolonged progression-free survival (PFS) and OS in unresected stage IIIA NSCLC patients [48]. Moreover, ICI has become a promising treatment in perioperative patients with NSCLC. The IMpower 010 trial demonstrated that atezolizumab after adjuvant platinum-based chemotherapy significantly prolonged DFS in postoperative patients with PD-L1 (SP263) positive stage II–IIIA NSCLC (HR, 0.66; 95%CI, 0.50–0.88) [6], but there were no survival benefits in patients without PD-L1 expression (HR, 0.97; 95%CI, 0.72–1.31). Neoadjuvant chemotherapy has not become a standard perioperative treatment in patients with NSCLC because it can lead to increased perioperative complications [49]. However, there are many clinical trials of neoadjuvant chemotherapy using ICIs, and neoadjuvant immunotherapy is a promising treatment [50]. The Checkmate 816 trial showed that neoadjuvant nivolumab plus platinum-based chemotherapy achieved a significantly longer event-free survival (HR, 0.63; 97.38%CI, 0.43–0.91; $p = 0.005$) and a higher pathological complete response rate (odds ratio, 13.94; 99%CI, 3.49–55.75) compared with neoadjuvant platinum-based chemotherapy alone in patients with stage IB–IIIA NSCLC [51]. However, neoadjuvant chemotherapy in patients with NSCLC can induce severe adverse events preoperatively that may cause surgery to be postponed or canceled. In the Checkmate 816 trial, definitive surgery was canceled in 16% of patients included in the nivolumab plus chemotherapy arm.

The reasons for canceled surgery were disease progression (7%), AEs (1%), or other scenarios (8%). Patient selection by appropriate biomarkers is important in both the adjuvant and neoadjuvant settings.

3. Current Biomarker Candidates for Perioperative Patients with NSCLC

Many previous studies have attempted to identify useful biomarkers for adjuvant chemotherapy, but none have yet been established in clinical practice.

Numerous studies have reported that signatures based on gene expression are prognostic factors in patients with NSCLC [11–22]. However, none of these signatures are ready for clinical application as they require statistical validation and reproducibility of the signatures. In addition, their actual medical utility and medical cost are unknown. It is also difficult to standardize the quantification methods and set cutoff levels because most studies have been based on microarray analysis of mRNA expression levels [11–22]. There is no consensus regarding the usefulness of genetic analysis in determining a treatment strategy for patients with postoperative lung cancer.

High expression of ERCC1 was reported to be a prognostic factor in patients with early-stage NSCLC who had received surgery alone [23]. DNA repair capacity is strongly associated with cisplatin resistance. In particular, the ERCC1 protein is considered to play an important role in nucleotide excision repair [24]. Therefore, several studies have investigated the association between ERCC1 expression and the efficacy of adjuvant platinum-based chemotherapy. A previous study suggested that ERCC1 was related to the resistance of NSCLC to cisplatin-based chemotherapy [24]. It included patients with completely resected NSCLC and found that patients with ERCC1-negative tumors benefited from adjuvant cisplatin-based chemotherapy but patients with ERCC1-positive tumors did not [24]. However, another study that performed immunohistochemical analysis of patients in two independent phase 3 trials was unable to validate ERCC1 protein expression as a predictive marker for the efficacy of adjuvant-chemotherapy [25]. Therefore, the usefulness of ERCC1 expression has not been established in therapeutic decision-making for patients with completely resected NSCLC.

Previous studies have verified the prognostic and predictive effects of the tumor suppressor gene tumor protein p53 gene (TP53) in patients with completely resected NSCLC. TP53 is considered to have important roles in the prevention and suppression of abnormal cell proliferation through multiple mechanisms, including cell cycle arrest, apoptosis, and DNA repair [52–54]. The Lung Adjuvant Cisplatin Evaluation Biomarker (LACE-Bio) pooled analysis demonstrated that TP53 mutations were marginally predictive of OS benefits from adjuvant platinum-based chemotherapy [54]. However, a study including 197 NSCLC patients enrolled in a randomized trial of postoperative radiation therapy and chemotherapy showed that TP53 mutations and increased expression of P53 protein were not significant prognostic factors in resected stage II–IIIA NSCLC [55]. A previous study suggested that HOXA9 promoter methylation was a prognostic factor that, in combination with mRNA and miRNA-based biomarkers, could identify patients with stage I adenocarcinoma at high risk of recurrence [11]. However, its usefulness is unclear for patients with completely resected NSCLC who have received adjuvant chemotherapy.

ICIs targeting PD-1/PD-L1 have improved the survival of patients with many types of cancer. PD-L1 is currently the most commonly used biomarker for selecting patients who would receive clinical benefits from anti-PD-1/PD-L1 antibodies [56]. Several studies have examined the relationship between PD-L1 expression and the benefit of postoperative adjuvant chemotherapy. A recent study suggested that PD-L1 expression in tumor cells is associated with improved survival with adjuvant chemotherapy (HR, 3.02; 95%CI, 1.69–5.40) [57]. In contrast, the LACE-Bio study showed that neither tumor nor immune cell PD-L1 expression is predictive of clinical benefits from adjuvant chemotherapy [58]. Therefore, it is controversial whether PD-L1 expression in tumor cells is a biomarker for adjuvant chemotherapy in patients with completely resected NSCLC.

Recent studies have attempted a method of verifying cancer characteristics and prognosis by detecting tumor cells and tumor-derived DNA in the blood. Detection and quantification of circulating tumor DNA (ctDNA) by personalized mutation detection panels or cancer personalized profiling by deep sequencing (CAPP-Seq) may help to detect MRD that cannot be detected by imaging [59–61]. A recent study showed that postoperative ctDNA positivity is significantly associated with shorter recurrence-free survival. In patients with completely resected stage II–III NSCLC, patients with postoperative ctDNA positivity received benefits from adjuvant chemotherapy, whereas those with postoperative ctDNA negativity had a low risk of relapse without adjuvant chemotherapy [62]. However, its usefulness may be limited in patients with early-stage NSCLC because ctDNA levels in the blood are reported to be associated with tumor size and stage. A study that included 640 cases of various types of cancer showed that ctDNA levels were 100 times higher in stage IV than in stage I disease [63]. The detection sensitivity of ctDNA in early-stage NSCLC is considered to be an issue that requires addressing. CAPP-Seq is a comprehensive mutation analysis method for measurement of ctDNA that is considered to have high sensitivity and may help to detect recurrence of lung cancer in postoperative patients with NSCLC in the future [64]. However, it remains unclear whether measurement of ctDNA using CAPP-Seq is useful as a biomarker for the efficacy of adjuvant chemotherapy in patients with NSCLC. Further studies are needed for the practical use of ctDNA measurement in early-stage NSCLC.

4. ACTN4 as a Biomarker for Evaluation of Metastatic Ability

Even if the primary tumor is completely removed grossly, microscopic metastases may remain that cannot be detected by diagnostic imaging. Therefore, indicators of tumor malignancy and high metastatic ability may be useful candidate biomarkers in assessing patient suitability for postoperative adjuvant chemotherapy. Cancer metastasis advances in a multiple-step process. Cancer cells break through the basement membrane, invade the extracellular matrix, and intravasate through the endothelium into the vascular and lymphatic systems to finally establish distant metastatic sites [65–68]. The dynamic assembly of the actin cytoskeleton plays an important role in the formation processes of cancer metastases. ACTN4 was isolated as a novel isoform of alpha-actinin, which is the actin-binding protein [26,28]. Alpha-actinin has several isotypes in humans, and ACTN4 is classified as the non-muscle type of alpha-actinin [26,28]. Non-muscle types of alpha-actinin, including ACTN4, are related to cell adhesion and cell migration. ACTN-4 has been reported to show increased protein expression in several types of cancers, such as colorectal cancer, pancreatic cancer, ovarian cancer, oral squamous cell carcinoma [29,69–72], salivary gland carcinoma [73], and lung cancer [28,74–76]. Cancer cells at the invasive front of the primal site have high migration and metastatic ability. These cells lose their epithelial cell characteristics, resulting in epithelial–mesenchymal transition [77,78]. Cancer cells at the invasive front show increased expression of ACTN4 protein and EMT-like changes in colorectal cancer tissues [71]. In an in vitro study using cell lines of lung adenocarcinoma, a decrease of ACTN4 expression by siRNA reduced metastatic ability [32]. A previous study showed that siRNA suppression of ACTN-4 protein expression diminished cell protrusion associated with cancer invasion in colon cancer cells [27]. In pancreatic cancer cells, siRNA knockdown of ACTN4 reduced the invasive potential of cancer cells [27]. These results show that ACTN4 is associated with the migration and invasion of cancer cells and plays an important role in the metastasis of cancer. Moreover, ACTN4 directly regulates cell motility by remodeling the actin cytoskeleton [26]. These preclinical studies suggest that ACTN4 may indicate the metastatic ability and malignancy of cancer. Figure 1 shows the possible roles of ACTN4 in cancer metastasis and invasion. ACTN4 mediates the cytoskeleton to sites of cell adhesion and is modulated to enable cell migration [26,79]. ACTN4 has also been reported to induce epithelial–mesenchymal transition (EMT) through upregulation of Snail, which is a transcriptional repressor of E-cadherin expression and one of the main inducers of EMT [80]. Moreover, Snail upregulated by ACTN4 induces cell migration and cancer invasion via Snail-mediated matrix metalloproteinase-9 expression. ACTN4 is involved in the stabilization of β-catenin. The accumulation of β-catenin induced by ACTN4 upregulates cyclin D1 and c-myc, leading to tumorigenesis [81]. Nuclear factor-kappa B (NF-κB) is a transcription factor that regulates cell proliferation, cell differentiation, cellular immunity, and apoptosis [82]. Actinin-4 is related to the transcriptional activity of NF-κB and the NFκB pathway promotes tumor-cell proliferation and survival [83]. NF-κB also plays an important role in both the induction and maintenance of EMT [84]. Further studies are needed to identify the molecular mechanisms of ACTN4 in cancer metastasis and invasion in more detail.

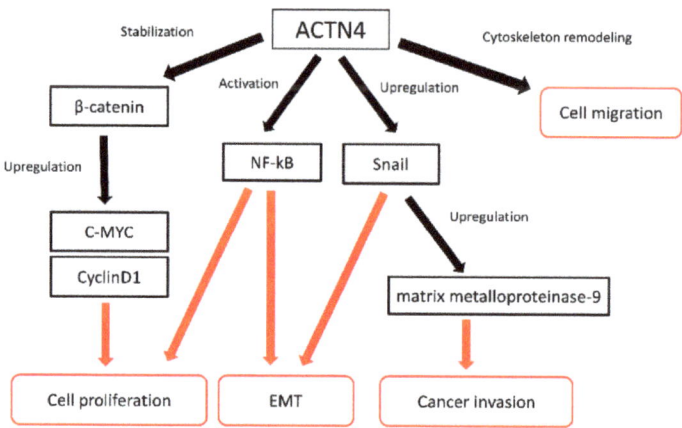

Figure 1. Functions of ACTN4 in cancer metastasis and invasion.

Recent studies using clinical specimens have also examined the usefulness of evaluating ACTN4 in NSCLC. Among these, Miura et al. reported that increased expression of ACTN4 mRNA may be a biomarker for adjuvant chemotherapy in patients with stage IB–II NSCLC. They reported that in a subgroup of patients with increased expression of ACTN4 mRNA, the OS of patients treated with adjuvant cisplatin plus vinorelbine was significantly longer than that of patients who underwent observation without adjuvant chemotherapy (HR, 0.273; 95%CI, 0.079–0.952) [32]. In another study, ACTN4 protein expression was reported to be a promising biomarker in patients with completely resected stage II–IIIA lung adenocarcinoma. In an ACTN4 immunohistochemistry (IHC)-positive subgroup, the OS of patients with adjuvant platinum-based chemotherapy was significantly longer than that of patients without adjuvant platinum-based chemotherapy (HR, 0.307; 95%CI, 0.107–0.882). The five-year relapse-free survival (RFS) rate was 56.5% in patients with adjuvant platinum-based chemotherapy and 33.5% in those without adjuvant platinum-based chemotherapy. In the ACTN4 IHC-negative subgroup, however, there was no significant difference between patients with and without adjuvant platinum-based chemotherapy [33].

Moreover, recent studies have suggested the usefulness of ACTN4 for the evaluation of patients with early-stage lung adenocarcinoma. Even in patients with stage I lung adenocarcinoma, some have recurrence and poor prognosis after curative surgery. ACTN4 gene amplification is determined by fluorescence in situ hybridization (FISH) in cancer tissues and has been shown to be a prognostic factor in several cancers. Noro et al. reported that ACTN4 gene amplification was a promising biomarker for predicting the prognosis of chemo-naive patients with stage I adenocarcinoma of the lung, with 5-year DFS and OS rates of patients with ACTN4 gene amplification of 37% and 64%, respectively. In contrast, the 5-year DFS and OS rates of patients without ACTN4 gene amplification were 86% and 92%, respectively [85]. In addition to its potential as a prognostic factor, ACTN4 gene amplification may also be a predictive biomarker for adjuvant UFT therapy in patients with completely resected stage I lung adenocarcinoma. In a retrospective study that included a total of 1136 patients with stage I adenocarcinoma, a subgroup analysis in patients aged ≥ 65 years showed that RFS was significantly longer in the adjuvant UFT therapy group than in the observational group in the *ACTN4* gene amplification positive cohort (HR, 0.084; 95%CI, 0.009–0.806) (Figure 2A) [34]. Among patients who did not receive adjuvant UFT therapy, those with *ACTN4* gene amplification negative had a longer RFS than those with *ACTN4* gene amplification positive (HR, 0.475; 95%CI, 0.239–0.946) (Figure 2B). In contrast, there was no difference in RFS between the adjuvant UFT therapy group and the observational group among *ACTN4* gene amplification negative patients (HR, 0.923; 95%CI, 0.566–1.506) (Figure 2C).

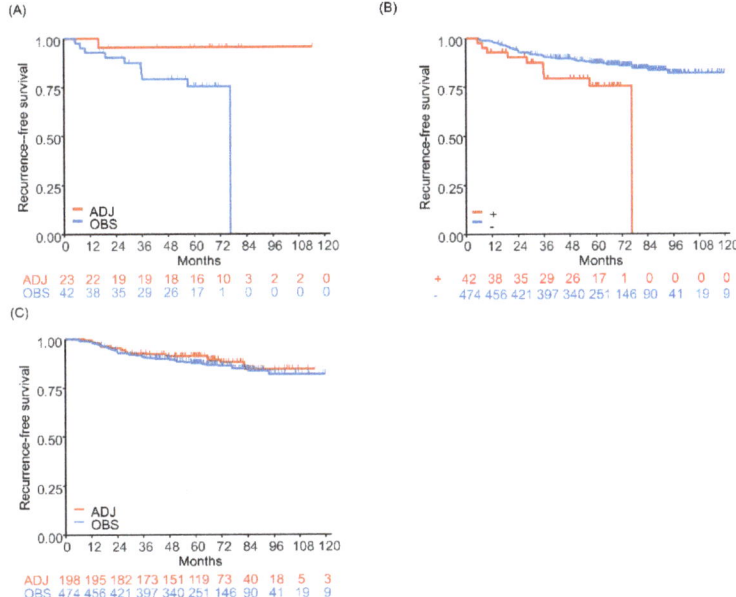

Figure 2. Analyses of patients aged ≥65 years with stage I adenocarcinoma who received adjuvant tegafur/uracil (UFT) therapy or underwent observation. (**A**) comparison of RFS between the adjuvant UFT therapy group and the observational group in patients who were *actinin-4 (ACTN4)* gene amplification positive, (**B**) comparison of RFS between *ACTN4* gene amplification negative and positive patients in the observational group, and (**C**) comparison of RFS between the adjuvant UFT therapy group and the observational group (Noro, R. et al., 2022 [34]).

Evaluation of ACTN4 may be beneficial in patients with lung adenocarcinoma as well as those with lung squamous cell carcinoma. The mRNA expression of ACTN4 evaluated by quantitative real-time PCR was a factor significantly associated with cancer-specific mortality in patients with stage I–II lung squamous cell carcinoma (HR, 2.68; 95%CI, 1.21–5.92) [86].

Table 1 summarizes the findings of previous studies that have examined the usefulness of ACTN4 as a predictive or prognostic biomarker in patients with completely resected carcinoma of the lung. These findings suggest that ACTN4 is a promising candidate biomarker for decision-making in postoperative adjuvant chemotherapy in stage I as well as stage II–III patients with NSCLC.

Table 1. Previous studies of ACTN4 in patients with early-stage non-small cell lung cancer.

	Histology	Stage	Adjuvant Chemotherapy	Evaluation Methods
Miura et al. (2016) [32]	NSCLC	IB-II	CDDP + VNR	mRNA expression
Shiraishi et al. (2017) [33]	Ad	II-IIIA	CDDP + VNR	Protein expression
Noro et al. (2021) [34]	Ad	IA/IB	UFT	Gene amplification
Miyanaga et al. (2013) [75]	HGNT	resected	Not specified	cDNA sequencing
Noro et al. (2013) [85]	Ad	IA-IB	Not specified	Gene amplification
Noro et al. (2017) [86]	Sq	I-II	Not specified	Gene expression
Yamagata et al. (2003) [87]	NSCLC	resected	Not specified	cDNA microarrays

Footnotes: Ad, adenocarcinoma; CDDP, cisplatin; cDNA, complementary DNA; HGNT, high-grade neuroendocrine tumor; NSCLC, non-small cell lung cancer; mRNA, messenger RNA; Sq, squamous cell carcinoma; UFT, tegafur/uracil; VNR, vinorelbine.

The curves in Figure 3 were created using a Kaplan–Meier plotter, which can assess the relationship between gene expression and survival in a variety of cancers, including lung cancer (https://kmplot.com/analysis/ (accessed on 24 May 2022) [88]. The sources are the Gene Expression Omnibus (GEO), European Genome-phenome Archive (EGA), and The Cancer Genome Atlas (TCGA) databases. Figure 3A,B shows that among lung adenocarcinoma patients, the OS of patients with high ACTN4 is significantly shorter than that of those with low ACTN4. Figure 3C,D shows that among lung squamous cell carcinoma patients, the OS of patients with high ACTN4 is significantly shorter than in those with low ACTN4. These results indicate that ACTN4 is a useful prognostic marker in patients with non-small cell lung cancer regardless of histology.

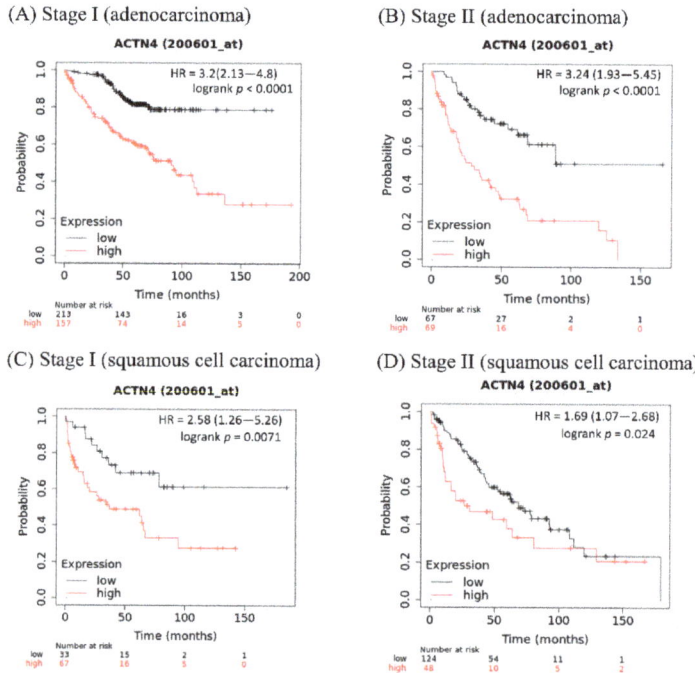

Figure 3. Kaplan–Meier curves showing overall survival in patients with lung cancer (actinin-4 expression high versus low). Overall survival in patients with (**A**) stage I lung adenocarcinoma, (**B**) stage II lung adenocarcinoma, (**C**) stage I lung squamous cell carcinoma, and (**D**) stage II lung squamous cell carcinoma.

5. Summary of the Advantages and Limitations of Perioperative Biomarkers

Table 2 summarizes the advantages and limitations of candidate biomarkers for the efficacy of adjuvant chemotherapy in lung cancer patients. ERCC1 and TP53 may indicate sensitivity to chemotherapeutic agents including cisplatin rather than MRD [24,52]. Likewise, PD-L1 expression is a predictor of ICI efficacy but not MRD [56]. Therefore, ERCC1, TP53, and PD-L1 may be difficult to use when deciding whether to perform adjuvant chemotherapy, although those biomarkers can be useful for selecting chemotherapeutic agents for perioperative treatment. In contrast, ACTN4 can be useful for decision-making for adjuvant chemotherapy because it indicates tumor metastatic potential and cancer invasiveness rather than sensitivity to specific chemotherapeutic agents [26,28]. CtDNA testing may also be a useful method for predicting postoperative MRD. However, medical cost is one of the challenges regarding its clinical application, as ctDNA testing may increase out-of-pocket expenses for patients [61]. ACTN4 can be evaluated by relatively simple and inexpensive methods such as real-time PCR, IHC, and FISH [32–34]. By combining ACTN4 with factors related to sensitivity to certain drugs, such as ERCC1 and PD-L1, it may be possible to provide more appropriate treatment for perioperative patients with lung cancer. The utility of ACTN4 needs to be verified in clinical trials.

Table 2. Advantages and limitations of perioperative biomarker candidates.

Biomarker	Function	Advantage	Limitation
Gene expression signature	Gene combinations for poor prognosis and poor chemotherapeutic response	More accurate prognostication of a signature from multiple genes compared with individual genes alone	Statistical validation and reproducibility of the signatures/Not a predictor for MRD
ERCC1	Removal of DNA intrastrand crosslinks by nucleotide excision repair	Predictor for the efficacy of cisplatin	Negative results in randomized phase III clinical trials/Not a predictor for MRD
TP53	Prevention and suppression of abnormal cell proliferation through mechanisms including cell cycle arrest, apoptosis, and DNA repair	One of the most frequently mutated genes in lung cancer regardless of histologic type	Not a predictor for MRD
PD-L1	Binding to its receptor PD-1 expressed by T cells and other immune cells to regulate immune responses	Predictor for the efficacy of anti-PD-1/PD-L1 antibody	Not a predictor for MRD
ctDNA	Tumor-derived DNA released in the blood	Possibility of MRD detection	Cost/Not a predictor for the efficacy of the specific chemotherapeutic agents
ACTN4	Involvement in cancer invasion and metastatic potential	Evaluating tumor metastatic potential and cancer invasiveness	Not a predictor for the efficacy of specific chemotherapeutic agents

Footnotes: ACTN4, actinin-4; ctDNA, circulating tumor DNA; ERCC1, excision repair cross-complementation group 1; MRD, minimal residual disease; PD-1, programmed cell death 1; PD-L1, programmed death-ligand 1; TP53, tumor protein p53 gene.

6. Conclusions

In this review, we have outlined the circumstances under which adjuvant chemotherapy is beneficial in NSCLC and discussed the biological roles of ACTN4 related to cancer invasion and metastases. Increased expression of ACTN4 protein and *ACTN4* gene amplification may be indicators of cancer invasive ability and metastatic ability in all patients with NSCLC. In patients with completely resected NSCLC, ACTN4 may be a useful biomarker of clinical benefit from adjuvant chemotherapy, which may lead to personalized adjuvant chemotherapy.

Author Contributions: Conceptualization, T.T., R.N. and K.H.; methodology, T.T., R.N., M.S. and K.H.; investigation, T.T. and R.N.; writing—original draft preparation, T.T. and R.N.; writing—review and editing, M.S. and K.H.; supervision, K.H. All authors have read and agreed to the published version of the manuscript.

Funding: This research received no external funding.

Acknowledgments: We are grateful to Cancer Science for allowing us to reuse figures from our previous articles.

Conflicts of Interest: R.N. and K.H. hold patents for predictive biomarkers with ACTN4 for cancers.

References

1. Miller, K.D.; Nogueira, L.; Mariotto, A.B.; Rowland, J.H.; Yabroff, K.R.; Alfano, C.M.; Jemal, A.; Kramer, J.L.; Siegel, R.L. Cancer treatment and survivorship statistics, 2019. *CA Cancer J. Clin.* **2019**, *69*, 363–385. [CrossRef]
2. Siegel, R.L.; Miller, K.D.; Jemal, A. Cancer statistics, 2019. *CA Cancer J. Clin.* **2019**, *69*, 7–34. [CrossRef]
3. Vansteenkiste, J.; Wauters, E.; Reymen, B.; Ackermann, C.J.; Peters, S.; De Ruysscher, D. Current status of immune checkpoint inhibition in early-stage NSCLC. *Ann. Oncol.* **2019**, *30*, 1244–1253. [CrossRef] [PubMed]
4. Goldstraw, P.; Chansky, K.; Crowley, J.; Rami-Porta, R.; Asamura, H.; Eberhardt, W.E.; Nicholson, A.G.; Groome, P.; Mitchell, A.; Bolejack, V.; et al. The IASLC Lung Cancer Staging Project: Proposals for Revision of the TNM Stage Groupings in the Forthcoming [Eighth] Edition of the TNM Classification for Lung Cancer. *J. Thorac. Oncol.* **2016**, *11*, 39–51. [CrossRef] [PubMed]
5. Pignon, J.-P.; Tribodet, H.; Scagliotti, G.V.; Douillard, J.-Y.; Shepherd, F.A.; Stephens, R.J.; Dunant, A.; Torri, V.; Rosell, R.; Seymour, L.; et al. Lung adjuvant cisplatin evaluation: A pooled analysis by the LACE Collaborative Group. *J. Clin. Oncol.* **2008**, *26*, 3552–3559. [CrossRef] [PubMed]
6. Felip, E.; Altorki, N.; Zhou, C.; Csőszi, T.; Vynnychenko, I.; Goloborodko, O.; Luft, A.; Akopov, A.; Martinez-Marti, A.; Kenmotsu, H.; et al. Adjuvant atezolizumab after adjuvant chemotherapy in resected stage IB-IIIA non-small-cell lung cancer [IMpower010]: A randomised; multicentre; open-label; phase 3 trial. *Lancet* **2021**, *398*, 1344–1357. [CrossRef]
7. Wu, Y.-L.; Tsuboi, M.; He, J.; John, T.; Grohe, C.; Majem, M.; Goldman, J.W.; Laktionov, K.; Kim, S.-W.; Kato, T.; et al. Osimertinib in Resected EGFR-Mutated Non-Small-Cell Lung Cancer. *N. Engl. J. Med.* **2020**, *383*, 1711–1723. [CrossRef]
8. Ng, R.; Hasan, B.; Mittmann, N.; Florescu, M.; Shepherd, F.A.; Ding, K.; Butts, C.A.; Cormier, Y.; Darling, G.; Goss, G.D.; et al. Economic analysis of NCIC CTG JBR.10: A randomized trial of adjuvant vinorelbine plus cisplatin compared with observation in early stage non-small-cell lung cancer–a report of the Working Group on Economic Analysis, and the Lung Disease Site Group, National Cancer Institute of Canada Clinical Trials Group. *J. Clin. Oncol.* **2007**, *25*, 2256–2261.
9. Zafar, S.Y.; Peppercorn, J.M.; Schrag, D.; Taylor, D.H.; Goetzinger, A.M.; Zhong, X.; Abernethy, A.P. The financial toxicity of cancer treatment: A pilot study assessing out-of-pocket expenses and the insured cancer patient's experience. *Oncologist* **2013**, *18*, 381–390. [CrossRef] [PubMed]
10. Tran, G.; Zafar, S.Y. Financial toxicity and implications for cancer care in the era of molecular and immune therapies. *Ann. Transl. Med.* **2018**, *6*, 166. [CrossRef]
11. Robles, A.I.; Arai, E.; Mathé, E.A.; Okayama, H.; Schetter, A.J.; Brown, D.; Petersen, D.; Bowman, E.D.; Noro, R.; Welsh, J.A.; et al. An Integrated Prognostic Classifier for Stage I Lung Adenocarcinoma Based on mRNA, microRNA, and DNA Methylation Biomarkers. *J. Thorac. Oncol.* **2015**, *10*, 1037–1048.
12. Zuo, S.; Wei, M.; Zhang, H.; Chen, A.; Wu, J.; Wei, J.; Dong, J. A robust six-gene prognostic signature for prediction of both disease-free and overall survival in non-small cell lung cancer. *J. Transl. Med.* **2019**, *17*, 152. [PubMed]
13. Li, B.; Cui, Y.; Diehn, M.; Li, R. Development and Validation of an Individualized Immune Prognostic Signature in Early-Stage Nonsquamous Non-Small Cell Lung Cancer. *JAMA Oncol.* **2017**, *3*, 1529–1537. [CrossRef]
14. Shahid, M.; Choi, T.G.; Nguyen, M.N.; Matondo, A.; Jo, Y.H.; Yoo, J.Y.; Nguyen, N.N.Y.; Yun, H.R.; Kim, J.; Akter, S.; et al. An 8-gene signature for prediction of prognosis and chemoresponse in non-small cell lung cancer. *Oncotarget* **2016**, *7*, 86561–86572.
15. Xu, W.; Jia, G.; Davie, J.R.; Murphy, L.; Kratzke, R.; Banerji, S. A 10-Gene Yin Yang Expression Ratio Signature for Stage IA and IB Non-Small Cell Lung Cancer. *J. Thorac. Oncol.* **2016**, *11*, 2150–2160. [PubMed]
16. Leng, S.; Do, K.; Yingling, C.M.; Picchi, M.A.; Wolf, H.J.; Kennedy, T.C.; Feser, W.J.; Baron, A.E.; Franklin, W.A.; Brock, M.V.; et al. Defining a gene promoter methylation signature in sputum for lung cancer risk assessment. *Clin. Cancer Res.* **2012**, *18*, 3387–3395. [PubMed]
17. Chen, H.-Y.; Yu, S.-L.; Chen, C.-H.; Chang, G.-C.; Chen, C.-Y.; Yuan, A.; Cheng, C.-L.; Wang, C.-H.; Terng, H.-J.; Kao, S.-F.; et al. A five-gene signature and clinical outcome in non-small-cell lung cancer. *N. Engl. J. Med.* **2007**, *356*, 11–20.
18. Chen, D.-T.; Hsu, Y.-L.; Fulp, W.J.; Coppola, D.; Haura, E.B.; Yeatman, T.J.; Cress, W.D. Prognostic and predictive value of a malignancy-risk gene signature in early-stage non-small cell lung cancer. *J. Natl. Cancer Inst.* **2011**, *103*, 1859–1870.
19. Xie, Y.; Xiao, G.; Coombes, K.R.; Behrens, C.; Solis, L.M.; Raso, G.; Girard, L.; Erickson, H.S.; Roth, J.; Heymach, J.V.; et al. Robust gene expression signature from formalin-fixed paraffin-embedded samples predicts prognosis of non-small-cell lung cancer patients. *Clin. Cancer Res.* **2011**, *17*, 5705–5714. [PubMed]
20. Subramanian, J.; Simon, R. Gene expression-based prognostic signatures in lung cancer: Ready for clinical use? *J. Natl. Cancer Inst.* **2010**, *102*, 464–474.
21. Seike, M.; Yanaihara, N.; Bowman, E.D.; Zanetti, K.A.; Budhu, A.; Kumamoto, K.; Mechanic, L.E.; Matsumoto, S.; Yokota, J.; Shibata, T.; et al. Use of a cytokine gene expression signature in lung adenocarcinoma and the surrounding tissue as a prognostic classifier. *J. Natl. Cancer Inst.* **2007**, *99*, 1257–1269.

22. Okayama, H.; Kohno, T.; Ishii, Y.; Shimada, Y.; Shiraishi, K.; Iwakawa, R.; Furuta, K.; Tsuta, K.; Shibata, T.; Yamamoto, S.; et al. Identification of genes upregulated in ALK-positive and EGFR/KRAS/ALK-negative lung adenocarcinomas. *Cancer Res.* **2012**, *72*, 100–111. [PubMed]
23. Zheng, Z.; Chen, T.; Li, X.; Haura, E.; Sharma, A.; Bepler, G. DNA synthesis and repair genes RRM1 and ERCC1 in lung cancer. *N. Engl. J. Med.* **2007**, *356*, 800–808. [CrossRef] [PubMed]
24. Olaussen, K.A.; Dunant, A.; Fouret, P.; Brambilla, E.; André, F.; Haddad, V.; Taranchon, E.; Filipits, M.; Pirker, R.; Popper, H.H.; et al. DNA repair by ERCC1 in non-small-cell lung cancer and cisplatin-based adjuvant chemotherapy. *N. Engl. J. Med.* **2006**, *355*, 983–991.
25. Friboulet, L.; Olaussen, K.A.; Pignon, J.-P.; Shepherd, F.A.; Tsao, M.-S.; Graziano, S.; Kratzke, R.; Douillard, J.-Y.; Seymour, L.; Pirker, R.; et al. ERCC1 isoform expression and DNA repair in non-small-cell lung cancer. *N. Engl. J. Med.* **2013**, *368*, 1101–1110.
26. Honda, K.; Yamada, T.; Endo, R.; Ino, Y.; Gotoh, M.; Tsuda, H.; Yamada, Y.; Chiba, H.; Hirohashi, S. Actinin-4; a novel actin-bundling protein associated with cell motility and cancer invasion. *J. Cell Biol.* **1998**, *140*, 1383–1393. [PubMed]
27. Hayashida, Y.; Honda, K.; Idogawa, M.; Ino, Y.; Ono, M.; Tsuchida, A.; Aoki, T.; Hirohashi, S.; Yamada, T. E-cadherin regulates the association between beta-catenin and actinin-4. *Cancer Res.* **2005**, *65*, 8836–8845. [PubMed]
28. Honda, K. The biological role of actinin-4 [ACTN4] in malignant phenotypes of cancer. *Cell Biosci.* **2015**, *5*, 41. [PubMed]
29. Kikuchi, S.; Honda, K.; Tsuda, H.; Hiraoka, N.; Imoto, I.; Kosuge, T.; Umaki, T.; Onozato, K.; Shitashige, M.; Yamaguchi, U.; et al. Expression and gene amplification of actinin-4 in invasive ductal carcinoma of the pancreas. *Clin. Cancer Res.* **2008**, *14*, 5348–5356.
30. Yamamoto, S.; Tsuda, H.; Honda, K.; Onozato, K.; Takano, M.; Tamai, S.; Imoto, I.; Inazawa, J.; Yamada, T.; Matsubara, O. Actinin-4 gene amplification in ovarian cancer: A candidate oncogene associated with poor patient prognosis and tumor chemoresistance. *Mod. Pathol.* **2009**, *22*, 499–507.
31. Sugano, T.; Yoshida, M.; Masuda, M.; Ono, M.; Tamura, K.; Kinoshita, T.; Tsuda, H.; Honda, K.; Gemma, A.; Yamada, T. Prognostic impact of ACTN4 gene copy number alteration in hormone receptor-positive; HER2-negative; node-negative invasive breast carcinoma. *Br. J. Cancer* **2020**, *122*, 1811–1817.
32. Miura, N.; Kamita, M.; Kakuya, T.; Fujiwara, Y.; Tsuta, K.; Shiraishi, H.; Takeshita, F.; Ochiya, T.; Shoji, H.; Huang, W.; et al. Efficacy of adjuvant chemotherapy for non-small cell lung cancer assessed by metastatic potential associated with ACTN4. *Oncotarget* **2016**, *7*, 33165–33178.
33. Shiraishi, H.; Fujiwara, Y.; Kakuya, T.; Tsuta, K.; Motoi, N.; Miura, N.; Watabe, Y.; Watanabe, S.-I.; Noro, R.; Nagashima, K.; et al. Actinin-4 protein overexpression as a predictive biomarker in adjuvant chemotherapy for resected lung adenocarcinoma. *Biomark. Med.* **2017**, *11*, 721–731. [PubMed]
34. Noro, R.; Honda, K.; Nagashima, K.; Motoi, N.; Kunugi, S.; Matsubayashi, J.; Takeuchi, S.; Shiraishi, H.; Okano, T.; Kashiro, A.; et al. Alpha-actinin-4 [ACTN4] gene amplification is a predictive biomarker for adjuvant chemotherapy with tegafur/uracil in stage I lung adenocarcinomas. *Cancer Sci.* **2022**, *113*, 1002–1009. [CrossRef] [PubMed]
35. Arriagada, R.; Bergman, B.; Dunant, A.; Le Chevalier, T.; Pignon, J.-P.; Vansteenkiste, J.; International Adjuvant Lung Cancer Trial Collaborative Group. Cisplatin-based adjuvant chemotherapy in patients with completely resected non-small-cell lung cancer. *N. Engl. J. Med.* **2004**, *350*, 351–360.
36. Douillard, J.-Y.; Rosell, R.; De Lena, M.; Carpagnano, F.; Ramlau, R.; Gonzáles-Larriba, J.L.; Grodzki, T.; Pereira, J.R.; Le Groumellec, A.; Lorusso, V.; et al. Adjuvant vinorelbine plus cisplatin versus observation in patients with completely resected stage IB-IIIA non-small-cell lung cancer [Adjuvant Navelbine International Trialist Association [ANITA]]: A randomised controlled trial. *Lancet Oncol.* **2006**, *7*, 719–727.
37. Winton, T.; Livingston, R.; Johnson, D.; Rigas, J.; Johnston, M.; Butts, C.; Cormier, Y.; Goss, G.; Inculet, R.; Vallieres, E.; et al. Vinorelbine plus cisplatin vs. observation in resected non-small-cell lung cancer. *N. Engl. J. Med.* **2005**, *352*, 2589–2597. [PubMed]
38. Hamada, C.; Tsuboi, M.; Ohta, M.; Fujimura, S.; Kodama, K.; Imaizumi, M.; Wada, H. Effect of postoperative adjuvant chemotherapy with tegafur-uracil on survival in patients with stage IA non-small cell lung cancer: An exploratory analysis from a meta-analysis of six randomized controlled trials. *J. Thorac. Oncol.* **2009**, *4*, 1511–1516. [PubMed]
39. Hamada, C.; Tanaka, F.; Ohta, M.; Fujimura, S.; Kodama, K.; Imaizumi, M.; Wada, H. Meta-analysis of postoperative adjuvant chemotherapy with tegafur-uracil in non-small-cell lung cancer. *J. Clin. Oncol.* **2005**, *23*, 4999–5006.
40. Kelly, K.; Altorki, N.K.; Eberhardt, W.E.E.; O'Brien, M.E.R.; Spigel, D.R.; Crinò, L.; Tsai, C.-M.; Kim, J.-H.; Cho, E.K.; Hoffman, P.C.; et al. Adjuvant Erlotinib Versus Placebo in Patients with Stage IB-IIIA Non-Small-Cell Lung Cancer [RADIANT]: A Randomized; Double-Blind; Phase III Trial. *J. Clin. Oncol.* **2015**, *33*, 4007–4014. [PubMed]
41. Zhong, W.-Z.; Wang, Q.; Mao, W.-M.; Xu, S.-T.; Wu, L.; Shen, Y.; Liu, Y.-Y.; Chen, C.; Cheng, Y.; Xu, L.; et al. Gefitinib versus vinorelbine plus cisplatin as adjuvant treatment for stage II-IIIA [N1-N2] EGFR-mutant NSCLC [ADJUVANT/CTONG1104]: A randomised; open-label; phase 3 study. *Lancet Oncol.* **2018**, *19*, 139–148. [CrossRef]
42. Tada, H.; Mitsudomi, T.; Misumi, T.; Sugio, K.; Tsuboi, M.; Okamoto, I.; Iwamoto, Y.; Sakakura, N.; Sugawara, S.; Atagi, S.; et al. Randomized Phase III Study of Gefitinib Versus Cisplatin Plus Vinorelbine for Patients with Resected Stage II-IIIA Non-Small-Cell Lung Cancer with EGFR Mutation [IMPACT]. *J. Clin. Oncol.* **2022**, *40*, 231–241. [CrossRef] [PubMed]
43. Reck, M.; Rodríguez-Abreu, D.; Robinson, A.G.; Hui, R.; Csőszi, T.; Fülöp, A.; Gottfried, M.; Peled, N.; Tafreshi, A.; Cuffe, S.; et al. Pembrolizumab versus Chemotherapy for PD-L1-Positive Non-Small-Cell Lung Cancer. *N. Engl. J. Med.* **2016**, *375*, 1823–1833. [CrossRef] [PubMed]

44. Gandhi, L.; Rodríguez-Abreu, D.; Gadgeel, S.; Esteban, E.; Felip, E.; De Angelis, F.; Domine, M.; Clingan, P.; Hochmair, M.J.; Powell, S.F.; et al. Pembrolizumab plus Chemotherapy in Metastatic Non-Small-Cell Lung Cancer. *N. Engl. J. Med.* **2018**, *378*, 2078–2092. [CrossRef]
45. Socinski, M.A.; Jotte, R.M.; Cappuzzo, F.; Orlandi, F.; Stroyakovskiy, D.; Nogami, N.; Rodríguez-Abreu, D.; Moro-Sibilot, D.; Thomas, C.A.; Barlesi, F.; et al. Atezolizumab for First-Line Treatment of Metastatic Nonsquamous NSCLC. *N. Engl. J. Med.* **2018**, *378*, 2288–2301. [CrossRef]
46. Hellmann, M.D.; Paz-Ares, L.; Bernabe Caro, R.; Zurawski, B.; Kim, S.-W.; Carcereny Costa, E.; Park, K.; Alexandru, A.; Lupinacci, L.; de la Mora Jimenez, E.; et al. Nivolumab plus Ipilimumab in Advanced Non-Small-Cell Lung Cancer. *N. Engl. J. Med.* **2019**, *381*, 2020–2031. [CrossRef]
47. Paz-Ares, L.; Ciuleanu, T.-E.; Cobo, M.; Schenker, M.; Zurawski, B.; Menezes, J.; Richardet, E.; Bennouna, J.; Felip, E.; Juan-Vidal, O.; et al. First-line nivolumab plus ipilimumab combined with two cycles of chemotherapy in patients with non-small-cell lung cancer [CheckMate 9LA]: An international; randomised; open-label; phase 3 trial. *Lancet Oncol.* **2021**, *22*, 198–211. [CrossRef]
48. Antonia, S.J.; Villegas, A.; Daniel, D.; Vicente, D.; Murakami, S.; Hui, R.; Kurata, T.; Chiappori, A.; Lee, K.H.; de Wit, M.; et al. Overall Survival with Durvalumab after Chemoradiotherapy in Stage III NSCLC. *N. Engl. J. Med.* **2018**, *379*, 2342–2350. [CrossRef]
49. Blumenthal, G.M.; Bunn, P.A., Jr.; Chaft, J.E.; McCoach, C.E.; Perez, E.A.; Scagliotti, G.V.; Carbone, D.P.; Aerts, H.J.W.L.; Aisner, D.L.; Bergh, J.; et al. Current Status and Future Perspectives on Neoadjuvant Therapy in Lung Cancer. *J. Thorac. Oncol.* **2018**, *13*, 1818–1831. [CrossRef]
50. Soh, J.; Hamada, A.; Fujino, T.; Mitsudomi, T. Perioperative Therapy for Non-Small Cell Lung Cancer with Immune Checkpoint Inhibitors. *Cancers* **2021**, *13*, 4035. [CrossRef]
51. Forde, P.M.; Spicer, J.; Lu, S.; Provencio, M.; Mitsudomi, T.; Awad, M.M.; Felip, E.; Broderick, S.R.; Brahmer, J.R.; Swanson, S.J.; et al. Neoadjuvant Nivolumab plus Chemotherapy in Resectable Lung Cancer. *N. Engl. J. Med.* **2022**, *386*, 1973–1985. [CrossRef]
52. Kandioler, D.; Stamatis, G.; Eberhardt, W.; Kappel, S.; Zöchbauer-Müller, S.; Kührer, I.; Mittlböck, M.; Zwrtek, R.; Aigner, C.; Bichler, C.; et al. Growing clinical evidence for the interaction of the p53 genotype and response to induction chemotherapy in advanced non-small cell lung cancer. *J. Thorac. Cardiovasc. Surg.* **2008**, *135*, 1036–1041. [CrossRef]
53. Scoccianti, C.; Vesin, A.; Martel, G.; Olivier, M.; Brambilla, E.; Timsit, J.-F.; Tavecchio, L.; Brambilla, C.; Field, J.K.; Hainaut, P.; et al. Prognostic value of TP53; KRAS and EGFR mutations in nonsmall cell lung cancer: The EUELC cohort. *Eur. Respir. J.* **2012**, *40*, 177–184. [CrossRef]
54. Ma, X.; Le Teuff, G.; Lacas, B.; Tsao, M.S.; Graziano, S.; Pignon, J.-P.; Douillard, J.-Y.; Le Chevalier, T.; Seymour, L.; Filipits, M.; et al. Prognostic and Predictive Effect of TP53 Mutations in Patients with Non-Small Cell Lung Cancer from Adjuvant Cisplatin-Based Therapy Randomized Trials: A LACE-Bio Pooled Analysis. *J. Thorac. Oncol.* **2016**, *11*, 850–861. [CrossRef] [PubMed]
55. Schiller, J.H.; Adak, S.; Feins, R.H.; Keller, S.M.; Fry, W.A.; Livingston, R.B.; Hammond, M.E.; Wolf, B.; Sabatini, L.; Jett, J.; et al. Lack of prognostic significance of p53 and K-ras mutations in primary resected non-small-cell lung cancer on E4592: A Laboratory Ancillary Study on an Eastern Cooperative Oncology Group Prospective Randomized Trial of Postoperative Adjuvant Therapy. *J. Clin. Oncol.* **2001**, *19*, 448–457. [CrossRef]
56. Doroshow, D.B.; Bhalla, S.; Beasley, M.B.; Sholl, L.M.; Kerr, K.M.; Gnjatic, S.; Wistuba, I.I.; Rimm, D.L.; Tsao, M.S.; Hirsch, F.R. PD-L1 as a biomarker of response to immune-checkpoint inhibitors. *Nat. Rev. Clin. Oncol.* **2021**, *18*, 345–362. [CrossRef]
57. Gross, D.J.; Chintala, N.K.; Vaghjiani, R.G.; Grosser, R.; Tan, K.S.; Li, X.; Choe, J.; Li, Y.; Aly, R.G.; Emoto, K.; et al. Tumor and Tumor-Associated Macrophage Programmed Death-Ligand 1 Expression Is Associated with Adjuvant Chemotherapy Benefit in Lung Adenocarcinoma. *J. Thorac. Oncol.* **2022**, *17*, 89–102. [CrossRef]
58. Tsao, M.S.; Le Teuff, G.; Shepherd, F.A.; Landais, C.; Hainaut, P.; Filipits, M.; Pirker, R.; Le Chevalier, T.; Graziano, S.; Kratze, R.; et al. PD-L1 protein expression assessed by immunohistochemistry is neither prognostic nor predictive of benefit from adjuvant chemotherapy in resected non-small cell lung cancer. *Ann. Oncol.* **2017**, *28*, 882–889. [CrossRef]
59. Ohara, S.; Suda, K.; Sakai, K.; Nishino, M.; Chiba, M.; Shimoji, M.; Takemoto, T.; Fujino, T.; Koga, T.; Hamada, A.; et al. Prognostic implications of preoperative versus postoperative circulating tumor DNA in surgically resected lung cancer patients: A pilot study. *Transl. Lung Cancer Res.* **2020**, *9*, 1915–1923. [CrossRef] [PubMed]
60. Chaudhuri, A.A.; Chabon, J.J.; Lovejoy, A.F.; Newman, A.M.; Stehr, H.; Azad, T.D.; Khodadoust, M.S.; Esfahani, M.S.; Liu, C.L.; Zhou, L.; et al. Early Detection of Molecular Residual Disease in Localized Lung Cancer by Circulating Tumor DNA Profiling. *Cancer Discov.* **2017**, *7*, 1394–1403. [CrossRef] [PubMed]
61. Abbosh, C.; Birkbak, N.J.; Wilson, G.A.; Jamal-Hanjani, M.; Constantin, T.; Salari, R.; Le Quesne, J.; Moore, D.A.; Veeriah, S.; Rosenthal, R.; et al. Phylogenetic ERCC1 analysis depicts early-stage lung cancer evolution. *Nature* **2017**, *545*, 446–451. [CrossRef]
62. Qiu, B.; Guo, W.; Zhang, F.; Lv, F.; Ji, Y.; Peng, Y.; Chen, X.; Bao, H.; Xu, Y.; Shao, Y.; et al. Dynamic recurrence risk and adjuvant chemotherapy benefit prediction by ctDNA in resected NSCLC. *Nat. Commun.* **2021**, *12*, 6770. [CrossRef] [PubMed]
63. Bettegowda, C.; Sausen, M.; Leary, R.J.; Kinde, I.; Wang, Y.; Agrawal, N.; Bartlett, B.R.; Wang, H.; Luber, B.; Alani, R.M.; et al. Detection of circulating tumor DNA in early- and late-stage human malignancies. *Sci. Transl. Med.* **2014**, *6*, 224ra24. [CrossRef]
64. Newman, A.M.; Bratman, S.V.; To, J.; Wynne, J.F.; Eclov, N.C.W.; Modlin, L.A.; Liu, C.L.; Neal, J.W.; Wakelee, H.A.; Merritt, R.E.; et al. An ultrasensitive method for quantitating circulating tumor DNA with broad patient coverage. *Nat. Med.* **2014**, *20*, 548–554. [CrossRef]
65. Kedrin, D.; van Rheenen, J.; Hernandez, L.; Condeelis, J.; Segall, J.E. Cell motility and cytoskeletal regulation in invasion and metastasis. *J. Mammary Gland Biol. Neoplasia* **2007**, *12*, 143–152. [CrossRef] [PubMed]

66. Otey, C.A.; Carpen, O. Alpha-actinin revisited: A fresh look at an old player. *Cell Motil. Cytoskelet.* **2004**, *58*, 104–111. [CrossRef] [PubMed]
67. Palmer, T.D.; Ashby, W.J.; Lewis, J.D.; Zijlstra, A. Targeting tumor cell motility to prevent metastasis. *Adv. Drug Deliv. Rev.* **2011**, *63*, 568–581. [CrossRef]
68. Fidler, I.J. The pathogenesis of cancer metastasis: The 'seed and soil' hypothesis revisited. *Nat. Rev. Cancer.* **2003**, *3*, 453–458. [CrossRef] [PubMed]
69. Meng, X.; Matsumoto, F.; Mori, T.; Miura, N.; Ino, Y.; Onidani, K.; Kobayashi, K.; Matsuzaki, Y.; Yoshimoto, S.; Ikeda, K.; et al. BP180 Is a Prognostic Factor in Head and Neck Squamous Cell Carcinoma. *Anticancer Res.* **2021**, *41*, 1089–1099. [CrossRef]
70. Kakuya, T.; Mori, T.; Yoshimoto, S.; Watabe, Y.; Miura, N.; Shoji, H.; Onidani, K.; Shibahara, T.; Honda, K. Prognostic significance of gene amplification of ACTN4 in stage I and II oral tongue cancer. *Int. J. Oral Maxillofac. Surg.* **2017**, *46*, 968–976. [CrossRef] [PubMed]
71. Honda, K.; Yamada, T.; Hayashida, Y.; Idogawa, M.; Sato, S.; Hasegawa, F.; Ino, Y.; Ono, M.; Hirohashi, S. Actinin-4 increases cell motility and promotes lymph node metastasis of colorectal cancer. *Gastroenterology* **2005**, *128*, 51–62. [CrossRef] [PubMed]
72. Yamamoto, S.; Tsuda, H.; Honda, K.; Kita, T.; Takano, M.; Tamai, S.; Inazawa, J.; Yamada, T.; Matsubara, O. Actinin-4 expression in ovarian cancer: A novel prognostic indicator independent of clinical stage and histological type. *Mod. Pathol.* **2007**, *20*, 1278–1285. [CrossRef] [PubMed]
73. Watabe, Y.; Mori, T.; Yoshimoto, S.; Nomura, T.; Shibahara, T.; Yamada, T.; Honda, K. Copy number increase of ACTN4 is a prognostic indicator in salivary gland carcinoma. *Cancer Med.* **2014**, *3*, 613–622. [CrossRef]
74. Honda, K. Development of Biomarkers to Predict Recurrence by Determining the Metastatic Ability of Cancer Cells. *J. Nippon Med. Sch.* **2022**, *89*, 24–32. [CrossRef]
75. Miyanaga, A.; Honda, K.; Tsuta, K.; Masuda, M.; Yamaguchi, U.; Fujii, G.; Miyamoto, A.; Shinagawa, S.; Miura, N.; Tsuda, H.; et al. Diagnostic and prognostic significance of the alternatively spliced ACTN4 variant in high-grade neuroendocrine pulmonary tumours. *Ann. Oncol.* **2013**, *24*, 84–90. [CrossRef] [PubMed]
76. Honda, K.; Yamada, T.; Seike, M.; Hayashida, Y.; Idogawa, M.; Kondo, T.; Ino, Y.; Hirohashi, S. Alternative splice variant of actinin-4 in small cell lung cancer. *Oncogene* **2004**, *23*, 5257–5262. [CrossRef]
77. Morris, H.T.; Machesky, L.M. Actin cytoskeletal control during epithelial to mesenchymal transition: Focus on the pancreas and intestinal tract. *Br. J. Cancer* **2015**, *112*, 613–620. [CrossRef]
78. López-Novoa, J.M.; Nieto, M.A. Inflammation and EMT: An alliance towards organ fibrosis and cancer progression. *EMBO Mol. Med.* **2009**, *1*, 303–314. [CrossRef] [PubMed]
79. Shao, H.; Travers, T.; Camacho, C.J.; Wells, A. The carboxyl tail of alpha-actinin-4 regulates its susceptibility to m-calpain and thus functions in cell migration and spreading. *Int. J. Biochem. Cell Biol.* **2013**, *45*, 1051–1063. [CrossRef]
80. Ma, S.Y.; Park, J.-H.; Jung, H.; Ha, S.-M.; Kim, Y.; Park, D.H.; Lee, D.H.; Lee, S.; Chu, I.-H.; Jung, S.Y.; et al. Snail maintains metastatic potential, cancer stem-like properties, and chemoresistance in mesenchymal mouse breast cancer TUBO–P2J cells. *Oncol. Rep.* **2017**, *38*, 1867–1876. [CrossRef]
81. An, H.-T.; Yoo, S.; Ko, J. α-Actinin-4 induces the epithelial-to-mesenchymal transition and tumorigenesis via regulation of Snail expression and β-catenin stabilization in cervical cancer. *Oncogene* **2016**, *35*, 5893–5904. [CrossRef]
82. Xia, L.; Tan, S.; Zhou, Y.; Lin, J.; Wang, H.; Oyang, L.; Tian, Y.; Liu, L.; Su, M.; Wang, H.; et al. Role of the NFκB-signaling pathway in cancer. *OncoTargets Ther.* **2018**, *11*, 2063–2073. [CrossRef] [PubMed]
83. Zhao, X.; Hsu, K.-S.; Lim, J.H.; Bruggeman, L.A.; Kao, H.-Y. α-Actinin 4 potentiates nuclear factor κ-light-chain-enhancer of activated B-cell (NF-κB) activity in podocytes independent of its cytoplasmic actin binding function. *J. Biol. Chem.* **2015**, *290*, 338–349. [CrossRef] [PubMed]
84. Huber, M.A.; Azoitei, N.; Baumann, B.; Grünert, S.; Sommer, A.; Pehamberger, H.; Kraut, N.; Beug, H.; Wirth, T. NF-kappaB is essential for epithelial-mesenchymal transition and metastasis in a model of breast cancer progression. *J. Clin. Investig.* **2004**, *114*, 569–581. [CrossRef]
85. Noro, R.; Honda, K.; Tsuta, K.; Ishii, G.; Maeshima, A.M.; Miura, N.; Furuta, K.; Shibata, T.; Tsuda, H.; Ochiai, A.; et al. Distinct outcome of stage I lung adenocarcinoma with ACTN4 cell motility gene amplification. *Ann. Oncol.* **2013**, *24*, 2594–2600. [CrossRef] [PubMed]
86. Noro, R.; Ishigame, T.; Walsh, N.; Shiraishi, K.; Robles, A.I.; Ryan, B.M.; Schetter, A.J.; Bowman, E.D.; Welsh, J.A.; Seike, M.; et al. A Two-Gene Prognostic Classifier for Early-Stage Lung Squamous Cell Carcinoma in Multiple Large-Scale and Geographically Diverse Cohorts. *J. Thorac. Oncol.* **2017**, *12*, 65–76. [CrossRef]
87. Yamagata, N.; Shyr, Y.; Yanagisawa, K.; Edgerton, M.; Dang, T.P.; Gonzalez, A.; Nadaf, S.; Larsen, P.; Roberts, J.R.; Nesbitt, J.C.; et al. A training-testing approach to the molecular classification of resected non-small cell lung cancer. *Clin. Cancer Res.* **2003**, *9*, 4695–4704.
88. Lánczky, A.; Győrffy, B. Web-Based Survival Analysis Tool Tailored for Medical Research [KMplot]: Development and Implementation. *J. Med. Internet Res.* **2021**, *23*, e27633. [CrossRef]

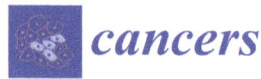 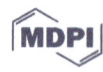

Article

Gene Expression Analysis Links Autocrine Vasoactive Intestinal Peptide and ZEB1 in Gastrointestinal Cancers

Ishani H. Rao [1], Edmund K. Waller [1], Rohan K. Dhamsania [2] and Sanjay Chandrasekaran [3],*

1. Department of Hematology and Medical Oncology, Emory University School of Medicine, Atlanta, GA 30322, USA
2. Philadelphia College of Osteopathic Medicine (PCOM)-Georgia Campus, Suwanee, GA 30024, USA
3. Harold C. Simmons Cancer Center, University of Texas Southwestern Medical Center, Dallas, TX 75390, USA
* Correspondence: sanjay.chandrasekaran@utsouthwestern.edu

Simple Summary: The downstream signaling mechanisms and importance of the autocrine secretion of the vasoactive intestinal peptide (VIP) in cancer remains poorly understood. We hypothesized that VIP expression may promote cancer-associated signaling pathways. We analyzed gene sequencing data from cancer and healthy tissues based on the co-expression data of the VIP with 760 cancer-related genes. We identified a meaningful and novel association between the VIP and transcription factor ZEB1 in healthy and malignant human gastrointestinal tissues. ZEB1 is a known regulator of cancer EMT (epithelial–mesenchymal transition). Gene set analysis further supports the overlap in the EMT and cell cycle pathways. Our results identify a potentially novel function of the autocrine VIP as an important signaling peptide and biomarker of ZEB1-mediated EMT.

Abstract: VIP (vasoactive intestinal peptide) is a 28-amino acid peptide hormone expressed by cancer and the healthy nervous system, digestive tract, cardiovascular, and immune cell tissues. Many cancers express VIP and its surface receptors VPAC1 and VPAC2, but the role of autocrine VIP signaling in cancer as a targetable prognostic and predictive biomarker remains poorly understood. Therefore, we conducted an in silico gene expression analysis to study the mechanisms of autocrine VIP signaling in cancer. VIP expression from TCGA PANCAN tissue samples was analyzed against the expression levels of 760 cancer-associated genes. Of the 760 genes, 10 (MAPK3, ZEB1, TEK, NOS2, PTCH1 EIF4G1, GMPS, CDK2, RUVBL1, and TIMELESS) showed statistically meaningful associations with the VIP (Pearson's R-coefficient > |0.3|; $p < 0.05$) across all cancer histologies. The strongest association with the VIP was for the epithelial–mesenchymal transition regulator ZEB1 in gastrointestinal malignancies. Similar positive correlations between the VIP and ZEB1 expression were also observed in healthy gastrointestinal tissues. Gene set analysis indicates the VIP is involved in the EMT and cell cycle pathways, and a high VIP and ZEB1 expression is associated with higher median estimate and stromal scores These findings uncover novel mechanisms for VIP- signaling in cancer and specifically suggest a role for VIP as a biomarker of ZEB1-mediated EMT. Further studies are warranted to characterize the specific mechanism of this interaction.

Keywords: VIP; ZEB1; cancer; EMT; gastrointestinal cancers

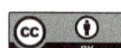

Citation: Rao, I.H.; Waller, E.K.; Dhamsania, R.K.; Chandrasekaran, S. Gene Expression Analysis Links Autocrine Vasoactive Intestinal Peptide and ZEB1 in Gastrointestinal Cancers. *Cancers* **2023**, *15*, 3284. https://doi.org/10.3390/cancers15133284

Academic Editors: Daniel L. Pouliquen and Cristina Núñez González

Received: 30 May 2023
Revised: 12 June 2023
Accepted: 19 June 2023
Published: 22 June 2023

Copyright: © 2023 by the authors. Licensee MDPI, Basel, Switzerland. This article is an open access article distributed under the terms and conditions of the Creative Commons Attribution (CC BY) license (https://creativecommons.org/licenses/by/4.0/).

1. Introduction

Vasoactive Intestinal Peptide (VIP) is the final 28-amino acid (AA) product following multiple processing steps starting from prepro-VIP, a 170 AA precursor peptide [1,2] to which VIP primarily binds and signals through using two GPCRs (G-protein coupled receptors), VPAC1 and VPAC2 [3]. VIP, VPAC1, and VPAC2 are all broadly expressed in multiple healthy tissue types, in particular, tissues of the nervous system, digestive tract, and the respiratory, cardiovascular, and immune systems [4,5], and physiologically, VPAC/VIP signaling regulates embryonal development and growth, neuronal and epithelial cell signaling, gut absorption and motility, endocrine-mediated glycemia and circadian rhythms, immune cell responses, and carcinogenesis [6,7]. In the immune system, the VIP functions as a Type 2 cytokine [8]. VPAC1 is constitutively expressed in various immune cell populations, including T lymphocytes, macrophages, and dendritic cells [1,9]. Studies using transgenic mice have demonstrated that Th2 CD4+ T cells up-regulate VIP expression upon antigen presentation, while Th1 CD4+ T cells do not [10].

The importance of autocrine VIP as a biomarker or therapeutic target in cancer has remained elusive for many years. An in vitro study of >400 human primary tumors, tumor metastases, and normal tissues using subtype selective VPAC receptor autoradiography has established that most cancers express VPAC, with VPAC1 being the predominant receptor subtype in cancers and healthy tissues [11]. In clinical studies, radiolabeled-VIP binds VPAC and detects primary and metastatic tumors in a variety of cancer histologies [12,13], and serum VIP levels are > two-fold higher in patients with colon adenocarcinoma [14,15].

To date, the primary function of autocrine VIP signaling was thought to drive cancer cell proliferation. Mechanistically, VIP binds to surface VPAC1 and VPAC2 and generates downstream signals through adenylate cyclase to catalyze cyclic AMP (cAMP) synthesis and protein kinase A (PKA) activation [16]. The PKA phosphorylation of the CREB (cAMP-response element binding) transcription factor subsequently activates oncogenes such as c-Myc to drive cancer proliferation. In practice, in vitro studies with exogenous VIP or the pharmacologic inhibition of VIP signaling using VPAC1 and VPAC2 peptide antagonists have shown mixed results. No consistent increase in the proliferation rates of colon and pancreatic cancer cell lines was seen when adding exogenous VIP to cancer cells in vitro, and, in certain cell lines, exogenous VIP even inhibited growth [14]. Similarly, the pharmacologic inhibition of VIP signaling using VPAC1 and VPAC2 peptide antagonists in vitro demonstrated variable anti-tumor responses depending on cancer histology and the cell line tested, with positive responses primarily seen in pancreatic, colorectal, gastric, and breast cancer models [5,17–21]. Recent studies showed exogenous VIP feeds back to induce EGFR (epidermal growth factor receptor) and HER2 (human epidermal growth factor receptor 2) phosphorylation in breast cancer cells and inhibits the apoptotic effects of the RAS/RAF inhibitor sorafenib on cancer stem cells, suggesting there remain unknown downstream mechanisms of VIP [22–25].

The consistent co-expression of VIP and VPAC in cancer and the availability of radiotracers to follow the VIP/VPAC as predictive or prognostic biomarkers, coupled with the ability to inhibit VIP signaling via VPAC1 and VPAC2 peptide antagonists, supports the need to further characterize the VIP signaling landscape and determine its importance in the properties of cancer that have been described as the "hallmarks of cancer" [24,25]. In this exploratory analysis, we utilized an in silico gene expression model to uncover new downstream signaling pathways of VIP in cancer and corroborate these pathways in analyses of healthy tissues.

2. Materials and Methods

Gene association and expression: Cancer mRNA expression data for VIP and Pearson's correlation (R) for VIP versus 760 other genes (gene panel based on the Nanostring nCounter® Tumor Signaling 360™ profiling panel) were abstracted from the TCGA (The Cancer Genome Atlas) PANCAN dataset using the University of California Santa Cruz (UCSC) Xena platform and recorded into Microsoft Excel by cancer hallmark (per Nanostring designation) (Supplemental Table S1) [26–28]. The date of cutoff for data abstraction was 1 December 2020 and of the 12,839 samples available for analysis, 2036 null values were excluded (Supplemental Figure S1.1). Individual tissue sample mRNA expression levels and R coefficients for VIP and 10 identified lead genes were further abstracted for all TCGA tumor histologies. Histologies were also organized into sub-groups by the tissue germ layer of origin (ectoderm, endoderm, and mesoderm) (Supplemental Table S2). Healthy tissue gene expression data was obtained from the Genotype-Tissue Expression (GTEx) Project on 19 April 2023 (https://www.gtexportal.org/home/ (19 April 2023)) [29]. Cancer cell line-specific gene expression data was downloaded on 4/19/23 from the CCLE (cancer cell line encyclopedia) using the DepMap resource (Public Expression Dataset 22Q4) (https://depmap.org/portal (accessed on 19 April 2023)).

Statistical analysis: The strength of association between VIP and comparator genes' expression data from the TCGA, GTEX, and CCLE datasets was determined using a Pearson's correlation test (R). For initial screening, R-coefficients > |0.3| and corresponding p-value < 0.05 were considered statistically meaningful [30]. Gene expression data (RNA-Log2(norm_count+1)) for VIP and ZEB1 in healthy (GTEX) and cancer (TCGA) tissues were analyzed per a Mann–Whitney U test for non-parametric data with $p < 0.05$ defined as statistically significant using GraphPad Prism (v9.5.1).

VIP and ZEB1 Expression and Cancer Pathway Activity: Gene set analysis was performed to assess the pathway activity of VIP and ZEB1 in gastrointestinal malignancies, including COAD (colon adenocarcinoma), ESCA (esophageal carcinoma), PAAD (pancreatic adenocarcinoma), and STAD (stomach adenocarcinoma). The analysis was conducted using the GSCA (Gene Set Cancer Analysis) tool, as previously described [31], with pathway activity scores assigned in ten critical cancer-related pathways (TSC/mTOR, RTK, RAS/MAPK, PI3K/AKT, hormone ER, hormone AR, EMT, DNA damage response, cell cycle, and apoptosis) based on a total of 7876 TCGA samples across 32 different cancer types. Pathway activity was determined by stratifying samples into high and low-expression groups based on the median gene expression, and a score was then calculated using a student t-test, with p-values adjusted by the false discovery rate (FDR). Reported results were considered significant when the FDR was <0.05, indicating a low likelihood of false positives.

Estimate, Stromal, and Immune Scoring: Estimate, stromal, and immune scores were used to compare tumor purity, stromal cell presence, and immune cell infiltration in stomach adenocarcinoma samples based on VIP and ZEB1 high vs. low tumor expression using the ESTIMATE scoring system, as previously described (https://bioinformatics.mdanderson.org/estimate/index.html (accessed on 8 June 2023)) [32]. A total of 377 of the 415 STAD samples with scoring available were evaluable (nulls removed and primary tumor only). The median estimate, stromal, and immune scores were analyzed per the Mann–Whitney U test for non-parametric data with $p < 0.05$ defined as statistically significant using GraphPad Prism (v9.5.1)

3. Results

3.1. VIP Expression in Cancer

The protein expression of VIP, VPAC1, and VPAC2 was investigated using immunohistochemistry data from the Human Protein Atlas (HPA) (Figure 1) [33,34]. Consistent with previous research [11], the HPA protein analysis revealed that VPAC1 is expressed in nearly all cancer histologies. In fact, VPAC1 expression was observed in over 70% of tissue samples from breast, carcinoid, head and neck, ovarian, and pancreatic cancers. On the other hand, the expression of VIP varied among different tumor histologies, with several histologies showing no detectable protein expression. However, it is noteworthy that many of the VIP non-expressing histologies still exhibited the expression of VPAC1 or VPAC2 receptors. For example, cancers of the breast, endometrium, prostate, testis, urothelium/bladder, and melanoma showed an expression of VPAC1 or VPAC2 despite lacking VIP expression. The differential expression patterns of VIP and its receptors across different histologies suggest distinct roles and potential interactions between VIP-receptor signaling and other pathways in cancer. Therefore, we undertook further investigations to elucidate the functional significance of these observations in the context of specific cancers.

To further characterize the signaling landscape, VIP mRNA expression was compared against a panel of 760 cancer-pertinent genes across all evaluable tissue samples in the TCGA PANCAN database. The selected gene panel was based on the Nanostring nCounter® Tumor Signaling 360™ testing panel [28]. A total of 285 genes showed positive R associations with VIP expression, while 475 were negatively associated (Figure 2A). Only ~10% of each cohort of positively or negatively associated genes demonstrated an

$R > |0.2|$ (25/285 positive correlation, 52/475 negative correlation). Based on our prespecified cutoff of $R > |0.3|$, five positively correlated and five negatively correlated lead genes were identified (positive correlation: MAPK3, ZEB1, NOS2, TEK, and PTCH1; negative correlation: EIF4G1, GMPS, CDK2, RUVBL1, and TIMELESS) (all $p < 0.05$, Supplemental Figure S1.2).

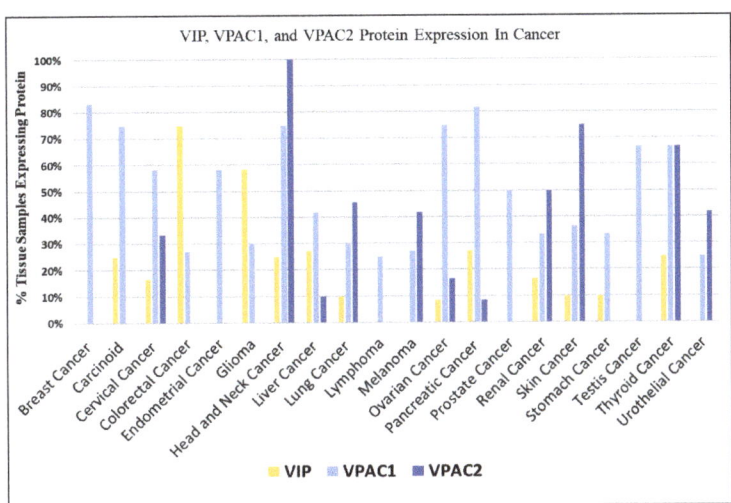

Figure 1. Protein expression of VIP and VIP Receptors In Cancer: VIP expression is highest in gliomas and colorectal, pancreas, thyroid cancers. VPAC1 is generally expressed on all cancer types and VPAC2 expression is limited to certain cancer types including those of the head and neck, lung, skin, kidney, thyroid, bladder, and melanoma.

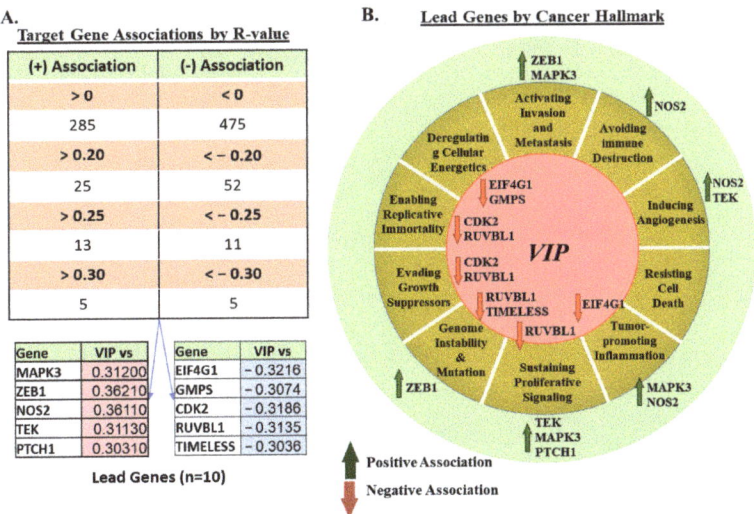

Figure 2. 10 Lead Genes Identified and Associated Cancer Hallmarks: (**A**) 10 lead-genes identified with R values $> |0.3|$ for the entire analyzed dataset. (**B**) Further analysis by cancer hallmark shows potential associations of VIP with hallmarks other than proliferative signaling.

3.2. mRNA Expression of VIP Associated Genes by Cancer Hallmark and Tissue Histology

To provide functional context to our findings, we also examined the association of the genes of interest with the pathways involved in the cancer hallmarks. Eight genes (CPA3, FAM30A, FOXP3, HDC, HSD11B1, PNIC, SH2D1A, and TCL1A) were excluded due to their primary involvement in the functions of non-malignant immune cells. Amongst the 752 genes remaining, the majority are involved in cancer hallmarks for activating sustaining proliferative signaling (n = 223), tumor-promoting inflammation (n = 178), invasion and metastasis (n = 146), and avoiding immune destruction (n = 122), with some overlap in certain genes across multiple cancer hallmarks (Supplemental Figure S1.3). Further focusing on lead gene functions, mapping by cancer hallmark, shows that VIP may be involved in the up- or down-regulation of genes relevant to nearly all cancer hallmarks (other than resisting cell death), with the higher number of lead gene associations seen in the hallmark pathway of "sustaining proliferative signaling" (RUVBL1, TEK, MAPK3, and PTCH1) (Figure 2B).

To explore the cancer histologies where the associations between VIP and lead genes are most significant, we employed increasingly stringent R-coefficient cutoffs ($> |0.4|$ and $> |0.5|$). The R-coefficients between VIP and each lead gene were determined for all assessable samples within each TCGA cancer histology (Supplemental Figure S2). When using $R > |0.4|$, nine out of the ten lead genes exhibited histology-specific associations with VIP. Among them, TEK showed the highest number of histology-specific associations (n = 13), followed by ZEB1 (n = 8) (Figure 3). When further increasing the cutoff to $R > |0.5|$, only four out of the ten lead genes retained significant associations with VIP. These genes were ZEB1, TEK, GMPS, and TIMELESS. These associations showed histologic overlap in cancers of the gastrointestinal tract (STAD and COAD), lung (LUSC), and kidney (KICH). Notably, the strongest association observed was between VIP and ZEB1 in stomach adenocarcinoma ($R = 0.76$, Figure 4A). These findings highlight the cancer histologies where the association between the expression of VIP and lead genes is particularly meaningful, based on progressively stricter R-coefficient criteria. The strong association between VIP and ZEB1 in stomach adenocarcinoma warranted further investigation.

Gene	# Histologies R > |0.4|	Histologies	# Histologies R > |0.5|	Histologies	TCGA Cancer Abbreviations
MAPK3	1	LGG	0		- LUSC: Lung squamous cell carcinoma
ZEB1	8	READ, COAD, ESCA, PAAD, STAD, UCEC, KICH, KIRC	5	READ, COAD, ESCA, STAD, UCEC	- BRCA: Breast invasive carcinoma - LGG: Brain Lower Grade Glioma
NOS2	1	MESO	0	-	- READ: Rectum adenocarcinoma
TEK	13	BRCA, LUSC, READ, COAD, ESCA, LUAD, PAAD, STAD, THYM, UCEC, KICH, KIRP, MESO	6	LUSC, COAD, PAAD, STAD, THYM, KICH	- LUAD: Lung adenocarcinoma - STAD: Stomach adenocarcinoma - THYM: Thymoma - THCA: Thyroid Carcinoma
PTCH1	0	-	0	-	- COAD: Colon adenocarcinoma
EIF4G1	3	THCA, UCEC, KICH	0	-	- ESCA: Esophageal carcinoma
GMPS	6	BRCA, LUSC, LUAD, STAD, THCA, KICH,	2	LUSC, KICH	- UCEC: Uterine Corpus Endometrial Carcinoma - CHOL: Cholangiocarcinoma
CDK2	1	CHOL, LGG	0	-	- LIHC: Liver hepatocellular carcinoma
RUVBL1	5	BRCA, LGG, LUSC, STAD, THYM	0	-	- PAAD: Pancreatic adenocarcinoma
TIMELESS	5	BRCA, LUSC, ESCA, STAD, TGCT	1	STAD	- MESO: Mesothelioma - KICH: Kidney chromophobe - KIRP: Kidney renal papillary cell carcinoma - KIRC: Kidney renal clear cell carcinoma - TGCT: Testicular Germ Cell Tumor

Figure 3. Lead Gene associations by tumor histology and increasing R-value Strength: Lead genes with corresponding histologies by increasing R-value strength. At $R > |0.5|$, only 4/10 lead genes retain meaningful associations with VIP.

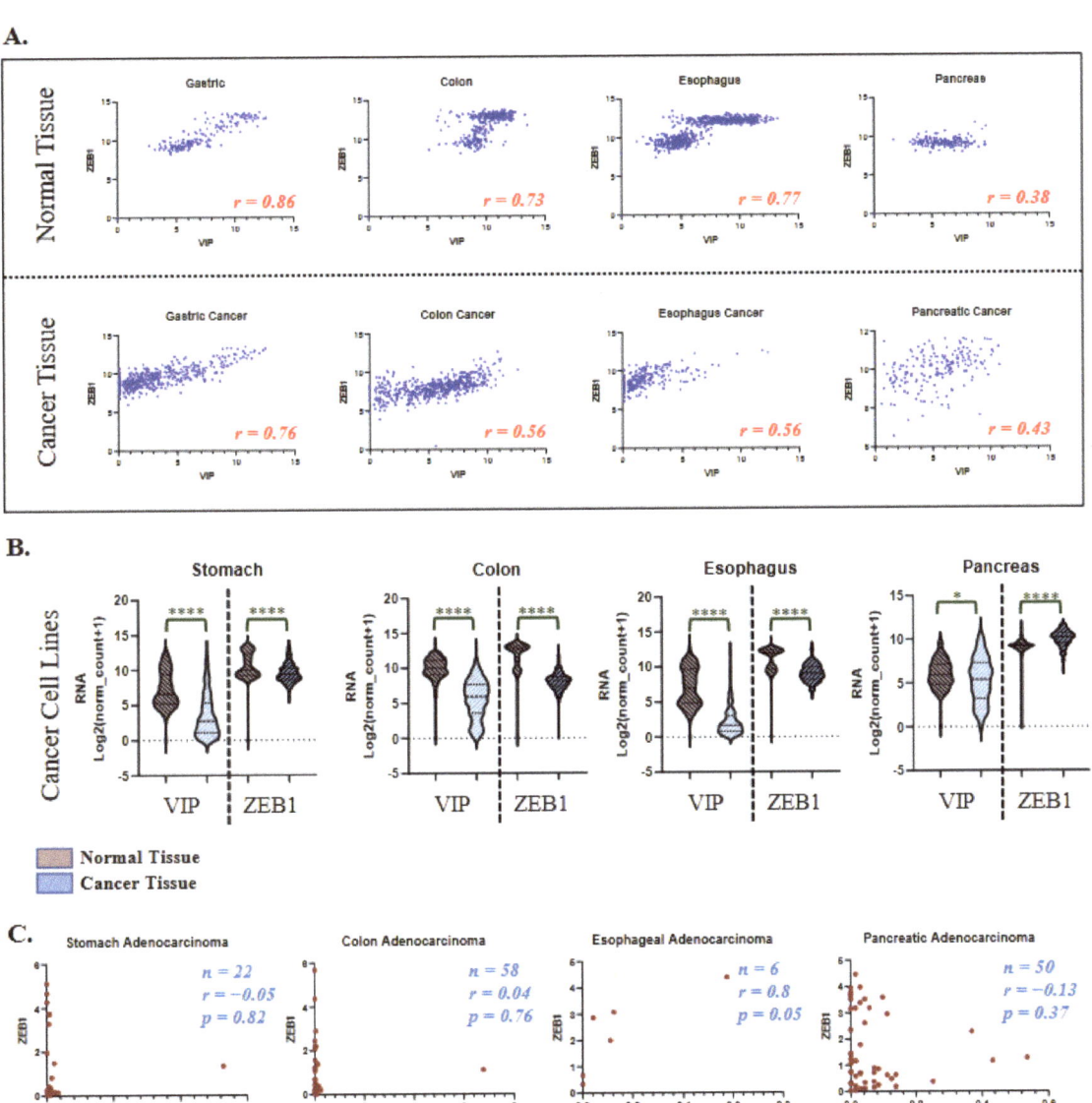

Figure 4. VIP and ZEB1 mRNA expression in gastrointestinal cancer and health tissues: (**A**) Similar VIP vs ZEB1 associations are seen in gastric, colon, esophageal, and pancreatic cancer (TCGA) and healthy (GTEX) tissues ($p < 0.0001$ for all analyses). (**B**) Total mRNA expression of VIP and ZEB1 is reduced in cancers of the stomach, colon, and esophagus ($p < 0.0001$ (****)), increased ZEB1 in cancer tissue ($p < 0.0001$), and similar in the pancreas for VIP $p = 0.012$ (*). (**C**) VIP and ZEB1 mRNA expression (log2(TPM+1)) in human gastric (stomach), colon, and pancreatic adenocarcinoma cancer cell lines (CCLE) does not show meaningful expression correlations. Positive correlation is seen in esophageal cell lines ($R = 0.8$, $p = 0.05$).

Given the known importance of VIP in embryogenesis, we also sub-grouped individual cancer histologies by germ layer of origin and looked for germ layer-specific expression associations (Supplemental Figure S3A, Supplemental Table S2). In this context, we also evaluated whether cross-reactive peptide signaling influenced our findings. The PACAP (pituitary adenylate cyclase-activating polypeptide) peptide shares 67% homology with VIP and is also able to bind to VPAC1 and VPAC2, in addition to its specific PAC1 receptor (Supplemental Figure S3B) [5,35]. Associations between lead genes and VIP or PACAP stratified by germinal layer did not indicate confounding functional overlap between VIP and PACAP. Germinal layer findings for VIP revealed tumors of ectodermal and mesodermal origin demonstrated correlations with $R > |0.4|$ with non-meaningful $R < |0.2|$ signals seen in PTCH1 (mesoderm) and GMPS, CDK2, RUVBL1, and TIMELESS (endoderm).

3.3. VIP and ZEB1 Expression in Healthy Tissue and Cancer Cell Lines

Given the compelling association between VIP and ZEB1 identified in gastrointestinal malignancies, especially of the stomach and colon, we tested VIP and ZEB1 expression in their corresponding healthy tissues. The healthy gastrointestinal tissue expression of VIP and ZEB1 was analyzed using the GTEX dataset [29]. Healthy gastric, colon, esophageal, and pancreatic tissues had R coefficients between VIP and ZEB1, an expression similar to those seen in TCGA cancer tissues ($p < 0.0001$ for all analyses) (Figure 4A). The biphasic distribution of VIP/ZEB1 (low) vs. VIP/ZEB1 (high) seen in the colon and esophageal tissues is thought to be related to the differences in the presence of mucosal and submucosal tissue in the samples. VIP expression in healthy pancreatic tissue is likely more susceptible to hormonal regulation of the endocrine pancreatic tissue, supporting the findings of variable VIP expression with somewhat consistent ZEB1 expression.

To determine if VIP and ZEB1 expression is up-regulated or down-regulated in cancer vs. healthy tissue, the total mRNA levels of VIP and ZEB1 between healthy and cancer tissue were compared. VIP and ZEB1 expression were both lower in stomach, colon, and esophageal cancer tissue compared to healthy tissue ($p < 0.0001$, Figure 4B). There were minimally significant differences in VIP expression between normal and pancreatic cancer tissue ($p = 0.012$) and increased ZEB1 expression in cancer tissue. We next analyzed associations between VIP and ZEB1 expression in the human stomach, colon, esophageal, and pancreatic adenocarcinoma cell lines from the CCLE (cancer cell line encyclopedia) using the DepMap resource. Interestingly, the cell line expression data did not recapitulate the VIP and ZEB1 associations seen in healthy and cancer tissues and showed only a statistically significant association between VIP and ZEB1 in a limited number of esophageal adenocarcinoma cases ($p = 0.05$) (Figure 4C).

3.4. Gene Set Analysis of VIP and ZEB1

The consistent association between VIP and ZEB1 expression in both healthy and cancerous tissues suggests a potential linkage of the signaling pathways of these two genes. To investigate this further, gene set analysis (GSA) was conducted in colon, gastric, esophageal, and pancreatic cancers using the GSCA tool for the following cancer-related pathways: TSC/mTOR, RTK, RAS/MAPK, PI3K/AKT, hormone ER, hormone AR, EMT, DNA damage response, cell cycle, and apoptosis. GSA revealed that VIP and ZEB1 had activating effects on EMT and inhibitory effects on the cell cycle pathway in both colon and gastric cancers. Additionally, in gastric cancer, VIP and ZEB1 showed inhibitory effects on the apoptosis pathway (FDR < 0.05, Figure 5A, Supplemental Table S3). Comparisons between the high and low tissue expression of VIP and ZEB1 were performed based on the GSA results, focusing on the EMT and cell cycle pathways in gastric and colon cancer (Figure 5B). These findings indicate that VIP and ZEB1 may jointly influence the EMT and cell cycle pathways in gastric and colon cancers. Moreover, the inhibitory effects on the apoptosis pathway observed in gastric cancer suggest potential roles for VIP and ZEB1 in modulating cell survival mechanisms in this specific cancer type.

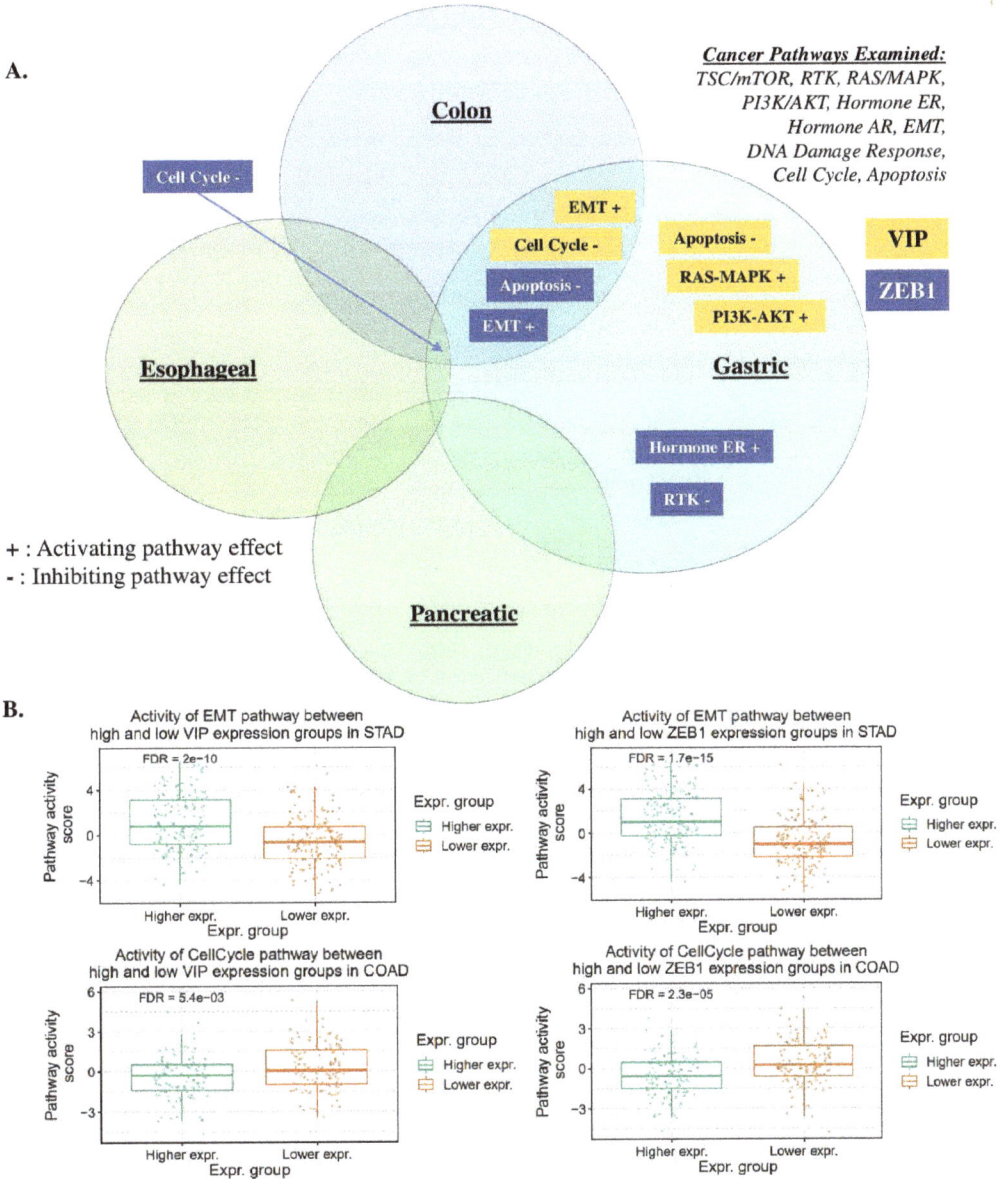

Figure 5. Gene Set Analysis of VIP and ZEB1 in colon, esophageal, gastric, and pancreatic cancers: (**A**) VIP and ZEB1 share activating effects on EMT and inhibitory effects on cell cycle in gastric and colon cancer. No pathway effects seen in pancreatic cancer (**B**) Representative box plots showing impact of high vs low VIP and ZEB1 expression in gastric and colon cancer in EMT activation and cell cycle inhibition (FDR < 0.25).

3.5. Estimate, Stromal, and Immune Scoring

VIP is also known to exert paracrine effects in cancer by supporting the immunosuppressive activity of CD4+CD25+ regulatory T cells and tolerogenic dendritic cells [8,36]. In vivo studies have demonstrated that treatment with VPAC peptide antagonists can reverse these immune effects and down-regulate T cell expression of the inhibitory marker PD-1, promote cytotoxic T cell differentiation and expansion, and enhance intratumoral T cell infiltration, ultimately leading to tumor elimination [15,37–39], and we have recently shown that inhibiting VIP in murine pancreatic cancer models improves the response to T cell checkpoint inhibitors [15]. To determine if the VIP and ZEB1 associations seen in our analysis were confounded by immune cell-mediated paracrine VIP, we compared whether high versus low VIP and ZEB1 expression correlated with tumor purity, stromal tissue presence, or immune cell infiltration using the estimate, stromal, and immune scores, respectively. ZEB1 and VIP high-expressing tumors (n = 189) were associated with higher median estimate and stromal scores, with high expression most associated with positive scores (Figure 6A,B). Median immune scores were positive for low and high ZEB1 and VIP expression, with higher scores associated with increased VIP and ZEB1 expression (Figure 6C).

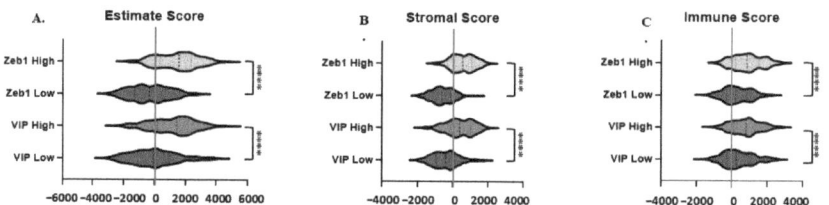

Figure 6. Estimate, Stromal, and Immune scores grouped by low versus high VIP and ZEB1 Expression: (**A**) Median Estimate score for ZEB1 high (1569) and ZEB1 low (−348.7) and VIP high (1428) and VIP low (−66.05) (**B**). Median Stromal score for ZEB1 high (568.2) and ZEB1 low (−621.5) and VIP high (387.2) and VIP low (−397.6) (**C**). Median Immune score for ZEB1 high (864) and ZEB1 low (215) and VIP high (814.2) and VIP low (264.1). $p < 0.0001$ for all comparisons (****).

4. Discussion

To comprehensively characterize the signaling landscape of autocrine VIP in cancer, we conducted an *in silico* gene expression analysis. Determining the downstream effects of VIP in cancer is crucial to understanding its role as a circulating biomarker and VPAC as a diagnostic, prognostic, or predictive target. The utility of radiolabeled-VIP and the development of VIP-targeted theranostics is severely limited by this lack of understanding.

Comprehensive gene expression studies of cancer are valuable when studying peptides such as VIP. The VIP sequence is highly conserved across mammals and rarely mutated in cancers, in support of a critical role for VIP-signaling in normal physiology [2]. Furthermore, protein expression studies, including techniques such as Western blot and immunohistochemistry (IHC), may not fully capture peptide expression data due to limiting factors such as the multiple cleavage steps of the prepro peptide, variability in the antibody binding, and the short half-life of the peptide.

Among the initial screening panel of 760 genes, our *in silico* model identified 10 lead genes that showed strong associations with VIP expression. Some of these genes, such as MAPK, NOS2, CDK2, and TIMELESS, have been previously associated with VIP in non-cancer models [40–43]. However, our analysis also revealed several novel associations, the most compelling being the association with the ZEB1 transcription factor.

The association between VIP and ZEB1 in gastrointestinal tissues appears to be present in both healthy and malignant tissues. ZEB1 is a well-characterized transcription factor known to play a role in the regulation of epithelial–mesenchymal transition (EMT) in cancer [44]. EMT is a process in which primary tumor cells down-regulate the expression of structural and cell adhesion molecules, such as cytokeratin and E-cadherin, and lose their epithelial markers to acquire a more aggressive, spindle cell-like mesenchymal phenotype to drive tumor metastasis and distant invasion [45].

Detecting the early signs of EMT and targeting the process pharmacologically has been a long-standing focus of cancer research, but the heterogeneity across multiple cancer histologies and redundant downstream signaling pathways involved in E-cadherin loss have limited the success of these efforts. Transcription factors critical to EMT, including ZEB1, STAT, SNAIL, and TWIST, are not ideal targets for pharmacological interventions or readily assessed through imaging techniques. Therefore, identifying upstream cell surface targets such as VPAC1 or VPAC2 could aid in the development of EMT-targeted cancer therapies [45]. Recently, Colangelo et al. uncovered an axis between TIMELESS and ZEB1 in colorectal cancers, demonstrating that the loss of TIMELESS promotes tumor progression and poor prognosis by inducing ZEB1 expression and EMT. These findings align with the negative correlation we observed between VIP and TIMELESS in our analysis [46].

However, the current study has some design limitations. The 760-gene panel used is a limited dataset, however, this selection was deliberate to focus on well-elucidated genes with known functions in cancer to facilitate the further translation of our findings. The under-representation of certain histologies in the TCGA dataset may have led to histology-specific errors and potential missed associations due to a smaller sample size. The initial screening of lead genes by R > {0.3} may appear to be a less stringent threshold, however, this was done only when evaluating the VIP-gene associations across all TCGA histologies and samples. Of note, all R in the initial screen were < {0.4}.

Findings from in silico analyses can be challenging to translate into in vitro studies or in vivo therapies. The divergent findings in VIP and ZEB1 expression associations between tissues (healthy and malignant) and cancer cell lines highlight the need for future studies in both settings. Factors such as culture conditions may affect VIP, ZEB1, and EMT-related phenotypes in vitro. Heterogeneity in the tumor microenvironment and between sequenced samples may also affect data interpretation, however, the estimate, stromal, and immune scoring data support that our findings are not confounded by the paracrine effects of immune cell infiltrates and are cancer cell and cancer stroma dependent. The differences seen by the cancer-mediated stromal cell presence may also indicate why the patterns vary between healthy tissues and cancer tissues.

The identified association between ZEB1 and VIP expression may not be causal. However, the consistent association of the expression levels for these genes across multiple cancer histologies, healthy tissues, and gene set analyses indicates potential significance and warrants further investigation. Furthermore, while the transition from a proliferative to invasive phenotype is considered fundamental to EMT, our findings that VIP is involved in both processes support more recent arguments that EMT and, conversely, MET (mesenchymal–epithelial transition) represent a continuum of states and not discrete phenotypes [47].

Taken together, the VIP–VPAC axis offers a widely expressed and targetable biomarker in cancer. The presence of VPAC in both VIP-expressing and non-expressing tissues suggests that cancers may be simultaneously susceptible to both autocrine and paracrine VIP effects. Whether targeting VPAC can be diagnostic, prognostic, and/or predictive remains to be fully explored. Our findings indicate that in gastrointestinal malignancies, further in vitro and in vivo validation is necessary to elucidate the mechanism of interaction between VIP and ZEB1 and to determine how VIP supports ZEB1-mediated EMT involved in tumor invasion and metastasis.

5. Conclusions

We performed hypothesis-generating in silico analyses of associations of autocrine VIP gene expression with gene targets and pathways in cancer. We identified a potential novel association of the VIP–VPAC axis with ZEB1 expression in gastrointestinal malignancies. Further studies are necessary to understand how inhibiting or activating the VIP–VPAC axis may serve as a prognostic biomarker of cancer metastasis or a predictive biomarker for response to VIP-targeted therapies on EMT in gastrointestinal malignancies.

Supplementary Materials: The following supporting information can be downloaded at: https://www.mdpi.com/article/10.3390/cancers15133284/s1, Supplemental Figure S1: Analyzed sample numbers, p-values, and pertinent cancer hallmarks for the 760 target gene panel; Supplemental Figure S2: Heat map of R-values for lead gene associations by cancer histology; Supplemental Figure S3: Heat map of lead gene associations by tissue germ layer; Supplemental Table S1: R-Values in target gene set by cancer hallmark with heat map; Supplemental Table S2. TCGA tumor histologies and abbreviations by germ layer; and Supplemental Table S3: Gene set analysis data for VIP and ZEB1.

Author Contributions: Conceptualization, S.C. and I.H.R.; methodology, S.C., I.H.R. and R.K.D.; software, S.C.; formal analysis, S.C., I.H.R. and E.K.W.; investigation, I.H.R.; resources, S.C. and E.K.W.; data curation, S.C.; writing—original draft preparation, I.H.R. and R.K.D.; writing—review and editing, S.C., I.H.R. and E.K.W.; visualization, S.C.; supervision, S.C.; project administration, I.H.R.; funding acquisition, S.C. and E.K.W. All authors have read and agreed to the published version of the manuscript.

Funding: These studies were supported by funding from the Winship Cancer Institute Elkin Fellowship (SC), NIH T32 CA160040 (SC), and Abraham J. and Phyllis Katz Foundation (EKW).

Institutional Review Board Statement: Not applicable.

Informed Consent Statement: Not applicable.

Data Availability Statement: TCGA data can be accessed via UCSC Xena at (http://xena.ucsc.edu/) (accessed on 1 December 2020)). Healthy tissue data are available at the GTEX portal (https://www.gtexportal.org/home/ (accessed on 19 April 2023)). Cancer cell line data are available through the cancer cell line encyclopedia (CCCLE) available via the DepMap resource (https://depmap.org/portal (accessed on 19 April 2023)).

Acknowledgments: The results are based upon data generated from the TCGA Research Network: https://www.cancer.gov/tcga (accessed on 1 December 2020)). The TCGA data used for the analyses were obtained from the UCSC Xena Portal (https://xena.ucsc.edu (accessed on 1 December 2020)). The Genotype-Tissue Expression (GTEx) Project was supported by the Common Fund of the Office of the Director of the National Institutes of Health, and by NCI, NHGRI, NHLBI, NIDA, NIMH, and NINDS. The healthy tissue data used for the analyses described in this manuscript were obtained from the GTEx Portal on 19 April 2023.

Conflicts of Interest: E.K.W. holds intellectual property covering VIP antagonists and is a founder and equity partner in Cambium Oncology. The other authors have no financial conflict of interest.

References

1. Delgado, M.; Pozo, D.; Ganea, D. The Significance of Vasoactive Intestinal Peptide in Immunomodulation. *Pharmacol. Rev.* **2004**, *56*, 249–290. [CrossRef]
2. Ng, S.Y.L.; Chow, B.K.C.; Kasamatsu, J.; Kasahara, M.; Lee, L.T.O. Agnathan VIP, PACAP and Their Receptors: Ancestral Origins of Today's Highly Diversified Forms. *PLoS ONE* **2012**, *7*, e44691. [CrossRef]
3. Harmar, A.J.; Arimura, A.; Gozes, I.; Journot, L.; Laburthe, M.; Pisegna, J.R.; Rawlings, S.R.; Robberecht, P.; Said, S.I.; Sreedharan, S.P.; et al. International Union of Pharmacology. XVIII. Nomenclature of receptors for vasoactive intestinal peptide and pituitary adenylate cyclase-activating polypeptide. *Pharmacol. Rev.* **1998**, *50*, 265–270.
4. Dickson, L.; Finlayson, K. VPAC and PAC receptors: From ligands to function. *Pharmacol. Ther.* **2009**, *121*, 294–316. [CrossRef]
5. Moody, T.W.; Nuche-Berenguer, B.; Jensen, R.T. VIP/PACAP, and their receptors and cancer. *Curr. Opin. Endocrinol. Diabetes Obes.* **2016**, *23*, 38–47. [CrossRef]
6. Iwasaki, M.; Akiba, Y.; Kaunitz, J.D. Recent advances in vasoactive intestinal peptide physiology and pathophysiology: Focus on the gastrointestinal system. *F1000Research* **2019**, *8*, 1629. [CrossRef]
7. Fabricius, D.; Karacay, B.; Shutt, D.; Leverich, W.; Schafer, B.; Takle, E.; Thedens, D.; Khanna, G.; Raikwar, S.; Yang, B.; et al. Characterization of Intestinal and Pancreatic Dysfunction in VPAC1-Null Mutant Mouse. *Pancreas* **2011**, *40*, 861–871. [CrossRef]
8. Delgado, M.; Ganea, D. Vasoactive intestinal peptide: A neuropeptide with pleiotropic immune functions. *Amino Acids* **2013**, *45*, 25–39. [CrossRef]
9. Smalley, S.G.R.; Barrow, P.A.; Foster, N. Immunomodulation of innate immune responses by vasoactive intestinal peptide (VIP): Its therapeutic potential in inflammatory disease. *Clin. Exp. Immunol.* **2009**, *157*, 225–234. [CrossRef]
10. Vassiliou, E.; Jiang, X.; Delgado, M.; Ganea, D. TH2 Lymphocytes Secrete Functional VIP upon Antigen Stimulation. *Arch. Physiol. Biochem.* **2001**, *109*, 365–368. [CrossRef]

1. Reubi, J.C.; Läderach, U.; Waser, B.; Gebbers, J.O.; Robberecht, P.; Laissue, J.A. Vasoactive intestinal peptide/pituitary adenylate cyclase-activating peptide receptor subtypes in human tumors and their tissues of origin. *Cancer Res* **2000**, *60*, 3105–3112. [PubMed]
2. Virgolini, I.; Raderer, M.; Kurtaran, A.; Angelberger, P.; Yang, Q.; Radosavljevic, M.; Leimer, M.; Kaserer, K.; Li, S.; Kornek, G.; et al. 123I-vasoactive intestinal peptide (VIP) receptor scanning: Update of imaging results in patients with adenocarcinomas and endocrine tumors of the gastrointestinal tract. *Nucl. Med. Biol.* **1996**, *23*, 685–692. [CrossRef] [PubMed]
3. Virgolini, I. Mack Forster Award Lecture Receptor nuclear medicine: Vasointestinal peptide and somatostatin receptor scintigraphy for diagnosis and treatment of tumour patients. *Eur. J. Clin. Investig.* **1997**, *27*, 793–800. [CrossRef] [PubMed]
4. Hejna, M.; Hamilton, G.; Brodowicz, T.; Haberl, I.; Fiebiger, W.C.; Scheithauer, W.; Virgolini, I.; Köstler, W.J.; Oberhuber, G.; Raderer, M. Serum levels of vasoactive intestinal peptide (VIP) in patients with adenocarcinomas of the gastrointestinal tract. *Anticancer. Res.* **2001**, *21*, 1183–1187.
5. Ravindranathan, S.; Passang, T.; Li, J.-M.; Wang, S.; Dhamsania, R.; Ware, M.B.; Zaidi, M.Y.; Zhu, J.; Cardenas, M.; Liu, Y.; et al. Targeting vasoactive intestinal peptide-mediated signaling enhances response to immune checkpoint therapy in pancreatic ductal adenocarcinoma. *Nat. Commun.* **2022**, *13*, 6418. [CrossRef] [PubMed]
6. Harmar, A.J.; Fahrenkrug, J.; Gozes, I.; Laburthe, M.; May, V.; Pisegna, J.R.; Vaudry, D.; Vaudry, H.; Waschek, J.A.; Said, S.I. Pharmacology and functions of receptors for vasoactive intestinal peptide and pituitary adenylate cyclase-activating polypeptide: IUPHAR Review 1. *Br. J. Pharmacol.* **2012**, *166*, 4–17. [CrossRef]
7. Laburthe, M.; Rousset, M.; Chevalier, G.; Boissard, C.; Dupont, C.; Zweibaum, A.; Rosselin, G. Vasoactive intestinal peptide control of cyclic adenosine $3':5'$-monophosphate levels in seven human colorectal adenocarcinoma cell lines in culture. *Cancer Res.* **1980**, *40*, 2529–2533.
8. Laburthe, M.; Rousset, M.; Boissard, C.; Chevalier, G.; Zweibaum, A.; Rosselin, G. Vasoactive intestinal peptide: A potent stimulator of adenosine $3':5'$-cyclic monophosphate accumulation in gut carcinoma cell lines in culture. *Proc. Natl. Acad. Sci. USA* **1978**, *75*, 2772–2775. [CrossRef]
9. Moody, T.W.; Hill, J.M.; Jensen, R.T. VIP as a trophic factor in the CNS and cancer cells. *Peptides* **2003**, *24*, 163–177. [CrossRef]
10. Moody, T.W.; Zia, F.; Draoui, M.; Brenneman, D.E.; Fridkin, M.; Davidson, A.; Gozes, I. A vasoactive intestinal peptide antagonist inhibits non-small cell lung cancer growth. *Proc. Natl. Acad. Sci. USA* **1993**, *90*, 4345–4349. [CrossRef]
11. Moody, T.W.; Leyton, J.; Chan, D.; Brenneman, D.C.; Fridkin, M.; Gelber, E.; Levy, A.; Gozes, I. VIP receptor antagonists and chemotherapeutic drugs inhibit the growth of breast cancer cells. *Breast Cancer Res. Treat.* **2001**, *68*, 55–64. [CrossRef] [PubMed]
12. Valdehita, A.; Bajo, A.M.; Schally, A.V.; Varga, J.L.; Carmena, M.J.; Prieto, J.C. Vasoactive intestinal peptide (VIP) induces transactivation of EGFR and HER2 in human breast cancer cells. *Mol. Cell. Endocrinol.* **2009**, *302*, 41–48. [CrossRef] [PubMed]
13. Sastry, K.S.; Chouchane, A.I.; Wang, E.; Kulik, G.; Marincola, F.M.; Chouchane, L. Cytoprotective effect of neuropeptides on cancer stem cells: Vasoactive intestinal peptide-induced antiapoptotic signaling. *Cell Death Dis.* **2017**, *8*, e2844. [CrossRef] [PubMed]
14. Hanahan, D.; Weinberg, R.A. Hallmarks of cancer: The next generation. *Cell* **2011**, *144*, 646–674. [CrossRef] [PubMed]
15. Hanahan, D. Hallmarks of Cancer: New Dimensions. *Cancer Discov.* **2022**, *12*, 31–46. [CrossRef]
16. The Cancer Genome Atlas n.d. Available online: https://www.cancer.gov/about-nci/organization/ccg/research/structural-genomics/tcga (accessed on 1 January 2020).
17. Goldman, M.J.; Craft, B.; Hastie, M.; Repečka, K.; McDade, F.; Kamath, A.; Banerjee, A.; Luo, Y.; Rogers, D.; Brooks, A.N.; et al. Visualizing and interpreting cancer genomics data via the Xena platform. *Nat. Biotechnol.* **2020**, *38*, 675–678. [CrossRef]
18. Nanostring Tumor Signaling 360 n.d. Available online: https://nanostring.com/support-documents/tumor-signaling-360-panel/ (accessed on 1 January 2020).
19. Carithers, L.J.; Moore, H.M. The Genotype-Tissue Expression (GTEx) Project. *Biopreservation Biobanking* **2015**, *13*, 307–308. [CrossRef]
20. Schober, P.; Boer, C.; Schwarte, L.A. Correlation Coefficients: Appropriate Use and Interpretation. *Anesth. Analg.* **2018**, *126*, 1763–1768. [CrossRef]
21. Liu, C.-J.; Hu, F.-F.; Xie, G.-Y.; Miao, Y.-R.; Li, X.-W.; Zeng, Y.; Guo, A.-Y. GSCA: An integrated platform for gene set cancer analysis at genomic, pharmacogenomic and immunogenomic levels. *Brief. Bioinform.* **2023**, *24*, bbac558. [CrossRef]
22. Yoshihara, K.; Shahmoradgoli, M.; Martínez, E.; Vegesna, R.; Kim, H.; Torres-Garcia, W.; Treviño, V.; Shen, H.; Laird, P.W.; Levine, D.A.; et al. Inferring tumour purity and stromal and immune cell admixture from expression data. *Nat. Commun.* **2013**, *4*, 2612. [CrossRef]
23. The Human Protein Atlas, n.d. Available online: https://www.proteinatlas.org/ (accessed on 1 January 2020).
24. Uhlén, M.; Fagerberg, L.; Hallström, B.M.; Lindskog, C.; Oksvold, P.; Mardinoglu, A.; Sivertsson, Å.; Kampf, C.; Sjöstedt, E.; Asplund, A.; et al. Proteomics. Tissue-Based Map of the Human Proteome. *Science* **2015**, *347*, 1260419. [CrossRef] [PubMed]
25. Vaudry, D.; Falluel-Morel, A.; Bourgault, S.; Basille, M.; Burel, D.; Wurtz, O.; Fournier, A.; Chow, B.K.C.; Hashimoto, H.; Galas, L.; et al. Pituitary Adenylate Cyclase-Activating Polypeptide and Its Receptors: 20 Years after the Discovery. *Pharmacol. Rev.* **2009**, *61*, 283–357. [CrossRef] [PubMed]
26. Gonzalez-Rey, E.; Chorny, A.; Fernandez-Martin, A.; Ganea, D.; Delgado, M. Vasoactive intestinal peptide generates human tolerogenic dendritic cells that induce CD4 and CD8 regulatory T cells. *Blood* **2006**, *107*, 3632–3638. [CrossRef] [PubMed]

37. Li, J.-M.; Petersen, C.T.; Li, J.-X.; Panjwani, R.; Chandra, D.J.; Giver, C.R.; Blazar, B.R.; Waller, E.K. Modulation of Immune Checkpoints and Graft-versus-Leukemia in Allogeneic Transplants by Antagonizing Vasoactive Intestinal Peptide Signaling. *Cancer Res.* **2016**, *76*, 6802–6815. [CrossRef] [PubMed]
38. Petersen, C.T.; Hassan, M.; Morris, A.B.; Jeffery, J.; Lee, K.; Jagirdar, N.; Staton, A.D.; Raikar, S.S.; Spencer, H.T.; Sulchek, T.; et al. Improving ex vivo T cell expansion from DLBCL patients for T cell therapies via antagonism of PI3K δ and VIP. *Blood* **2017**, *130*, 3195.
39. Petersen, C.T.; Hassan, M.; Morris, A.B.; Jeffery, J.; Lee, K.; Jagirdar, N.; Staton, A.D.; Raikar, S.S.; Spencer, H.T.; Sulchek, T.; et al. Improving T-cell expansion and function for adoptive T-cell therapy using ex vivo treatment with PI3Kδ inhibitors and VIP antagonists. *Blood Adv.* **2018**, *2*, 210–223. [CrossRef]
40. Fernández, M.; Sánchez-Franco, F.; Palacios, N.; Sánchez, I.; Cacicedo, L. IGF-I and vasoactive intestinal peptide (VIP) regulate cAMP-response element-binding protein (CREB)-dependent transcription via the mitogen-activated protein kinase (MAPK) pathway in pituitary cells: Requirement of Rap1. *J. Mol. Endocrinol.* **2005**, *34*, 699–712. [CrossRef]
41. MacEachern, S.J.; Patel, B.A.; Keenan, C.M.; Dicay, M.; Chapman, K.; McCafferty, D.-M.; Savidge, T.C.; Beck, P.L.; MacNaughton, W.K.; Sharkey, K.A. Inhibiting Inducible Nitric Oxide Synthase in Enteric Glia Restores Electrogenic Ion Transport in Mice With Colitis. *Gastroenterology* **2015**, *149*, 445–455.e3. [CrossRef]
42. Anderson, P.; Gonzalez-Rey, E. Vasoactive Intestinal Peptide Induces Cell Cycle Arrest and Regulatory Functions in Human T Cells at Multiple Levels. *Mol. Cell. Biol.* **2010**, *30*, 2537–2551. [CrossRef]
43. Muraro, N.; Pírez, N.; Ceriani, M. The circadian system: Plasticity at many levels. *Neuroscience* **2013**, *247*, 280–293. [CrossRef]
44. Caramel, J.; Ligier, M.; Puisieux, A. Pleiotropic Roles for ZEB1 in Cancer. *Cancer Res.* **2018**, *78*, 30–35. [CrossRef] [PubMed]
45. Davis, F.M.; Stewart, T.A.; Thompson, E.W.; Monteith, G.R. Targeting EMT in cancer: Opportunities for pharmacological intervention. *Trends Pharmacol. Sci.* **2014**, *35*, 479–488. [CrossRef] [PubMed]
46. Colangelo, T.; Carbone, A.; Mazzarelli, F.; Cuttano, R.; Dama, E.; Nittoli, T.; Albanesi, J.; Barisciano, G.; Forte, N.; Palumbo, O.; et al. Loss of circadian gene Timeless induces EMT and tumor progression in colorectal cancer via Zeb1-dependent mechanism. *Cell Death Differ.* **2022**, *29*, 1552–1568. [CrossRef] [PubMed]
47. Yang, J.; Antin, P.; Berx, G.; Blanpain, C.; Brabletz, T.; Bronner, M.; Campbell, K.; Cano, A.; Casanova, J.; Christofori, G.; et al. Guidelines and definitions for research on epithelial–mesenchymal transition. *Nat. Rev. Mol. Cell Biol.* **2020**, *21*, 341–352, Correction in *Nat. Rev. Mol. Cell Biol.* **2021**, *22*, 834. [CrossRef] [PubMed]

Disclaimer/Publisher's Note: The statements, opinions and data contained in all publications are solely those of the individual author(s) and contributor(s) and not of MDPI and/or the editor(s). MDPI and/or the editor(s) disclaim responsibility for any injury to people or property resulting from any ideas, methods, instructions or products referred to in the content.

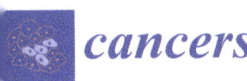

Review

The Entanglement between Mitochondrial DNA and Tumor Metastasis

Qiwei Wu [1], Hsiang-i Tsai [2], Haitao Zhu [1,2,*] and Dongqing Wang [1,*]

1. Department of Medical Imaging, The Affiliated Hospital of Jiangsu University, Zhenjiang 212001, China; 2211913036@stmail.ujs.edu.cn
2. Laboratory of Radiology, The Affiliated Hospital of Jiangsu University, Zhenjiang 212001, China; tsaihsiangi88@163.com
* Correspondence: haitaozhu@ujs.edu.cn (H.Z.); wangdongqing71@163.com (D.W.); Tel.: +86-138-6139-0259 (D.W.)

Simple Summary: Mitochondrial dysfunction is one of the main features of cancer cells. As genetic material in mitochondria, mitochondrial DNA (mtDNA) variations and dysregulation of mitochondria-encoded genes have been shown to correlate with survival outcomes in cancer patients. Cancer metastasis is often a major cause of treatment failure, which is a multi-step cascade process. With the development of gene sequencing and in vivo modeling technology, the role of mtDNA in cancer metastasis has been continuously explored. Our review systematically provides a summary of the multiple roles of mtDNA in cancer metastasis and presents the broad prospects for mtDNA in cancer prediction and therapy.

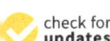

Citation: Wu, Q.; Tsai, H.-i.; Zhu, H.; Wang, D. The Entanglement between Mitochondrial DNA and Tumor Metastasis. *Cancers* 2022, *14*, 1862. https://doi.org/10.3390/cancers14081862

Academic Editors: Daniel L. Pouliquen and Cristina Núñez González

Received: 13 March 2022
Accepted: 1 April 2022
Published: 7 April 2022

Publisher's Note: MDPI stays neutral with regard to jurisdictional claims in published maps and institutional affiliations.

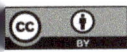

Copyright: © 2022 by the authors. Licensee MDPI, Basel, Switzerland. This article is an open access article distributed under the terms and conditions of the Creative Commons Attribution (CC BY) license (https://creativecommons.org/licenses/by/4.0/).

Abstract: Mitochondrial DNA, the genetic material in mitochondria, encodes essential oxidative phosphorylation proteins and plays an important role in mitochondrial respiration and energy transfer. With the development of genome sequencing and the emergence of novel in vivo modeling techniques, the role of mtDNA in cancer biology is gaining more attention. Abnormalities of mtDNA result in not only mitochondrial dysfunction of the the cancer cells and malignant behaviors, but regulation of the tumor microenvironment, which becomes more aggressive. Here, we review the recent progress in the regulation of cancer metastasis using mtDNA and the underlying mechanisms, which may identify opportunities for finding novel cancer prediction and therapeutic targets.

Keywords: mitochondrial DNA; tumor progression; metastasis; immune escape

1. Introduction

Tumor metastasis accounts for the overwhelming number of deaths in cancer patients. Tumor metastasis is a multi-step process [1], including the invasion, migration and adhesion of tumor cells; immune escape; and repopulation in the second location. An increasing number of underlying molecular mechanisms that are involved in tumor metastasis progression are being revealed. Among these factors, the role of mitochondrial DNA (mtDNA) and the related mitochondrial dysfunction have attracted significant attention.

From tumorigenesis to metastasis, cancer cells depend on metabolic reprogramming to survive [2]. Warburg proposed that unlike normal cells, cancer cells do not need to rely on the oxidative phosphorylation (OXPHOS) system to generate ATP. Even under aerobic conditions, cancer cells can convert glucose into lactic acid through glycolysis and produce ATP [3]. We call this theory the Warburg effect or aerobic glycolysis, which has become a biochemical marker of cancer. The unlimited proliferation ability of cancer cells results in their craving for ATP and metabolites. Mitochondria are crucial for oxidizing glucose, fats and amino acids to release energy through the tricarboxylic acid (TCA) cycle and OXPHOS [4], which is thought to be the "energy factory" of cancer cells [5]. The transfer mitochondria from aggressively growing tumors to less aggressive tumors can cause an increase in tumor aggressiveness, indicating the critical role of mitochondria in determining the cancer cell biology [6]. With the in-depth study of the mitochondrial genome, more evidence has revealed the relationship between mtDNA abnormalities and many diseases, especially cancer. Moreover, the alterations of genes encoding mitochondrial components are associated with increased cancer risk, and may even become carcinogenic factors [7].

As the core component of mitochondrial, mtDNA encodes 13 OXPHOS-system-related protein complexes (complex I, III-V) subunits [8], which drives mitochondrial respiration and energy production [9]. Mitochondrial dysfunction has previously been reported to enhance the tumorigenicity and metastatic potential of lung and breast cancer cells [10–12]. Mutations in mtDNA (for example, insertion of the MT-ND6 gene) can disrupt the function of complex I, leading to an increase in ROS, while the corresponding tendency for metastasis is also increased [10,13]. This obstacle also leads to the upregulation of glycolysis and metastasis-related gene transcription [13]. The altered function of complex I in metastasis was subsequently reconfirmed in the MDA-MB-231 breast cancer cell line, and its increased metastatic potential appeared to be associated with mutations in MT-ND6 (C12084T) and MT-ND5 (A13966G). The missense and nonsense mutations in MT-ND6 enhanced tumor invasion and migration, as also demonstrated in the A549 lung cancer cell line [14]. Therefore, mtDNA is an important factor in tumor initiation and progression [6,15,16].

As more in-depth studies of mitochondrial-encoded factors emerge, this may lead to exciting advances in targeting mtDNA to inhibit tumor metastasis. This review summarizes the structure and function of the mitochondrial genome and the relationship between mtDNA and tumor metastasis. Our goal is to establish a framework in related fields and address the role of the mitochondrial genome in tumor metastasis.

2. mtDNA

2.1. Structures of mtDNA

The special form of deoxyribonucleic acid is mtDNA. It is the only genetic material outside the nucleus that can be copied, transcribed and translated independently [17]. Human mtDNA is a circular-shaped, double-stranded DNA measuring about 16,569 bp. The mtDNA includes a G-enriched inner light strand (L-strand) and a C-enriched heavy strand (H-strand) [9,18]. Human mtDNA is a genetically compact genome with no introns, which overlaps in some regions. It encodes 2 rRNAs (16S RNA, 12S RNA) and 22 tRNAs for protein synthesis, as well as 13 peptides for electron transfer and oxidative phosphorylation. In addition to these coding areas, mtDNA also consists of a non-coding region, the displacement (D)-loop, which participates in the regulation of mtDNA replication transcription [19] (Figure 1).

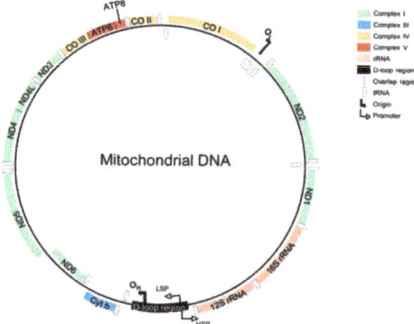

Figure 1. The structure of mtDNA. It encodes 2 rRNAs and 22 tRNAs for protein synthesis, as well as 13 peptides for electron transfer and oxidative phosphorylation. Except for these coding areas, mtDNA has a non-coding region located in the displacement (D)-loop, which participates in the regulation of mtDNA replication transcription. The genes coding for subunits of OXPHOS complex I are ND1-ND6. The gene encoding for cytochrome B of complex III is abbreviated as Cyt B. Genes for

cytochrome c oxidase (complex IV) are CO I-CO III. Additionally, the subunits of complex V are ATPase 6 and 8, abbreviated as A6 and A8, respectively. The two ribosomal RNAs encoded by mtDNA are 12S and 16S. Except for these coding areas, mtDNA has a non-coding region located in the displacement (D)-loop, which participates in the regulation of mtDNA replication transcription. The displacement loop is represented as the D-loop and contains sequences for the initiation of replication and transcription, including the origin of heavy-strand replication (O_H). The light-strand replication's origin is indicated by O_L. The position of the light-strand promoter is shown as LSP and the position of the heavy-strand promotor as HSP.

2.2. Characteristics and Maintenance of mtDNA

Almost every base of mtDNA is involved in gene construction, meaning any mutation would affect an important functional region of the genome [9]. Furthermore, mtDNA has its own unique biological environment and properties: (1) The mtDNA is vulnerable to ROS damage due to its lack of histone protection [20,21]. (2) The mtDNA has a high mutation rate [22,23], which may be due to its relatively naive protection and repair mechanisms. Currently, mtDNA damage can usually only be repaired via base excision repair (BER), homologous recombination (HR) and microhomology-mediated end joining (MMEJ) [24]. (3) Due to its small molecular mass and the absence of introns, mtDNA shows continuous synthesis throughout the cell cycle, although this is not synchronized with the cell cycle and mainly occurs in the S and G2 phases, which makes the dynamic process more susceptible to interference by external factors. (4) It has a high copy number. In many cells, the volume of mtDNA is higher than needed to maintain oxidative phosphorylation. Furthermore, the poor proofreading ability of DNA polymerase and the easy formation of a hairpin structure in the RNA transfer position results in the mtDNA replication process being more prone to mistakes. Although its replication is independent of nDNA replication, the trans-acting factors, copy number and integrity of mtDNA are closely regulated and encoded by nDNA. The nDNA-encoded polymerase g (POLG) and mitochondrial transposition factor A (TFAM) [25] are necessary to maintain the copy number and integrity of mtDNA [26–28]. Moreover, these proteins bind to the D-loop region of mtDNA, forming NUCLEOIDS, which are considered to be units of mtDNA transmission and inheritance [29]. TFAM is also the main component that initiates and drives mtDNA packaging and the NUCLEOIDS structure, and is directly proportional to the mtDNA copy number [30]. Therefore, mtDNA could bind to form complexes with TFAM rather than being naked as previously thought [29,31].

The mtDNA copy number may also have an unknown regulatory mechanism. As mitochondria divide randomly in daughter cells, there may be two conditions during cell division: homoplasmy (the same genotype) and heteroplasmy (coexistence of wild-type and mutant mitochondrial genomes) [32]. Normally, all mtDNA in a cell should be identical. In heterogeneous cells, owing to the different mitochondrial genomes in each cell, the ratio of mutants to wild-type mitochondria determines whether the cell is deficient of energy; that is, when the mutation reaches a certain ratio, an impaired phenotype occurs and lead to diseases, which is called the threshold effect [33]. The threshold level is dependent on the tissue type, metabolic requirements and copy number of remaining WT mtDNA (aberrant mitochondrial function in aging and cancer). It has also been shown that a decrease in mtDNA replication machinery or enhanced mitophagy results in a lower mtDNA copy number [34]. Meanwhile, doxorubicin (Dox)-induced mitochondrial phagocytosis in cardiomyocytes resulted in a decrease in the copy number of mitochondrial DNA [35]. This suggests that mitophagy is quite important in mtDNA copy number regulation, which needs to be demonstrated by further studies. As a multi-genome with strict control over the copy number, the regulatory mechanism of the mtDNA copy number remains unclear. It seems to be controlled by cell-specific mechanisms and regulated by various internal environmental stressors.

2.3. The Release of mtDNA

Mitochondrial dynamics play an important role in the nuclear distribution of mtDNA, cristae reorganization and the mitochondrial pro-apoptotic state [36]. The deletion of mitochondrial TFAM significantly altered the packaging and distribution of mtDNA and induced mtDNA release into the cytoplasm, which was considered to be "cytoplasmic mtDNA stress" [37]. Furthermore, studies have shown that mtDNA can be released from apoptotic mitochondria. BAX/BAK is activated during apoptosis, whereby large BAX/BAK pores appear on the outer membrane of mitochondria, while the inner membrane of mitochondria can herniate into the cytoplasm and carry mtDNA [38,39]. Mitochondrial membrane damage and mitochondrial division can also cause the release of mtDNA into the cytoplasm. When the mitochondria are subjected to stress in a variety of ways, mtDNA breaks into fragments and then binds to the voltage-dependent anion channel (VDAC) in the outer membrane of the mitochondria. This leads to the aggregation of multiple VDAC monomers and the formation of a pore in the middle through which mtDNA can escape [40]. In conclusion, changes in mitochondrial morphology and dynamics can promote the release of mtDNA. The release of mtDNA and its vulnerability to damage have been found to be involved in tumorigenesis and progression.

3. mtDNA and Tumor Metastasis

Tumor metastasis is a series of invasive and metastatic cascades in which tumor cells detonate from the original tumor to reach surrounding or distal tissues to form new lesions. It is the result of the interaction between tumor cells and the tumor microenvironment [41]. Metastasis is the main cause of death in tumor patients, with most patients dying from the spread of the cancer rather than the primary tumor [42]. The process of tumor metastasis mainly goes through five stages: (1) local detachment of tumor cells and invasion of surrounding tissues (resistance to anoikis) (anoilis: loss of cell adhesion to the ECM and lead to apoptosis); (2) intravasation, where tumor cells enter the blood or lymphatic system; (3) tumor cell transport and survival in the circulatory system; (4) exudate leakage from circulation into distal tissues; (5) colonization, to form metastatic foci. Obstruction of any of these steps would prevent metastasis (Figure 2).

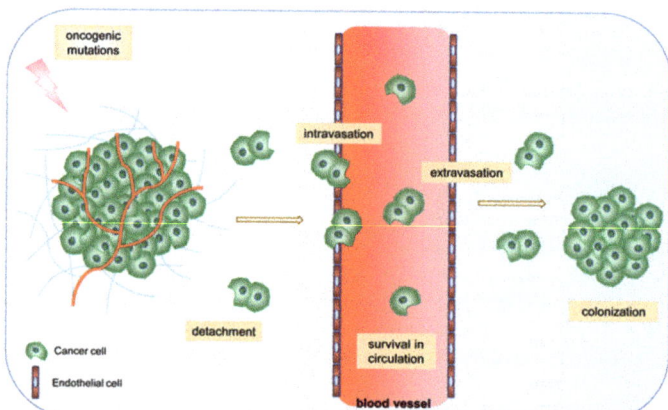

Figure 2. Steps of tumor metastasis. The process of tumor metastasis mainly goes through five stages: (1) local detachment of tumor cells and invasion of surrounding tissues (resistance to anoikis); (2) intravasation, where tumor cells enter the blood or lymphatic system; (3) tumor cell transport and survival in the circulatory system; (4) exudate leakage from circulation into distal tissues; (5) colonization, to form metastatic foci. Obstruction of any of these steps would prevent the formation of the metastasis. As early as 1889, Stephen Paget first proposed the seed and soil hypothesis, which has been widely recognized as the critical theory for tumor metastasis.

To date, there is no clear evidence of a definitive relationship between mtDNA and tumor metastasis, but some non-random changes in the mitochondrial genome associated with tumor progression have been reported in many tumor types [14,43,44]. We reviewed the literature on mtDNA alterations that cause or are associated with metastatic mutations, and there is considerable evidence that mtDNA alterations can accelerate tumor progression by enhancing the invasiveness and metastatic potential of tumor cells. Studies have supposed that replacing mtDNA from poorly metastatic tumor cells with mtDNA from highly metastatic tumor cells in mice via cytoplasmic hybrid (cybrid) technology could result in better metastatic capacity [45]. Thus, mtDNA alterations have an important role in enhancing a tumor's metastatic capacity. This was consistent with the conclusion by Amanda E. Brinker [46]. They used a novel mouse model, a mitochondrial nuclear exchange model termed MNX, to verify whether the mitochondrial genome affects the tumor incubation period and metastasis efficiency. The mitochondrial haplotype altered the tumorigenicity and metastasis of breast cancer in an oncogenic driver-dependent manner [46]. As expected, there was an inherently strong relationship between mtDNA and tumor metastasis. Here, we summarize the role played by mtDNA in the various stages of tumor metastasis.

3.1. mtDNA during Cancer Cell Anti-Anoikis

Metastasis is not caused by the random survival of cells shed by the primary tumors, but by the selective growth of specialized subsets of highly metastatic cells [47]. Metastatic cells can be generated through clonal evolution or clonal selection, and mutational genetic drivers within tumor cells confer proliferative and invasive properties [48]. Loss of cell adhesion to the ECM leads to apoptosis, called anoikis. Resistance to anoikis is a prerequisite for tumor metastasis. Deletion of mtDNA in prostate epithelial PNT1A cells was demonstrated to prevent anoikis and promote the migratory capacity of basement membrane proteins via the upregulation of p85 and p110 phosphatidylinositol 3-kinase (PI3K) subunits [49]. Inhibition of PI3K, siRNA-mediated Akt2 depletion and mtDNA reconstitution were sufficient to restore the sensitivity of tumor cells to anoikis and reduce their migration. In addition, Akt2 activation induced glucose transporter 1 (GLUT1) expression, glucose uptake and lactate production, which is a common phenotypic change in tumor cells [49]. Unlike normal cells, due to the Warburg effect, tumor cells are resistant to anoikis. Tumor cells show restricted OXPHOS and ROS before detachment [50]. Pyruvate dehydrogenase kinase (PDK) is an important mitochondrial enzyme in glucose metabolism. High expression of PDK can block OXPHOS, promote the Warburg effect [51] and mitigate excessive ROS produced by glucose oxidation. To some extent, it protects tumor cells from ROS-induced anoikis to promote metastasis [52].

In addition, cancer stem cells (CSCs) present in the primary tumor can be resistant to anoikis and have an inherent tendency to metastasize. Both clonal selection and CSCs may synergistically produce cells with metastatic ability. In breast cancer, a decrease in mtDNA can promote the production of breast cancer stem cells, thereby promoting breast cancer metastasis. Similarly, mtDNA deficiency may induce stem-cell-like properties in ovarian cancer in different ways in vitro, leading to different tumor behavior [53]. Compared to non-cancerous tissues, the mtDNA copy number was shown to be relatively reduced in lung, gastric, breast, renal cell, colorectal and prostate cancers, while mtDNA oxidative damage was increased [54–59]. A decreased mtDNA copy number was also found to be associated with metastasis to Ewing's sarcoma [60] and shorter survival in astrocytoma patients [61]. The mutations of mtDNA may be accompanied by decreased respiratory enzyme complex activity and mitochondrial dysfunction, leading to a malignant phenotype of the tumor [62]. It is interesting that the increased mtDNA copy number has also been reported to be associated with increased malignancy of tumors. The mtDNA copy number was increased in pancreatic, head and neck, esophageal and other cancers [63–65]. In these tumors, a higher mtDNA copy number indicated higher biosynthetic activity and energy activity, which was beneficial for cancer cells to achieve efficient adaption to the microenvironment. Furthermore, mitochondrial dysfunction caused by mtDNA mutations was also shown to promote the cell remodeling of cancer cells. The acquisition of mtDNA from host cells partially restored mitochondrial function in tumor cells, reestablishing the respiration to promote tumor growth. Lung metastatic tumor cells then exhibited complete restoration of respiratory function. These results indicated that the process of mtDNA transfer from host cells in the tumor microenvironment to tumor cells with impaired respiratory function overcame the pathophysiological process of mtDNA damage and supported the high plasticity of tumor cells [66].

3.2. mtDNA during Cancer Cell Intravasation or Extravasation

The rapid proliferation of tumor cells leads to tumor ischemia and hypoxia, which directly stimulates angiogenesis and promotes the secretion of cytokines such as matrix metalloproteinase-9 (MMP9), C-X-C motif chemokine ligand 12 (CXCL12) and Wnt7B by various cells, especially tumor cells. These cytokines also promote the proliferation of endothelial cells, angiogenesis and an increase in vascular permeability [67]. The neoplastic endothelial cells express high-adhesion molecules and connect to the original vascular endothelial cells, allowing continued vascular extension. In the initial stage of tumor metastasis, tumors locally infiltrate into the vascular or lymphatic system. Tumor cells can be activated by inflammatory signals and invade the matrix by secreting proteases that degrade extracellular matrix proteins. The tumor cells enter the neovascularization and then metastatic spread occurs with the extension of the vessels. Lung cancer cells carrying the 13885insC mutation of the mtDNA ND6 subunit had a higher spontaneous metastasis potential [13]. A PCR array analysis revealed a higher level of vascular endothelial growth factor (VEGF), CCL7 and other metastasis-associated genes. The increase in VEGF levels was obviously an important factor in stimulating tumor blood vessel growth. CCL7 was shown to recruit monocytes to promote tumor cell invasion, migration and infiltration by stimulating tumor angiogenesis. In primary tumors, tumor cells produced VEGF and fibroblast growth factor 1 (FGF1) to increase vascular density. Interactions with endothelial cells through VEGF and matrix metalloproteinase-1 (MMP1) signaling pathways enhanced vascular permeability, which provided favorable conditions for tumor metastasis [68]. During the process of extravasation, tumor cells could initiate metastasis by adhering to endothelial cells through various adhesion factors, while neutrophils could enhance tumor cell adhesion and transendothelial migration through the integrin–intercellular adhesion molecule-1 (ICAM-1) signaling pathway [69]. In ovarian cancer cells with a reduced mtDNA copy number, the upregulation of gene expression related to tumor metastasis and angiogenesis more powerfully confirmed the role of mtDNA in promoting tumor angiogenesis [53]. Neonatal tumor vessels provided essential oxygen and nutrients for tumor growth and metastasis. In contrast to normal vessels, tumor vessels were characterized by discontinuous pericyte coverage, an incomplete vascular matrix and high permeability [70] (Figure 3a). It has been reported that endogenous bacterial endotoxin lipopolysaccharides in sepsis can activate Gasdermin D and form mitochondrial pores to release mtDNA into the cytoplasm, which may cause the activation of the cGAS-STING pathway and suppress YAP signaling, thereby inhibiting the proliferation of endothelial cells [71]. Endothelial cells play a significant role in tumor metastasis. It is speculated that as a DAMP, mtDNA can promote tumor metastasis by inhibiting endothelial cell proliferation and mediating endothelial cell dysfunction in tumor cells.

Endothelial cells and pericytes constitute the physical barrier of tumor vessels, but some pericytes could be activated or undergo pericyte fibroblast transformation, leading to the loss of barrier function to promote tumor metastasis [72]. This makes the tumor vessels more susceptible to leakage, allowing tumor cells to colonize and metastasize directly into the vessels without going through a complex invasive process. However, it is interesting to note that in diabetic patients, palmitic acid (PA) treatment can induce damage to endothelial cells to release mtDNA and activate the cGAS-STING-IRF3 pathway in the cytoplasm, leading to upregulation of macrophage stimulating 1 (MST1), inactivation of

Yes-associated protein (YAP) and inhibition of angiogenesis [73]. This is contrary to the situation in tumors, and the specific reasons still need to be further explored.

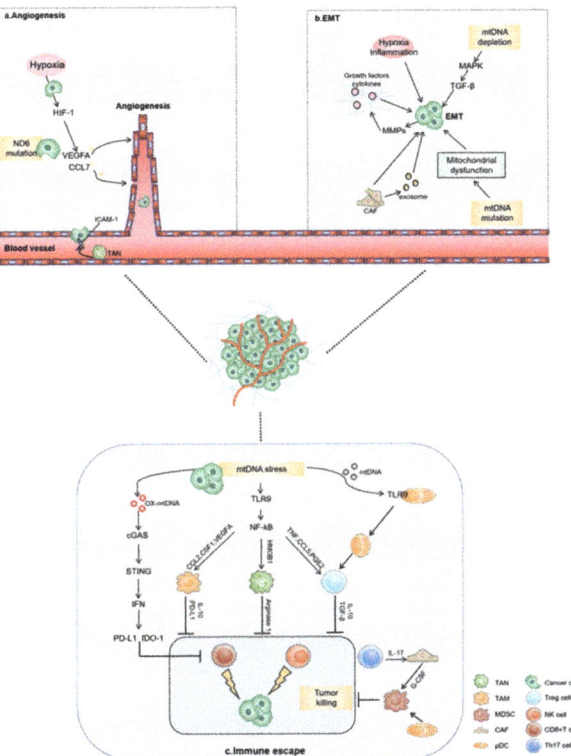

Figure 3. The association between mtDNA and tumor metastasis. (**a**) Angiogenesis is a rate-limiting factor in tumor growth. Cancer cells carrying the 13885insC mutation of the ND6 subunit have higher spontaneous metastasis potential. A PCR array analysis showed higher levels of VEGF, CCL7 and other metastasis-associated genes. The increase in VEGF and CCL7 levels is obviously an important factor in stimulating tumor blood vessel growth to promote tumor cell invasion, migration and infiltration. (**b**) EMT is a process in which the epithelial tumor cells lose adhesion ability and cause the migration of mesenchymal cells to promote metastasis and drug resistance. The mtDNA depletion can lead to a loss of characteristic epithelial cell features and to a mesenchymal phenotype being gained. The RAF/MAPK signaling pathway is highly activated and accompanied by the expression of TGF-β. The above suggest that the tumor cells acquire higher invasiveness. The mutations of mtDNA may be accompanied by decreased respiratory enzyme complex activity and mitochondrial dysfunction, which leads to the malignant phenotype of the tumor. (**c**) Tumor immune escape is a critical step in tumor metastasis and malignant progression. Oxidized mtDNA can be released into the cytoplasm, which induces IFN signals through cGAS-STING-TBK1, thereby upregulating the expression of PD-L1 and IDO-1 to inhibit the activation of T cells. It has been reported that mtDNA stress in HCC cells with increased mitochondrial division significantly increases CCL2 production by activating the TLR9-mediated NF-κB signaling pathway, thereby promoting TAM recruitment and polarization and consequently promoting tumor progression. Mitochondrial DAMP (including mtDNA) can activate neutrophils to generate NETs, which have been shown to promote cancer-related formation and are associated with accelerated metastasis. Immature pDC can recognize the CpG sequence on mtDNA through TLR9, and can induce the production of CD4$^+$CD25$^+$Treg cells after activation and maturation. Treg cells secrete cytokines IL10 and TGF-β, which produce powerful immunosuppressive functions.

In addition to affecting the tumor vasculature, mtDNA has been significantly associated with the epithelial–mesenchymal transition (EMT) process in tumor cells. EMT is a process in which the epithelial tumor cells lose their adhesion ability and cause the migration of mesenchymal cells to promote metastasis and drug resistance [74]. Tumor cells could activate the EMT process, undergoing significant cytoskeleton reconstruction and phenotypic changes. Tumor cells transform into the mesenchymal state, then secrete various extracellular matrix-degrading enzymes to promote their infiltration into blood vessels and lymphatic vessels [75]. Depletion of mtDNA has led to the loss of epithelial cell features and a mesenchymal phenotype being gained [76]. For example, in human prostate cancer cells (LNCaP) and breast cancer cells (MCF-7), deletion of mtDNA led to the activation of the RAF/MAPK signaling pathway. This process was also accompanied by the expression of transforming growth factor-beta (TGF-β) and type I TGF-beta receptor (TGF-βRI) [77]. All of these indications suggested that the tumor cells had acquired higher invasiveness [77]. Similarly, in breast cancer, a reduced mtDNA content in human mammary epithelial cells (HMECs) activated calcineurin-dependent mitochondrial retrograde signaling pathways that induced EMT-like reprogramming [78]. The TGF-β-EMT signal was activated in single breast tumor motile cells during this period, and was transferred to distal organs through hematogenous spread [79]. It is also noteworthy that the reduction in mtDNA also promoted the generation of breast cancer stem cells. Both these changes could promote the development of metastatic breast cancer [78]. On the contrary, the relatively high copy number of mtDNA was associated with low protein expression of E-cadherin and high expression of Vimentin in TE1 esophageal squamous cell carcinoma (ESCC) cells. The high mtDNA copy number appeared to contribute to the high bioenergetic function of mitochondria and provided favorable conditions for the invasion of esophageal cancer [80]. In colorectal cancer cells (SW620), the high expression of TFAM and mtDNA encoded ND6 and cytochrome c oxidase subunit II (COX-II), together with the high expression levels of the EMT markers N-cadherin and Vimentin, which may confer an advantage for the migration and invasion in CRCs [62]. EMT could be regulated by various signaling pathways, including TGF, HIF, Snail and Notch pathways [81]. It has been shown that TGF-β could convert mouse mammary epithelial NMUMG cells into an invasive fibroblastoid phenotype [82]. Subsequently, TGF-β has been proven to induce EMT in varieties cell lines, meaning it is considered to be a major EMT inducer. The inhibition of the TGF-β pathway in mesenchymal mouse colon carcinoma CT26 cell lines reduced invasion and metastatic formation in xenograft tumors [83]. The same phenomenon of EMT gene signal activation was be verified in diseases other than cancer. Aldosterone reduced the expression of PGC-1α to increase its acetylation and injure the mtDNA. It induced mitochondrial dysfunction and EMT to promote renal tubulointerstitial fibrosis [84] (Figure 3b). This also provided us with a new direction to prevent the metastasis of tumor cells through EMT.

3.3. mtDNA during Cancer Cell Survival in the Circulatory System

Tumor cells are shed from tumor tissue into the circulatory system for distant metastasis, but most of the scattered cells are not viable [85,86]. Disseminated cells are placed under extreme stress (from the immune system, ROS, hypoxia, hypotrophy and matrix changes), which greatly increases the pressure on their survival from one organ to another [6]. Studies have reported that the increased antioxidant capacity of tumor cells helps them survive after they shed from the tumor. In lung cancer mouse models, antioxidants can reduce oxidative stress and promote tumor progression [87]. Mutations in the mtDNA ATP synthase subunit 6 gene (MTATP6) can mediate resistance to apoptosis and promote survival in tumor cells [88]. When tumor cells were subjected to external stress or attack, mitochondrial released mtDNA to initiate their own protection programs to face the threats. At this point, a group of genes known as interferon stimulated gene (ISGs) came into play to protect their own nDNA, which was also the reason for the chemotherapy resistance of melanoma [37]. The mtDNA could also affect the level of p-glycoprotein (P-gp) and anti-apoptotic molecules such as Bcl-2, while P-gp is known to play an important role in mediating multi-drug resistance (MDR) in tumors [89,90]. Various evidence has indicated that aberrant mtDNA greatly enhanced the ability of tumor cells to cope with different threats, ensuring their survival in harsh environments and promoting metastasis. Hypoxia is widespread in tumor tissues [91], and overcoming hypoxic conditions is very important for tumor cell survival and metastasis [92]. Under hypoxic conditions, HMGB1 could mediate the binding of mtDNA and TLR9, thereby activating the protumorigenic signaling pathways to promote the growth and metastasis of hepatocellular carcinoma cells (HCC) [92]. In cancer cells with mutation in the mtDNA ND6 subunit G13997A, the expression of HIF1-α and MCL-1 was increased [19,93]. HIF1-α is one of the main regulators that adapt to hypoxia, and MCL-1 is an anti-apoptotic factor under hypoxia. Therefore, the high expression of these genes enabled tumor cells to survive under harsh conditions and effectively induce metastasis [94]. HIF-1 also regulates lactate dehydrogenase (LDH), monocarboxylate transporter (MCT) and other glycolytic enzymes, which is conducive to glycolytic conversion [95,96]. Furthermore, it can upregulate PDK, an inhibitor of pyruvate dehydrogenase (PDH), to inhibit the oxidative metabolism and promote metastasis [97]. Once tumor cells enter the circulatory system they became circulating tumor cells (CTCs), and they have to alter their metabolism in response to changes in environmental stress, especially hemodynamic shear stresses [98]. For example, compared to primary tumor cells, CTCs from breast cancer were mainly dependent on OXPHOS and increased ATP production. The transcriptional coactivator PGC-1α may play an important role in this. Overexpression of PGC-1α could promote the mitochondrial OXPHOS and enhance the invasion ability of breast cancer cells [99]. Some experiments have designed a variety of heterogeneous m.8993 T > G mutations in the mitochondrial gene MT-ATP6, which is called mTUNE line [100,101]. It has been shown that high levels of heterogeneity caused mTUNE cells to undergo glycolysis and metabolic conversion, while low levels of heterogeneity did not occur [102], suggesting that high heterogeneity levels of mtDNA mutations can promote tumor growth and metastasis.

During the various steps of metastasis, tumor cells are exposed to the immune system and recognized and killed by immune cells. However, tumors and their metastatic derivatives have developed strategies to overcome immune mechanisms. Tumor cells are able to induce the body to generate immunosuppressive cells and humoral suppressive factors, and are able to reprogram tumor-infiltrating immune cells to differentiate into immunosuppressive cells during metastasis [103]. CTCs can secrete LDH5 and cause ADAM10-mediated shedding of NKG2D ligand MICA/MICB, which prevents the identification and elimination of cells by NK-cell-mediated lysis [104]. Otherwise the immunosuppressive cells suppress the function of CD8$^+$ T cells and NK cells by secreting cytokines such as EGF, TNF-α, CXCL12, IL-10 and IL-6, thereby ensuring the survival of tumor cells [105]. Previously, mtDNA was thought to affect inflammation and immune responses. It can activate the cGAS-STING pathway, triggering the innate immune system and eliciting the type I IFN response [38,39]. We generally assume that the activation of SING should enhance the anti-tumor immunity of the body. However, advanced tumor necrosis was found to release DAMP, while mitochondrial DAMP (including mtDNA) could activate neutrophils to generate neutrophilic extracellular traps (NETs) [106], which have been shown to promote cancer-related formation and are associated with accelerated metastasis [107]. The depletion of CD8$^+$ T cells and NK cells could increase tumor metastasis without affecting the progression of the primary tumor [108]. CD8$^+$ T cells restrict the metastatic growth of cancer cells from the primary tumor; when MERTK, a tyrosine kinase receptor that inhibits NK cells activation, is inhibited, NK cells have the ability to reject metastatic tumor cells [109,110]. Mitochondrial Lon protease (LON) is a chaperone and DNA-binding protein. When LON is overexpressed in oral cancer, oxidized mtDNA is released into the cytoplasm, which then induces interferon (IFN) signals through cGAS-STING-TBK1. This upregulates the expression of programmed cell death ligand 1 (PD-L1) and indoleamine2,3-dioxygenase1 (IDO-1), which inhibits the activation of T cells [111].

3.4. mtDNA in Cancer Cell Colonization

Tumor cells produce a variety of soluble factors that can induce the formation of a non-maturing pre-metastatic tumor microenvironment at new organ tissue sites or non-in situ tumor sites in the same organ. Micrometastasis foci are formed when tumor cells arrive and colonize in the pre-metastatic microenvironment. With the exception of tumor cells, various cell types mix in the tumor microenvironment, such as fibroblasts, adipocytes, endothelial cells and myocytes. In prostate cancer, mtDNA mutations in potentially bone-metastatic cells may preferentially alter the bone and bone matrix microenvironment. These mtDNA mutations increase the secretion and expression of fibroblast growth factor 1 (FGF-1) and focal adhesion kinase (FAK) to promote prostate cancer bone metastasis [112]. Tumor cells could recruit immunosuppressive cells such as myeloid-derived suppressor cells (MDSCs), tumor-associated macrophages (TAMs), regulatory T cells (Tregs), T helper 17 cells (Th17) and tumor-associated neutrophils (TANs) to the primary and secondary tumor sites, creating an immunosuppressive microenvironment. It has been reported that mtDNA stress in HCC cells with increased mitochondrial division significantly induced the increase in CCL2 production by activating the TLR9-mediated NF-κB signaling pathway. CCL2 could promote the recruitment and polarization of TAMs, consequently advancing the progression of HCC [113]. By secreting cytokines to promote the recruitment and polarization of TAM, HCC cells can induce the formation of the immunosuppressive microenvironment and promote tumor cell metastasis and colonization [114]. Analogously, IL-1β induced IL17 expression in γδ T cells, leading to systemic granulocyte colony-stimulating factor (G-CSF)-dependent expansion and neutrophil polarization, inhibiting the function of $CD8^+$ T cells and promoting tumor metastasis. In addition to recruiting immunosuppressive cells, tumors can also regulate the function of immunosuppressive cells to enhance metastasis [115]. For instance, tumor-derived factors such as galectin-1 can promote systemic immunosuppression by regulating the clonal expansion and function of Treg, thereby enhancing breast cancer metastasis [116]. Additionally, tumor-infiltrating plasmacytoid dendritic cells (pDCs) could increase MDSCs and Tregs in transplanted breast cancer tissues and reduce the cytotoxicity of $CD8^+$ T cells to promote tumor bone metastasis [117] (Figure 3c). Immature pDC recognized the CpG sequence on mtDNA through TLR9 [118], and then induced the generation of $CD4^+CD25^+$Treg cells after activation and maturation. Treg cells secrete cytokines IL10 and TGF-β, which produce powerful immunosuppressive functions. We inferred that mtDNA exerts an immunosuppressive effect by enabling pDC maturation. Inhibition of cytosolic DNA sensing is a strategy that tumor cells use for immune evasion [119]. The mtDNA induced by myocardial infarction could inhibit the secretion of IL-6 and TNF-α in granulocytes, which may account for the patients' susceptibility to infection after injury or myocardial infarction [120]. The equal reaction may also occur in tumor patients. The mtDNA reduced the secretion of cytokines such as IL-6, decreasing the body's anti-tumor immune capacity and promoting the progress of the tumor. Furthermore, fascin, a type of actin, promotes metastatic colonization in lung cancer by enhancing metabolic stress resistance and mitochondrial OXPHOS. Fascin was directly recruited to mitochondria in response to metabolic stress to stabilize mitochondrial actin filaments (mtF-actin). Mechanistically, Fascin and mtF-actin controlled the balance of mtDNA to promote mitochondrial OXPHOS. The results suggested that the dysregulated actin cytoskeleton in metastatic lung cancer could be targeted to realign mitochondrial metabolism and prevent metastatic recurrence [121].

4. Future Prospects

4.1. mtDNA as a Potential Indicator for Cancer Diagnosis

Furthermore, mtDNA affects the occurrence and progression of tumor. Large-scale data from the International Cancer Genome Consortium (ICGC) and the Cancer Genome Atlas (TCGA) have confirmed that approximately 60% of solid tumors have at least one mtDNA mutation [122–124]. Additionally, mtDNA is connected with the mitochondrial inner membrane, which is rich in lipids, and the relatively high ratio of fat to DNA in the mitochondria makes mtDNA extremely sensitive to liposoluble substances. As a result, lipophilic carcinogens often tend to choose mtDNA as their primary site for binding and attack. Compared to nDNA, carcinogens prefer mtDNA, causing mtDNA mutations [125]. Endogenous damage factors such as oxygen free radicals produced by tumor cells can easily attack mtDNA. Additionally, mtDNA is susceptible to mutation after being attacked, which in turn disturbs the respiratory chain and affects the normal mitochondrial oxidative phosphorylation system and metabolic reprogramming [10,13]. Furthermore, mtDNA mutations lead to respiratory chain disorders that can increase the level of ROS, which in turn generate new mtDNA mutations, forming a vicious cycle. When mtDNA mutations accumulate to a certain extent, they can trigger cancer and promote its metastasis and other malignant processes. Additionally, one of the pathogenesis mechanisms of cancer is the inhibition of cell apoptosis. Mitochondria can regulate cell apoptosis well, whereas mtDNA mutations can lead to mitochondrial dysfunction. Therefore, this can inhibit cell apoptosis to accelerate the formation of cancer. Furthermore, mtDNA mutations are considered to be an early event of tumorigenesis. In addition to mtDNA mutations, alterations in copy number, transcription and expression levels of mtDNA may also be important causes of cancer occurrence and metastasis. The alterations in the amount of mtDNA in tumor cells may be associated with a loss of mtDNA replication ability. The amounts of mtDNA vary in different tumors, and even at different stages of the same tumor. In breast cancer, mtDNA decreased during stage 0-II and increased during stage II-IV, suggesting that mtDNA can be used as an indicator for breast cancer risk assessment [126]. Some studies have found that changes in mtDNA can be used as an indicator to assess tumor aggressiveness, and mtDNA plays a unique role in the treatment of a variety of cancers [127]. Recently, some researchers have analyzed the mtDNA defects in triple-negative breast cancer (TNBC) and divided TNBC into different invasive subgroups [128]. Based on the differences in mtDNA in patient tumor cells, the risk of the patient could be better evaluated, thereby providing more appropriate treatment options for the patient [128]. When exposed to physical or biochemical damage, mitochondrial dynamics are changed, followed by the release of mtDNA, which randomly integrate with nDNA through the nuclear membrane. Accordingly, the stability of the nuclear genome and cellular energy metabolism is altered, causing malignant transformation of cells. Although there was not enough evidence to show a direct link between mtDNA and tumorigenesis or metastasis, all of the indications suggested that mtDNA is at least involved in the mechanism of tumorigenesis and development, and that it may be a potential indicator for early diagnosis of cancer, or even a marker for cancer metastasis; this still needs to be further explored. If we can summarize the characteristics of mtDNA mutation between tumorigenesis and metastasis, this may provide a great direction for the early diagnosis of cancer and the prediction of tumor aggressiveness.

4.2. mtDNA as a Therapeutic Target for Cancer

Surgery, radiotherapy and chemotherapy have always been referred to as the three major traditional treatments for cancer, although targeted molecular therapy is not a new term. The role of mtDNA in inflammation and innate immunity means it can influence the sensitivity of tumor cells to radiotherapy and chemotherapy. Changes in mtDNA itself may also lead to malignant changes in cells. HeLa cells in cervical cancer showed increased radiosensitivity after mtDNA deletion [129], while most of other cancer cells (e.g., lung cancer A549 cell) showed significant radioresistance after mtDNA deletion. Apoptosis is considered to be one of the major forms of radiotherapy, while cell lines lacking mtDNA have shown greater resistance to apoptosis, mediating their radioresistance. Nevertheless, the increased radiosensitivity of the HeLa cell line with mtDNA deletion may be due to its infection by human papillomavirus and subsequently the inactivated p53 gene [130]. Ionizing radiation could upregulate the mRNA and protein expression of TFAM, while inhibition of TFAM could increase the radiation sensitivity of tumor cells. Similarly, mtDNA has also been found to affect the sensitivity of tumor cells to chemotherapy. In prostate cancer, the chemotherapeutic drug BMD188 (a fatty-acid-containing hydroxamic acid) was also effective against multi-drug-resistant cancer cells, but its action was dependent on the mitochondrial respiratory chain to induce apoptosis, whereas tumor cells with defective mtDNA demonstrated significant resistance to BMD188 [131]. In MDA-MB-231 cells with mtDNA deletion, the amount and volume of mitochondria increased, the mitochondrial cristae showed air-like changes (vacuolation) and the sensitivity to chemotherapy drugs was decreased. NADH dehydrogenase subunit 4 (MT-ND4) mutations made cells resistant to paclitaxel carboplatin therapy [132]. Both radiotherapy and chemotherapy can disrupt the mitochondrial structure, leading to mutations or the release of mtDNA. This could affect the level of ROS and adjust the tolerance of cells to radiotherapy and chemotherapy. Using mtDNA as the therapeutic target to sensitize radiotherapy and chemotherapy or reverse the malignant transformation of tumors and inhibit tumor metastasis may be a new avenue for clinical treatment.

5. Conclusions

Tumor cells exhibit genetic instability and are prone to mutations, deletions and translocations. Extensive research has been conducted on changes in the nDNA of tumor cells, while the exploration of mtDNA changes has only been noticed in recent years. Although there is much evidence that mtDNA plays an important role in cancer, there is still much debate about mtDNA's role in tumors. It is not yet clear whether it acts as a promoter, a bystander, a terminator or an accomplice in tumor progression. Furthermore, mtDNA may be able to affect different signal transduction mechanisms and changes in energy metabolism, and the production of ROS is involved in tumor development and progression. However, the specific role of mtDNA in cancer has not been discovered, and there are many complex links between mtDNA and cancer and its treatment. As an important organelle, mitochondrial participates in a variety of important physiological functions, such as energy generation and signal exchange. Additionally, mtDNA, the mitochondrial genome, plays a regulatory role in inter-mitochondrial, intra-cellular and inter-cellular communication. Due to the complexity and redundancy of the mitochondrial genome, it still needs to be further explored. In this review, we summarized the role of mtDNA in tumor metastasis and proposed certain directions for mtDNA research. With the deepening understanding of mtDNA, its mtDNA is becoming more promising. It is expected to be used as a cancer detection index and therapeutic target to improve the prognosis and treatment of patients.

Author Contributions: Q.W. wrote the manuscript and prepared the figures of the manuscript. H.-i.T. revised the manuscript. H.Z. and D.W. finalized the manuscript together. All authors have read and agreed to the published version of the manuscript.

Funding: This research was funded by National Natural Science Foundation of China (grant numbers 82071984), the Social Development Foundation of Jiangsu Province (grant numbers BK20191223), Young Medical Talents of Jiangsu (grant numbers QNRC2016833), Six Talent Peals project of Jiangsu Province (grant numbers WSW-039), Six for One Project of Jiangsu Province (grant numbers LGY201809 and the Social Development Foundation of Zhenjiang City (grant numbers SH2020031).

Conflicts of Interest: The authors declare no conflict of interests.

Abbreviations

BER	Base excision repair
CSCs	Cancer stem cells
CTCs	Circulating tumor cells
CXCL 12	C-X-C motif chemokine ligand 12
Cybrid	Cytoplasmic hybrid
ESCC	Esophageal squamous cell carcinoma
FAK	Focal adhesion kinase

FGF-1	Fibroblast growth factor 1
G-CSF	Granulocyte-colony-stimulating factor
GLUT 1	Glucose transporter 1
HCC	Hepatocellular carcinoma cells
HR	Homologous recombination
ICAM-1	Integrin/intercellular adhesion molecule-1
IDO-1	Indoleamine2,3-dioxygenase1
ISGs	Interferon-stimulated gene
LDH	Lactate dehydrogenase
MCT	Monocarboxylate transporter
MDR	Multidrug resistance
MMEJ	Microhomology-mediated end joining
MMP 9	Matrix metalloproteinase-9
MST 1	Macrophage-stimulating 1
mtDNA	Mitochondrial DNA
NETs	Neutrophilic extracellular traps
OXPHOS	Oxidative phosphorylation
PA	Palmitic acid
PDK	Pyruvate dehydrogenase kinase
PD-L1	Programmed cell death ligand 1
PI3K	Phosphatidylinositol 3-kinase
POLG	Polymerase g
TAMs	Tumor-associated macrophage
TANs	Tumor-associated neutrophils
Tregs	Regulatory T cells
TCA	Tricarboxylic acid
TFAM	Transposition factor A
TGF-β	Transforming growth factor-beta
VDAC	Voltage-dependent anion channel
VEGF	Vascular endothelial growth factor
YAP	Yes-associated protein

References

1. Yuzhalin, A.; Lim, S.; Kutikhin, A.; Gordon-Weeks, A. Dynamic matrisome: ECM remodeling factors licensing cancer progression and metastasis. *Biochim. Biophys. Acta Rev. Cancer* **2018**, *1870*, 207–228. [CrossRef] [PubMed]
2. Martínez-Reyes, I.; Chandel, N. Cancer metabolism: Looking forward. *Nat. Rev. Cancer* **2021**, *21*, 669–680. [CrossRef] [PubMed]
3. Warburg, O.; Wind, F.; Negelein, E. The Metabolism of Tumors in the Body. *J. Gen. Physiol* **1927**, *8*, 519–530. [CrossRef] [PubMed]
4. Nagase, H.; Watanabe, T.; Koshikawa, N.; Yamamoto, S.; Takenaga, K.; Lin, J. Mitochondria: Endosymbiont bacteria DNA sequence as a target against cancer. *Cancer Sci.* **2021**, *112*, 4834–4843. [CrossRef]
5. Wallace, D. Mitochondrial genetic medicine. *Nat. Genet.* **2018**, *50*, 1642–1649. [CrossRef]
6. Scheid, A.D.; Beadnell, T.C.; Welch, D.R. Roles of mitochondria in the hallmarks of metastasis. *Br. J. Cancer* **2021**, *124*, 124–135. [CrossRef] [PubMed]
7. Gammage, P.A.; Frezza, C. Mitochondrial DNA: The overlooked oncogenome? *BMC Biol.* **2019**, *17*, 1–10. [CrossRef]
8. Carew, J.; Zhou, Y.; Albitar, M.; Carew, J.; Keating, M.; Huang, P. Mitochondrial DNA mutations in primary leukemia cells after chemotherapy: Clinical significance and therapeutic implications. *Leukemia* **2003**, *17*, 1437–1447. [CrossRef]
9. Anderson, S.; Bankier, A.T.; Barrell, B.G.; de Bruijn, M.H.; Coulson, A.R.; Drouin, J.; Eperon, I.C.; Nierlich, D.P.; Roe, B.A.; Sanger, F.; et al. Sequence and organization of the human mitochondrial genome. *Nature* **1981**, *290*, 457–465. [CrossRef]
10. Ishikawa, K.; Takenaga, K.; Akimoto, M.; Koshikawa, N.; Yamaguchi, A.; Imanishi, H.; Nakada, K.; Honma, Y.; Hayashi, J. ROS-generating mitochondrial DNA mutations can regulate tumor cell metastasis. *Science* **2008**, *320*, 661–664. [CrossRef] [PubMed]
11. Ishikawa, K.; Hayashi, J. A novel function of mtDNA: Its involvement in metastasis. *Ann. N. Y. Acad. Sci.* **2010**, *1201*, 40–43. [CrossRef] [PubMed]
12. Imanishi, H.; Hattori, K.; Wada, R.; Ishikawa, K.; Fukuda, S.; Takenaga, K.; Nakada, K.; Hayashi, J. Mitochondrial DNA mutations regulate metastasis of human breast cancer cells. *PLoS ONE* **2011**, *6*, e23401. [CrossRef] [PubMed]
13. Koshikawa, N.; Akimoto, M.; Hayashi, J.; Nagase, H.; Takenaga, K. Association of predicted pathogenic mutations in mitochondrial ND genes with distant metastasis in NSCLC and colon cancer. *Sci. Rep.* **2017**, *7*, 1–11. [CrossRef] [PubMed]
14. Yuan, Y.; Wang, W.; Li, H.; Yu, Y.; Tao, J.; Huang, S.; Zeng, Z. Nonsense and missense mutation of mitochondrial ND6 gene promotes cell migration and invasion in human lung adenocarcinoma. *BMC Cancer* **2015**, *15*, 1–10. [CrossRef]

15. Zimmermann, F.; Mayr, J.; Neureiter, D.; Feichtinger, R.; Alinger, B.; Jones, N.; Eder, W.; Sperl, W.; Kofler, B. Lack of complex I is associated with oncocytic thyroid tumours. *Br. J. Cancer* **2009**, *100*, 1434–1437. [CrossRef] [PubMed]
16. Pereira, L.; Soares, P.; Máximo, V.; Samuels, D. Somatic mitochondrial DNA mutations in cancer escape purifying selection and high pathogenicity mutations lead to the oncocytic phenotype: Pathogenicity analysis of reported somatic mtDNA mutations in tumors. *BMC Cancer* **2012**, *12*, 1–10. [CrossRef] [PubMed]
17. Nissanka, N.; Moraes, C. Mitochondrial DNA heteroplasmy in disease and targeted nuclease-based therapeutic approaches. *EMBO Rep.* **2020**, *21*, e49612. [CrossRef]
18. Berglund, A.; Navarrete, C.; Engqvist, M.; Hoberg, E.; Szilagyi, Z.; Taylor, R.; Gustafsson, C.; Falkenberg, M.; Clausen, A. Nucleotide pools dictate the identity and frequency of ribonucleotide incorporation in mitochondrial DNA. *PLoS Genet.* **2017**, *13*, e1006628. [CrossRef] [PubMed]
19. Wallace, D. Mitochondrial diseases in man and mouse. *Science* **1999**, *283*, 1482–1488. [CrossRef]
20. Kornberg, R.D. Chromatin structure: A repeating unit of histones and DNA. *Science* **1974**, *184*, 868–871. [CrossRef] [PubMed]
21. Yakes, F.M.; Van Houten, B. Mitochondrial DNA damage is more extensive and persists longer than nuclear DNA damage in human cells following oxidative stress. *Proc. Natl Acad. Sci. USA* **1997**, *94*, 514–519. [CrossRef] [PubMed]
22. Lynch, M.; Koskella, B.; Schaack, S. Mutation pressure and the evolution of organelle genomic architecture. *Science* **2006**, *311*, 1727–1730. [CrossRef] [PubMed]
23. Johnson, A.A.; Johnson, K.A. Exonuclease proofreading by human mitochondrial DNA polymerase. *J. Biol. Chem.* **2001**, *276*, 38097–38107. [CrossRef]
24. Allkanjari, K.; Baldock, R. Beyond base excision repair: An evolving picture of mitochondrial DNA repair. *Biosci. Rep.* **2021**, *41*. [CrossRef] [PubMed]
25. Young, M.J.; Copeland, W.C. Human mitochondrial DNA replication machinery and disease. *Curr. Opin. Genet. Dev.* **2016**, *38*, 52–62. [CrossRef] [PubMed]
26. Naviaux, R.K.; Nguyen, K.V. POLG mutations associated with Alpers' syndrome and mitochondrial DNA depletion. *Ann. Neurol.* **2004**, *55*, 706–712. [CrossRef] [PubMed]
27. Ekstrand, M.I.; Falkenberg, M.; Rantanen, A.; Park, C.B.; Gaspari, M.; Hultenby, K.; Rustin, P.; Gustafsson, C.M.; Larsson, N.G. Mitochondrial transcription factor A regulates mtDNA copy number in mammals. *Hum. Mol. Genet.* **2004**, *13*, 935–944. [CrossRef] [PubMed]
28. Guo, J.; Zheng, L.; Liu, W.; Wang, X.; Wang, Z.; Wang, Z.; French, A.J.; Kang, D.; Chen, L.; Thibodeau, S.N.; et al. Frequent truncating mutation of TFAM induces mitochondrial DNA depletion and apoptotic resistance in microsatellite-unstable colorectal cancer. *Cancer Res.* **2011**, *71*, 2978–2987. [CrossRef]
29. Bonawitz, N.D.; Clayton, D.A.; Shadel, G.S. Initiation and beyond: Multiple functions of the human mitochondrial transcription machinery. *Mol. Cell* **2006**, *24*, 813–825. [CrossRef]
30. Stiles, A.R.; Simon, M.T.; Stover, A.; Eftekharian, S.; Khanlou, N.; Wang, H.L.; Magaki, S.; Lee, H.; Partynski, K.; Dorrani, N.; et al. Mutations in TFAM, encoding mitochondrial transcription factor A, cause neonatal liver failure associated with mtDNA depletion. *Mol. Genet. Metab.* **2016**, *119*, 91–99. [CrossRef]
31. Parisi, M.A.; Clayton, D.A. Similarity of human mitochondrial transcription factor 1 to high mobility group proteins. *Science* **1991**, *252*, 965–969. [CrossRef] [PubMed]
32. Taylor, R.W.; Turnbull, D.M. Mitochondrial DNA mutations in human disease. *Nat. Rev. Genet.* **2005**, *6*, 389–402. [CrossRef] [PubMed]
33. Rossignol, R.; Faustin, B.; Rocher, C.; Malgat, M.; Mazat, J.P.; Letellier, T. Mitochondrial threshold effects. *Biochem. J.* **2003**, *370*, 751–762. [CrossRef] [PubMed]
34. Špaček, T.; Pavluch, V.; Alán, L.; Capková, N.; Engstová, H.; Dlasková, A.; Berková, Z.; Saudek, F.; Ježek, P. Nkx6.1 decline accompanies mitochondrial DNA reduction but subtle nucleoid size decrease in pancreatic islet β-cells of diabetic Goto Kakizaki rats. *Sci. Rep.* **2017**, *7*, 1–15. [CrossRef] [PubMed]
35. Yin, J.; Guo, J.; Zhang, Q.; Cui, L.; Zhang, L.; Zhang, T.; Zhao, J.; Li, J.; Middleton, A.; Carmichael, P.; et al. Doxorubicin-induced mitophagy and mitochondrial damage is associated with dysregulation of the PINK1/parkin pathway. *Toxicol. Vitr.* **2018**, *51*, 1–10. [CrossRef] [PubMed]
36. Guerrero-Castillo, S.; van Strien, J.; Brandt, U.; Arnold, S. Ablation of mitochondrial DNA results in widespread remodeling of the mitochondrial complexome. *EMBO J.* **2021**, *40*, e108648. [CrossRef]
37. West, A.P.; Khoury-Hanold, W.; Staron, M.; Tal, M.C.; Pineda, C.M.; Lang, S.M.; Bestwick, M.; Duguay, B.A.; Raimundo, N.; MacDuff, D.A.; et al. Mitochondrial DNA stress primes the antiviral innate immune response. *Nature* **2015**, *520*, 553–557. [CrossRef]
38. Rongvaux, A.; Jackson, R.; Harman, C.C.; Li, T.; West, A.P.; de Zoete, M.R.; Wu, Y.; Yordy, B.; Lakhani, S.A.; Kuan, C.-Y.; et al. Apoptotic caspases prevent the induction of type I interferons by mitochondrial DNA. *Cell* **2014**, *159*, 1563–1577. [CrossRef]
39. White, M.J.; McArthur, K.; Metcalf, D.; Lane, R.M.; Cambier, J.C.; Herold, M.J.; van Delft, M.F.; Bedoui, S.; Lessene, G.; Ritchie, M.E.; et al. Apoptotic caspases suppress mtDNA-induced STING-mediated type I IFN production. *Cell* **2014**, *159*, 1549–1562. [CrossRef]

40. McArthur, K.; Whitehead, L.W.; Heddleston, J.M.; Li, L.; Padman, B.S.; Oorschot, V.; Geoghegan, N.D.; Chappaz, S.; Davidson, S.; San Chin, H.; et al. BAK/BAX macropores facilitate mitochondrial herniation and mtDNA efflux during apoptosis. *Science* **2018**, *359*, eaao6047. [CrossRef]
41. Aziz, M.; Agarwal, K.; Dasari, S.; Mitra, A. Productive Cross-Talk with the Microenvironment: A Critical Step in Ovarian Cancer Metastasis. *Cancers* **2019**, *11*, 1608. [CrossRef] [PubMed]
42. Al-Hajj, M.; Wicha, M.; Benito-Hernandez, A.; Morrison, S.; Clarke, M. Prospective identification of tumorigenic breast cancer cells. *Proc. Natl. Acad. Sci. USA* **2003**, *100*, 3983–3988. [CrossRef] [PubMed]
43. Gill, J.; Piskounova, E.; Morrison, S. Cancer, Oxidative Stress, and Metastasis. *Cold Spring Harb. Symp. Quant. Biol.* **2016**, *81*, 163–175. [CrossRef]
44. Kenny, T.; Germain, D. mtDNA, Metastasis, and the Mitochondrial Unfolded Protein Response (UPR). *Front. Cell Dev. Biol.* **2017**, *5*, 37. [CrossRef]
45. Petros, J.A.; Baumann, A.K.; Ruiz-Pesini, E.; Amin, M.B.; Sun, C.Q.; Hall, J.; Lim, S.; Issa, M.M.; Flanders, W.D.; Hosseini, S.H.; et al. mtDNA mutations increase tumorigenicity in prostate cancer. *Proc. Natl. Acad. Sci. USA* **2005**, *102*, 719–724. [CrossRef]
46. Brinker, A.; Vivian, C.; Koestler, D.; Tsue, T.; Jensen, R.; Welch, D. Mitochondrial Haplotype Alters Mammary Cancer Tumorigenicity and Metastasis in an Oncogenic Driver-Dependent Manner. *Cancer Res.* **2017**, *77*, 6941–6949. [CrossRef] [PubMed]
47. Firoozbakht, F.; Rezaeian, I.; D'agnillo, M.; Porter, L.; Rueda, L.; Ngom, A. An Integrative Approach for Identifying Network Biomarkers of Breast Cancer Subtypes Using Genomic, Interactomic, and Transcriptomic Data. *J. Comput. Biol.* **2017**, *24*, 756–766. [CrossRef] [PubMed]
48. Rycaj, K.; Li, H.; Zhou, J.; Chen, X.; Tang, D. Cellular determinants and microenvironmental regulation of prostate cancer metastasis. *Semin. Cancer Biol.* **2017**, *44*, 83–97. [CrossRef] [PubMed]
49. Moro, L.; Arbini, A.; Yao, J.; di Sant'Agnese, P.; Marra, E.; Greco, M. Mitochondrial DNA depletion in prostate epithelial cells promotes anoikis resistance and invasion through activation of PI3K/Akt2. *Cell Death Differ.* **2009**, *16*, 571–583. [CrossRef] [PubMed]
50. Missiroli, S.; Perrone, M.; Genovese, I.; Pinton, P.; Giorgi, C. Cancer metabolism and mitochondria: Finding novel mechanisms to fight tumours. *EBioMedicine* **2020**, *59*, 102943. [CrossRef] [PubMed]
51. Zhang, W.; Zhang, S.; Hu, X.; Tam, K. Targeting Tumor Metabolism for Cancer Treatment: Is Pyruvate Dehydrogenase Kinases (PDKs) a Viable Anticancer Target? *Int. J. Biol. Sci.* **2015**, *11*, 1390–1400. [CrossRef] [PubMed]
52. Yu, D.; Liu, C.; Guo, L. Mitochondrial metabolism and cancer metastasis. *Ann. Transl. Med.* **2020**, *8*, 904. [CrossRef] [PubMed]
53. Huang, R.; Wang, J.; Zhong, Y.; Liu, Y.; Stokke, T.; Trope, C.; Nesland, J.; Suo, Z. Mitochondrial DNA Deficiency in Ovarian Cancer Cells and Cancer Stem Cell-like Properties. *Anticancer Res.* **2015**, *35*, 3743–3753.
54. Simonnet, H.; Alazard, N.; Pfeiffer, K.; Gallou, C.; Béroud, C.; Demont, J.; Bouvier, R.; Schägger, H.; Godinot, C. Low mitochondrial respiratory chain content correlates with tumor aggressiveness in renal cell carcinoma. *Carcinogenesis* **2002**, *23*, 759–768. [CrossRef] [PubMed]
55. Wu, C.; Yin, P.; Hung, W.; Li, A.; Li, S.; Chi, C.; Wei, Y.; Lee, H. Mitochondrial DNA mutations and mitochondrial DNA depletion in gastric cancer. *Genes Chromosom. Cancer* **2005**, *44*, 19–28. [CrossRef] [PubMed]
56. Lee, H.; Yin, P.; Lin, J.; Wu, C.; Chen, C.; Wu, C.; Chi, C.; Tam, T.; Wei, Y. Mitochondrial genome instability and mtDNA depletion in human cancers. *Ann. N. Y. Acad. Sci.* **2005**, *1042*, 109–122. [CrossRef] [PubMed]
57. Tseng, L.; Yin, P.; Chi, C.; Hsu, C.; Wu, C.; Lee, L.; Wei, Y.; Lee, H. Mitochondrial DNA mutations and mitochondrial DNA depletion in breast cancer. *Genes Chromosom. Cancer* **2006**, *45*, 629–638. [CrossRef] [PubMed]
58. Cui, H.; Huang, P.; Wang, Z.; Zhang, Y.; Zhang, Z.; Xu, W.; Wang, X.; Han, Y.; Guo, X. Association of decreased mitochondrial DNA content with the progression of colorectal cancer. *BMC Cancer* **2013**, *13*, 1–7. [CrossRef] [PubMed]
59. Tu, H.; Gu, J.; Meng, Q.H.; Kim, J.; Davis, J.W.; He, Y.; Wagar, E.A.; Thompson, T.C.; Logothetis, C.J.; Wu, X. Mitochondrial DNA copy number in peripheral blood leukocytes and the aggressiveness of localized prostate cancer. *Oncotarget* **2015**, *6*, 41988–41996. [CrossRef] [PubMed]
60. Yu, M.; Wan, Y.; Zou, Q. Decreased copy number of mitochondrial DNA in Ewing's sarcoma. *Clin. Chim. Acta* **2010**, *411*, 679–683. [CrossRef]
61. Correia, R.L.; Oba-Shinjo, S.M.; Uno, M.; Huang, N.; Marie, S.K. Mitochondrial DNA depletion and its correlation with TFAM, TFB1M, TFB2M and POLG in human diffusely infiltrating astrocytomas. *Mitochondrion* **2011**, *11*, 48–53. [CrossRef] [PubMed]
62. Lin, C.; Liu, L.; Ou, L.; Pan, S.; Lin, C.; Wei, Y. Role of mitochondrial function in the invasiveness of human colon cancer cells. *Oncol. Rep.* **2018**, *39*, 316–330. [CrossRef] [PubMed]
63. Kim, M.; Clinger, J.; Masayesva, B.; Ha, P.; Zahurak, M.; Westra, W.; Califano, J. Mitochondrial DNA quantity increases with histopathologic grade in premalignant and malignant head and neck lesions. *Clin. Cancer Res.* **2004**, *10*, 8512–8515. [CrossRef] [PubMed]
64. Jiang, W.; Masayesva, B.; Zahurak, M.; Carvalho, A.; Rosenbaum, E.; Mambo, E.; Zhou, S.; Minhas, K.; Benoit, N.; Westra, W.; et al. Increased mitochondrial DNA content in saliva associated with head and neck cancer. *Clin. Cancer Res.* **2005**, *11*, 2486–2491. [CrossRef] [PubMed]
65. Lin, C.; Chang, S.; Wang, L.; Chou, T.; Hsu, W.; Wu, Y.; Wei, Y. The role of mitochondrial DNA alterations in esophageal squamous cell carcinomas. *J. Thorac. Cardiovasc. Surg.* **2010**, *139*, 189–197. [CrossRef] [PubMed]

66. Tan, A.; Baty, J.; Dong, L.; Bezawork-Geleta, A.; Endaya, B.; Goodwin, J.; Bajzikova, M.; Kovarova, J.; Peterka, M.; Yan, B.; et al. Mitochondrial genome acquisition restores respiratory function and tumorigenic potential of cancer cells without mitochondrial DNA. *Cell Metab.* **2015**, *21*, 81–94. [CrossRef]
67. Li, X.; Li, Y.; Lu, W.; Chen, M.; Ye, W.; Zhang, D. The Tumor Vessel Targeting Strategy: A Double-Edged Sword in Tumor Metastasis. *Cells* **2019**, *8*, 1602. [CrossRef] [PubMed]
68. Mehlen, P.; Puisieux, A. Metastasis: A question of life or death. *Nat. Rev. Cancer* **2006**, *6*, 449–458. [CrossRef]
69. Maishi, N.; Hida, K. Tumor endothelial cells accelerate tumor metastasis. *Cancer Sci.* **2017**, *108*, 1921–1926. [CrossRef] [PubMed]
70. Siemann, D. The unique characteristics of tumor vasculature and preclinical evidence for its selective disruption by Tumor-Vascular Disrupting Agents. *Cancer Treat. Rev.* **2011**, *37*, 63–74. [CrossRef] [PubMed]
71. Huang, L.; Hong, Z.; Wu, W.; Xiong, S.; Zhong, M.; Gao, X.; Rehman, J.; Malik, A. mtDNA Activates cGAS Signaling and Suppresses the YAP-Mediated Endothelial Cell Proliferation Program to Promote Inflammatory Injury. *Immunity* **2020**, *52*, 475–486. [CrossRef]
72. Fidler, I. The pathogenesis of cancer metastasis: The 'seed and soil' hypothesis revisited. *Nat. Rev. Cancer* **2003**, *3*, 453–458. [CrossRef] [PubMed]
73. Yuan, L.; Mao, Y.; Luo, W.; Wu, W.; Xu, H.; Wang, X.; Shen, Y. Palmitic acid dysregulates the Hippo-YAP pathway and inhibits angiogenesis by inducing mitochondrial damage and activating the cytosolic DNA sensor cGAS-STING-IRF3 signaling mechanism. *J. Biol. Chem.* **2017**, *292*, 15002–15015. [CrossRef]
74. Lavin, D.; Tiwari, V. Unresolved Complexity in the Gene Regulatory Network Underlying EMT. *Front. Oncol.* **2020**, *10*, 554. [CrossRef]
75. Vasaikar, S.; Deshmukh, A.; den Hollander, P.; Addanki, S.; Kuburich, N.; Kudaravalli, S.; Joseph, R.; Chang, J.; Soundararajan, R.; Mani, S. EMTome: A resource for pan-cancer analysis of epithelial-mesenchymal transition genes and signatures. *Br. J. Cancer* **2021**, *124*, 259–269. [CrossRef] [PubMed]
76. Chiu, H.; Li, C.; Yiang, G.; Tsai, A.; Wu, M. Epithelial to Mesenchymal Transition and Cell Biology of Molecular Regulation in Endometrial Carcinogenesis. *J. Clin. Med.* **2019**, *8*, 439. [CrossRef]
77. Naito, A.; Cook, C.; Mizumachi, T.; Wang, M.; Xie, C.; Evans, T.; Kelly, T.; Higuchi, M. Progressive tumor features accompany epithelial-mesenchymal transition induced in mitochondrial DNA-depleted cells. *Cancer Sci.* **2008**, *99*, 1584–1588. [CrossRef]
78. Guha, M.; Srinivasan, S.; Ruthel, G.; Kashina, A.; Carstens, R.; Mendoza, A.; Khanna, C.; Van Winkle, T.; Avadhani, N. Mitochondrial retrograde signaling induces epithelial-mesenchymal transition and generates breast cancer stem cells. *Oncogene* **2014**, *33*, 5238–5250. [CrossRef]
79. Giampieri, S.; Manning, C.; Hooper, S.; Jones, L.; Hill, C.; Sahai, E. Localized and reversible TGFbeta signalling switches breast cancer cells from cohesive to single cell motility. *Nat. Cell Biol.* **2009**, *11*, 1287–1296. [CrossRef]
80. Lin, C.; Lee, H.; Lee, S.; Shen, Y.; Wang, L.; Chen, Y.; Wei, Y. High mitochondrial DNA copy number and bioenergetic function are associated with tumor invasion of esophageal squamous cell carcinoma cell lines. *Int. J. Mol. Sci.* **2012**, *13*, 11228. [CrossRef]
81. Lu, J.; Tan, M.; Cai, Q. The Warburg effect in tumor progression: Mitochondrial oxidative metabolism as an anti-metastasis mechanism. *Cancer Lett.* **2015**, *356*, 156–164. [CrossRef]
82. Oft, M.; Peli, J.; Rudaz, C.; Schwarz, H.; Beug, H.; Reichmann, E. TGF-beta1 and Ha-Ras collaborate in modulating the phenotypic plasticity and invasiveness of epithelial tumor cells. *Genes Dev.* **1996**, *10*, 2462–2477. [CrossRef]
83. Oft, M.; Heider, K.; Beug, H. TGFbeta signaling is necessary for carcinoma cell invasiveness and metastasis. *Curr. Biol.* **1998**, *8*, 1243–1252. [CrossRef]
84. Yuan, Y.; Chen, Y.; Zhang, P.; Huang, S.; Zhu, C.; Ding, G.; Liu, B.; Yang, T.; Zhang, A. Mitochondrial dysfunction accounts for aldosterone-induced epithelial-to-mesenchymal transition of renal proximal tubular epithelial cells. *Free Radic. Biol. Med.* **2012**, *53*, 30–43. [CrossRef] [PubMed]
85. Welch, D.; Hurst, D. Defining the Hallmarks of Metastasis. *Cancer Res.* **2019**, *79*, 3011–3027. [CrossRef]
86. Weiss, L. Metastatic inefficiency. *Adv. Cancer Res.* **1990**, *54*, 159–211. [CrossRef]
87. Anastasiou, D.; Poulogiannis, G.; Asara, J.; Boxer, M.; Jiang, J.; Shen, M.; Bellinger, G.; Sasaki, A.; Locasale, J.; Auld, D.; et al. Inhibition of pyruvate kinase M2 by reactive oxygen species contributes to cellular antioxidant responses. *Science* **2011**, *334*, 1278–1283. [CrossRef] [PubMed]
88. Shidara, Y.; Yamagata, K.; Kanamori, T.; Nakano, K.; Kwong, J.Q.; Manfredi, G.; Oda, H.; Ohta, S. Positive contribution of pathogenic mutations in the mitochondrial genome to the promotion of cancer by prevention from apoptosis. *Cancer Res.* **2005**, *65*, 1655–1663. [CrossRef]
89. Ahmed-Belkacem, A.; Pozza, A.; Macalou, S.; Boumendjel, A.; Di Pietro, A. Inhibitors of cancer cell multidrug resistance mediated by breast cancer resistance protein (BCRP/ABCG2). *Anti-Cancer Drugs* **2006**, *17*, 239–243. [CrossRef]
90. Stouch, T.R.; Gudmundsson, O. Progress in understanding the structure-activity relationships of P-glycoprotein. *Adv. Drug Deliv. Rev.* **2002**, *54*, 315–328. [CrossRef]
91. Finger, E.; Giaccia, A. Hypoxia, inflammation, and the tumor microenvironment in metastatic disease. *Cancer Metastasis Rev.* **2010**, *29*, 285–293. [CrossRef]
92. Liu, Y.; Yan, W.; Tohme, S.; Chen, M.; Fu, Y.; Tian, D.; Lotze, M.; Tang, D.; Tsung, A. Hypoxia induced HMGB1 and mitochondrial DNA interactions mediate tumor growth in hepatocellular carcinoma through Toll-like receptor 9. *J. Hepatol.* **2015**, *63*, 114–121. [CrossRef]

93. Koshikawa, N.; Maejima, C.; Miyazaki, K.; Nakagawara, A.; Takenaga, K. Hypoxia selects for high-metastatic Lewis lung carcinoma cells overexpressing Mcl-1 and exhibiting reduced apoptotic potential in solid tumors. *Oncogene* **2006**, *25*, 917–928. [CrossRef] [PubMed]
94. Ishikawa, K.; Imanishi, H.; Takenaga, K.; Hayashi, J. Regulation of metastasis; mitochondrial DNA mutations have appeared on stage. *J. Bioenerg. Biomembr.* **2012**, *44*, 639–644. [CrossRef] [PubMed]
95. Denko, N. Hypoxia, HIF1 and glucose metabolism in the solid tumour. *Nat. Rev. Cancer* **2008**, *8*, 705–713. [CrossRef]
96. Singh, D.; Arora, R.; Kaur, P.; Singh, B.; Mannan, R.; Arora, S. Overexpression of hypoxia-inducible factor and metabolic pathways: Possible targets of cancer. *Cell Biosci.* **2017**, *7*, 1–9. [CrossRef] [PubMed]
97. Tello, D.; Balsa, E.; Acosta-Iborra, B.; Fuertes-Yebra, E.; Elorza, A.; Ordóñez, Á.; Corral-Escariz, M.; Soro, I.; López-Bernardo, E.; Perales-Clemente, E.; et al. Induction of the mitochondrial NDUFA4L2 protein by HIF-1α decreases oxygen consumption by inhibiting Complex I activity. *Cell Metab.* **2011**, *14*, 768–779. [CrossRef]
98. Mohme, M.; Riethdorf, S.; Pantel, K. Circulating and disseminated tumour cells-mechanisms of immune surveillance and escape. *Nat. Rev. Clin. Oncol.* **2017**, *14*, 155–167. [CrossRef]
99. LeBleu, V.; O'Connell, J.; Herrera, K.G.; Wikman, H.; Pantel, K.; Haigis, M.; de Carvalho, F.; Damascena, A.; Chinen, L.D.; Rocha, R.; et al. PGC-1α mediates mitochondrial biogenesis and oxidative phosphorylation in cancer cells to promote metastasis. *Nat. Cell Biol.* **2014**, *16*, 992–1003. [CrossRef]
100. Gammage, P.A.; Minczuk, M. Enhanced Manipulation of Human Mitochondrial DNA Heteroplasmy In Vitro Using Tunable mtZFN Technology. *Methods Mol. Biol.* **2018**, *1867*, 43–56. [CrossRef] [PubMed]
101. Gammage, P.A.; Gaude, E.; Van Haute, L.; Rebelo-Guiomar, P.; Jackson, C.B.; Rorbach, J.; Pekalski, M.L.; Robinson, A.J.; Charpentier, M.; Concordet, J.P.; et al. Near-complete elimination of mutant mtDNA by iterative or dynamic dose-controlled treatment with mtZFNs. *Nucleic Acids Res.* **2016**, *44*, 7804–7816. [CrossRef]
102. Gaude, E.; Schmidt, C.; Gammage, P.A.; Dugourd, A.; Blacker, T.; Chew, S.P.; Saez-Rodriguez, J.; O'Neill, J.S.; Szabadkai, G.; Minczuk, M.; et al. NADH Shuttling Couples Cytosolic Reductive Carboxylation of Glutamine with Glycolysis in Cells with Mitochondrial Dysfunction. *Mol. Cell* **2018**, *69*, 581–593. [CrossRef] [PubMed]
103. Yaguchi, T.; Sumimoto, H.; Kudo-Saito, C.; Tsukamoto, N.; Ueda, R.; Iwata-Kajihara, T.; Nishio, H.; Kawamura, N.; Kawakami, Y. The mechanisms of cancer immunoescape and development of overcoming strategies. *Int. J. Hematol.* **2011**, *93*, 294–300. [CrossRef] [PubMed]
104. Crane, C.; Austgen, K.; Haberthur, K.; Hofmann, C.; Moyes, K.; Avanesyan, L.; Fong, L.; Campbell, M.; Cooper, S.; Oakes, S.; et al. Immune evasion mediated by tumor-derived lactate dehydrogenase induction of NKG2D ligands on myeloid cells in glioblastoma patients. *Proc. Natl. Acad. Sci. USA* **2014**, *111*, 12823–12828. [CrossRef] [PubMed]
105. Smith, H.; Kang, Y. The metastasis-promoting roles of tumor-associated immune cells. *J. Mol. Med.* **2013**, *91*, 411–429. [CrossRef] [PubMed]
106. Hazeldine, J.; Dinsdale, R.; Harrison, P.; Lord, J. Traumatic Injury and Exposure to Mitochondrial-Derived Damage Associated Molecular Patterns Suppresses Neutrophil Extracellular Trap Formation. *Front. Immunol.* **2019**, *10*, 685. [CrossRef] [PubMed]
107. Yang, L.; Liu, Q.; Zhang, X.; Liu, X.; Zhou, B.; Chen, J.; Huang, D.; Li, J.; Li, H.; Chen, F.; et al. DNA of neutrophil extracellular traps promotes cancer metastasis via CCDC25. *Nature* **2020**, *583*, 133–138. [CrossRef]
108. Bidwell, B.; Slaney, C.; Withana, N.; Forster, S.; Cao, Y.; Loi, S.; Andrews, D.; Mikeska, T.; Mangan, N.; Samarajiwa, S.; et al. Silencing of Irf7 pathways in breast cancer cells promotes bone metastasis through immune escape. *Nat. Med.* **2012**, *18*, 1224–1231. [CrossRef] [PubMed]
109. Eyles, J.; Puaux, A.; Wang, X.; Toh, B.; Prakash, C.; Hong, M.; Tan, T.; Zheng, L.; Ong, L.; Jin, Y.; et al. Tumor cells disseminate early, but immunosurveillance limits metastatic outgrowth, in a mouse model of melanoma. *J. Clin. Investig.* **2010**, *120*, 2030–2039. [CrossRef]
110. Paolino, M.; Choidas, A.; Wallner, S.; Pranjic, B.; Uribesalgo, I.; Loeser, S.; Jamieson, A.; Langdon, W.; Ikeda, F.; Fededa, J.; et al. The E3 ligase Cbl-b and TAM receptors regulate cancer metastasis via natural killer cells. *Nature* **2014**, *507*, 508–512. [CrossRef] [PubMed]
111. Cheng, A.; Cheng, L.; Kuo, C.; Lo, Y.; Chou, H.; Chen, C.; Wang, Y.; Chuang, T.; Cheng, S.; Lee, A. Mitochondrial Lon-induced mtDNA leakage contributes to PD-L1-mediated immunoescape via STING-IFN signaling and extracellular vesicles. *J. Immunother. Cancer* **2020**, *8*, e001372. [CrossRef]
112. Arnold, R.S.; Sun, C.Q.; Richards, J.C.; Grigoriev, G.; Coleman, I.M.; Nelson, P.S.; Hsieh, C.L.; Lee, J.K.; Xu, Z.; Rogatko, A.; et al. Mitochondrial DNA mutation stimulates prostate cancer growth in bone stromal environment. *Prostate* **2009**, *69*, 1–11. [CrossRef]
113. Bao, D.; Zhao, J.; Zhou, X.; Yang, Q.; Chen, Y.; Zhu, J.; Yuan, P.; Yang, J.; Qin, T.; Wan, S.; et al. Mitochondrial fission-induced mtDNA stress promotes tumor-associated macrophage infiltration and HCC progression. *Oncogene* **2019**, *38*, 5007–5020. [CrossRef]
114. Ye, L.; Chen, W.; Bai, X.; Xu, X.; Zhang, Q.; Xia, X.; Sun, X.; Li, G.; Hu, Q.; Fu, Q.; et al. Hypoxia-Induced Epithelial-to-Mesenchymal Transition in Hepatocellular Carcinoma Induces an Immunosuppressive Tumor Microenvironment to Promote Metastasis. *Cancer Res.* **2016**, *76*, 818–830. [CrossRef]
115. Yang, P.; Li, Q.; Feng, Y.; Zhang, Y.; Markowitz, G.; Ning, S.; Deng, Y.; Zhao, J.; Jiang, S.; Yuan, Y.; et al. TGF-β-miR-34a-CCL22 signaling-induced Treg cell recruitment promotes venous metastases of HBV-positive hepatocellular carcinoma. *Cancer Cell* **2012**, *22*, 291–303. [CrossRef] [PubMed]

116. Dalotto-Moreno, T.; Croci, D.; Cerliani, J.; Martinez-Allo, V.; Dergan-Dylon, S.; Méndez-Huergo, S.; Stupirski, J.; Mazal, D.; Osinaga, E.; Toscano, M.; et al. Targeting galectin-1 overcomes breast cancer-associated immunosuppression and prevents metastatic disease. *Cancer Res.* **2013**, *73*, 1107–1117. [CrossRef]
117. Sawant, A.; Hensel, J.; Chanda, D.; Harris, B.; Siegal, G.; Maheshwari, A.; Ponnazhagan, S. Depletion of plasmacytoid dendritic cells inhibits tumor growth and prevents bone metastasis of breast cancer cells. *J. Immunol.* **2012**, *189*, 4258–4265. [CrossRef] [PubMed]
118. Pazmandi, K.; Agod, Z.; Kumar, B.V.; Szabo, A.; Fekete, T.; Sogor, V.; Veres, A.; Boldogh, I.; Rajnavolgyi, E.; Lanyi, A.; et al. Oxidative modification enhances the immunostimulatory effects of extracellular mitochondrial DNA on plasmacytoid dendritic cells. *Free Radic. Biol. Med.* **2014**, *77*, 281–290. [CrossRef]
119. Xu, M.; Pu, Y.; Han, D.; Shi, Y.; Cao, X.; Liang, H.; Chen, X.; Li, X.; Deng, L.; Chen, Z.; et al. Dendritic Cells but Not Macrophages Sense Tumor Mitochondrial DNA for Cross-priming through Signal Regulatory Protein α Signaling. *Immunity* **2017**, *47*, 363–373. [CrossRef] [PubMed]
120. Yao, X.; Carlson, D.; Sun, Y.; Ma, L.; Wolf, S.E.; Minei, J.P.; Zang, Q.S. Mitochondrial ROS Induces Cardiac Inflammation via a Pathway through mtDNA Damage in a Pneumonia-Related Sepsis Model. *PLoS ONE* **2015**, *10*, e0139416. [CrossRef] [PubMed]
121. Lin, S.; Huang, C.; Gunda, V.; Sun, J.; Chellappan, S.; Li, Z.; Izumi, V.; Fang, B.; Koomen, J.; Singh, P.; et al. Fascin Controls Metastatic Colonization and Mitochondrial Oxidative Phosphorylation by Remodeling Mitochondrial Actin Filaments. *Cell Rep.* **2019**, *28*, 2824–2836. [CrossRef] [PubMed]
122. Yuan, Y.; Ju, Y.S.; Kim, Y.; Li, J.; Wang, Y.; Yoon, C.J.; Yang, Y.; Martincorena, I.; Creighton, C.J.; Weinstein, J.N.; et al. Comprehensive molecular characterization of mitochondrial genomes in human cancers. *Nat. Genet.* **2020**, *52*, 342–352. [CrossRef] [PubMed]
123. Stewart, J.B.; Alaei-Mahabadi, B.; Sabarinathan, R.; Samuelsson, T.; Gorodkin, J.; Gustafsson, C.M.; Larsson, E. Simultaneous DNA and RNA Mapping of Somatic Mitochondrial Mutations across Diverse Human Cancers. *PLoS Genet.* **2015**, *11*, e1005333. [CrossRef]
124. Ju, Y.S.; Alexandrov, L.B.; Gerstung, M.; Martincorena, I.; Nik-Zainal, S.; Ramakrishna, M.; Davies, H.R.; Papaemmanuil, E.; Gundem, G.; Shlien, A.; et al. Origins and functional consequences of somatic mitochondrial DNA mutations in human cancer. *elife* **2014**, *3*, e02935. [CrossRef]
125. Greaves, L.C.; Reeve, A.K.; Taylor, R.W.; Turnbull, D.M. Mitochondrial DNA and disease. *J. Pathol.* **2012**, *226*, 274–286. [CrossRef] [PubMed]
126. Keseru, J.S.; Soltesz, B.; Lukacs, J.; Marton, E.; Szilagyi-Bonizs, M.; Penyige, A.; Poka, R.; Nagy, B. Detection of cell-free, exosomal and whole blood mitochondrial DNA copy number in plasma or whole blood of patients with serous epithelial ovarian cancer. *J. Biotechnol.* **2019**, *298*, 76–81. [CrossRef] [PubMed]
127. Salas, A.; Yao, Y.G.; Macaulay, V.; Vega, A.; Carracedo, A.; Bandelt, H.J. A critical reassessment of the role of mitochondria in tumorigenesis. *PLoS Med.* **2005**, *2*, e296. [CrossRef] [PubMed]
128. Guha, M.; Srinivasan, S.; Raman, P.; Jiang, Y.; Kaufman, B.A.; Taylor, D.; Dong, D.; Chakrabarti, R.; Picard, M.; Carstens, R.P.; et al. Aggressive triple negative breast cancers have unique molecular signature on the basis of mitochondrial genetic and functional defects. *Biochim. Biophys. Acta Mol. Basis Dis.* **2018**, *1864*, 1060–1071. [CrossRef]
129. Saori, K.; Daisaku, T.; Keiko, W.; Junichi, H.; Kazushige, H.; Makoto, A. Role of Mitochondrial DNA in Cells Exposed to Irradiation: Generation of Reactive Oxygen Species (ROS) is Required for G2 Checkpoint upon Irradiation. *J. Health Sci.* **2005**, *21*, 385–393.
130. Campbell, C.T.; Kolesar, J.E.; Kaufman, B.A. Mitochondrial transcription factor A regulates mitochondrial transcription initiation, DNA packaging, and genome copy number. *Biochim. Biophys. Acta* **2012**, *1819*, 921–929. [CrossRef]
131. Joshi, B.; Li, L.; Taffe, B.G.; Zhu, Z.; Wahl, S.; Tian, H.; Ben-Josef, E.; Taylor, J.D.; Porter, A.T.; Tang, D.G. Apoptosis induction by a novel anti-prostate cancer compound, BMD188 (a fatty acid-containing hydroxamic acid), requires the mitochondrial respiratory chain. *Cancer Res.* **1999**, *59*, 4343–4355. [PubMed]
132. Guerra, F.; Perrone, A.M.; Kurelac, I.; Santini, D.; Ceccarelli, C.; Cricca, M.; Zamagni, C.; De Iaco, P.; Gasparre, G. Mitochondrial DNA mutation in serous ovarian cancer: Implications for mitochondria-coded genes in chemoresistance. *J. Clin. Oncol.* **2012**, *30*, e373–e378. [CrossRef] [PubMed]

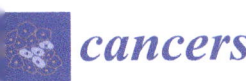

Article

Long-Chain Acyl Coenzyme A Dehydrogenase, a Key Player in Metabolic Rewiring/Invasiveness in Experimental Tumors and Human Mesothelioma Cell Lines

Daniel L. Pouliquen [1,*,†], Giacomo Ortone [2], Letizia Rumiano [2], Alice Boissard [3], Cécile Henry [3], Stéphanie Blandin [4], Catherine Guette [3], Chiara Riganti [2] and Joanna Kopecka [2,†]

1. Université d'Angers, Inserm, CNRS, Nantes Université, CRCI²NA, F-49000 Angers, France
2. Department of Oncology, University of Torino, via Santena 5/bis, 10126 Torino, Italy; giacomo.ortone@edu.unito.it (G.O.); letizia.rumiano@edu.unito.it (L.R.); chiara.riganti@unito.it (C.R.); joanna.kopecka@unito.it (J.K.)
3. Université d'Angers, ICO, Inserm, CNRS, Nantes Université, CRCI²NA, F-49000 Angers, France; alice.boissard@ico.unicancer.fr (A.B.); cecile.henry@ico.unicancer.fr (C.H.); catherine.guette@ico.unicancer.fr (C.G.)
4. CHU Nantes, CNRS, Inserm, BioCore, US16, SFR Bonamy, Nantes Université, F-44000 Nantes, France; stephanie.blandin@univ-nantes.fr
* Correspondence: daniel.pouliquen@inserm.fr; Tel.: +33-2-41-35-28
† These authors contributed equally to this work.

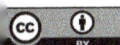

Citation: Pouliquen, D.L.; Ortone, G.; Rumiano, L.; Boissard, A.; Henry, C.; Blandin, S.; Guette, C.; Riganti, C.; Kopecka, J. Long-Chain Acyl Coenzyme A Dehydrogenase, a Key Player in Metabolic Rewiring/Invasiveness in Experimental Tumors and Human Mesothelioma Cell Lines. *Cancers* **2023**, *15*, 3044. https://doi.org/10.3390/cancers15113044

Academic Editor: Alfonso Baldi

Received: 12 May 2023
Revised: 30 May 2023
Accepted: 31 May 2023
Published: 3 June 2023

Copyright: © 2023 by the authors. Licensee MDPI, Basel, Switzerland. This article is an open access article distributed under the terms and conditions of the Creative Commons Attribution (CC BY) license (https://creativecommons.org/licenses/by/4.0/).

Simple Summary: This study aims to investigate mitochondrial metabolic differences between invasive and non-invasive malignant mesotheliomas in order to find new biomarkers for invasive properties and new potential actionable targets with the goal of improving the diagnosis and treatment of such tumors, which are highly resistant to current treatments.

Abstract: Cross-species investigations of cancer invasiveness are a new approach that has already identified new biomarkers which are potentially useful for improving tumor diagnosis and prognosis in clinical medicine and veterinary science. In this study, we combined proteomic analysis of four experimental rat malignant mesothelioma (MM) tumors with analysis of ten patient-derived cell lines to identify common features associated with mitochondrial proteome rewiring. A comparison of significant abundance changes between invasive and non-invasive rat tumors gave a list of 433 proteins, including 26 proteins reported to be exclusively located in mitochondria. Next, we analyzed the differential expression of genes encoding the mitochondrial proteins of interest in five primary epithelioid and five primary sarcomatoid human MM cell lines; the most impressive increase was observed in the expression of the long-chain acyl coenzyme A dehydrogenase (ACADL). To evaluate the role of this enzyme in migration/invasiveness, two epithelioid and two sarcomatoid human MM cell lines derived from patients with the highest and lowest overall survival were studied. Interestingly, sarcomatoid vs. epithelioid cell lines were characterized by higher migration and fatty oxidation rates, in agreement with ACADL findings. These results suggest that evaluating mitochondrial proteins in MM specimens might identify tumors with higher invasiveness. Data are available via ProteomeXchange with the dataset identifier PXD042942.

Keywords: malignant mesothelioma; metabolism; mitochondria; long-chain specific acyl-CoA dehydrogenase; fatty acid β-oxidation; biomarker

1. Introduction

The role of mitochondria, at the crossroads of many studies related to cancer invasiveness, has been extensively investigated over the last fifteen years [1]. Their involvement in motility and invasion, microenvironment, plasticity, and colonization was recently reviewed [2]. Since the pioneering work of Ishikawa et al. demonstrating the role of mtDNA transfer in the acquisition of high metastatic potential [3], cancer cells were shown to acquire mitochondria from neighboring cells in order to acquire phenotypic characteristics, including stemness, representing a gain of function for tumors, i.e., enhancing their invasive properties [4]. The interplay between mitochondrial dynamics and extracellular matrix (ECM) remodeling was emphasized [5], and the molecular mechanisms linking dysregulated fission/fusion to tumor progression and metastasis were deciphered [6]. Together with an updated view of the effects of mitochondria dysfunction on tumor glycolysis [7], these important breakthroughs are having a profound impact on new therapeutic strategies aiming at overcoming hypoxic and chemorefractory tumors [8]. Finally, the upregulation of mitochondrial proteins involved both in ATP production and drug resistance [9], and/or immune-resistance [10] could lead to new therapies. In parallel, all these studies could also shed light on new biomarkers for better predictions of cancer chemosensitivity [11].

In this context, proteomics-based investigations provide crucial insights into the role of mitochondrial proteome rewiring [11–13]. The development of high-throughput proteomics techniques, combined with the use of experimental models of increasing invasiveness, has led to the identification of new proteins of interest both in rats and humans [14]. Given this methodological background, in this study, we aim to focus on mitochondrial proteins, which appear to play an important role in metabolic rewiring and the invasiveness process, both in experimental tumor models and tumor cells from patients.

2. Materials and Methods

2.1. Collection of Rat Tumor Tissues for Proteomic Analyses

The formalin-fixed paraffin embedded (FFPE) tissue samples used in this study were collected from the same groups of Fisher F344 rats with four different experimental mesotheliomas at increasing stages of invasiveness, as previously described [15]. To generate the tumors, the experimental procedures used for in vivo manipulations at the Unité Thérapeutique Expérimentale de l'Institut de Recherche en Santé de l'Université de Nantes (UTE-IRS UN) between 2011 and 2015 followed the European Union guidelines for the care and use of laboratory animals in research (approval #01257.03 from the French Ministry of Higher Education and Research (MESR)). The rats were purchased from Charles River Laboratories (L'Arbresle, 69210, France), and the experiments were approved by the ethics committee for animal experiments (CEEA) of the Pays de la Loire Region and registered under the number 2011.38. The non-invasive M5-T2, mildly invasive F4-T2, moderately invasive F5-T1 and deeply invasive M5-T1 tumors were collected after intraperitoneal injection of 3×10^6 cells of the corresponding cell lines (https://technology-offers.inserm-transfert.com/offer/, accessed on 30 January 2023, recorded as RT00418, RT00419, RT00421 and RT00417, respectively) into syngeneic rats.

2.2. Proteomic Analyses

For each sample analyzed, four or five 20-μm-thick sections of tumor tissue were scratched with a scalpel and collected in a 1.5-mL Eppendorf® microtube. Next, all the material collected was deparaffinized in three successive xylene washes and then rehydrated in 100%, 95%, 70% and 50% ethanol solutions. The pellets were vacuum-dried, and the dried tissues resuspended in 200 μL of Rapigest SF (Waters, Milford, MA, USA). Dithiothreitol (AppliChem, Darmstadt, Germany) was then added (5 mM final concentration), and the samples were incubated in a thermo shaker at 95 °C for one hour before being sonicated twice (ultrasonic processor 75185, Bioblock Scientific, Illkirch, France). Cystein residues were alkylated by adding 200 mM S-Methyl methanethiosulfonate at 37 °C (10 mM final concentration). Sequencing-grade trypsin was added at a ratio ≥ 2 μg mm^{-3} tissue (at 37 °C overnight). The reaction was stopped with formic acid (9% final concentration, incubation at 37 °C for one hour), and the acid-treated samples were centrifuged at 16,000× g for 10 min. After removing the salts from the supernatant, the peptides were collected in a new Eppendorf® microtube using C18 STAGE tips, and their concentration finally determined using the Micro BCA™ Protein Assay Kit (Thermo Fisher Scientific, St Herblain,

France). The rat spectral library, SWATH-MS analysis, peptide identification, and relative quantification were performed as previously described [15]. The statistical analysis of the SWATH data set and peak extraction output data matrix from PeakView were imported into MarkerView (v.2, AB Sciex Pte, Ltd., Framingham, MA, USA) for data normalization and relative protein quantification. Proteins with a statistical p-value < 0.05, estimated by MarkerView, were considered to be differentially expressed under different conditions.

2.3. Histology and Immuno-Histochemical Analyses

The FFPE blocs were cut with a Leica RM2255 microtome (Leica Biosystems, Nussloch, Germany). Areas of interest for both proteomic and histological analyses were selected based on examination of sections of all samples stained with hematoxylin phloxine saffron (HPS), scanned on a Nanozoomer 2.0 HT Hamamatsu. For immuno-histochemistry, tumor sections were stained with anti-ACADL NBP2-92854 polyclonal antibody (Novus Biologicals, Centennial, CO, USA).

2.4. Chemicals

Cell line culture medium and fetal bovine serum (FBS) were from Invitrogen Life Technologies (Carlsbad, CA, USA). Cell culture plasticware was from Falcon (Becton Dickinson, Hongkong, China). A BCA Kit from Sigma Chemical Co. (Saint Louis, MO, USA) was used to determine protein contents. Reagents for electrophoresis were bought from Bio-Rad Laboratories. All the other reagents, unless otherwise specified, were purchased from Sigma Chemical Co.

2.5. Cells

Ten primary human MM cell lines (5 epithelioid and 5 sarcomatoid), obtained during diagnostic thoracoscopies, were collected from the S. Antonio e Biagio e Cesare Arrigo Hospital Biological Bank of Malignant Mesothelioma (Alessandria, Italy) after obtaining written informed consent. The local Ethics Committees approved the study (#9/11/2011; #126/2016). Primary MM cells were used until passage 10. Table 1 contains clinical and pathological data of the MM patients. Primary MM cells were cultured in HAM's F12 medium and supplemented with 10% v/v fetal FBS and 100 U/mL penicillin-100 µg/mL streptomycin.

Table 1. Origin and characteristics of human mesothelioma cell lines.

UNP (Number)	Histotype	Gender	Age (Years)	Asbestos Exposure	First Line of Treatment	Second Line of Treatment	TTP (Months)	OS (Months)
1	Epithelioid	M	74	Unknown	Carbo + Pem	No	7	11
2	Epithelioid	F	58	Yes	Carbo + Pem	Pem	6	13
3	Epithelioid	M	76	Unknown	CisPt + Pem	No	3	8
4	Epithelioid	M	68	Yes	Carbo + Pem	Pem	4	9
5	Epithelioid	F	84	Yes	CisPt + Pem	No	7	8
6	Sarcomatoid	M	80	Yes	Carbo + Pem	Trabectedin	3	5
7	Sarcomatoid	F	78	Unknown	Pem	No	4	6
8	Sarcomatoid	M	69	Yes	Carbo + Pem	Trabectedin	7	10
9	Sarcomatoid	F	74	Unknown	Carbo + Pem	No	5	7
10	Sarcomatoid	M	78	Yes	Carbo + Pem	Trabectedin	4	9

UNP: unknown patient; M: male; F: female; Carbo: carboplatin; Pem: pemetrexed; CisPt: cisplatin; TTP: time to progression; OS: overall survival.

2.6. Immunoblotting

Cells were rinsed with lysis buffer (150 mM NaCl; 1.0% Nonidet P-40; 50 mM Tris-Cl; pH 7.4), supplemented with the protease inhibitor cocktail, sonicated and centrifuged (13,000× g, for 10 min at 4 °C). Then, 20 µg of proteins were probed with antibodies ACADL (ab152160, Abcam, Cambridge, UK), GAPDH (sc-47724, Santa Cruz Biotechnology Inc.,

Dallas, TX, USA) and then with secondary antibodies conjugated with peroxidase (Bio-Rad Laboratories, Hercules, CA, USA). After washing blots with Tris-buffered saline/Tween 0.01% v/v, blots were developed with enhanced chemiluminescence (Bio-Rad Laboratories) and visualized using a ChemiDoc™ Touch Imaging System device (Bio-Rad Laboratories).

2.7. Mitochondria Isolation

Cells were washed twice with PBS, then lysed in 0.8 mL of mitochondria lysis buffer (50 mM TRIS, 100 mM KCl, 5 mM $MgCl_2$, 1 mM EDTA and 1.8 mM ATP, pH 7.2) mixed with protease inhibitor cocktail set III (100 µL). PMSF (100 µL) and NaF (25 µL). Cells were scraped and collected in an Eppendorf® tube and then sonicated twice for 10 s at 40% power. Subsequently, samples were centrifuged at 2000 rpm for 1 min at 4 °C. The supernatant was collected into a new series of Eppendorf® tubes and centrifuged again at 13,000 rpm for 5 min at 4 °C. Pellets containing mitochondria were washed with 0.4 mL of mitochondria lysis buffer and centrifuged at 13,000 rpm for 5 min at 4 °C. Subsequently, the supernatant was aspirated and the pellets resuspended in 0.2 mL of mitochondria resuspension buffer (Sucrose 250 mM, K_2HPO_4 15 mM, $MgCl_2$ 2 mM and EDTA 0.5 mM, pH 7.2). The resuspended mitochondria were then divided into two parts: one part was used to measure mitochondria protein content using a BCA kit (Sigma, Saint Louis, MO, USA), and the other was divided into 50 µL aliquots and stored at -80 °C until use.

2.8. ETC (Electron Transport Chain from Complex I to Complex III)

The electron transport between complexes I and III was measured in mitochondrial extracts obtained previously. In particular, 10 µL of mitochondria samples were put in a 96-well plate, together with 160 µL of buffer A (5 mM KH_2PO_4, 5 mM of $MgCl_2$, 5% w/v bovine serum albumin, pH 7.2), 100 µL of buffer B (50 mM KH_2PO_4, 5 mM $MgCl_2$, 5% w/v serum bovine albumin, 0.05% saponin, pH 7.5) and freshly added 0.12 mM of cytochrome c-oxidized form and 0.2 mM of NaN_3. After waiting 5 min to equilibrate the plate at room temperature, 30 µL of NADH (0.15 mM and diluted in buffer B) was added to each well. The reaction then started, and the absorbance was read at 550 nm for 6 min, with 1 read every 15 s. Considering only the linear part of the curve and calculating results in accordance with Lambert-Beer equations, the results obtained were expressed as nmoles of cytochrome C reduced/min/mg mitochondrial protein.

2.9. ATP

ATP quantities were measured following the Sigma-Aldrich protocol 213-579-1. First 50 µL of ATP assay mix (lyophilized powder containing luciferase, luciferin, $MgSO_4$, DTT, EDTA, BSA and tricine buffer salts, pH 7.8) was added to a vial for 3 min. Then, 50 µL of sample (mitochondria extract obtained as described in the previous steps) was rapidly added and the quantity of light was measured in a black 96-well plate in a microplate reader. The results were expressed as nmols of ATP/mg mitochondrial.

2.10. β-Oxidation of Fatty Acid

Assays were performed using the fatty acid complete oxidation kit (ab222944; Abcam, Cambridge, UK) as per the manufacturer's instructions. Cells were plated at 40,000 cells per well in a 96-well plate with 200 µL of medium per well and left overnight to equilibrate. The cells were washed twice with prewarmed FA-free measurement media, incubated with FA measurement media (150 µM FAO-Conjugate; 0.5 mM L-Carnitine) with extracellular O_2 consumption reagent (ab197243; Abcam, Cambridge, UK) and then sealed with mineral oil. The fluorescence signal was read in a microplate reader (Ex/Em = 380/650 nM). The results were expressed as pmoles of O_2/min.

2.11. Scratch Assay

Cells were plated at 1×10^6 cells per well in a 6-well plate. After 24 h, scratches using a 20–200 µL pipette tip were made. Cell migration was calculated measuring distance (in µM) between the cells at T0 (immediately after the scratch) and T1 (24 h after the scratch) and dividing it by 24 h. The results were expressed as µM/h.

2.12. Real Time PCR (RT-PCR)

Total RNA was extracted using VWR Life Science RiboZol™ RNA Extraction Reagent (VWR Life Science, Radnor, PA, USA) and reverse-transcribed using the iScriptTM cDNA Synthesis Kit (Bio-Rad Laboratories). qRT-PCR was carried out using SYBR Green Supermix (Bio-Rad Laboratories). qPrimerDepot software (http://primerdepot.nci.nih.gov/, accessed on 13 september 2022) was used to obtain the desired PCR primers (Supplementary Table S1). Gene Expression Quantitation software (Bio-Rad Laboratories) was used to assess relative gene expression levels.

2.13. Statistical Analysis

All data in the text and figures are provided as means ± SEM. The results were analyzed using a one-way ANOVA and Tukey test. $p < 0.05$ was considered significant.

3. Results

3.1. Mitochondrial Biomarkers Involved in the Acquisition of Invasiveness in Rat Mesotheliomas

To identify a set of mitochondrial proteins involved in the acquisition of tumor invasiveness, we analyzed the proteomes of four experimental models of mesothelioma grown in immunocompetent F344 rats presenting increasing stages of invasiveness. For each tumor type, 1300 proteins were detected, and the comparison of abundance levels for the three invasive tumors ((1) mildly invasive F4-T2, (2) moderately invasive F5-T1 and (3) deeply invasive M5-T1)) versus (4) the noninvasive tumor M5-T2 (Figure 1) produced a list of 433 proteins satisfying the condition $p < 0.05$. The full list of genes encoding these proteins, together with their full names, is given in Supplementary Table S2.

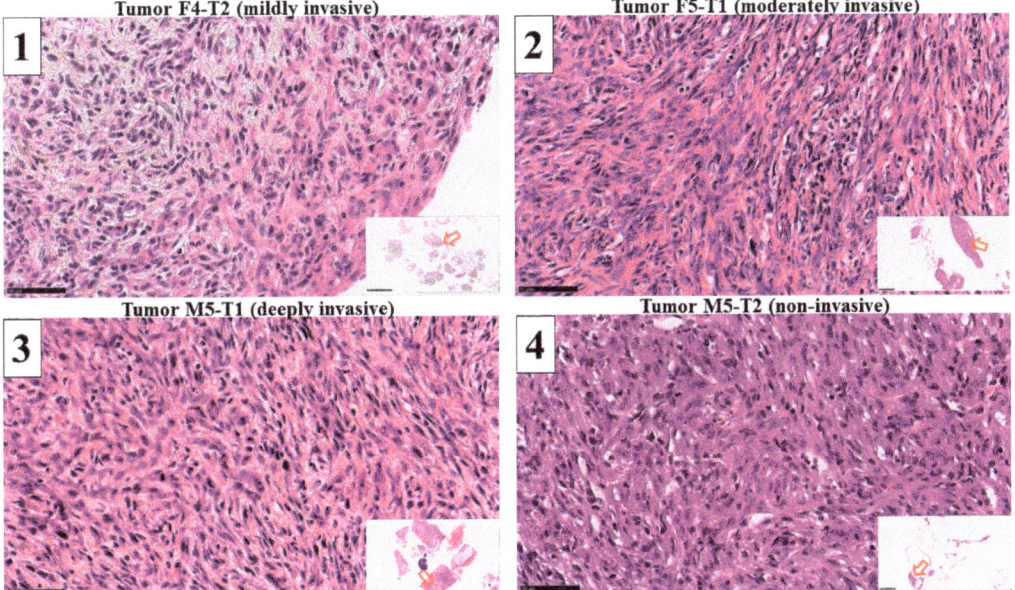

Figure 1. Histological features of the four experimental rat mesothelioma tumor models. HPS staining, ×400 (the scale bar represents 50 µm). Inserts (bottom right corner) represent general views (the scale bars represent 5 mm (left column) or 2.5 mm (right column)), with the open red arrows showing the location of the magnified areas.

In a second step, the subcellular extracellular locations of these proteins were recorded on https://www.proteinatlas.org (accessed on 29 September 2022), and 36 proteins exclusively or mainly located in mitochondria were identified. A list of mitochondrial proteins exhibiting significant abundance changes (increase or decrease in [1 + 2 + 3] vs. 4) is shown in Table 2.

Table 2. Mitochondrial proteins exhibiting significant abundance changes ($p < 0.05$) in the three invasive rat malignant mesothelioma tumors relative to the non-invasive tumor. # According to www.uniprot.org for Rattus norvegicus. * Protein location not restricted to mitochondria. ↑ Increased abundance, ↓ decreased abundance.

Code #	Gene #	Full Name #	[1 + 2 + 3] vs. 4
ACADL	Acadl	Long-chain specific acyl-CoA dehydrogenase, mitochondrial	↑
AL7A1 *	Aldh7a1	Alpha-aminoadipic semialdehyde dehydrogenase	↑
ATP5H	Atp5h	ATP synthase subunit d, mitochondrial	↑
ATPO	Atp5o	ATP synthase subunit O, mitochondrial	↑
BCAT2 *	Bcat2	Branched-chain-amino-acid aminotransferase, mitochondrial	↑
COX2	Mtco2	Cytochrome c oxidase subunit 2	↑
COX5B	Cox5b	Cytochrome c oxidase subunit 5B, mitochondrial	↑
CX6C2	Cox6c2	Cytochrome c oxidase subunit 6C-2	↑
EFTU	Tufm	Elongation factor Tu, mitochondrial	↑
HCD2	Hsd17b10	3-hydroxyacyl-CoA dehydrogenase type-2	↑
IDH3A	Idh3a	Isocitrate dehydrogenase [NAD] subunit alpha, mitochondrial	↑
IDH3B	Idh3b	Isocitrate dehydrogenase [NAD] subunit beta, mitochondrial	↑
KAD2	Ak2	Adenylate kinase 2, mitochondrial	↑
MDHM	Mdh2	Malate dehydrogenase, mitochondrial	↑
MYG1 *	Myg1	UPF0160 protein MYG1, mitochondrial	↑
OAT *	Oat	Ornithine aminotransferase, mitochondrial	↑
PHB	Phb	Prohibitin	↑
PHB2	Phb2	Prohibitin-2	↑
SSBP	Ssbp1	Single-stranded DNA-binding protein, mitochondrial	↑
TRAP1	Trap1	Heat shock protein 75 kDa, mitochondrial	↑
ACADS	Acads	Short-chain specific acyl-CoA dehydrogenase, mitochondrial	↓
ACON	Aco2	Aconitate hydratase, mitochondrial	↓
CISY *	Cs	Citrate synthase, mitochondrial	↓
DECR *	Decr1	2, 4 dienoyl-CoA reductase, mitochondrial	↓
GSTP1 *	Gstp1	Glutathione S-transferase P	↓
HCDH	Hadh	Hydroxyacyl-CoA dehydrogenase, mitochondrial	↓
IVD *	Ivd	Isovaleryl-CoA dehydrogenase, mitochondrial	↓
MGST1 *	Mgst1	Microsomal glutathione S-transferase 1	↓
ODO2	Dlst	Dihydrolipoyllysine-residue succinyltransferase component of 2-oxoglutarate dehydrogenase complex, mitochondrial	↓
PRDX3	Prdx3	Thioredoxin-dependent peroxide reductase, mitochondrial	↓
RMD3 *	Rmdn3	Regulator of microtubule dynamics protein 3	↓
S10AA	S100a10	Protein S100-A10	↓
SUOX	Suox	Sulfite oxidase, mitochondrial	↓
THTM	Mpst	3-mercaptopyruvate sulfurtransferase	↓
THTR	Tst	Thiosulfate sulfurtransferase	↓
TIM9	Timm9	Mitochondrial import inner membrane translocase subunit Tim9	↓

Twenty-six proteins were reported to be exclusively located in mitochondria, including 17 concerned with the most dramatic changes (13 increased and 4 decreased, with $p < 0.01$) and involved in 11 main biological functions. Among the proteins increasing in abundance with invasiveness, two were involved in fatty acid β-oxidation (FAO), encoded by *Acadl* [16] and *Hsd17b10* (Table 1 and Figure 2A) [17], and one in adenine nucleotide metabolism (encoded by *Ak2*) [18]. This list also included two subunits of ATP synthase, with the first being one of the F0 membrane-spanning components (proton channel) (encoded by

Atp5h) [19] and the second being part of the connector linking the F1 catalytic core to F0 (encoded by *Atp5o*) [20]. Other increased proteins corresponded to two subunits of the cytochrome c oxidase (encoded by *Mtco2, Cox5b, Cox6c2*) [21], a chaperone regulating cellular stress responses (encoded by *Trap1*), two subunits of the isocitrate dehydrogenase (encoded by *Idh3a* and *Idh3b*) [22] and the malate dehydrogenase (encoded by *Mdh2*) [23], and two mitochondrial scaffolding/chaperone proteins (encoded by *Phb* and *Phb2*) [24]. The last two increased proteins participate in protein translation in mitochondria and contribute to mitochondrial genome stability and biogenesis (encoded by *Tufm* and *Ssbp1*, respectively) [25,26]. Of the four main proteins decreasing in abundance with invasiveness, two represented enzymes of sulfur metabolism (encoded by *Suox* and *Mpst*) [27], one was a peroxide reductase playing a role in protection against oxidative stress (encoded by *Prdx3*) [28] and the other modulated ion channels and receptors (encoded by *S100a10*) [29].

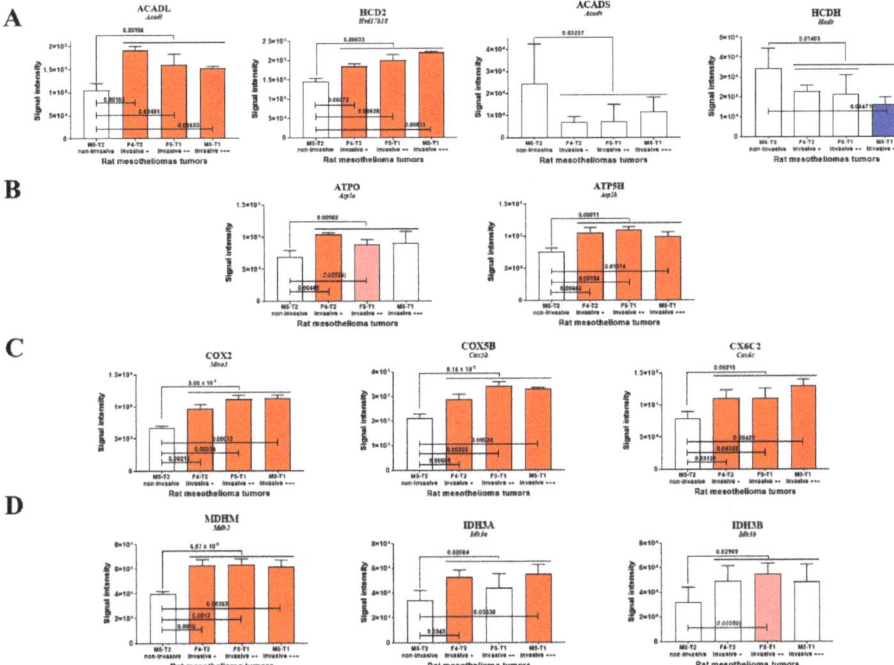

Figure 2. Abundance changes with invasiveness, main mitochondrial proteins. (**A**) FAO enzymes. (**B**) ATP synthase subunits. (**C**) Cytochrome oxidase subunits. (**D**) TCA enzymes. Red bars represent increase and blue bars decrease, with light colors used for tendencies. Protein codes (for *rattus norvegicus*) are put in upper case and bold, and gene names in italics.

Of the enzymes involved in mitochondrial FAO and detected in proteomic analyses, the long-chain acyl coenzyme A dehydrogenase (encoded by *Acadl*) exhibited the most dramatic changes, with a significant increase being observed for each individual invasive tumor (1 vs. 4, 2 vs. 4, 3 vs. 4) (Figure 2A). Another enzyme in this metabolic pathway, also involved in branched-amino acid catabolism and encoded by *Hsd17b10*, exhibited a similar pattern of increase with invasiveness (Figure 2A). Conversely, for two additional enzymes in this pathway (encoded by *Acads*, and *Hadh*), invasiveness was associated with a decrease, while no significant change was observed for each individual comparison, i.e., 1 vs. 4, 2 vs. 4, and 3 vs. 4 for ACADS (Figure 2A).

The evolution in ACADL and HCD2 levels was associated with a parallel increase in two subunits of ATP synthase (Figure 2B) and three subunits of cytochrome oxidase

(Figure 2C), suggesting a link with ATP production and flux within the electron transport chain. A similar increased level of two enzymes in the tricarboxylic cycle, i.e., malate dehydrogenase 2 and isocitrate dehydrogenase, also tended to demonstrate its involvement in the invasiveness process (Figure 2D).

3.2. Immuno-Histochemical Study of ACADL Distribution in Rat Tumors

Examination of ACADL expression by IHC in the four tumor models revealed pronounced differences with the level of invasiveness. The non-invasive tumor (M5-T2) was characterized by the absence of staining (Figure 3A). In contrast, the mildly invasive F4-T2 (Figure 3B) and moderately invasive F5-T1 (Figure 3C) tumors exhibited a weak, homogeneous distribution of ACADL expression within the tumor tissues. The most striking feature was the strong staining observed in the deeply invasive M5-T1 tumor (Figure 3D). Moreover, ACADL expression appeared heterogeneous within the tumor, with some areas showing intense staining in external parts of the tumor, as shown on high magnification views (Figure 3E).

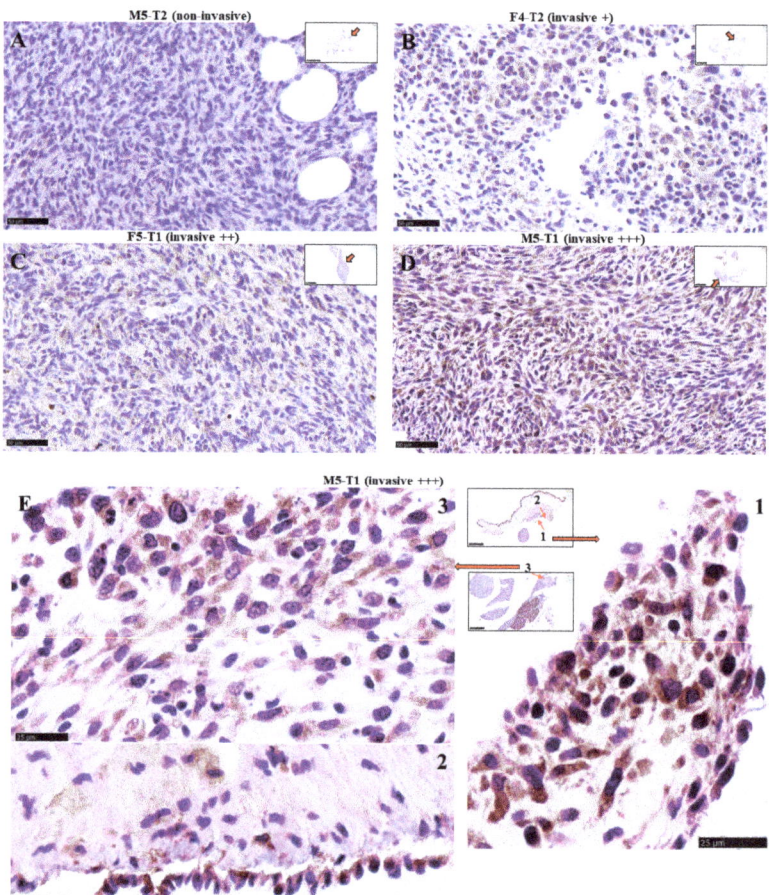

Figure 3. Distribution of *ACADL* expression in rat mesothelioma tumors. (**A–D**) Comparison of overall IHC staining with increasing invasiveness, ×400 (the scale bars represent 50 µm). (**E**) Magnifications of areas of intense staining in the most aggressive, M5-T1 tumor (the scale bars represent 25 µm).

3.3. Fatty Acid β-Oxidation Supports Cell Invasiveness in Human Primary Mesothelioma Cell Lines

Next, to determine whether our findings on rat mesothelioma tumors could be confirmed in human malignant mesothelioma (MM), we analyzed the differential expression of genes encoding the different mitochondrial proteins of interest listed above (in Section 3.1, Table 1) in five primary sarcomatoid and five primary epithelioid mesothelioma cell lines. Interestingly, the most impressive increase was observed in the expression of *ACADL*. Other highly expressed genes in sarcomatoid mesothelioma cell lines were two ATP synthase subunits (*ATP5H*, *ATPO*), *MTCO2*, *COX5B*, *COX 6C2*, *IDH3A*, *IDH3B* and *TIMM9* (Figure 4A). These findings confirm proteomic data obtained in rat tumors. To evaluate the role of ACADL in the migration/invasiveness of mesothelioma cells, we chose two primary epithelioid mesothelioma cell lines (UP1, UP2) and two primary sarcomatoid mesothelioma cell lines (UP 6, UP 7) derived from patients with the highest and lowest OS, respectively (Table 1), which were therefore indicative of higher or lower invasive properties. In agreement with this finding, primary mesothelioma cells were characterized by low and high migration rates, respectively (Figure 4B,C). Migration of primary mesothelioma cells, evaluated with a scratch assay, was inhibited by addition of etomoxir, a drug that blocks FAO (Figure 4B,C). Primary sarcomatoid mesothelioma cell lines have higher expression of *ACADL* mRNA (Figure 5A) and protein (Figure 5B), accompanied by higher activity of FAO in comparison with epithelioid mesothelioma cell lines (Figure 6A). Etomoxir did not change *ACADL* expression (Figure 5A,B) but it functionally inhibited FAO in the primary sarcomatoid mesothelioma cell lines (Figure 6). A higher FAO rate (Figure 6A) fuels the electron transport chain, which works faster (Figure 6B) and causes higher ATP production (Figure 6C). In addition to higher FAO, primary sarcomatoid mesothelioma cell lines have more active mitochondrial respiratory complexes and produce more ATP. All these metabolic processes are inhibited by etomoxir (Figure 6). Altogether, these data confirm that FAO supports ATP production through electron transport chain activity, providing energy for cell migration/invasiveness in sarcomatoid mesothelioma tumors.

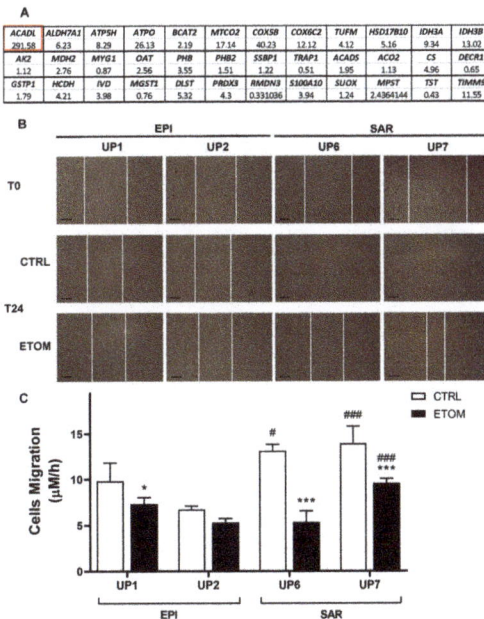

Figure 4. Different expressions of mitochondrial genes between epithelioid and sarcomatoid MM cells. (**A**) Mitochondrial gene expression in 10 primary MM cell lines (Table 1) derived from two

different histopathological subtypes, i.e., epithelioid (EPI, $n = 5$) and sarcomatoid (SAR, $n = 5$), was analyzed with real time PCR. Data are expressed as relative mean fold increase SAR vs. EPI MM cells. (**B**,**C**) MPM epithelioid (EPI UP1 and EPI UP2), and sarcomatoid (SAR UP6 and SAR UP7) cells were grown to confluence, then scratched and incubated for 24 h in fresh medium (CTRL) or medium with 10 µM of etomoxir (ETOM). (**B**) Representative bright-field images immediately after the scratch and after 24 h. (**C**) Cell migration. Data are presented as means ± SEM ($n = 3$). * $p < 0.05$, *** $p < 0.001$: ETOM treated cells vs. CTRL cells; # $p < 0.05$, ### $p < 0.001$: SAR cells vs. EPI cells. Scale bar is 100 µm.

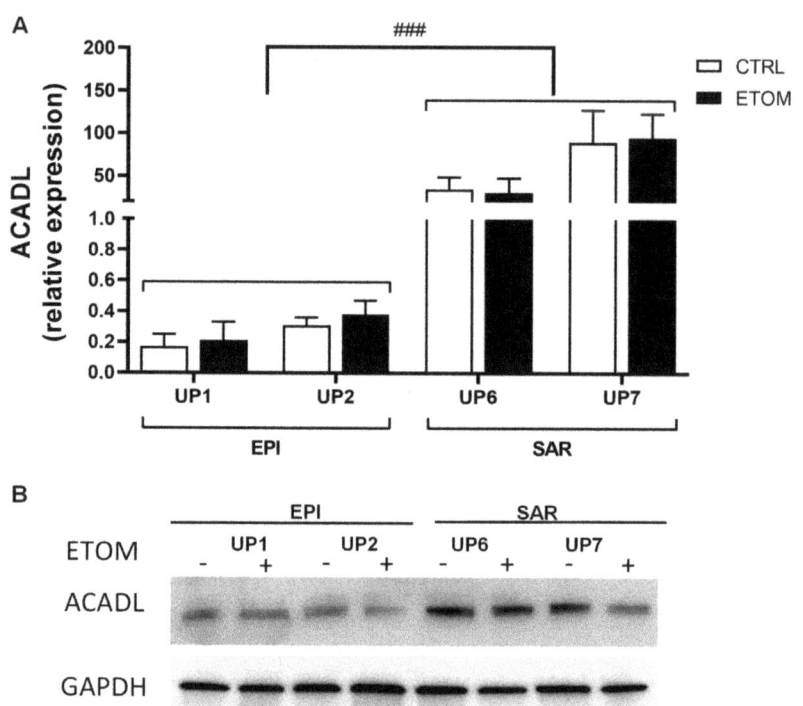

Figure 5. Sarcomatoid MPM cells have higher expression of *ACADL* compared with epithelioid MM cells. Primary MM cells derived from two different histopathological subtypes, i.e., epithelioid (EPI UP1 and UP2) and sarcomatoid (SAR UP6 and UP7), were incubated in fresh medium (CTRL), or in medium with 10 µm of etomoxir (ETOM) for 24 h then used for measurements. (**A**) *ACADL* mRNA levels were measured with RT-PCR, in triplicate. Data are presented as means ± SEM ($n = 3$). ### $p < 0.001$: SAR cells vs. EPI cells. (**B**) *ACADL* protein was measured with immunoblotting in primary MM cell lines. GAPDH was used as a loading control. The figure is representative of one out of three experiments with similar results. The uncropped blots and molecular weight markers are shown in Supplementary Figure S1.

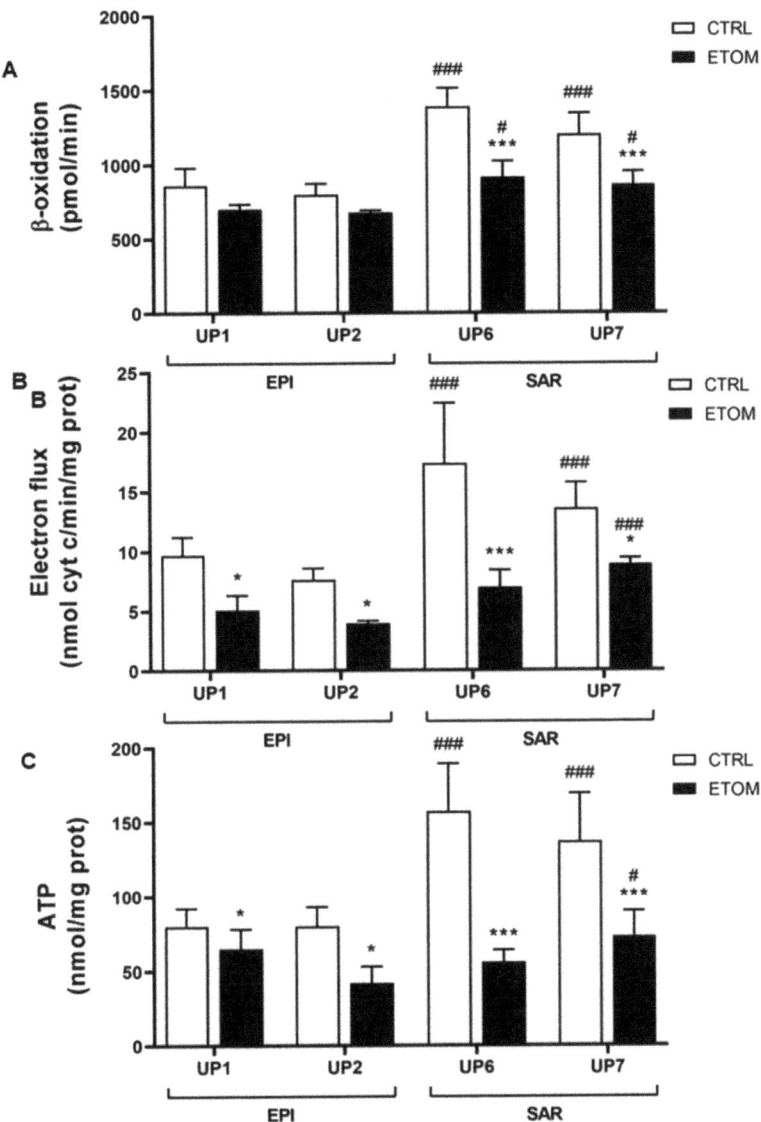

Figure 6. Sarcomatoid MM cells have more active mitochondrial metabolism compared with epithelioid MM cells. Primary MM cells derived from two different histopathological subtypes, i.e., epithelioid (EPI UP1 and UP2) and sarcomatoid (SAR UP6 and SAR UP7), were grown in fresh medium (CTRL) or in medium with 10 µM of etomoxir for 24 h and then used for the following analysis. (**A**) Fatty acid β-oxidation was measured with fluorimetric assay in triplicate. Data are presented as means ± SEM ($n = 3$). *** $p < 0.001$: ETOM treated cells vs. CTRL cells; # $p < 0.05$, ### $p < 0.001$: SAR cells vs. EPI cells. (**B**) The electron flux between Complex I and III was measured spectrophotometrically in triplicate. Data are expressed as means ± SEM ($n = 3$). * $p < 0.05$, *** $p < 0.001$: ETOM treated cells vs. CTRL cells, ### $p < 0.001$: SAR cells vs. EPI cells. (**C**) ATP release was measured with a chemiluminescence-based assay in duplicate. Data are expressed as means ± SEM ($n = 3$). * $p < 0.05$, *** $p < 0.001$: ETOM treated cells vs. CTRL cells; # $p < 0.05$, ### $p < 0.001$: SAR cells vs. EPI cells.

4. Discussion

Cross-species investigations have provided new insights into universal mechanisms in biology, improving, for example, our understanding of oncogenic signatures in breast cancer development in humans and dogs [30]. Applied to proteomic analyses in cancer, common biomarkers of invasiveness have been identified in rat and human mesotheliomas [14]. Genomic analyses have also pointed to markers which are useful for the diagnosis and prognosis of hepatocellular carcinomas in both species [31]. To date, cross-species comparisons of important findings relevant to mitochondria have been very limited, focusing, for example, on detecting heteroplasmy [32]. In this study, we identified several biomarkers of interest that appear to play an important role in metabolic rewiring and invasiveness in both human and rat mesotheliomas.

As biosynthetic hubs, mitochondria consume a variety of different fuels to generate energy in the form of ATP for cancer cells, where fatty acid oxidation plays an important role [33]. Although most cancer researchers initially focused on glycolysis, glutaminolysis and fatty acid synthesis, the relevance of fatty acid oxidation in the metabolic reprogramming of cancer cells was extensively reviewed 10 years ago, and its role in NADPH production was emphasized [34]. Linked to this statement, our results revealed a consistent finding regarding the FAO enzyme *ACADL*, observed both in humans and rats, and associated with the acquisition of invasive properties, i.e., higher expression of *ACADL* was initially found to be positively correlated to prostate cancer progression [35].

Our data also agreed with the work of Yu et al. showing that *ACADL* was overexpressed both in cell lines and clinical specimens, being related to esophageal squamous cell carcinoma progression and poor prognosis [16]. Another close FAO enzyme, which is encoded by *HSD17B10*, is also involved in branched amino acid catabolism and steroid metabolism. Our data are in line with previously published reports emphasizing its upregulation in invasive tumors. For example, Salas et al. showed its predictive value in the response to chemotherapy in osteosarcomas [17]. Its overexpression also accelerated cell growth, enhanced cell respiration and increased cellular resistance to cell death in pheochromocytoma [36]. Finally, and even more interestingly, Condon et al. found that *HSD17B10* was one of the six genes impacting the mTORC1 pathway [37], which is dysregulated and activated in cancer cells to drive survival, neovascularization and invasion [38].

Interestingly, the increased β-oxidation rate, electron flux and ATP production observed in human sarcomatoid mesothelioma cell lines were all consistent with the increased expression of ATP synthase subunits, cytochrome *c* oxidase subunits, abundance changes in these proteins in rat tumors, and with our observations concerning the long-chain acyl coenzyme A dehydrogenase. Fiorillo et al. have highlighted the fact that ATP-high cancer cells are phenotypically the most aggressive, with enhanced stem-like properties, multi-drug resistance potential and an increased capacity for cell migration, invasion and metastasis [9]. Wang et al. also pointed out that high ATP expression was linked to poor prognosis in glioblastoma, clear cell renal cell carcinoma and ovarian, prostate, and breast cancers [39]. Moreover, an additional role of ATP synthase in the formation of the permeability transition pore (PTP) was also recently reported as representing a mechanism controlling tumor cell death [40]. In this process, our findings also tend to confirm the important role of the subunit *d* of ATP synthase (encoded by (*Atp5h/ATP5H*), linked to the work by Chang et al., who reported the involvement of the overexpression of this subunit in venous invasion, distant metastasis of colon cancer and, finally, poor survival [41].

Within the enzymes of mitochondrial metabolism involved in cancer progression, besides isocitrate dehydrogenase and malate dehydrogenase, subunits of the cytochrome *c* oxidase (complex IV of the respiratory chain) such as COX5B have also been reported [42]. Our results agreed with previously published literature on the impact of its high expression on tumor invasiveness and poor prognosis in patients with breast cancer [43]. More recently, further insights have confirmed its tremendous role as a growth-promoting gene, both in hepatoma [44] and colorectal cancer [45]. Interestingly, the combined upregulation of COX5B and ATP5H was also reported by Yusenko et al. in renal oncocytomas [19]. Another subunit of the cytochrome *c* oxidase, COX6C, also upregulated in relation to invasiveness in our study, appeared to be differentially expressed in various cancers [46]. Notably, Jang et al. detected it in extracellular vesicles (EV) in the plasma of metastatic melanoma and ovarian and breast cancer patients, suggesting that the classic EV production and mitochondrial pathways are interconnected [47]. In that study, an additional crucial observation was the presence of another inner mitochondrial membrane protein in these EVs [47], encoded by *MTCO2*. These breakthroughs are consistent with both the increased abundance of SODM and the expression of this gene that we found in the most invasive rat tumors as well as in human mesothelioma cell lines. Linked to the tremendous increase in ACADL, the greater abundance and expression of the two subunits of isocitrate dehydrogenase tend to confirm previous observations regarding the central role of the TCA cycle in metabolic reprogramming and tumor invasiveness. Laurenti and Tennant have previously reviewed the impact of its dysregulation in cancers in association with hypoxia and increased intracellular levels of ROS [48]. Moreover, as shown by Zeng et al., the aberrant expression of *IDH3A*, which represented an upstream activator of HIF-1, promoted tumor growth and angiogenesis in various cancer types [22].

In addition to the dramatic changes observed in ACADL associated with tumor invasiveness, we also identified another protein involved in the mitochondrial translation machinery, i.e., *TUFM*. This observation, which is consistent with the higher abundance and expression of proteins involved in mtDNA maintenance, may be relevant to data from several existing reports. For example, Cruz et al. found this protein in a list of five candidate biomarkers of drug-resistant ovarian cancer [49]. Interestingly, the mitochondrial translation pathway is required for increased electron transport chain activity [50], and its inhibition plays a part in sensitizing renal cell carcinoma to chemotherapy [25]. Chatla et al. demonstrated that TUFM was required for increased mitochondrial biosynthesis [51]. Moreover, the authors of that work suggested the existence of a link with another elevated mitochondrial protein found in our study, i.e., encoded by *ALDH7A1*. ALDH7A1 is an enzyme which mechanistically appeared to provide cells with protection against various forms of stress through multiple pathways [52]. It is involved in stem cell pathways [53,54], and the link between its high expression and tumor invasiveness has been clearly established through the works of van den Hoogen et al. [55] and Giacalone et al. [56] in prostate cancer and lung cancer, respectively. Interestingly, in good agreement with our findings, Lee et al. also demonstrated its relationship with lipid catabolism as an energy source in pancreatic cancer cells [57]. ALDH7A1 was first known as antiquitin; the study of its subcellular localization revealed its presence in cytosol in addition to mitochondria [58]. Finally, an intriguing feature of this enzyme, which resonates with the latter observation, was presented in a recent work by Babbi et al., i.e., the central role played by this protein, which is also present in the nucleus, is to interact with 23 other proteins in IntAct and 62 in BioGRID, while *ALDH7A1* represents one of the most frequent genes in KEGG metabolic pathways [59].

5. Conclusions

In conclusion, starting from a proteomic approach and following on with ad hoc biological validation, we identified significant differences between non-invasive and invasive mesotheliomas, developed in both rats and patient-derived cells, in terms of the expression of mitochondrial proteins. This suggests that mitochondrial activity plays an important role in cancer. In particular, ACADL and subunits of ATP synthase are highly expressed in invasive rat mesotheliomas, as well as in more aggressive human sarcomatoid mesothelioma cells, which have more active FAO, electron chain transport and ATP synthesis, supporting their growth and invasiveness. Evaluating mitochondrial proteins in MM specimens might help to identify tumors with higher invasiveness and new potential targets that could be explored to improve the treatment of this disease.

Supplementary Materials: The following supporting information can be downloaded at: https://www.mdpi.com/article/10.3390/cancers15113044/s1, Table S1: Primers for gene expression analysis; Table S2: Proteins with increased abundance (I) or decreased abundance (D); Figure S1: The original whole blot of Figure 5.

Author Contributions: Conceptualization, D.L.P., J.K. and C.R.; methodology, validation, G.O. and L.R.; Preparation of samples for proteomics, D.L.P., A.B. and C.H.; Preparation of samples and immuno-histochemistry, S.B.; Software, validation, C.G.; formal analysis, G.O. and L.R.; data curation, D.L.P. and J.K.; writing—original draft preparation, D.L.P. and J.K.; writing—review and editing, D.L.P., J.K. and C.R.; supervision, D.L.P., J.K., C.R. and C.G.; funding acquisition D.L.P., J.K. and C.R. All authors have read and agreed to the published version of the manuscript.

Funding: This research was funded by the Italian Association of Cancer Research (IG21408 to C.R.), Fondazione Cassa di Risparmio di Torino (ID 2020.1648 to J.K., ID 2021.05556 to C.R.). This research was conducted with the support of the "Mobilité internationale pour la recherche" (Mir program of the University of Angers) between the Universities of Angers (France) and Turin (Italy) in 2020–2021 and 2021–2022.

Institutional Review Board Statement: Experiments on F344 rats were conducted at the UTE-IRS UN facility (Nantes Université) following the European Union guidelines for the care and use of laboratory rodents in research protocols. The research was approved by the Ethics Committee for Animal Experiments (CEEA) of the Pays de la Loire Region (2011.38) and #0125703 of the French Ministry of Higher Education and Research (MESR). For the research on ten primary human mesothelioma cell lines, the local Ethics Committees approved the study "PROMESO—Studio prospettico per la determinazione di marcatori prognostici/predittivi e nuove strategie terapeutiche nel mesothelioma pleurico malign (MPM) utilizzando un approcio traslazionale" (#9/11/2011; #126/2016).

Informed Consent Statement: Informed consent was obtained from all subjects involved in the study.

Data Availability Statement: The data can be shared up on request.

Acknowledgments: We thank Costanzo Costamagna for the technical support. We are grateful to all the staff at the Animal Facility (UTE-IRS UN) at Nantes University for the excellent care of the rats during the experiments. We also acknowledge the IBISA MicroPICell facility (Biogenouest), a member of the national infrastructure France-Bioimaging supported by the French national research agency (ANR-10-INBS-04).

Conflicts of Interest: The authors declare no conflict of interest.

Abbreviations

MM, malignant mesothelioma; ACADL, long-chain acyl coenzyme A dehydrogenase; ECM, extracellular matrix; FAO, fatty acid b-oxidation.

References

1. Faubert, B.; Solmonson, A.; DeBerardinis, R.J. Metabolic reprogramming and cancer progression. *Science* **2020**, *368*, eaaw5473. [CrossRef]
2. Scheid, A.D.; Beadnell, T.C.; Welch, D.R. Roles of mitochondria in the hallmarks of metastasis. *Br. J. Cancer* **2021**, *124*, 124–135. [CrossRef]
3. Ishikawa, K.; Takenaga, K.; Akimoto, M.; Koshikawa, N.; Yamaguchi, A.; Imanishi, H.; Nakada, K.; Honma, Y.; Hayashi, J.-I. ROS-generating mitochondrial DNA mutations can regulate tumor cell metastasis. *Science* **2008**, *320*, 661–664. [CrossRef]
4. Zampieri, L.X.; Silva-Almeida, C.; Rondeau, J.D.; Sonveaux, P. Mitochondrial transfer in cancer: A comprehensive review. *Int. J. Mol. Sci.* **2021**, *22*, 3245. [CrossRef]
5. Yanes, B.; Rainero, E. The interplay between cell-extracellular matrix interaction and mitochondria dynamics in cancer. *Cancers* **2022**, *14*, 1433. [CrossRef] [PubMed]
6. Boulton, D.P.; Caino, M.C. Mitochondrial fission and fusion in tumor progression to metastasis. *Front. Cell Dev. Biol.* **2022**, *10*, 849962. [CrossRef] [PubMed]
7. Bononi, G.; Masoni, S.; Di Bussolo, V.; Tuccinardi, T.; Granchi, C.; Minutolo, F. Historical perspective of tumor glycolysis: A century with Otto Warburg. *Semin. Cancer Biol.* **2022**, *86*, 325–333. [CrossRef]
8. Akman, M.; Belisario, D.C.; Salaroglio, I.C.; Kopecka, J.; Donadelli, M.; De Smaele, E.; Riganti, C. Hypoxia, endoplasmic reticulum stress and chemoresistance: Dangerous liaisons. *J. Exp. Clin. Cancer Res.* **2021**, *40*, 28. [CrossRef] [PubMed]

9. Fiorillo, M.; Ózsvári, B.; Sotgia, F.; Lisanti, M.P. High ATP production fuels cancer drug resistance and metastasis: Implications for mitochondrial ATP depletion therapy. *Front. Oncol.* **2021**, *11*, 740720. [CrossRef]
10. Kopecka, J.; Gazzano, E.; Castella, B.; Salaroglio, I.C.; Mungo, E.; Massaia, M.; Riganti, C. Mitochondrial metabolism: Inducer or therapeutic target in tumor immune-resistance? *Semin. Cell Dev. Biol.* **2020**, *98*, 80–89. [CrossRef] [PubMed]
11. Xie, L.; Zhou, T.; Xie, Y.; Bode, A.M.; Cao, Y. Mitochondria-shaping proteins and chemotherapy. *Front. Oncol.* **2021**, *11*, 769036. [CrossRef]
12. Concolino, A.; Olivo, E.; Tammè, L.; Fiumara, C.; De Angelis, M.T.; Quaresima, B.; Agosti, V.; Costanzo, F.S.; Cuda, G.; Scumaci, D. Proteomics analysis to assess the role of mitochondria in BRCA1-mediated breast tumorigenesis. *Proteomes* **2018**, *6*, 16. [CrossRef] [PubMed]
13. Arif, T.; Stern, O.; Pittala, S.; Chalifa-Caspi, V.; Shoshan-Barmatz, V. Rewiring of cancer cell metabolism by mitochondrial VDAC1 depletion results in time-dependent tumor reprogramming: Glioblastoma as a proof of concept. *Cells* **2019**, *8*, 1330. [CrossRef] [PubMed]
14. Nader, J.S.; Boissard, A.; Henry, C.; Valo, I.; Verrièle, V.; Grégoire, M.; Coqueret, O.; Guette, C.; Pouliquen, D.L. Cross-species proteomics identifies CAPG and SBP1 as crucial invasiveness biomarkers in rat and human malignant mesothelioma. *Cancers* **2020**, *12*, 2430. [CrossRef]
15. Nader, J.S.; Abadie, J.; Deshayes, S.; Boissard, A.; Blandin, S.; Blanquart, C.; Boisgerault, N.; Coqueret, O.; Guette, C.; Grégoire, M.; et al. Characterization of increasing stages of invasiveness identifies stromal/cancer cell crosstalk in rat models of mesothelioma. *Oncotarget* **2018**, *9*, 16311–16329. [CrossRef]
16. Yu, D.-L.; Li, H.-W.; Wang, Y.; Li, C.-Q.; You, D.; Jiang, L.; Song, Y.-P.; Li, X.-H. Acyl-CoA dehydrogenase long chain expression is associated with esophageal squamous cell carcinoma progression and poor prognosis. *OncoTargets Ther.* **2018**, *11*, 7643–7653. [CrossRef]
17. Salas, S.; Jézéquel, P.; Campion, L.; Deville, J.-L.; Chibon, F.; Bartoli, C.; Gentet, J.-C.; Charbonnel, C.; Gouraud, W.; Voutsinos-Porche, B.; et al. Molecular characterization of the response to chemotherapy in conventional osteosarcomas: Predictive value of HSD17B10 and IFITM2. *Int. J. Cancer* **2009**, *125*, 851–860. [CrossRef]
18. Klepinin, A.; Zhang, S.; Klepinina, L.; Rebane-Klemm, E.; Terzic, A.; Kaambre, T.; Dzeja, P. Adenylate kinase and metabolic signaling in cancer cells. *Front. Oncol.* **2020**, *10*, 660. [CrossRef]
19. Yusenko, M.V.; Ruppert, T.; Kovacs, G. Analysis of differentially expressed mitochondrial proteins in chromophobe renal cell carcinomas and renal oncocytomas by 2-D gel electrophoresis. *Int. J. Biol. Sci.* **2010**, *6*, 213–224. [CrossRef] [PubMed]
20. Wiebringhaus, R.; Pecoraro, M.; Neubauer, H.A.; Trachtova, K.; Trimmel, B.; Wieselberg, M.; Pencik, J.; Egger, G.; Krall, C.; Moriggl, R.; et al. Proteomic analysis identifies NDUFS1 and ATP5O as novel markers for survival outcome in prostate cancer. *Cancers* **2021**, *13*, 6036. [CrossRef]
21. Lamb, R.; Ozsvari, B.; Bonuccelli, G.; Smith, D.L.; Pestell, R.G.; Martinez-Outschoorn, U.E.; Clarke, R.B.; Sotgia, F.; Lisanti, M.P. Dissecting tumor metabolic heterogeneity: Telomerase and large cell size metabolically define a sub-population of stem-like, mitochondrial-rich, cancer cells. *Oncotarget* **2015**, *6*, 21892–21905. [CrossRef]
22. Zeng, L.; Morinibu, A.; Kobayashi, M.; Zhu, Y.; Wang, X.; Goto, Y.; Yeom, C.J.; Zhao, T.; Hirota, K.; Shinomiya, K.; et al. Aberrant IDH3α expression promotes malignant tumor growth by inducing HIF-1-mediated metabolic reprogramming and angiogenesis. *Oncogene* **2015**, *34*, 4758–4766. [CrossRef] [PubMed]
23. Liu, Q.; Harvey, C.T.; Geng, H.; Xue, C.; Chen, V.; Beer, T.M.; Qian, D.Z. Malate dehydrogenase 2 confers docetaxel resistance via regulations of JNK signaling and oxidative metabolism. *Prostate* **2013**, *73*, 1028–1037. [CrossRef] [PubMed]
24. Bavelloni, A.; Piazzi, M.; Raffini, M.; Faenza, I.; Blalock, W.L. Prohibitin 2: At a communications crossroads. *IUBMB Life* **2015**, *67*, 239–254. [CrossRef]
25. Wang, B.; Ao, J.; Yu, D.; Rao, T.; Ruan, Y.; Yao, X. Inhibition of mitochondrial translation effectively sensitizes renal cell carcinoma to chemotherapy. *Biochem. Biophys. Res. Commun.* **2017**, *490*, 767–773. [CrossRef]
26. Xu, S.; Wu, Y.; Chen, Q.; Cao, J.; Hu, K.; Tang, J.; Sang, Y.; Lai, F.; Wang, L.; Zhang, R.; et al. hSSB1 regulates both the stability and the transcriptional activity of p53. *Cell Res.* **2013**, *23*, 423–435. [CrossRef] [PubMed]
27. Murphy, B.; Bhattacharya, R.; Mukherjee, P. Hydrogen sulfide signaling in mitochondria and disease. *FASEB J.* **2019**, *33*, 13098–13125. [CrossRef] [PubMed]
28. Ismail, T.; Kim, Y.; Lee, H.; Lee, D.-S.; Lee, H.-S. Interplay between mitochondrial peroxiredoxins and ROS in cancer development and progression. *Int. J. Mol. Sci.* **2019**, *20*, 4407. [CrossRef]
29. Seo, J.-S.; Svenningsson, P. Modulation of ion channels and receptors by p11 (S100A10). *Trends Pharmacol. Sci.* **2020**, *41*, 487–497. [CrossRef]
30. Kim, T.-M.; Yang, S.; Seung, B.-J.; Lee, S.; Kim, D.; Ha, Y.-J.; Seo, M.-k.; Kim, K.-K.; Kim, H.S.; Cheong, J.-H.; et al. Cross-species oncogenic signatures of breast cancer in canine mammary tumors. *Nat. Commun.* **2020**, *11*, 3616. [CrossRef]
31. Al-Harazi, O.; Kaya, I.H.; Al-Eid, M.; Alfantoukh, L.; Al Zahrani, A.S.; Al Sebayel, M.; Kaya, N.; Colak, D. Identification of gene signature as diagnostic and prognostic blood biomarker for early hepatocellular carcinoma using integrated cross-species transcriptomic and network analyses. *Front. Genet.* **2021**, *12*, 710049. [CrossRef] [PubMed]
32. Rensch, T.; Villar, D.; Horvath, J.; Odom, D.T.; Flicek, P. Mitochondrial heteroplasmy in vertebrates using ChIP-sequencing data. *Genome Biol.* **2016**, *17*, 139. [CrossRef]

33. Spinelli, J.B.; Haigis, M.C. The multifaceted contributions of mitochondria to cellular metabolism. *Nat. Cell Biol.* **2018**, *20*, 745–754. [CrossRef]
34. Carracedo, A.; Cantley, L.C.; Pandolfi, P.P. Cancer metabolism: Fatty acid oxidation in the limelight. *Nat. Rev. Cancer* **2013**, *13*, 227–232. [CrossRef]
35. Xie, B.-X.; Zhang, H.; Wang, J.; Pang, B.; Wu, R.-Q.; Qian, X.-L.; Yu, L.; Li, S.-H.; Shi, Q.-G.; Huang, C.-F.; et al. Analysis of differentially expressed genes in LNCaP prostate cancer progression model. *J. Androl.* **2011**, *32*, 170–182. [CrossRef]
36. Carlson, E.A.; Marquez, R.T.; Du, F.; Wang, Y.; Xu, L.; Yan, S.S. Overexpression of 17b-hydroxysteroid dehydrogenase type 10 increases pheochromocytoma cell growth and resistance to cell death. *BMC Cancer* **2015**, *15*, 166. [CrossRef] [PubMed]
37. Condon, K.J.; Orozco, J.M.; Adelman, C.H.; Spinelli, J.B.; van der Helm, P.W.; Roberts, J.M.; Kunchok, T.; Sabatini, D.M. Genome-wide CRISPR screens reveal multitiered mechanisms through which mTORC1 senses mitochondrial dysfunction. *Proc. Natl. Acad. Sci. USA* **2021**, *118*, e2022120118. [CrossRef]
38. Braun, C.; Weichhart, T. mTOR-dependent immunometabolism as Achilles' heel of anticancer therapy. *Eur. J. Immunol.* **2021**, *51*, 3161–3175. [CrossRef] [PubMed]
39. Wang, T.; Ma, F.; Qian, H.-l. Defueling the cancer: ATP synthase as an emerging target in cancer therapy. *Mol. Ther. Oncolytics* **2021**, *23*, 82–95. [CrossRef]
40. Galber, C.; Acosta, M.J.; Minervini, G.; Giorgio, V. The role of mitochondrial ATP synthase in cancer. *Biol. Chem.* **2020**, *401*, 1199–1214. [CrossRef]
41. Chang, H.J.; Lee, M.R.; Hong, S.-H.; Yoo, B.C.; Shin, Y.-K.; Jeong, J.Y.; Lim, S.-B.; Choi, H.S.; Park, J.-G. Identification of mitochondrial F_0F_1-ATP synthase involved in liver metastasis of colorectal cancer. *Cancer Sci.* **2007**, *98*, 1184–1191. [CrossRef]
42. Gaude, E.; Frezza, C. Defects in mitochondrial metabolism and cancer. *Cancer Metab.* **2014**, *2*, 10. [CrossRef]
43. Gao, S.-P.; Sun, H.-F.; Fu, W.-Y.; Li, L.-D.; Zhao, Y.; Chen, M.-T.; Jin, W. High expression of COX5B is associated with poor prognosis in breast cancer. *Future Oncol.* **2017**, *13*, 1711–1719. [CrossRef]
44. Chu, Y.-D.; Lin, W.-R.; Lin, Y.-H.; Kuo, W.-H.; Tseng, C.-J.; Lim, S.-N.; Huang, Y.-L.; Huang, S.-C.; Wu, T.-J.; Lin, K.-H.; et al. COX5B-mediated bioenergetic alteration regulates tumor growth and migration by modulating AMPK-UHMK1-ERK cascade in hepatoma. *Cancers* **2020**, *12*, 1646. [CrossRef]
45. Chu, Y.-D.; Lim, S.-N.; Yeh, C.-T.; Lin, W.-R. COX5B-mediated bioenergetic alterations modulate cell growth and anticancer drug susceptibility by orchestrating claudin-2 expression in colorectal cancers. *Biomedicines* **2022**, *10*, 60. [CrossRef]
46. Tian, B.-X.; Sun, W.; Wang, S.-H.; Liu, P.-J.; Wang, Y.-C. Differential expression and clinical significance of COX6C in human diseases. *Am. J. Transl. Res.* **2021**, *13*, 1–10.
47. Jang, S.C.; Crescitelli, R.; Cvjetkovic, A.; Belgrano, V.; Bagge, R.O.; Sundfeldt, K.; Ochiya, T.; Kalluri, R.; Lötvall, J. Mitochondrial protein enriched extracellular vesicles discovered in human melanoma tissues can be detected in patient plasma. *J. Extracell. Vesicles* **2019**, *8*, 1635420. [CrossRef]
48. Laurenti, G.; Tennant, D.A. Isocitrate dehydrogenase (IDH), succinate dehydrogenase (SDH), fumarate hydratase (FH): Three players for one phenotype in cancer? *Biochem. Soc. Trans.* **2016**, *44*, 1111–1116. [CrossRef]
49. Cruz, I.N.; Coley, H.M.; Kramer, H.B.; Madhuri, T.K.; Safuwan, N.A.M.; Angelino, A.R.; Yang, M. Proteomics analysis of ovarian cancer cell lines and tissues reveals drug resistance-associated proteins. *Cancer Genom. Proteom.* **2017**, *14*, 35–52. [CrossRef]
50. Norberg, E.; Lako, A.; Chen, P.-H.; Stanley, I.A.; Zhou, F.; Ficarro, S.B.; Chapuy, B.; Chen, L.; Rodig, S.; Shin, D.; et al. Differential contribution of the mitochondrial translation pathway to the survival of diffuse large B-cell lymphoma subsets. *Cell Death Differ.* **2017**, *24*, 251–262. [CrossRef]
51. Chatla, S.; Du, W.; Wilson, A.F.; Meetei, A.R.; Pang, Q. *Fancd2*-deficient hematopoietic stem and progenitor cells depend on augmented mitochondrial translation for survival and proliferation. *Stem Cell Res.* **2019**, *40*, 101550. [CrossRef]
52. Brocker, C.; Cantore, M.; Failli, P.; Vasiliou, V. Aldehyde dehydrogenase 7A1 (ALDH7A1) attenuates reactive aldehyde and oxidative stress induced cytotoxicity. *Chem. Biol. Interact.* **2011**, *191*, 269–277. [CrossRef]
53. Prabhu, V.V.; Lulla, A.R.; Madhukar, N.S.; Ralff, M.D.; Zhao, D.; Kline, C.L.B.; Van den Heuvel, A.P.; Lev, A.; Garnett, M.J.; McDermott, U.; et al. Cancer stem cell-related gene expression as a potential biomarker of response for first-in-class imipridone ONC201 in solid tumors. *PLoS ONE* **2017**, *12*, e0180541. [CrossRef]
54. Bizzaro, V.; Belvedere, R.; Milone, M.R.; Pucci, B.; Lombardi, R.; Bruzzese, F.; Popolo, A.; Parente, L.; Budillon, A.; Petrella, A. Annexin A1 is involved in the acquisition and maintenance of a stem cell-like/aggressive phenotype in prostate cancer cells with acquired resistance to zoledronic acid. *Oncotarget* **2015**, *6*, 25074–25092. [CrossRef]
55. Van den Hoogen, C.; van der Horst, G.; Cheung, H.; Buijs, J.T.; Pelger, R.C.M.; van der Pluijm, G. The aldehyde dehydrogenase enzyme 7A1 is functionally involved in prostate cancer bone metastasis. *Clin. Exp. Metastasis* **2011**, *28*, 615–625. [CrossRef] [PubMed]
56. Giacalone, N.J.; Den, R.B.; Eisenberg, R.; Chen, H.; Olson, S.J.; Massion, P.P.; Carbone, D.P.; Lu, B. ALDH7A1 expression is associated with recurrence in patients with surgically resected non-small-cell lung carcinoma. *Future Oncol.* **2013**, *9*, 737–745. [CrossRef]
57. Lee, J.-S.; Lee, H.; Woo, S.M.; Jang, H.; Jeon, Y.; Kim, H.Y.; Song, J.; Lee, W.J.; Hong, E.K.; Park, S.-J.; et al. Overall survival of pancreatic ductal adenocarcinoma is doubled by *Aldh7a1* deletion in the KPC mouse. *Theranostics* **2021**, *11*, 3472–3488. [CrossRef] [PubMed]

68. Wong, J.W.-Y.; Chan, C.-L.; Tang, W.-K.; Cheng, C.H.-K.; Fong, W.-P. Is antiquitin a mitochondrial enzyme? *J. Cell. Biochem.* **2010**, *109*, 74–81. [CrossRef]
69. Babbi, G.; Baldazzi, D.; Savojardo, C.; Martelli, P.L.; Casadio, R. Highlighting human enzymes active in different metabolic pathways and diseases: The case study of EC 1.2.3.1 and EC 2.3.1.9. *Biomedicines* **2020**, *8*, 250. [CrossRef]

Disclaimer/Publisher's Note: The statements, opinions and data contained in all publications are solely those of the individual author(s) and contributor(s) and not of MDPI and/or the editor(s). MDPI and/or the editor(s) disclaim responsibility for any injury to people or property resulting from any ideas, methods, instructions or products referred to in the content.

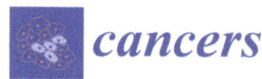 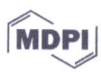

Article

CCR7 Mediates Cell Invasion and Migration in Extrahepatic Cholangiocarcinoma by Inducing Epithelial–Mesenchymal Transition

Mitsunobu Oba [1,2,†], Yoshitsugu Nakanishi [1,*,†], Tomoko Mitsuhashi [2], Katsunori Sasaki [1], Kanako C. Hatanaka [3,4], Masako Sasaki [5], Ayae Nange [3], Asami Okumura [3], Mariko Hayashi [1,2], Yusuke Yoshida [1,2], Takeo Nitta [1], Takashi Ueno [1], Toru Yamada [1], Masato Ono [1], Shota Kuwabara [1], Keisuke Okamura [1], Takahiro Tsuchikawa [1], Toru Nakamura [1], Takehiro Noji [1], Toshimichi Asano [1], Kimitaka Tanaka [1], Kiyoshi Takayama [5], Yutaka Hatanaka [3,4] and Satoshi Hirano [1]

1. Department of Gastroenterological Surgery II, Hokkaido University Faculty of Medicine, Sapporo 060-8638, Japan
2. Department of Surgical Pathology, Hokkaido University Hospital, Sapporo 060-8648, Japan
3. Research Division of Genome Companion Diagnostics, Hokkaido University Hospital, Sapporo 060-8648, Japan
4. Center for Development of Advanced Diagnostics (C-DAD), Hokkaido University Hospital, Sapporo 060-8648, Japan
5. NB Health Laboratory Co. Ltd., Sapporo 001-0021, Japan
* Correspondence: y.nakanishi@mac.com; Tel.: +81-11-706-7714; Fax: +81-11-706-7158
† These authors contributed equally to this work.

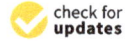

Citation: Oba, M.; Nakanishi, Y.; Mitsuhashi, T.; Sasaki, K.; Hatanaka, K.C.; Sasaki, M.; Nange, A.; Okumura, A.; Hayashi, M.; Yoshida, Y.; et al. CCR7 Mediates Cell Invasion and Migration in Extrahepatic Cholangiocarcinoma by Inducing Epithelial–Mesenchymal Transition. *Cancers* 2023, 15, 1878. https://doi.org/10.3390/cancers15061878

Academic Editors: Daniel L. Pouliquen and Cristina Núñez González

Received: 10 February 2023
Revised: 14 March 2023
Accepted: 15 March 2023
Published: 21 March 2023

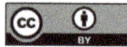

Copyright: © 2023 by the authors. Licensee MDPI, Basel, Switzerland. This article is an open access article distributed under the terms and conditions of the Creative Commons Attribution (CC BY) license (https://creativecommons.org/licenses/by/4.0/).

Simple Summary: Extrahepatic cholangiocarcinoma (EHCC) is an aggressive tumor. The five-year survival rate for patients who undergo surgical resection is only 20–40% due to recurrences. Therefore, elucidating the molecular mechanisms underlying invasion and metastasis in EHCC is crucial for developing adjuvant therapy. The epithelial–mesenchymal transition (EMT) contributes to the metastatic cascade in various tumors. C-C chemokine receptor 7 (CCR7) interacts with its ligand, chemokine (C-C motif) ligand 19 (CCL19), to promote EMT. The association between CCR7 expression and clinicopathological features and EMT status was examined via the immunohistochemical staining of tumor sections from 181 patients with perihilar cholangiocarcinoma. This association was then investigated in two EHCC cell lines. CCR7 mediates cell invasion and migration in EHCC by inducing EMT, which was abrogated by a CCR7 antagonist. CCR7 may be a potential target for adjuvant therapy in EHCC.

Abstract: The epithelial–mesenchymal transition (EMT) contributes to the metastatic cascade in various tumors. C-C chemokine receptor 7 (CCR7) interacts with its ligand, chemokine (C-C motif) ligand 19 (CCL19), to promote EMT. However, the association between EMT and CCR7 in extrahepatic cholangiocarcinoma (EHCC) remains unknown. This study aimed to elucidate the prognostic impact of CCR7 expression and its association with clinicopathological features and EMT in EHCC. The association between CCR7 expression and clinicopathological features and EMT status was examined via the immunohistochemical staining of tumor sections from 181 patients with perihilar cholangiocarcinoma. This association was then investigated in TFK-1 and EGI-1 EHCC cell lines. High-grade CCR7 expression was significantly associated with a large number of tumor buds, low E-cadherin expression, and poor overall survival. TFK-1 showed CCR7 expression, and Western blotting revealed E-cadherin downregulation and vimentin upregulation in response to CCL19 treatment. The wound healing and Transwell invasion assays revealed that the activation of CCR7 by CCL19 enhanced the migration and invasion of TFK-1 cells, which were abrogated by a CCR7 antagonist. These results suggest that a high CCR7 expression is associated with an adverse postoperative prognosis via EMT induction and that CCR7 may be a potential target for adjuvant therapy in EHCC.

Keywords: CCR7; CCL19; extrahepatic cholangiocarcinoma; epithelial–mesenchymal transition; tumor budding

1. Introduction

Extrahepatic cholangiocarcinoma (EHCC) and its subtypes, especially perihilar cholangiocarcinoma (PHCC), are aggressive tumors. PHCC is defined as a cancer that arises predominantly in the lobar extrahepatic bile ducts, distal to the segmental bile ducts, and proximal to the cystic duct [1]. The therapeutic gold standard for EHCC patients is complete tumor resection. However, due to the incidence of local or distant recurrences, the five-year survival rate for patients who underwent surgical resection is only 20–40% [2–4]. Moreover, PHCC, in particular, is often anatomically unresectable. Therefore, elucidating the mechanism of invasion and metastasis in EHCC is essential for developing adjuvant therapy for improving postoperative prognosis.

The epithelial–mesenchymal transition (EMT) is a crucial step in cancer progression [5,6]. It is a critical physiological process for embryonic development with phenotypic alterations, such as the loss of intercellular adhesion and cell polarity as well as acquisition of migratory and invasive abilities [7,8]. A hallmark of EMT is the downregulation of cell adhesion molecules, such as E-cadherin, and the upregulation of mesenchymal molecules, such as vimentin [7,8]. Aberrant EMT activation in malignant tumors can trigger tumor progression and metastasis [8]. However, the mechanism by which EMT occurs in EHCC remains unknown. Chemokines are a class of small molecule proteins that play significant roles in various physiological, pathological, and immunological responses when bound to their unique chemokine receptors on the cell surface. In the tumor microenvironment, chemokines and chemokine receptors play essential roles in tumor proliferation, invasion, and metastasis. C-C chemokine receptor type 7 (CCR7) is primarily expressed in B cells, naïve T cells, memory T cells, and mature dendritic cells and interacts with chemokine (C-C motif) ligand 19 (CCL19) [9] and CCL21 [10,11]. This interaction is vital for lymphocyte trafficking and lymph node homing [12,13]. Müller et al. first described the expression of CCR7 in the tumor microenvironment (in breast cancer) [9]. CCR7 expression in various tumors has been linked to tumor cell proliferation [14], invasion [15], angiogenesis [16], and metastasis [17]. Additionally, CCR7 induces EMT in the cells of breast [18], gastric [19], and pancreatic cancers [20]. Furthermore, CCR7 expression is correlated with poor prognosis in gastric cancer [21], esophageal squamous cell carcinoma [22], pancreatic cancer [23], urinary bladder cancer [24], and renal cell carcinoma [25]. Therefore, CCR7 overexpression in the tumor microenvironment is critical for cancer progression and metastasis. EHCC has a poor prognosis because it is metastasis-prone. To our knowledge, no study has assessed the frequency and impact of CCR7 expression in EHCC, which may be implicated in the molecular mechanisms underlying EMT, invasion, and metastasis.

The present study aimed to determine the impact of CCR7 expression on the clinicopathological features and postoperative survival of patients with EHCC and the relationship between CCR7 expression and EMT in human EHCC cell lines.

2. Materials and Methods

2.1. Patients

This study included patients ($n = 181$) with PHCC who underwent curative surgical resection between January 1995 and December 2016 at the Department of Gastroenterological Surgery II, Hokkaido University Hospital. Patients who received neoadjuvant chemotherapy or radiotherapy were excluded from the study. Clinical and pathological data of the patients were collected. Written informed consent was obtained from the patients and healthy volunteers from whom peripheral blood samples were collected to isolate peripheral blood mononuclear cells (PBMCs). This study was approved by the Hokkaido

University Institutional Review Board (No. 018-0137) and conducted in accordance with the guidelines of the institutional review board and the Declaration of Helsinki.

2.2. Tissue Preparation and Histopathology

After gross examination, all excised specimens were fixed in 10% buffered formalin and serially sectioned (3–6 mm). Subsequently, formalin-fixed paraffin-embedded blocks were sliced into 4 μm thick sections and stained for microscopic analysis with hematoxylin and eosin (H&E). Pathological primary tumor (pT) and regional lymph node metastasis were diagnosed as defined by the Cancer Staging Manual, 8th edition, American Joint Committee on Cancer (AJCC) [1].

2.3. Tissue Microarray

A tissue microarray [26] of all 181 samples was prepared for immunohistochemistry (IHC) staining. We first reviewed the archived H&E slides of all cases and selected a slide to determine two representative tumor areas (invasive front and center of the tumor) and one representative non-neoplastic area of the bile duct as an internal control. Subsequently, a manual tissue microarrayer (JF-4; Sakura Finetek, Tokyo, Japan) was used to inject 2.0 mm diameter needles into the corresponding sites on paraffin blocks. An experienced pathologist (T.M.) examined a section from each microarray stained with H&E, and evaluated the adequacy of tissue sampling and histopathological diagnosis.

2.4. Immunohistochemistry

Tissue sections were deparaffinized with xylene and rehydrated using a graded ethanol series. Heat-induced antigen retrieval was performed in a high-pH antigen retrieval buffer (BenchMark ULTRA; Roche, Basel, Switzerland). Endogenous peroxidase was blocked by incubation at 36 °C with 3% H_2O_2 for 4 min. Sections were subsequently labeled using the horseradish-peroxidase-labeled polymer method (Ventana ultraView DAB Universal Kit; Roche) and an automated immunostaining system (BenchMark ULTRA; Roche). Immunostained sections were counterstained with hematoxylin, dehydrated in ethanol, and cleared in xylene. Finally, sections were stained with anti-CCR7 (clone P-007, 1:100,000 dilution; NB Health Laboratory, Sapporo, Japan), anti-E-cadherin (clone 36, RTU, RRID: AB_397580; Ventana/Roche), and anti-vimentin (clone V9, RTU, RRID: AB_306239; Ventana/Roche) mouse monoclonal primary antibodies.

2.5. Assessment of Tumor Buds

Tumor buds, defined as dedifferentiated cancer cells or clusters of fewer than five cancer cells at the invasive front fields [27,28], reflect the ability of cells to migrate, invade, and metastasize. They are believed to undergo EMT and possess a mesenchymal phenotype [29–31]. We previously reported that the quantity of tumor buds at the invasive front fields reflects the EMT status and is associated with tumor invasion and metastasis in EHCC patients [32]. The tumor buds were counted in all 181 patients using previously described methods [32] to evaluate the association between their number and CCR7 expression. Using the International Tumor Budding Consensus Conference method, the tumor buds were counted on the H&E-stained slides containing whole tissue sections (Figure 1A,B) [26]. The H&E slide with the most significant tumor budding was selected for each patient. Tumor buds were counted in a single invasive front field at 200× magnification (0.785 mm^2), and the areas with the highest density of tumor buds were labeled hot spots [26].

2.6. IHC Scoring in TMA

We evaluated IHC staining based on the intensity and proportion of positive tumor cells in the TMA cores of 181 PHCC specimens and calculated the IHC score, previously reported as the "H score" [33]. The ordinal values for staining intensity are as follows: grade 0 (negative; Figure 1C), +1 (weak; Figure 1D), +2 (moderate; Figure 1E), and +3 (strong; Figure 1F). In CCR7, the staining intensity of tumor cells was regarded as strong (grade + 3) when the staining of the cytoplasm and tumor cell membranes was similar to that of the surrounding lymphocytes. Next, the percentage of each grade of tumor cells in each spot of the TMA core was estimated. Subsequently, the H scores of the samples were calculated as the product of the percentage of stained cells and corresponding staining intensity (0, 1, 2, or 3) as follows: H score = sum of (IHC staining grade × % of tumor cells with each IHC staining grade). For example, when the percentages of tumor cells with IHC staining grades of 0, +1, +2, and +3 on the spot were 10, 30, 35, and 25%, respectively, the H score of that spot was calculated as (0 × 10 + 1 × 30 + 2 × 35 + 3 × 25) = 175. E-cadherin and vimentin staining was assessed as described previously [32]. Briefly, the staining intensities of tumor buds were initially classified into three groups (grade 0 (negative; E-cadherin, Figure 1G; vimentin, Figure 1J), +1 (weak–moderate; E-cadherin, Figure 1H; vimentin, Figure 1K), and +2 (strong; E-cadherin, Figure 1I; vimentin, Figure 1L)), and the proportion of tumor cells with each grade on each spot of the TMA core was estimated. Subsequently, the H score was determined using the same formula as CCR7. Three researchers (M.O., Y.N., and T.M.), blinded to the clinical information of patients, independently examined and scored each case. Differences in interpretation were resolved by consensus among the three researchers.

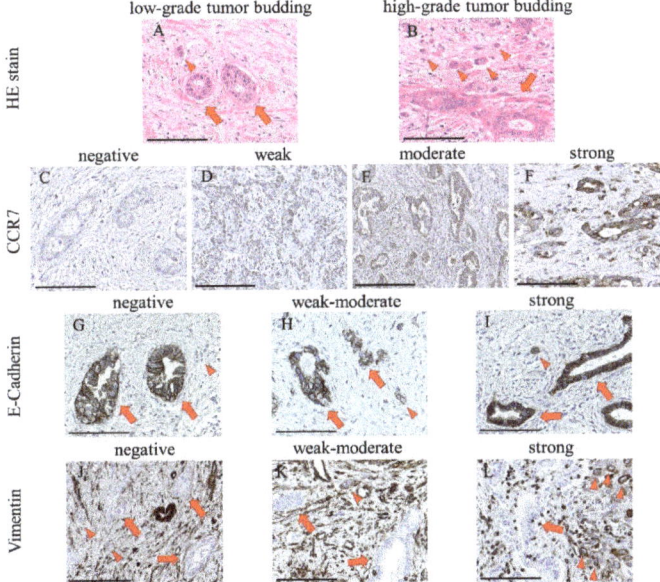

Figure 1. CCR7 expression and epithelial–mesenchymal transition status in perihilar cholangiocarcinoma. (**A,B**) Representative images of hematoxylin and eosin staining for low-grade (**A**) and high-grade (**B**) tumor budding from $n = 181$ samples. The arrows and arrowheads indicate neoplastic glandular structures and tumor bud cells, respectively. (**C–F**) Immunohistochemical detection of negative (**C**), weak (**D**), moderate (**E**), and strong (**F**) CCR7 expression in tumor cells. CCR7 protein was detected in the cytoplasm and cell membranes of tumor cells and the surrounding lymphocytes. The staining intensity of strongly stained tumor cells was comparable to that of the surrounding lymphocytes. The arrows and arrowheads indicate neoplastic glandular structures and lymphocytes, respectively. (**G–I**) E-cadherin was detected in the cell membrane of neoplastic glandular structures, while tumor bud cells showed negative (**G**), weak–moderate (**H**), or strong (**I**) staining for E-cadherin. The arrows and arrowheads indicate neoplastic glandular structures and tumor bud cells, respectively. (**J–L**) Vimentin was not expressed in neoplastic glandular structures, while tumor bud cells displayed negative (**J**), weak–moderate (**K**), or strong (**L**) staining for vimentin. The arrows and arrowheads indicate neoplastic glandular structures and tumor bud cells, respectively. Scale bar = 100 μm.

2.7. EMT Status in IHC Examination

We examined the association between the IHC staining scores for CCR7 expression in 181 PHCC specimens and EMT status defined by the combination of E-cadherin and vimentin IHC staining scores using TMA. EMT status was defined and each case was divided into three groups: (1) cases in which the epithelial status (Figure 1I,J) was high E-cadherin with low vimentin expression (E-high/V-low); (2) cases in which the intermediate status was low (E-low/V-low) or high (E-high/V-high) expression of E-cadherin and vimentin; and (3) cases in which the mesenchymal status (Figure 1G,L) was low E-cadherin with high vimentin expression (E-low/V-high). We also examined the association between the IHC staining H scores for CCR7 expression and the number of tumor buds. Median values established the boundaries between low and high H scores for E-cadherin and vimentin.

2.8. Cell Culture

Two human EHCC cell lines, TFK-1 and EGI-1, were used in this study. The cell lines were obtained from the RIKEN BioResource Center (RIKEN BRC, Tsukuba, Japan) and the German Collection of Microorganisms and Cell Cultures GmbH (DSMZ, Braunschweig, Germany), respectively. TFK-1 and EGI-1 were cultured in RPMI-1640 and EMEM supplemented with 4 mM L-glutamine and 2× MEM amino acids—both essential and non-essential. Next, 10% (v/v) fetal bovine serum (FBS), 100 U/mL penicillin, and 100 µg/mL streptomycin were added to each medium. All cell lines were cultured at a density of 0.5–2.0×10^6 cells/mL at 37 °C and 5% CO_2. Human peripheral blood aspirates were obtained by venipuncture from a healthy volunteer with written informed consent, and peripheral blood mononuclear cells (PBMCs) were separated by Ficoll density gradient centrifugation.

2.9. RNA Extraction and Reverse Transcription PCR

CCR7 mRNA levels were determined using reverse transcription (RT)-PCR. Total RNA was extracted using an RNeasy Plus Mini Kit (QIAGEN GmbH, Hilden, Germany) according to the manufacturer's instructions. Samples were quantified using a NanoDrop 2000c Spectrophotometer (Thermo Fisher Scientific, Waltham, MA, USA). cDNA was synthesized using the Super Script™ III First-Strand Synthesis System for RT-PCR (Invitrogen Life Technologies, Carlsbad, CA, USA) using 1.0 µg of RNA following the manufacturer's protocol. RT-PCR was performed using a GeneTouch Thermal Cycler (Hangzhou Bioer Technology, Hangzhou, China). The PCR conditions were as follows: initial denaturation at 94 °C for 2 min, followed by 33 cycles of denaturation at 98 °C for 10 s, annealing at 60 °C for 30 s, and extension at 68 °C for 30 s (CCR7), followed by 25 cycles of denaturation at 98 °C for 10 s and annealing and extension at 68 °C for 30 s (β-actin). The PCR was performed using KOD Plus Ver.2 (TOYOBO, Osaka, Japan) according to the manufacturer's instructions. Primers were synthesized at Eurofins Genomics (Tokyo, Japan) and were as follows: CCR7 sense, 5′-ACATCGGAGACAACACCACA-3′ and antisense, 5′-CATGCCACTGAAGAAGCTCA-3′; β-actin sense, 5′-CAACCGCGAGAAGATGACCC-3′ and antisense, 5′-GGAACCGCTCATTGCCAATGG-3′. RT-PCR products were visualized with ethidium bromide (0.5 µg/mL) using a ChemiDoc™ XRS Plus System (Bio-Rad Laboratories; Hercules, CA, USA). Quantitative analyses of data were carried out using TaqMan gene expression assays (CCR7 Assay ID: Hs01013469_m1, and ACTB Assay ID: Hs01060665_g1; Applied Biosystems/Thermo Fisher Scientific). The expression level of CCR7 mRNA was calculated using the ratio of CCR7 mRNA to β-actin mRNA.

2.10. Western Blot Analysis

The cells were cultured with or without 100 ng/mL CCL19 for 48 h. The harvested cells were suspended in lysis buffer containing 50 mM Tris-HCl (pH 8.0), 150 mM NaCl, 1% (v/v) Nonidet P-40 alternative, 0.1% (w/v) sodium dodecyl sulfate (SDS), 0.5% (w/v) sodium deoxycholate, and protease inhibitor cocktail (Promega, Madison, WI, USA) and lysed with sonication successively. The total protein was extracted by centrifugation.

The concentration of the extracted protein was determined using a TaKaRa BCA protein assay kit (Takara Bio, Kusatsu, Japan) following the manufacturer's instructions. For immunoblotting, cell lysates were loaded at a protein concentration of 20 μg per well. Proteins were separated by 7.5% sodium dodecyl sulfate-polyacrylamide gel electrophoresis (SDS-PAGE) and transferred to a polyvinylidene fluoride (PVDF) membrane (Immobilon-P Transfer Membrane; Merck Millipore, Darmstadt, Germany). The membrane was blocked with 5% (w/v) skimmed milk in Tris-buffered saline (50 mM Tris-HCl, 150 mM NaCl, pH 8.0) with Tween 20 (TBS-T). They were then probed with E-cadherin rabbit polyclonal antibody (1:10,000 dilution; Proteintech Group, Chicago, IL, USA) and vimentin rabbit polyclonal antibody (1:2000 dilution; Proteintech Group) for 90 min at 25 °C. After washing with TBS-T, they were incubated with anti-rabbit IgG antibodies conjugated to horseradish peroxidase (1:10,000 dilution; Jackson ImmunoResearch Laboratories, West Grove, PA, USA) for 60 min at 25 °C. For β-actin, the membranes were incubated with anti-β-actin IgG antibodies conjugated to horseradish peroxidase (1:10,000 dilution; Cell Signaling Technology, Danvers, MA, USA). After applying Amersham ECL Prime Western blotting Detection Reagent (GE Healthcare Limited, Buckinghamshire, UK), the protein bands were visualized using a chemiluminescent detection system (ChemiDoc™ XRS Plus System; Bio-Rad Laboratories). Thereafter, membranes were stripped with Western blotting stripping buffer (Takara Bio) and then washed and re-probed with the aforementioned antibodies. Semi-quantitative analyses of data were carried out using Image Lab™ 5.1 (Bio-Rad Laboratories). β-Actin was used as an endogenous loading control. The experiment was repeated thrice.

2.11. Wound Healing Assay

A Culture-Insert 2 well, which is a silicon gasket with two 70-μL wells (Ibidi, Grafelfing, Germany), was placed on a 24-well plate surface. The cells were added into each chamber (3.5×10^4 cells) and incubated until the cells grew to confluence. Subsequently, the Culture-Insert was removed gently, after which the cells were washed twice with PBS and then cultured in 500 μL serum-free medium with or without 100 ng/mL CCL19 (BioLegend, San Diego, CA, USA). Cell migration to close the gap was examined at 0, 24, and 48 h by microscopy. Areas of the initial gap and the part filled by migration were measured on the images, and the rate of migration area was calculated using the following formula:

Rate of migration area (%) = (area of the part filled by migration)/(area of initial gap).

The area was evaluated using a high-resolution imaging and analysis system, BZ-9000 (KEYENCE, Osaka, Japan). The experiment was performed in triplicate.

2.12. Cell Proliferation Assay

The cells were seeded at a density of 2000 cells/well in 96-well plates and incubated for 24 and 48 h with or without 100 ng/mL CCL19. Cell proliferation was assessed using a one-step Cell Counting Kit-8 (CCK-8; Dojindo Laboratories, Kumamoto, Japan). Following the manufacturer's instructions, 10 μL of CCK-8 solution was added to each well and incubated for 3 h. Finally, the absorbance at 450 and 650 nm was recorded using a SpectraMax 190 reader (Molecular Devices, San Jose, CA, USA). The experiment was repeated thrice.

2.13. Migration and Invasion Assay

Transwell® inserts (6.5 mm diameter, 8 μm pores; Corning Inc., Corning, NY, USA) were used to determine cell migration. For the invasion assay, Matrigel® invasion chambers (6.4 mm diameter, 8 μm pores; Corning Inc.) were used. Each cell resuspended in 200 μL of medium with or without 100 ng/mL CCL19 containing 1% FBS was added to the upper compartment of the chamber. In the migration assay, 5.0×10^4 cells of TFK-1 and 1.0×10^4 cells of EGI-1 were seeded. In the invasion assay, 1.0×10^5 TFK-1 and 1.0×10^4 EGI-1 cells were seeded. Afterward, 500 μL of each medium containing 10% FBS was placed into the lower chamber. In the migration assay, when required, each cell was preincubated for 6 h with 15 μg/mL human CCR7 antibody as a neutralizing antibody (clone 150503; R&D Systems, Minneapolis, MN, USA) or mouse monoclonal IgG as an isotype control (clone 20102; R&D Systems). After 48-h incubation, non-migrating cells on the upper surface of the membrane were removed with a cotton swab. The invading cells on the lower surface of the insert were stained with Diff-Quik stain (Sysmex Corporation, Kobe, Japan) and digitally photographed. The tumor cell invasion area was evaluated using a high-resolution imaging and analysis system, BZ-9000 (KEYENCE). Each experiment was performed in triplicate.

2.14. Statistical Analyses

Qualitative variables were analyzed using the chi-square test. Quantitative variables were analyzed using the one-way analysis of variance (ANOVA) to compare the differences between two or more groups. Comparisons between multiple groups were performed using analysis of variance with a post-hoc pairwise t-test. Correlations between CCR7 expression and the number of tumor buds were evaluated using Spearman's rank method. Overall survival (OS) was calculated using the median time between the date of surgery and the date of the last follow-up or death. The cut-off value of the CCR7 staining H score for discriminating postoperative OS was obtained using a recursive partitioning technique. Kaplan–Meier estimates of OS curves were compared using the log-rank test. In the multivariate analysis of OS, the significance of prognostic factors was investigated using Cox proportional hazards models. The significance level was set to $p < 0.05$, and the confidence interval was 95%. Statistical analysis was performed using JMP software for Windows (version 14.0; SAS Institute, Inc., Cary, NC, USA).

3. Results

3.1. CCR7 Expression Was Observed in PHCC Tumor Tissues

In the IHC examination (Figure 1), the CCR7 protein was detected in the cytoplasm and membranes of PHCC cells (Figure 1D–F). The medians (range) of the IHC H scores for CCR7, E-cadherin, and vimentin expression were 90 (0–300), 80 (0–200), and 0 (0–200), respectively. Histograms of the H scores for CCR7 expression are shown in Figure 2A. Based on a cut-off value of 170, the H-score of CCR7 expression was classified into two grades: low-grade, 0–169, and high-grade, ≥170. Based on their median values, the cut-off values for low or high H scores for E-cadherin and vimentin were 70 and 10, respectively.

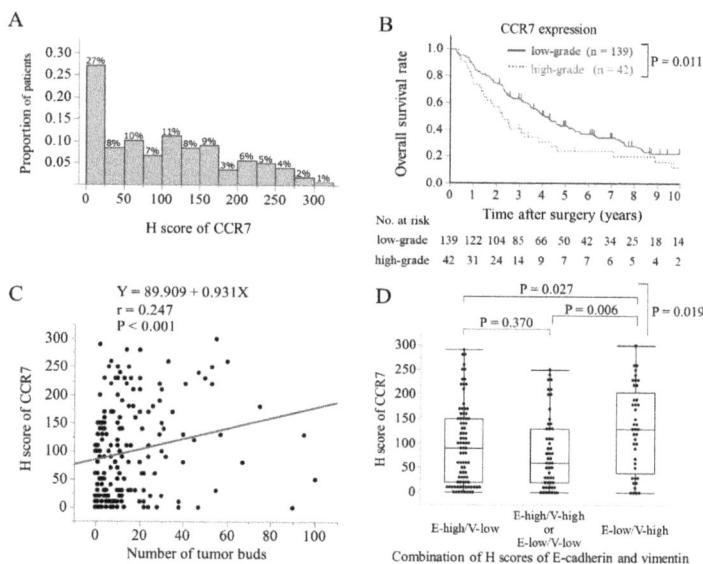

Figure 2. CCR7 expression was associated with poor prognosis and EMT status. (**A**) Histograms

displaying patient distribution according to IHC staining scores of CCR7 expression. (**B**) Kaplan–Meier survival curves for the 181 patients with perihilar cholangiocarcinoma based on CCR7 expression grade. According to the log-rank test, patients with high CCR7 expression had a significantly worse long-term overall survival rate than those with low CCR7 expression ($p = 0.011$). (**C**) The correlation between IHC staining scores for CCR7 expression and the number of tumor buds was assessed using Spearman's rank method. High CCR7 expression grade was associated with the number of tumor buds ($p < 0.001$). (**D**) The relationship between CCR7 expression and the combination of the H scores of E-cadherin (E) and vimentin (V) was assessed using an analysis of variance with post-hoc pairwise t-test. High-grade CCR7 expression correlated significantly with EMT status ($p = 0.019$).

3.2. Clinicopathological Features and Overall Survival Were Associated with CCR7 Expression

High-grade CCR7 expression was associated with poor histological differentiation ($p = 0.003$; chi-squared test) and microscopic venous invasion ($p = 0.036$; chi-squared test) (Table 1). The median (range) follow-up time after surgery was 40 (3–231) months. Table 2 summarizes the results of the univariate and multivariate analyses of the effects of clinicopathological factors on postoperative OS in 181 patients with PHCC. Patients with high-grade CCR7 expression exhibited a significantly worse OS than those with low CCR7 expression according to the log-rank test ($p = 0.011$; Figure 2B). Moreover, multivariate analysis identified CCR7 protein expression level (HR, 1.67, 95% CI, 1.10–2.48, $p = 0.017$) and pT and pN classification as the independent prognostic factors for OS in patients with PHCC.

Table 1. Comparison of the clinicopathological features among patients with different CCR7 expression grades ($n = 181$).

		CCR7 Expression Grades				
		Low-Grade ($n = 139$)		High-Grade ($n = 42$)		
Clinicopathological feature		n	(%)	n	(%)	p
Age	<70	66	(47.5)	27	(64.3)	0.055
	≥70	73	(52.5)	15	(35.7)	
Sex	Male	108	(77.7)	35	(83.3)	0.423
	Female	31	(22.3)	7	(16.7)	
Histological grade	G1	45	(32.4)	4	(9.5)	0.003
	G2	68	(48.9)	23	(54.8)	
	G3	26	(18.7)	15	(35.7)	
pT classification (AJCC, 8th edition)	T1	3	(2.2)	2	(4.8)	0.242
	T2	94	(67.6)	23	(54.8)	
	T3	25	(18.0)	7	(16.7)	
	T4	17	(12.2)	10	(23.8)	
pN classification (AJCC, 8th edition)	N0	75	(54.0)	24	(57.1)	0.674
	N1	55	(39.6)	14	(33.3)	
	N2	9	(6.5)	4	(9.5)	
pM classification (AJCC, 8th edition)	M0	137	(98.6)	41	(97.6)	0.688
	M1	2	(1.4)	1	(2.4)	
Microscopic lymphatic invasion	Absent	66	(47.5)	18	(42.9)	0.598
	Present	73	(52.5)	24	(57.1)	
Microscopic venous invasion	Absent	61	(43.9)	11	(26.2)	0.036
	Present	78	(56.1)	31	(73.8)	
Microscopic perineural invasion	Absent	11	(7.9)	6	(14.3)	0.235
	Present	128	(92.1)	36	(85.7)	
Invasive carcinoma at resected margin	Negative	124	(89.2)	34	(81.0)	0.176
	Positive	15	(10.8)	8	(19.1)	
Median survival time (years)		3.9		2.3		0.018

G1, well differentiated; G2, moderately differentiated; G3, poorly differentiated (according to the AJCC 8th edition). Low-grade, H-score of CCR7 staining 0–169; high-grade, H-score of CCR7 staining ≥170. AJCC, American Joint Committee on Cancer.

Table 2. Univariate and multivariate analyses of factors associated with the overall survival of the 181 patients with PHCC.

Variable		No. of Patients		Univariate		Multivariate	
		n	(%)	Median Survival (Months)	p	Relative Risk (95% CI)	p
Age (years)	<70	93	(51.4)	46	0.491		
	≥70	88	(48.6)	44			
Sex	Male	143	(79.0)	46	0.529		
	Female	38	(21.0)	44			
Histological grade	G1	49	(27.1)	56	0.221		
	G2	91	(50.3)	43			
	G3	41	(22.7)	28			
pT classification (AJCC, 8th edition)	T1	5	(2.8)	53	0.001	1	0.026
	T2	117	(64.6)	53		1.07 (0.39–4.45)	
	T3	32	(17.7)	30		1.70 (0.56–7.36)	
	T4	27	(14.9)	21		2.14 (0.71–9.30)	
pN classification (AJCC, 8th edition)	N0	99	(54.7)	76	<0.001	1	<0.001
	N1	69	(38.1)	29		2.32 (1.60–3.36)	
	N2	13	(7.2)	19		3.21 (1.54–6.16)	
pM classification (AJCC, 8th edition)	M0	178	(98.3)	46	0.011	1	0.265
	M1	3	(1.7)	16		2.27 (0.49–7.78)	
Microscopic lymphatic invasion	Absent	84	(46.4)	57	0.094		
	Present	97	(53.6)	30			
Microscopic venous invasion	Absent	72	(39.8)	53	0.009	1	0.183
	Present	109	(60.2)	32		1.30 (0.88–1.93)	
Microscopic perineural invasion	Absent	17	(9.4)	58	0.195		
	Present	164	(90.6)	43			
Invasive carcinoma at resected margin	Negative	158	(87.3)	49	<0.001	1	0.056
	Positive	23	(12.7)	21		1.66 (0.98–2.67)	
CCR7 expression grade	Low-grade	139	(76.8)	50	0.011	1	0.017
	High-grade	42	(23.2)	27		1.67 (1.10–2.48)	

PHCC, perihilar cholangiocarcinoma; G1, well differentiated; G2, moderately differentiated; G3, poorly differentiated (according to the AJCC 8th edition). Low-grade, H-score of CCR7 staining 0–169; high-grade, H-score of CCR7 staining ≥170. AJCC, American Joint Committee on Cancer; CCR7, C-C chemokine receptor type 7; CI, Confidence interval; PHCC, perihilar cholangiocarcinoma.

3.3. High CCR7 Expression Was Associated with EMT

The intensity of CCR7 expression was correlated with the number of tumor buds ($p < 0.001$, $r = 0.247$; Spearman's rank method; Figure 2C). The median (range) scores of CCR7 expression in epithelial status (E-high/V-low), intermediate status (E-low/V-low or E-high/V-high), and mesenchymal status (E-low/V-high) were 90 (0–290), 60 (0–250), and 130 (0–300), respectively. CCR7 expression was significantly higher in the mesenchymal state than that in the epithelial or intermediate states ($p = 0.019$, ANOVA; Figure 2D).

3.4. CCR7 Expression Was Observed in TFK-1 Cells

Before investigating the effect of the CCL19/CCR7 axis on the proliferation, migration, and invasion abilities of EHCC cells via EMT, we screened for endogenous CCR7 expression in TFK-1 and EGI-1. CCR7 mRNA was found in TFK-1 cells but not in EGI-1 cells (Figure 3A).

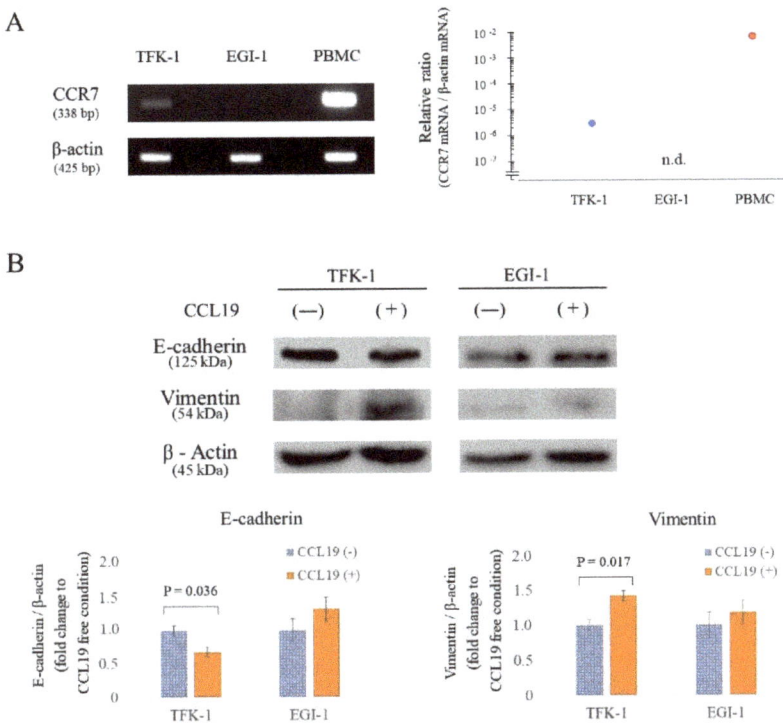

Figure 3. CCR7 expression and the effect of CCL19/CCR7 on EMT-related proteins in cholangiocarcinoma cells. (**A**) RT-PCR analysis of CCR7 mRNA expression in each cell line. CCR7 mRNA levels were standardized with respect to β-actin mRNA. CCR7 mRNA was detected in TFK-1 and PBMCs but not in EGI-1. n.d.; not detected. (**B**) Changes in E-cadherin and vimentin protein levels following treatment with 100 ng/mL CCL19 in each cell line were evaluated using Western blotting. TFK-1 cells showed significant downregulation of E-cadherin ($p = 0.036$) and upregulation of vimentin ($p = 0.017$) in response to CCL19 treatment (one-way ANOVA). Data were normalized to β-actin levels. n.d.; not detected. The uncropped blots are shown in Figure S1.

3.5. CCR7/CCL19 Axis Affects the Expression of EMT-Related Proteins

Western blot analyses were performed to determine the variation of E-cadherin and vimentin protein levels in each cell line following 100 ng/mL CCL19 treatment for 48 h. E-cadherin expression was significantly decreased ($p = 0.036$; Figure 3B), and vimentin expression was significantly increased ($p = 0.017$; Figure 3B) in TFK-1 cells after stimulation with CCL19. On the other hand, EGI-1 showed no significant change ($p > 0.05$; Figure 3B).

3.6. CCL19 Promotes Lateral Migration of TFK-1 Cells

The lateral migration ability and migration ability enhancement of each cell line following CCL19 treatment were investigated using an in vitro wound healing assay. As shown in Figure 4A, TFK-1 and EGI-1 cells showed slight migration. However, CCL19 treatment significantly enhanced the migration ability of TFK-1 cells at 48 h ($p = 0.035$). On the other hand, in the EGI-1 cells, CCL19 treatment did not show any effect ($p > 0.05$).

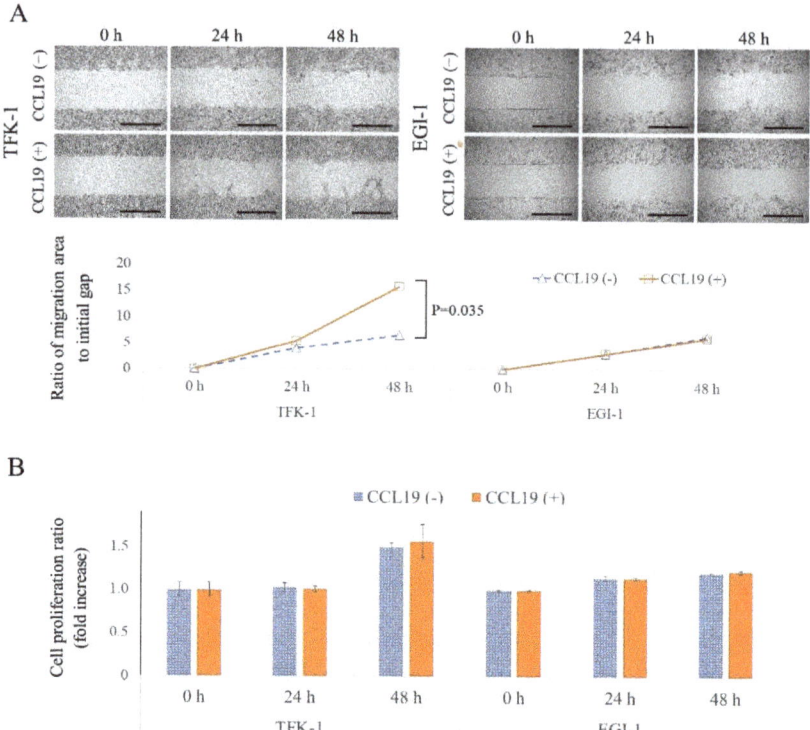

Figure 4. Effect of CCL19/CCR7 on migration and cell proliferation. (**A**) A wound healing assay was used to determine lateral migration ability with or without CCL19 (100 ng/mL) for 24 and 48 h. Migration was significantly enhanced by treatment with CCL19 in TFK-1 cells ($p = 0.035$, one-way ANOVA). Scale bar = 500 μm. (**B**) Cell proliferation assay showing the effect of CCL19 (100 ng/mL) treatment at 0, 24, and 48 h using the WST-8 method. Absorbance at 450 nm was measured against a reference wavelength of 650 nm. Each bar represents the mean ± SD of three independent experiments.

3.7. CCL19 Did Not Affect Cell Proliferation

In the wound healing assay, there is a possibility that the gap could be filled not only by cell migration but also by cell proliferation. Therefore, the degree of cell proliferation under the same culture conditions as the wound healing assay was evaluated. No enhancement in cell proliferation was observed with CCL19 treatment ($p > 0.05$; Figure 4B).

3.8. CCL19 Promotes the Migration and Invasion of TFK-1 Cells

The vertical migration and invasion abilities of each cell line, and enhancements in these abilities following CCL19 treatment, were investigated using Transwell® inserts and Matrigel® invasion chambers. CCL19 treatment significantly enhanced the migration and invasion abilities of TFK-1 cells at 48 h ($p = 0.016$, Figure 5A and $p < 0.001$, Figure 5B, respectively). However, in the EGI-1 cells, CCL19 treatment did not show any effect ($p > 0.05$; Figure 5A,B).

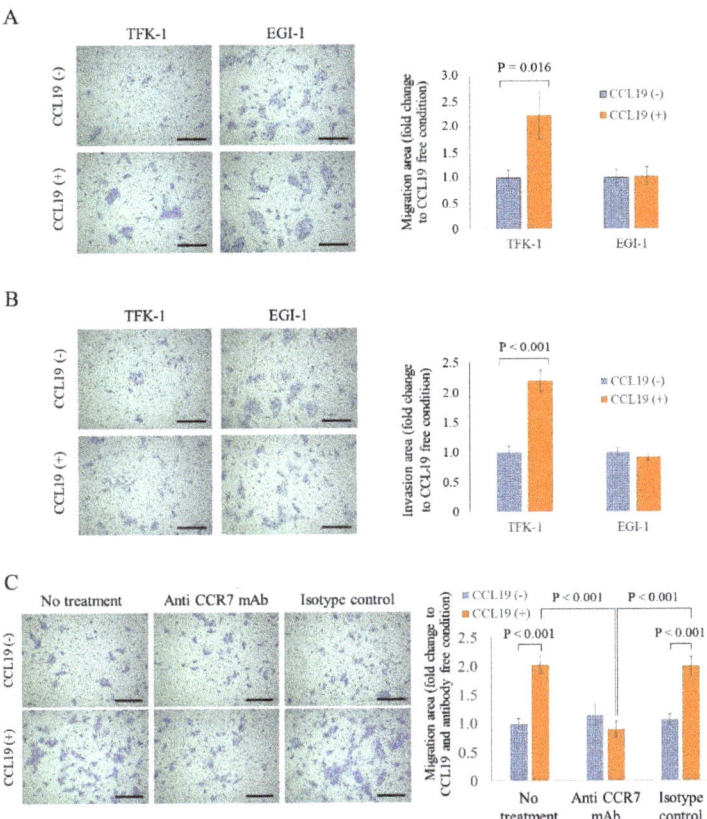

Figure 5. CCR7-dependent CCL19 promoted migration and invasion in cells. (**A**) The migration assay, used to determine the vertical migration ability for 48 h, showed that migration was significantly enhanced by treatment with CCL19 (100 ng/mL) in TFK-1 cells only ($p = 0.016$, one-way ANOVA). (**B**) The invasion assay, used to determine the invasion ability for 48 h, showed that invasion was significantly enhanced by treatment with CCL19 (100 ng/mL) in TFK-1 cells only ($p < 0.001$, one-way ANOVA). (**C**) A migration assay performed after preincubation of TFK-1 with 15 μg/mL anti-CCR7 antibodies for 6 h showed that anti-CCR7 antibody significantly suppressed CCL19-mediated migration ($p < 0.001$, one-way ANOVA). Panels on the left in (**A**–**C**) show representative images of cells at the end-point, while those on the right show the quantification of the area covered by the assayed cells. Scale bar = 100 μm. Each bar represents the mean ± SD of three independent experiments.

3.9. CCR7 Antagonist Inhibits CCL19-Mediated Migration of TFK-1 Cells

Next, we examined whether the enhanced migration of TFK-1 cells, stimulated upon CCL19 treatment, could be inhibited by using an anti-CCR7 antibody that could neutralize the effect of CCL19. Pretreatment with an anti-CCR7 antibody completely counteracted the CCL19-mediated migration of TFK-1 cells (Figure 5C). As a control, the IgG isotype control did not suppress the enhancement of CCL19-mediated migration.

4. Discussion

In the present study, we aimed to investigate the impact of CCR7 expression on the clinicopathological features and postoperative survival in patients with PHCC and the relationship between CCR7 expression and EMT status in human EHCC cell lines. The results of the clinicopathological examination showed that high-grade CCR7 expression was one of the most adverse postoperative prognostic factors in patients who underwent surgical resections for PHCC, and it was associated with a higher number of tumor buds and mesenchymal status (a combination of low E-cadherin and high vimentin expression). These results indicate that high CCR7 expression may be associated with poor OS via EMT in patients with PHCC.

Therefore, we investigated the association between CCR7 expression and EMT in human EHCC cell lines in vitro. Among the two human EHCC cell lines tested, CCR7 was detected in TFK-1 but not EGI-1. The CCR7/CCL19 interaction significantly enhanced lateral migration ability in the wound healing assay, along with vertical migration and invasion ability in the Transwell migration and invasion assays of TFK-1 cells. Notably, this effect was not observed in EGI-1 cells. Furthermore, neither cell line exhibited enhanced proliferation after the CCL19 treatment, suggesting that the cell filling observed in the wound healing assay was a result of enhanced migration rather than proliferation. Following treatment with CCL19, the epithelial marker E-cadherin was downregulated, whereas the mesenchymal marker vimentin was upregulated in TFK-1 cells. These results suggest that CCL19 induces EMT in human EHCC cells that are positive for CCR7.

Furthermore, we found that stimulation of TFK-1 cells with CCL19 increased cell migration, and the anti-CCR7 antibody significantly suppressed this increase. These results confirmed that CCR7 activation is responsible for increased migration, suggesting that CCR7 may be an effective therapeutic target. Beatriz et al. [34] revealed the efficacy of the anti-CCR7 antibody treatment against a xenograft human mantle cell lymphoma model in vivo. However, CCR7 is also responsible for the migration of CCR7-expressing cells, such as natural regulatory T cells or semi-mature dendritic cells, which are involved in immune tolerance [35,36]. Anti-CCR7 therapy may also suppress the migration of such physiological CCR7-expressing cells, and its immediate implementation in clinical practice needs to be carefully considered. In this regard, Winter et al. [37] demonstrated that the chronic deficiency of CCR7 could lead to autoimmune diseases. Because certain types of immunodeficiency may be induced with anti-CCR7 therapy, additional research is required to develop alternative strategies, such as targeting CCR7 exclusively in cancer cells or inhibiting CCR7-associated signal transduction pathways. In future clinical applications, anti-CCR7 antibodies may represent an adjunct therapy to enhance the efficacy of existing chemotherapy techniques, similar to anti-HER2 therapy in breast cancer. This may be particularly important if CCR7 expression is high in resected or biopsy specimens, as the combination of anti-CCR7 antibodies with gemcitabine or cisplatin may inhibit recurrence or promote response.

The present study had several limitations. First, in this retrospective study, samples were collected from a single Japanese center. Notably, a meta-analysis reported that the impact of high CCR7 expression on poor OS was more significant in Asian patients than that in Caucasians [38]. Therefore, a larger and more diverse sample must be analyzed to eliminate the risk of bias and validate the conclusions of this study. Second, IHC was utilized to evaluate clinical tumor samples. Although IHC staining has been widely used in several protein expression studies, it has disadvantages, such as disparities in technical procedures and scoring standards among facilities and studies. Therefore, a multi-institutional prospective study is required to confirm these results. Third, this study is focused on CCL19/CCR7 interactions, but another ligand of CCR7, CCL21, is similar to CCL19 and may also be relevant to the topic of this study. Although CCL19 is considered more efficient than CCL21 in activating ERK1/2 [39] related to EMT, the two ligands share only 32% amino acid identity and have ligand bias [40]. Therefore, there is a possibility that further knowledge will be obtained based on experiments involving CCL21. Fourth, the present study did not explore signaling pathways nor conduct in vivo experiments with animal models that provide a tumor microenvironment similar to that of humans.

5. Conclusions

The present study suggests that CCR7 mediates EMT progression, and high CCR7 expression is associated with a poor prognosis owing to EMT. Therefore, in the future, CCR7 could be a potential therapeutic target for PHCC adjuvant therapy.

Supplementary Materials: The following supporting information can be downloaded at: https://www.mdpi.com/article/10.3390/cancers15061878/s1, Figure S1: Western blot.

Author Contributions: M.O. (Mitsunobu Oba) and Y.N. conceptualized, designed, and performed the study and wrote the manuscript; T.M., M.H., Y.Y., T.N. (Takeo Nitta), T.U., T.Y., M.O. (Masato Ono) and S.K. performed pathological diagnosis; K.O., T.T., T.N. (Toru Nakamura), T.N. (Takehiro Noji), T.A., K.T. (Kimitaka Tanaka), K.T. (Kiyoshi Takayama), Y.H. and S.H. developed methodologies, reviewed and revised the manuscript; M.O. (Mitsunobu Oba), Y.N., M.H., Y.Y., T.N. (Takeo Nitta) and T.U. acquired, analyzed and interpreted the data; K.S., K.C.H., M.S., A.N. and A.O. provided technical and material support. All authors have read and agreed to the published version of the manuscript.

Funding: This research received no external funding.

Institutional Review Board Statement: This study was conducted in accordance with the Declaration of Helsinki and approved by the Institutional Review Board of Hokkaido University (protocol code No. 018-0137 and date of approval 18 December 2018).

Informed Consent Statement: Informed consent was obtained from all subjects involved in the study. Written informed consent has been obtained from the patients to publish this paper.

Data Availability Statement: The datasets generated and/or analyzed during the current study are not publicly available due to privacy reasons but are available from the corresponding author on reasonable request.

Acknowledgments: The authors are grateful to the Department of Gastroenterological Surgery II, Hokkaido University Faculty of Medicine for their scientific advice.

Conflicts of Interest: The authors declare no conflict of interest.

References

1. Amin, M.B.; Edge, S.; Greene, F.; Byrd, D.R.; Washington, M.K.; Brookland, R.K.; Washington, M.K.; Gershenwald, J.E.; Compton, C.C.; Hess, K.R.; et al. *AJCC Cancer Staging Manual*, 8th ed.; Springer: New York, NY, USA, 2016.
2. DeOliveira, M.L.; Cunningham, S.C.; Cameron, J.L.; Kamangar, F.; Winter, J.M.; Lillemoe, K.D.; Choti, M.A.; Yeo, C.J.; Schulick, R.D. Cholangiocarcinoma: Thirty-one-year experience with 564 patients at a single institution. *Ann. Surg.* **2007**, *245*, 755–762. [CrossRef]
3. van der Gaag, N.A.; Kloek, J.J.; de Bakker, J.K.; Musters, B.; Geskus, R.B.; Busch, O.R.C.; Bosma, A.; Gouma, D.J.; van Gulik, T.M. Survival analysis and prognostic nomogram for patients undergoing resection of extrahepatic cholangiocarcinoma. *Ann. Oncol.* **2012**, *23*, 2642–2649. [CrossRef] [PubMed]
4. Nakanishi, Y.; Okamura, K.; Tsuchikawa, T.; Nakamura, T.; Noji, T.; Asano, T.; Matsui, A.; Tanaka, K.; Murakami, S.; Ebihara, Y.; et al. Time to recurrence after surgical resection and survival after recurrence among patients with perihilar and distal cholangiocarcinomas. *Ann. Surg. Oncol.* **2020**, *27*, 4171–4180. [CrossRef] [PubMed]
5. Cao, H.; Xu, E.; Liu, H.; Wan, L.; Lai, M. Epithelial-mesenchymal transition in colorectal cancer metastasis: A system review. *Pathol. Res. Pract.* **2015**, *211*, 557–569. [CrossRef]
6. Sung, W.J.; Kim, H.; Park, K.K. The biological role of epithelial-mesenchymal transition in lung cancer (review). *Oncol. Rep.* **2016**, *36*, 1199–1206. [CrossRef]
7. Thiery, J.P.; Sleeman, J.P. Complex networks orchestrate epithelial-mesenchymal transitions. *Nat. Rev. Mol. Cell Biol.* **2006**, *7*, 131–142. [CrossRef]
8. Thiery, J.P.; Acloque, H.; Huang, R.Y.; Nieto, M.A. Epithelial-mesenchymal transitions in development and disease. *Cell* **2009**, *139*, 871–890. [CrossRef]
9. Müller, A.; Homey, B.; Soto, H.; Ge, N.; Catron, D.; Buchanan, M.E.; McClanahan, T.; Murphy, E.; Yuan, W.; Wagner, S.N.; et al. Involvement of chemokine receptors in breast cancer metastasis. *Nature* **2001**, *410*, 50–56. [CrossRef]
10. Willimann, K.; Legler, D.F.; Loetscher, M.; Roos, R.S.; Delgado, M.B.; Clark-Lewis, I.; Baggiolini, M.; Moser, B. The chemokine Slc is expressed in T cell areas of lymph nodes and mucosal lymphoid tissues and attracts activated T cells via Ccr7. *Eur. J. Immunol.* **1998**, *28*, 2025–2034. [CrossRef]
11. Ott, T.R.; Pahuja, A.; Nickolls, S.A.; Alleva, D.G.; Struthers, R.S. Identification of Cc chemokine Receptor 7 residues important for receptor activation. *J. Biol. Chem.* **2004**, *279*, 42383–42392. [CrossRef]

12. Dieu, M.C.; Vanbervliet, B.; Vicari, A.; Bridon, J.M.; Oldham, E.; Aït-Yahia, S.; Brière, F.; Zlotnik, A.; Lebecque, S.; Caux, C. Selective recruitment of immature and mature dendritic cells by distinct chemokines expressed in different anatomic sites. *J. Exp. Med.* **1998**, *188*, 373–386. [CrossRef]
13. Hirao, M.; Onai, N.; Hiroishi, K.; Watkins, S.C.; Matsushima, K.; Robbins, P.D.; Lotze, M.T.; Tahara, H. Cc chemokine Receptor-7 on dendritic cells is induced after interaction with apoptotic tumor cells: Critical role in migration from the tumor site to draining lymph nodes. *Cancer Res.* **2000**, *60*, 2209–2217. [PubMed]
14. Xu, Y.; Liu, L.; Qiu, X.; Jiang, L.; Huang, B.; Li, H.; Li, Z.; Luo, W.; Wang, E. CCL21/Ccr7 promotes G2/M phase progression via the erk pathway in human non-small cell lung cancer cells. *PLoS ONE* **2011**, *6*, e21119. [CrossRef] [PubMed]
15. Mo, M.; Zhou, M.; Wang, L.; Qi, L.; Zhou, K.; Liu, L.F.; Chen, Z.; Zu, X.B. CCL21/Ccr7 enhances the proliferation, migration, and invasion of human bladder cancer T24 cells. *PLoS ONE* **2015**, *10*, e0119506. [CrossRef] [PubMed]
16. Zhao, B.; Cui, K.; Wang, C.L.; Wang, A.L.; Zhang, B.; Zhou, W.Y.; Zhao, W.H.; Li, S. The chemotactic interaction between CCL21 and its receptor, Ccr7, facilitates the progression of pancreatic cancer via induction of angiogenesis and lymphangiogenesis. *J. Hepatobiliary Pancreat. Sci.* **2011**, *18*, 821–828. [CrossRef] [PubMed]
17. Liu, F.Y.; Safdar, J.; Li, Z.N.; Fang, Q.G.; Zhang, X.; Xu, Z.F.; Sun, C.F. Ccr7 regulates cell migration and invasion through Jak2/Stat3 in metastatic squamous cell carcinoma of the head and neck. *BioMed Res. Int.* **2014**, *2014*, 415375. [CrossRef]
18. Xu, B.; Zhou, M.; Qiu, W.; Ye, J.; Feng, Q. Ccr7 mediates human breast cancer cell invasion, migration by inducing epithelial-mesenchymal transition and suppressing apoptosis through Akt pathway. *Cancer Med.* **2017**, *6*, 1062–1071. [CrossRef]
19. Zhang, J.; Zhou, Y.; Yang, Y. Ccr7 pathway induces epithelial-mesenchymal transition through up-regulation of snail signaling in gastric cancer. *Med. Oncol.* **2015**, *32*, 467. [CrossRef]
20. Zhang, L.; Wang, D.; Li, Y.; Liu, Y.; Xie, X.; Wu, Y.; Zhou, Y.; Ren, J.; Zhang, J.; Zhu, H.; et al. CCL21/Ccr7 axis contributed to CD133+ pancreatic cancer stem-like cell metastasis via emt and erk/NF-κB pathway. *PLoS ONE* **2016**, *11*, e0158529. [CrossRef]
21. Ma, H.; Gao, L.; Li, S.; Qin, J.; Chen, L.; Liu, X.; Xu, P.; Wang, F.; Xiao, H.; Zhou, S.; et al. Ccr7 enhances Tgf-Beta1-Induced epithelial-mesenchymal transition and is associated with lymph node metastasis and poor overall survival in gastric cancer. *Oncotarget* **2015**, *6*, 24348–24360. [CrossRef]
22. Irino, T.; Takeuchi, H.; Matsuda, S.; Saikawa, Y.; Kawakubo, H.; Wada, N.; Takahashi, T.; Nakamura, R.; Fukuda, K.; Omori, T.; et al. Cc-chemokine receptor Ccr7: A key molecule for lymph node metastasis in esophageal squamous cell carcinoma. *BMC Cancer* **2014**, *14*, 291. [CrossRef]
23. Nakata, B.; Fukunaga, S.; Noda, E.; Amano, R.; Yamada, N.; Hirakawa, K. Chemokine receptor Ccr7 expression correlates with lymph node metastasis in pancreatic cancer. *Oncology* **2008**, *74*, 69–75. [CrossRef] [PubMed]
24. Xiong, Y.; Huang, F.; Li, X.; Chen, Z.; Feng, D.; Jiang, H.; Chen, W.; Zhang, X. CCL21/Ccr7 interaction promotes cellular migration and invasion via modulation of the Mek/ERK1/2 signaling pathway and correlates with lymphatic metastatic spread and poor prognosis in urinary bladder cancer. *Int. J. Oncol.* **2017**, *51*, 75–90. [CrossRef]
25. Xia, Y.; Liu, L.; Xiong, Y.; Bai, Q.; Wang, J.; Xi, W.; Qu, Y.; Xu, J.; Guo, J. Prognostic value of Cc-chemokine receptor seven expression in patients with metastatic renal cell carcinoma treated with tyrosine kinase inhibitor. *BMC Cancer* **2017**, *17*, 70. [CrossRef]
26. Lugli, A.; Kirsch, R.; Ajioka, Y.; Bosman, F.; Cathomas, G.; Dawson, H.; El Zimaity, H.; Fléjou, J.F.; Hansen, T.P.; Hartmann, A.; et al. Recommendations for reporting tumor budding in colorectal cancer based on the International Tumor Budding Consensus Conference (Itbcc) 2016. *Mod. Pathol.* **2017**, *30*, 1299–1311. [CrossRef] [PubMed]
27. Ueno, H.; Murphy, J.; Jass, J.R.; Mochizuki, H.; Talbot, I.C. Tumour 'budding' as an index to estimate the potential of aggressiveness in rectal cancer. *Histopathology* **2002**, *40*, 127–132. [CrossRef] [PubMed]
28. Ueno, H.; Mochizuki, H.; Hashiguchi, Y.; Shimazaki, H.; Aida, S.; Hase, K.; Matsukuma, S.; Kanai, T.; Kurihara, H.; Ozawa, K.; et al. Risk factors for an adverse outcome in early invasive colorectal carcinoma. *Gastroenterology* **2004**, *127*, 385–394. [CrossRef]
29. Prall, F. Tumour budding in colorectal carcinoma. *Histopathology* **2007**, *50*, 151–162. [CrossRef]
30. Karamitopoulou, E. Tumor budding cells, cancer stem cells and epithelial-mesenchymal transition-type cells in pancreatic cancer. *Front. Oncol.* **2012**, *2*, 209. [CrossRef]
31. Grigore, A.D.; Jolly, M.K.; Jia, D.; Farach-Carson, M.C.; Levine, H. Tumor budding: The name is EMT. Partial EMT. *J. Clin. Med.* **2016**, *5*, 51. [CrossRef]
32. Ogino, M.; Nakanishi, Y.; Mitsuhashi, T.; Hatanaka, Y.; Amano, T.; Marukawa, K.; Nitta, T.; Ueno, T.; Ono, M.; Kuwabara, S.; et al. Impact of tumour budding grade in 310 patients who underwent surgical resection for extrahepatic cholangiocarcinoma. *Histopathology* **2019**, *74*, 861–872. [CrossRef]
33. Bacus, S.; Flowers, J.L.; Press, M.F.; Bacus, J.W.; McCarty, K.S., Jr. The evaluation of estrogen receptor in primary breast carcinoma by computer-assisted image analysis. *Am. J. Clin. Pathol.* **1988**, *90*, 233–239. [CrossRef]
34. Somovilla-Crespo, B.; Alfonso-Pérez, M.; Cuesta-Mateos, C.; Carballo-de Dios, C.; Beltrán, A.E.; Terrón, F.; Pérez-Villar, J.J.; Gamallo-Amat, C.; Pérez-Chacón, G.; Fernández-Ruiz, E.; et al. Anti-Ccr7 therapy exerts a potent anti-tumor activity in a xenograft model of human mantle cell lymphoma. *J. Hematol. Oncol.* **2013**, *6*, 89. [CrossRef] [PubMed]
35. Förster, R.; Braun, A.; Worbs, T. Lymph node homing of T cells and dendritic cells via afferent lymphatics. *Trends Immunol.* **2012**, *33*, 271–280. [CrossRef] [PubMed]
36. Förster, R.; Davalos-Misslitz, A.C.; Rot, A. Ccr7 and its ligands: Balancing immunity and tolerance. *Nat. Rev. Immunol.* **2008**, *8*, 362–371. [CrossRef] [PubMed]

37. Winter, S.; Rehm, A.; Wichner, K.; Scheel, T.; Batra, A.; Siegmund, B.; Berek, C.; Lipp, M.; Höpken, U.E. Manifestation of spontaneous and early autoimmune gastritis in Ccr7-deficient mice. *Am. J. Pathol.* **2011**, *179*, 754–765. [CrossRef]
38. Zu, G.; Luo, B.; Yang, Y.; Tan, Y.; Tang, T.; Zhang, Y.; Chen, X.; Sun, D. Meta-analysis of the prognostic value of C-C chemokine receptor type 7 in patients with solid tumors. *Cancer Manag. Res.* **2019**, *11*, 1881–1892. [CrossRef]
39. Kohout, T.A.; Nicholas, S.L.; Perry, S.J.; Reinhart, G.; Junger, S.; Struthers, R.S. Differential desensitization, receptor phosphorylation, beta-arrestin recruitment, and ERK1/2 activation by the two endogenous ligands for the CC chemokine receptor 7. *J. Biol. Chem* **2004**, *279*, 23214–23222. [CrossRef]
40. Steen, A.; Larsen, O.; Thiele, S.; Rosenkilde, M.M. Biased and G protein-independent signaling of chemokine receptors. *Front. Immunol.* **2014**, *5*, 277. [CrossRef]

Disclaimer/Publisher's Note: The statements, opinions and data contained in all publications are solely those of the individual author(s) and contributor(s) and not of MDPI and/or the editor(s). MDPI and/or the editor(s) disclaim responsibility for any injury to people or property resulting from any ideas, methods, instructions or products referred to in the content.

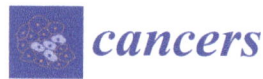 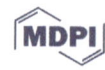

Article

Probing the Potential of Defense Response-Associated Genes for Predicting the Progression, Prognosis, and Immune Microenvironment of Osteosarcoma

Liangkun Huang [1,†], Fei Sun [1,†], Zilin Liu [1], Wenyi Jin [2], Yubiao Zhang [1], Junwen Chen [1], Changheng Zhong [1], Wanting Liang [3] and Hao Peng [1,*]

[1] Department of Orthopedics Surgery, Renmin Hospital of Wuhan University, Wuhan 430060, China; lkh1227@whu.edu.cn (L.H.)
[2] Department of Biomedical Sciences, College of Veterinary Medicine and Life Sciences, City University of Hong Kong, Kowloon Tong, Hong Kong SAR, China
[3] Department of Clinical Medicine, Xianyue Hospital of Xiamen Medical College, Xiamen 310058, China
* Correspondence: penghao0718@163.com
† These authors contributed equally to this work.

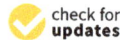

Citation: Huang, L.; Sun, F.; Liu, Z.; Jin, W.; Zhang, Y.; Chen, J.; Zhong, C.; Liang, W.; Peng, H. Probing the Potential of Defense Response-Associated Genes for Predicting the Progression, Prognosis, and Immune Microenvironment of Osteosarcoma. *Cancers* **2023**, *15*, 2405. https://doi.org/10.3390/cancers15082405

Academic Editors: Daniel L. Pouliquen and Cristina Núñez González

Received: 16 March 2023
Revised: 18 April 2023
Accepted: 19 April 2023
Published: 21 April 2023

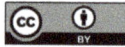

Copyright: © 2023 by the authors. Licensee MDPI, Basel, Switzerland. This article is an open access article distributed under the terms and conditions of the Creative Commons Attribution (CC BY) license (https://creativecommons.org/licenses/by/4.0/).

Simple Summary: Osteosarcoma (OS) is the most common primary orthopedic malignancy and typically affects children and young adults. Its lesions often metastasize to distant sites in the body, such as the lungs. Metastatic OS frequently recurs and has a poor prognosis. Our main objective of this study is to provide new insights into the clinical management of patients with osteosarcoma and to explore the risk factors affecting osteosarcoma metastasis. We established a biological marker consisting of three genes from the perspective of defense response for the first time to predict the prognosis of osteosarcoma and to discover new treatment methods. Our findings have implications for both the clinical management and future research of osteosarcoma.

Abstract: Background: The defense response is a type of self-protective response of the body that protects it from damage by pathogenic factors. Although these reactions make important contributions to the occurrence and development of tumors, the role they play in osteosarcoma (OS), particularly in the immune microenvironment, remains unpredictable. Methods: This study included the clinical information and transcriptomic data of 84 osteosarcoma samples and the microarray data of 12 mesenchymal stem cell samples and 84 osteosarcoma samples. We obtained 129 differentially expressed genes related to the defense response (DRGs) by taking the intersection of differentially expressed genes with genes involved in the defense response pathway, and prognostic genes were screened using univariate Cox regression. Least absolute shrinkage and selection operator (LASSO) penalized Cox regression and multivariate Cox regression were then used to establish a DRG prognostic signature (DGPS) via the stepwise method. DGPS performance was examined using independent prognostic analysis, survival curves, and receiver operating characteristic (ROC) curves. In addition, the molecular and immune mechanisms of adverse prognosis in high-risk populations identified by DGPS were elucidated. The results were well verified by experiments. Result: BNIP3, PTGIS, and ZYX were identified as the most important DRGs for OS progression (hazard ratios of 2.044, 1.485, and 0.189, respectively). DGPS demonstrated outstanding performance in the prediction of OS prognosis (area under the curve (AUC) values of 0.842 and 0.787 in the training and test sets, respectively, adj-p < 0.05 in the survival curve). DGPS also performed better than a recent clinical prognostic approach with an AUC value of only 0.674 [metastasis], which was certified in the subsequent experimental results. These three genes regulate several key biological processes, including immune receptor activity and T cell activation, and they also reduce the infiltration of some immune cells, such as B cells, CD8+ T cells, and macrophages. Encouragingly, we found that DGPS was associated with sensitivity to chemotherapeutic drugs including JNK Inhibitor VIII, TGX221, MP470, and SB52334. Finally, we verified the effect of BNIP3 on apoptosis, proliferation, and migration of osteosarcoma cells through experiments. Conclusions: This study elucidated the role and mechanism of BNIP3, PTGIS, and ZYX in OS progression and was well verified by the experimental results, enabling reliable prognostic means and treatment strategies to be proposed for OS patients.

Keywords: defense response; osteosarcoma; prognosis; metastasis; immune; therapy

1. Introduction

The defense response is the innate function of the body for resisting invasion by internal and external pathogenic factors, which appear with the existence of a foreign body or injury, and helps limit damage to the body or facilitate the promotion of injury recovery. A variety of pathogenic factors and foreign bodies often threaten the human body, and the results caused by the body's immune response may also result in damage to the body [1,2]. Immune cells are involved in constituting the tumor microenvironment (TME) from the early stage of tumor formation. Immune cells can recognize tumor-specific antigens and activate the immune system, and the coordination of natural and acquired immune cells can generate an efficient anti-tumor immune response, while tumor cells also have different immunosuppressive mechanisms to counteract the anti-tumor immune response [3]. At the same time, the body possesses a complete defense system that can protect it from potential damage by disease-causing agents. The body's defense response can influence tumorigenesis and progression. Several studies have identified an association between different tumors and defense response-related genes [4–7]. Defense response occurrence helps the body to kill tumor cells and prevents their escape [8–10]. Therefore, there is a close relationship between the development of both defense response-related genes and tumors.

Osteosarcoma (OS) is a malignant tumor that generally occurs in children and young adults [6,7]. Osteosarcoma often metastasizes to various parts of the body, including the lungs. Metastatic OS often relapses and the prognosis is generally poor [8]. As neoadjuvant chemotherapy and other therapies have developed in recent decades, the five-year survival rate of osteosarcoma has reached 70% [11]. However, the overall five-year survival rate for patients who are diagnosed with early lung metastasis is below 20% [12], and prognostic factors and appropriate treatment for metastatic OS patients have yet to be determined [13,14]. Therefore, exploring a new prognostic method to further improve the prognosis of osteosarcoma patients is essential.

A correlation may exist between the defense response of the body and tumor occurrence and development. A tumor is a foreign body that stimulates the human body to produce a corresponding defense response. There are many studies exploring the relationship between different tumors and the defense response, but there are few relevant studies in osteosarcoma. The aim of this study was to explore the potential correlation between the defense response of the body and osteosarcoma occurrence and development. A completely new prognostic prediction method and treatment strategy for osteosarcoma was obtained, and relevant experimental verification was conducted as a means of providing new ideas for osteosarcoma treatment and scientific research.

2. Materials and Methods

2.1. Data Collection

We obtained 84 osteosarcoma samples with both clinical information and transcriptomic data from the TARGET database (https://xena.ucsc.edu/, accessed on 6 April 2023), and we obtained microarray data for 12 MSC samples and 84 osteosarcoma samples from the GSE33383 dataset (GPL10295 platform) from the GEO database (https://www.ncbi.nlm.nih.gov/geo/, accessed on 6 April 2023). The collected clinical information included survival status, survival time, metastasis, sex, and age. The tumor samples in the TARGET database were randomly assigned to the training ($n = 50$) and test ($n = 34$) sets using R software (version 4.1.2).

2.2. Acquisition of Defense Response-Associated Differential Genes

We selected 12 mesenchymal stem cell samples and 84 osteosarcoma cell samples from the GPL10295 platform in dataset GSE33383 for differentially expressed gene (DEG) screening, and mesenchymal stem cell samples were selected as the control group for osteosarcoma samples. The R package "limma" was then used to identify DEGs in GSE33383; the criterion was determined by fold-change (set as 1) and adjusted p value (set as 0.05). The differentially expressed genes were used for GSEA analysis and they were found to be significantly enriched in the Gene Ontology (GO) DEFENSE RESPONSE pathway. In order to obtain DRGs, the gene set of this pathway was intersected with the differentially expressed genes. The R package "pheatmap"(version 1.0.12) was used to draw the DRG expression heatmaps of normal samples and tumor tissue samples.

2.3. Construction of a Prognostic DRGs Signature

The R package "survival" (version 3.5-5) was used to perform univariate Cox regression for each DRG using the survival data. Then, LASSO regression was performed to avoid overfitting. The optimal and minimum criteria for the penalty (λ) were selected with 10 times cross-validation. Then, we used multivariate Cox regression analysis to identify the prognostic DRGs, and DGPS was constructed. These prognosis-related DRGs were utilized to construct an equation (DGPS) to calculate risk scores of osteosarcoma samples: $RiskScore = \sum_{i=1}^{n} Coef_i^* X_i$, where $Coef_i^*$ represents the coefficient (risk factor values for different genes) and Xi represents the normalized count of the DRG (gene expression). Risk scores were calculated for each osteosarcoma sample based only on the expression of different DRGs (i.e., the equation described above), and the median risk score of all osteosarcoma samples was used as the basis for classifying risk subgroups as high-risk (above the median score) and low-risk (below the median score).

2.4. Validation of DGPS

The Kaplan–Meier (KM) method was used to demonstrate the survival prediction value of DGPS. The accuracy and diagnostic value of DGPS were assessed using ROC curves and AUC. Principal component analysis (PCA) was performed to verify DGPS, and the R package "scatterplot3d" was used for visualization. The consistency index (C-index) was used for predicting the precision of DGPS with R packages "dplyr", "survival", "pec", and "rms". The test group and all cohorts were used in the validation of this model.

2.5. Exploration of the Relationship between DGPS and Clinical Features

To assess the suitability of DGPS for osteosarcoma with various clinical features, we used univariate and multivariate Cox regression analyses on 84 osteosarcoma samples from the TARGET database (https://xena.ucsc.edu/, accessed on 6 April 2023) to explore the association between DGPS and gender, age, and metastasis in order to reveal their potential role in OS.

2.6. Nomogram Construction of DGPS and Clinical Characteristics

Univariate and multivariate Cox regression were performed on 84 osteosarcoma samples from the TARGET database (https://xena.ucsc.edu/, accessed on 6 April 2023) in order to study the independent prognostic role of DGPS. A nomogram was then developed using the R packages "regplot" (version 1.1), "rms" (version 6.6-0), and "survival" (version 3.5-5). A calibration curve was then constructed to verify its precision.

2.7. Exploration of the Relationship between Model Genes and OS Metastasis

A box plot was used to explore the relationship between BNIP3 and OS metastasis, and then ROC, AUC, and a correlation scatter diagram were used on 84 osteosarcoma samples from the TARGET database (https://xena.ucsc.edu/, accessed on 6 April 2023) to verify this relationship based on the R packages "ROCR" and "ggplot2." The expression level of BNIP3 in each tumor was studied using GEPIA.

2.8. Enrichment Analysis of Biologically Relevant Pathways

Then, we screened the DEGs among different risk subgroups using the R package "DESeq2" with the following limiting condition: log2 |folding change| > 1 and adjusted p value < 0.05. The database pathways of GO and Kyoto Encyclopedia of Genes and Genomes (KEGG) were explored to elucidate biologically relevant pathways using the R packages "clusterProfiler" (version 4.6.2), "org.Hs.eg.db" (version 3.16.0), and "enrichplot" (version 1.18.4).

2.9. Exploration of Immune Microenvironment Landscape

To explore the association between DGPS and the infiltration of immune microenvironment landscape, a single-sample gene set enrichment analysis (ssGSEA) algorithm in the R package "GSVA" was then used on 84 osteosarcoma samples from the TARGET database (https://xena.ucsc.edu/, accessed on 6 April 2023) to evaluate the infiltration and functional scoring of immune cells in osteosarcoma. Immune checkpoint correlation analysis was carried out using the R package "limma" (version 3.54.2).

2.10. Exploration of Drug Sensitivity

The sensitivity to chemotherapeutic drugs was represented by the half-maximal inhibitory concentration (IC50) of chemotherapeutic drugs. IC50 is a crucial indicator to access tumor response to therapy; a smaller IC50 indicates a higher sensitivity of tumor cells to this chemotherapeutic agent, and the opposite indicates a lower sensitivity. In order to assess the value of DGPS in the clinical management of OS and find suitable potential chemotherapeutic drugs for patients with osteosarcoma, the drug therapy response was evaluated for each patient using the R package "pRRophetic" (version 6) (the drug source was the 251 anticancer drugs in the R package "pRRophetic" (version 6)). This was accomplished by creating statistical models of gene expression and drug sensitivity data from cell lines in the Cancer Genome Project (CGP) and then applying these models to the oncogene expression levels in tumor samples to generate in vivo drug sensitivity predictions [15]. The IC50 values of different subgroups were then compared using the Wilcoxon signed-rank test.

2.11. Cell Culture

The human osteosarcoma cell line 143B (CRL-8303) was purchased from American Type Culture Collection (ATCC) and was cultured in Dulbecco's Modified Eagle's Medium (DMEM) under conditions of 5% CO_2 at 37 °C. The medium was supplemented with 10% fetal bovine serum (FBS), 100 IU/mL penicillin, and 100 mg/mL streptomycin [16].

2.12. Apoptosis Analysis by Flow Cytometry

Flow cytometry was used to detect cell apoptosis. The cells were washed twice with precooled PBS. Follow-up assays were carried out according to the instructions of the apoptosis kit. The collected cells were resuspended in a 10 mL centrifuge tube containing a $1\times$ binding buffer to make 1×10^6 cells/mL. 5 µL Annexin V/PI was used for staining at room temperature for 15 min. Eventually, 400 µL $1\times$ Binding Buffer was added to detect apoptosis of 143B cells by flow cytometry.

2.13. 5-Ethynyl-2′-Deoxyuridine (EdU) Experiment

The EyoClick EdU Cell Proliferation Kit with Alexa Fluor 594 was used to verify the proliferation ability of cells. 143B cells with BNP3 knocked out or overexpressed were seeded at a density of 5×10^4 cells/well in a 6-well plate covered with 24 mm × 24 mm coverslips and synchronized with pure medium for 12 h. The medium was completely replaced with MEM medium. The kit's instructions were followed for washing and fixation. The 143B cells were stained with apollo fluorescent board azide 594 under $CuSO_4$ for 30 min at 37 °C. After that, cell nuclei were stained with DAPI (10 µg/mL) for 10 min and washed with PBST to completely remove the unbound DAPI, the cover was removed, and the glass was secured. Fluorescence microscopy was used to observe the fluorescence staining of cells (Olympus, Japan).

2.14. Wound-Healing Assay

Osteosarcoma cells of different transfection types (4×10^5) were cultured on 6-well plates for 12 h to ensure 80% cell density was achieved. Artificial wounds were made using the tip of 200 µL pipette, and phosphate-buffered saline was used to wash the nutrient solution twice. Finally, 3~5 mL of the serum-free nutrient solution was added and the migration distance was measured at 0 and 24 h after injury.

2.15. Statistical Analysis

All statistical analysis was carried out using R software (version 4.1.2). RNA-seq transcriptome data were included in the TARGET (https://xena.ucsc.edu/, accessed on 6 April 2023) and GEO (https://www.ncbi.nlm.nih.gov/geo/, accessed on 6 April 2023) databases. The Wilcoxon rank sum test was applied to compare the differences between different risk subgroups of quantitative data. The criterion for a statistically significant difference was set at $p < 0.05$.

3. Results

3.1. Identification of Prognosis Related-DRGs

Differential gene analysis was performed using 12 normal samples and 84 osteosarcoma samples from the GSE33383 dataset as a method to obtain the differentially expressed genes in osteosarcoma (Figure 1A), and GSEA analysis showed that these genes were significantly enriched in the GOBP_DEFENSE_RESPONSE pathway (Figure 1B). From the search results of the relevant literature in PubMed Central, it was found that the number of studies on the GOBP_DEFENSE_RESPONSE pathway in the last 10 years demonstrated a significantly increasing trend (Figure 1C). In total, 129 DRGs were obtained from the intersection of the gene set of this pathway and the osteosarcoma DEGs (Figure 1D). Their expression in osteosarcoma and normal samples can be seen in the heatmap (Figure 1E).

3.2. DGPS Was Validated as an Independent Prognostic Factor of Osteosarcoma

We carried out univariate Cox regression analysis on these 129 DRGs and obtained 10 DRGs with prognostic value (Figure 2A). The correlation network map (Rcutoff = 0.2) found BNIP3 and ZYX to be at the center of 10 risk DRGs (Figure 2B). The 10 risk DRGs were selected by LASSO analysis (Figure 2C,D) before multivariate Cox analysis was executed, then we screened three DRGs to establish DGPS: RiskScore = 0.42* Expression PTGIS + 0.567* Expression BNIP3 − 1.477* Expression ZYX. We then distributed patients into different risk subgroups based on the median risk score. We carried out univariate and multivariate Cox regression analyses on risk scores and clinical characteristics as a means of assessing the predictive value of DGPS. Then, statistically significant differences were observed for risk score and metastasis (Figure 3A). Meanwhile, risk score and metastasis retained prognostic value for OS in multivariate Cox regression analysis (Figure 3B). The AUC values of the one-year, three-year, and five-year ROC curves reached 0.812, 0.799, and 0.842, respectively, showing accurate prediction of the survival rate of osteosarcoma patients at one, three, and five years by DGPS (Figure 3C). The ROC plots of DGPS and the clinical characteristics showed that the AUC values of DGPS were higher than those of all the other clinical characteristics (Figure 3D). The Kaplan–Meier survival curve showed significant differences in survival status among patients in different risk subgroups based on DGPS division (Figure 3E). The risk score distribution and survival status maps showed that among patients classified into different risk subgroups according to the median risk score, mortality was higher in the high-risk group (Figure 3F,G). The risk heatmap showed that BNIP3 and PTGIS were highly expressed in the high-risk group, while ZYX was highly expressed in the low-risk group (Figure 3H). A stratified subgroup analysis was then performed as a means of exploring the prognostic value of DGPS among all cohorts. We divided the entire cohort into various sets by gender, age (<14 and ≥14), and metastasis. Based on DGPS among different clinical groups, the KM survival curve indicated that the low-risk group had significantly higher overall survival compared to the high-risk group (Figure 4). These findings all demonstrated that DGPS could be an independent prognostic factor for use in the accurate prediction of OS patient prognosis.

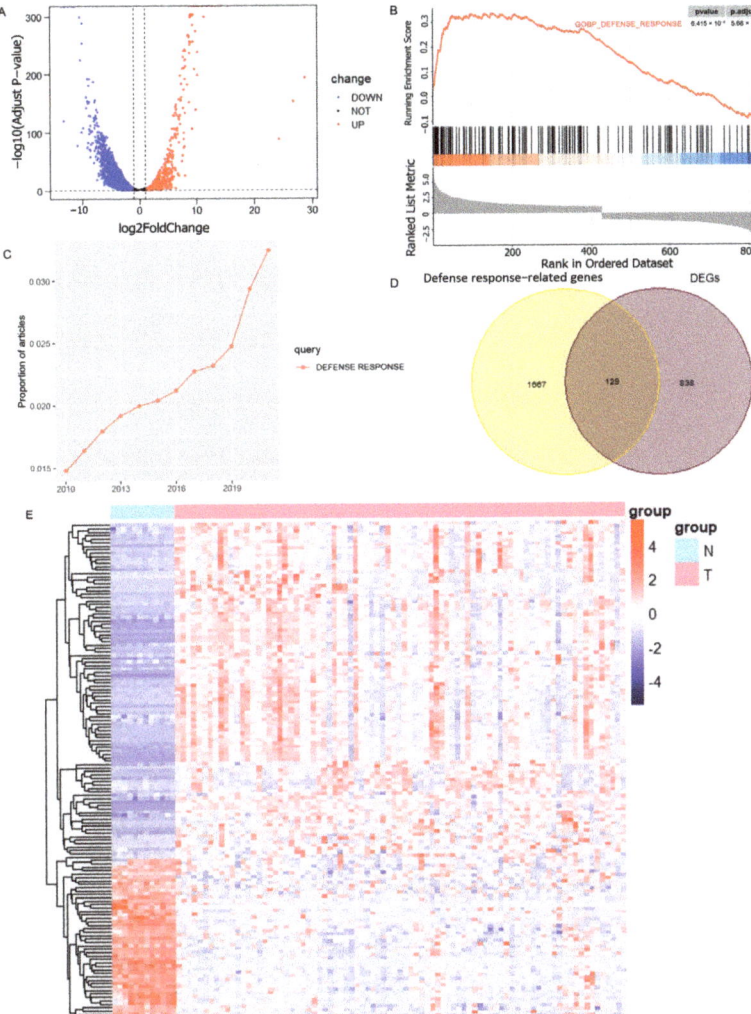

Figure 1. Screening of DEGs related to the defense response. (**A**) Volcano plot illustrating the DEGs in osteosarcoma and normal groups with the threshold set at $|logFC| \geq 1$ and adj-$p \leq 0.05$. (**B**) DEGs are significantly enriched in the GOBP_DEFENSE_RESPONSE pathway. (**C**) Trend in the number of studies on GOBP_DEFENSE_RESPONSE pathways in recent years. (**D**) DRGs obtained by taking the intersection of DEGs and GOBP_DEFENSE_RESPONSE pathway genes. (**E**) Heatmap showing the expression of DRGs in osteosarcoma samples and normal samples.

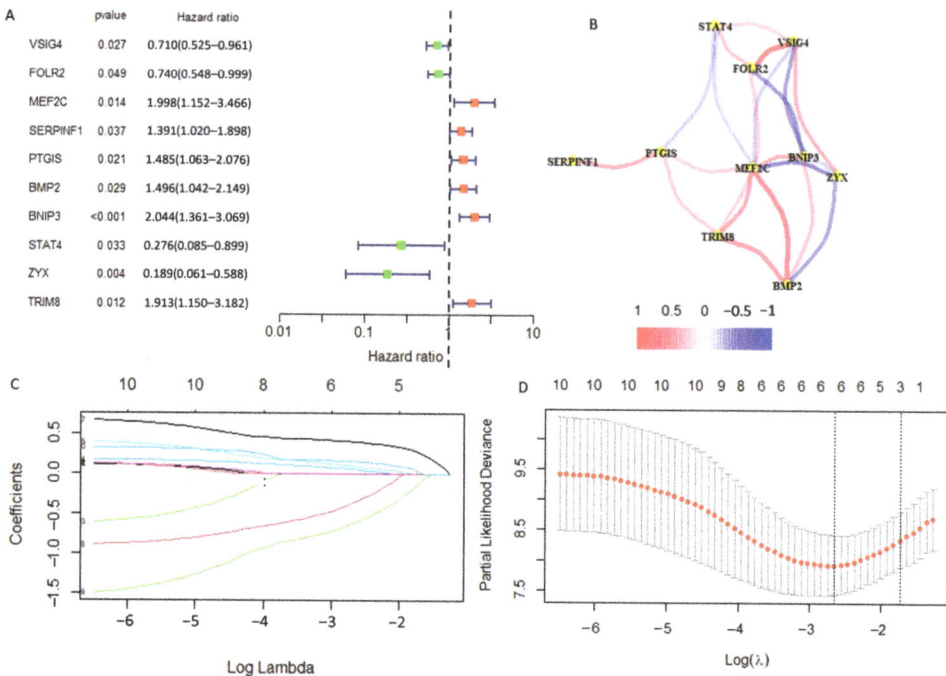

Figure 2. Obtaining DRGs associated with osteosarcoma prognosis. (**A**) Univariate Cox regression analysis for identifying prognostic DRGs. (**B**) Interaction network diagram of prognosis-related DRGs. (**C,D**) Lasso–Cox regression analysis was performed to construct prognostic prediction models.

3.3. Verification of DGPS

In order to verify the stability of DGPS, the test set and all cohorts were investigated using ROC, Kaplan–Meier survival curves, risk score distribution, survival status maps, and risk heatmaps. The AUC at one, three, and five years reached 0.879, 0.757, and 0.787 in the test set, respectively, and reached 0.815, 0.798, and 0.827 in the entire cohort, respectively (Figure 5A,B). The AUC value of DGPS was higher than that of the other clinical characteristics in the test set and all cohorts (Figure 5C,D). The KM survival curves of the test set and entire cohort showed that the low-risk group had a higher overall survival rate than the high-risk group (Figure 5E,F). The distribution of risk scores and the distribution of overall survival status and risk score were verified in the test set and all cohorts. (Figure 5G–J). The risk heatmaps of the test set and all cohorts showed that the risk genes were expressed at the same level in the high- and low-risk subgroups as in the training set (Figure 5K,L). PCA was carried out to explore the differences between different risk subgroups. DGPS divided different risk subgroups into two clusters, but there was no significant distinction based on the expression of 129 DRGs and all genes (Figure 6A–C). The box diagrams showed that the expression of BNIP3 and PTGIS was significantly lower in the low-risk group than in the high-risk group, while the opposite was true for the expression of ZYX (Figure 6D–F).

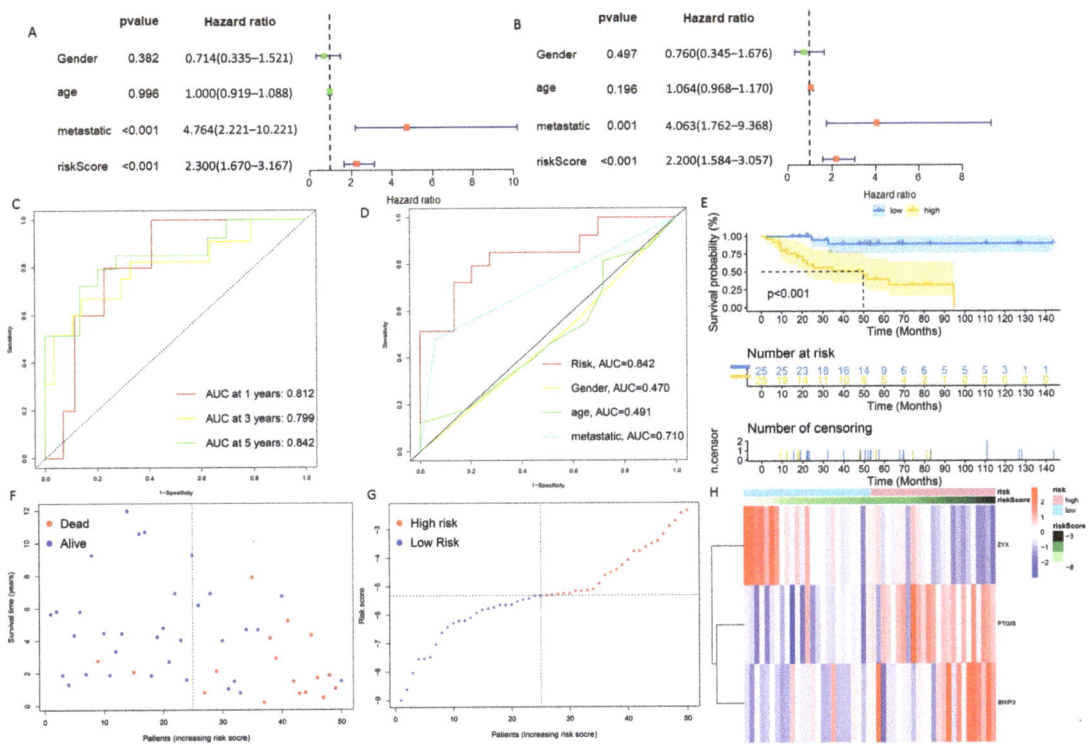

Figure 3. Evaluation of DGPS. (**A**) Univariate Cox analysis. Risk score and metastasis were statistically significant. (**B**) Multivariate Cox analysis. (**C**) ROC curve of DGPS in training group. (**D**) ROC demonstrating that the predictive accuracy of DGPS was superior to the other clinical parameters in the training set. (**E**) Kaplan–Meier curves of overall survival in the training set. (**F,G**) Distribution of risk scores and distribution of overall survival status and risk score in the training set. Blue: low risk; red: high risk. (**H**) Heatmap indicating the expression degrees of BNIP3, PTGIS, and ZYX in the training set. ROC curve, receiver operating characteristics curve; AUC, area under the curve; $p < 0.05$, statistically significant.

3.4. Construction and Verification of Nomogram

We constructed a nomogram to precisely predict the one-, three-, and five-year survival probability of OS (Figure 7A). The calibration curves indicated that the one-, three-, and five-year survival rates calculated by the nomogram were satisfactorily consistent with the actual OS patient survival rate (Figure 7B). In addition, the C-index indicated that the predictive accuracy of DGPS was better than that of other clinical features (Figure 7C). ROC curves constructed based on the nomogram at one, three, and five years showed that the nomogram had excellent prognostic predictive value (Figure 7D). The same tests showed good performance for both the test set and all cohorts (Figure 7E–L).

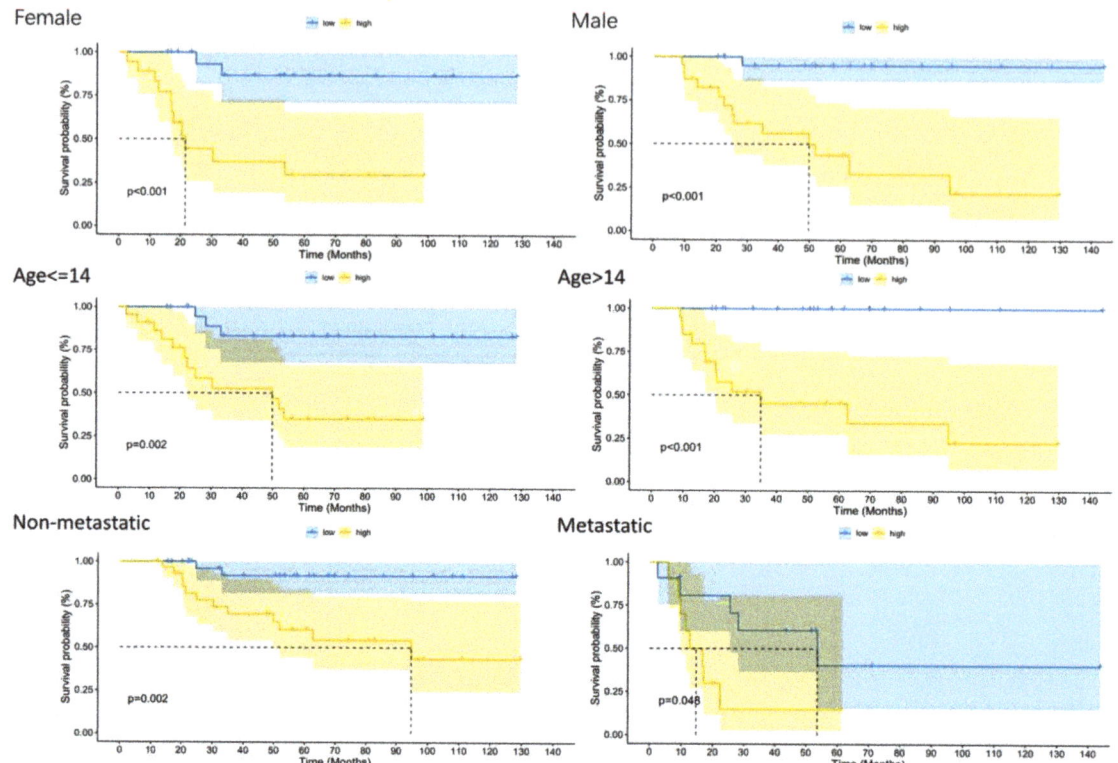

Figure 4. Kaplan–Meier plots depicting subgroup survival analyses stratified by gender, age, and metastasis.

3.5. Exploration of the Association of Tumor Metastasis with BNIP3

The expression of BNIP3 was detected in different metastatic subgroups. The box diagram results demonstrated that the expression of BNIP3 was significantly lower in the non-metastatic group than in the metastatic group (Figure 8A). The ROC curve in the training set demonstrated that the expression of BNIP3 had satisfactory accuracy for the prediction of tumor metastasis (Figure 8B), which was also verified in all cohorts (Figure 8C). In addition, the relationship between BNIP3 expression and OS metastasis-related gene expression can be seen in Figure 8D. BNIP3 was positively correlated with genes that promote osteosarcoma metastasis, such as MYC, NELL1, SAR1A, and PLOD2, and negatively correlated with genes that inhibit osteosarcoma metastasis, such as TNFAIP8L1 and TRIM22, which suggested that a certain association exists between BNIP3 expression and OS metastasis. Pan-cancer analysis performed in the GEPIA database showed that BNIP3 was lowly expressed in tumors such as CHOL and COAD and highly expressed in tumors such as KIRC and TGCT (Figure 8E,F). The top 20 genes with the strongest positive or negative correlations with BNIP3 expression were further screened for enrichment analysis, and the results showed that these genes were significantly enriched in pathways such as antigen processing and presentation of peptide antigen, regulation of angiogenesis, cellular response to hypoxia, gap junction channel activity, etc. (Figure 9A–C).

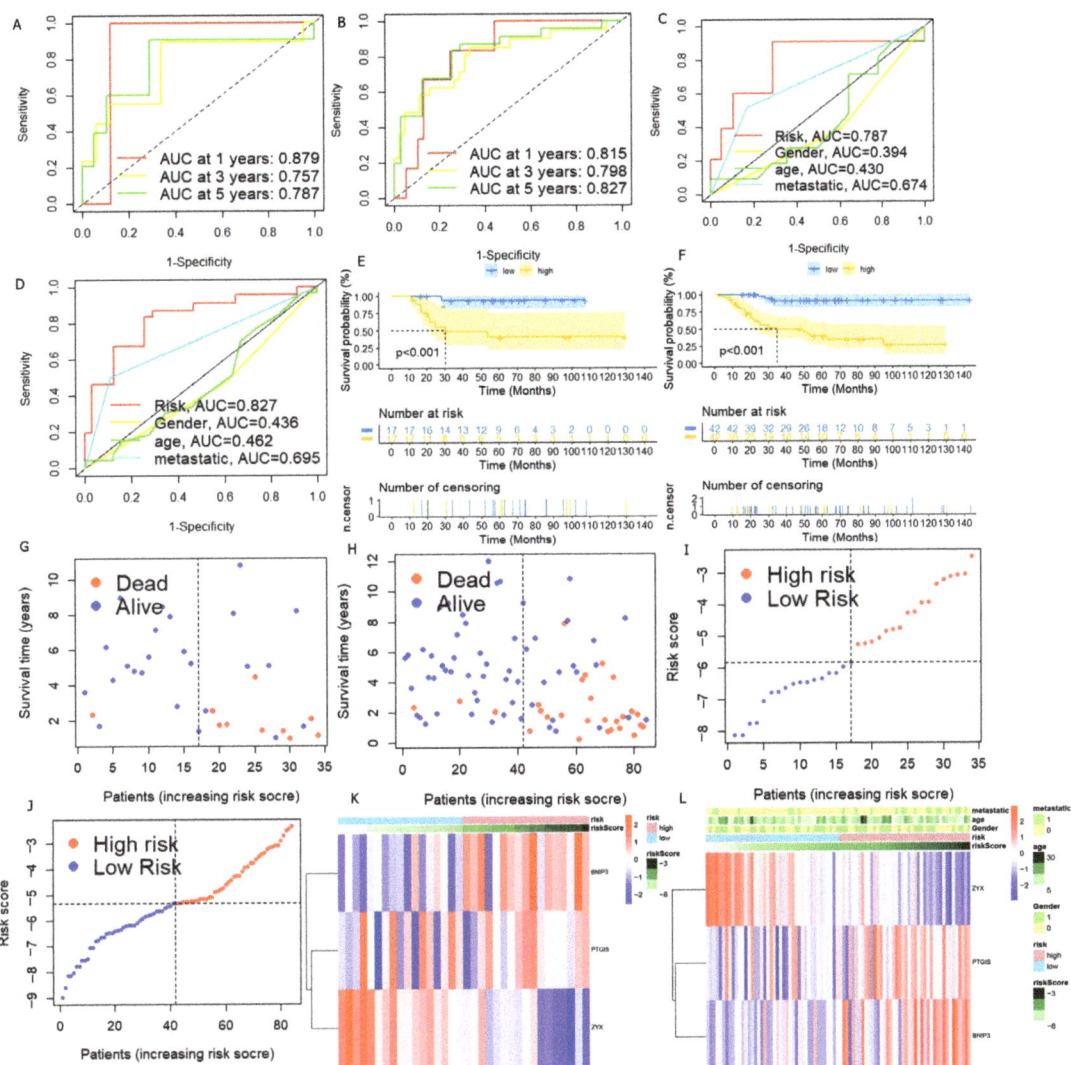

Figure 5. Verification of DGPS. ROC curve of DGPS in the test set (**A**) and in the entire cohort (**B**). ROC demonstrated that the predictive accuracy of DGPS was superior to that of other clinical characteristics in the test set (**C**) and in the entire cohort (**D**). Kaplan–Meier curves of overall survival (OS) in the test set (**E**) and in the entire cohort (**F**). Survival status of patients with osteosarcoma in the test set (**G,I**) and in the entire cohort (**H,J**). Blue: low risk; red: high risk. The heatmap indicates the expression degrees of BNIP3, PTGIS, and ZYX in the test set (**K**) and in the entire cohort (**L**).

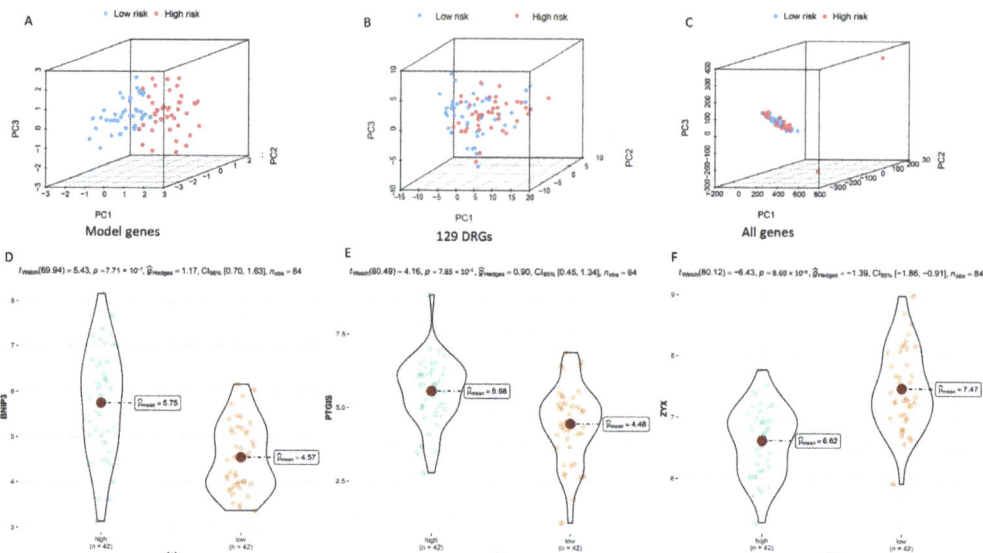

Figure 6. PCA plots depicting the distribution of samples based on the expression of model genes (**A**), DRGs (**B**), and all genes (**C**). Differential expression of model genes in the high- and low-risk groups is shown in box plots (**D–F**).

3.6. Enrichment Analysis of Biologically Relevant Pathways

We carried out GO and KEGG enrichment analyses to explore the biologically relevant functions and pathways between different risk subgroups, and we identified 3206 DEGs. In the biological process category, the genes were mainly enriched in T cell activation, B cell-mediated immunity, and leukocyte-mediated immunity. In the cellular component category, they were found to be mainly enriched in the external side of the plasma membrane, the apical part of the cell, etc. In the molecular function category, they were found to be primarily enriched in antigen binding, immune receptor activity, and passive transmembrane transporter activity (Figure 10A,C,E). KEGG enrichment analysis demonstrated that DEGs were primarily enriched in Th17 cell differentiation, Th1 and Th2 cell differentiation, the T cell receptor signaling pathway, etc. (Figure 10B,D,F).

3.7. Exploration of Relationship between Immune Microenvironment and DGPS

We carried out multiple immune assessment algorithms as a means of investigating the difference in the TME landscape of OS patients in different risk subgroups. From the ESTIMATE results, we found that patients in the low-risk group had higher stromal, immune, and ESTIMATE scores and lower tumor purity than the high-risk group (Figure 11A). We found that DGPS was associated with immune checkpoint-related gene expression, with the high-risk group showing high levels of expression of LAG3, CD274, CD27, CTLA4, etc. (Figure 11B). In addition, the immune cell differential analysis demonstrated that B cells, CD8+T cells, neutrophils, NK cells, pDCs, Th1 cells, Th2 cells, and TILs were significantly downregulated in the high-risk group (Figure 11C). Immune function analysis found that the low-risk group had higher immune function scores in categories such as CCR, checkpoint, T cell co-inhibition, etc. than the high-risk group (Figure 11D). The levels of immune characteristics were higher in the low-risk group than in the high-risk group (Figure 11E). The relationship between immune cells (Figure 12) and immune functions (Figure 13) with risk score and different risk subgroups was also explored. These results all indicated that DGPS had an association with the immune microenvironment and could reveal OS patient immunity status (Figure 14).

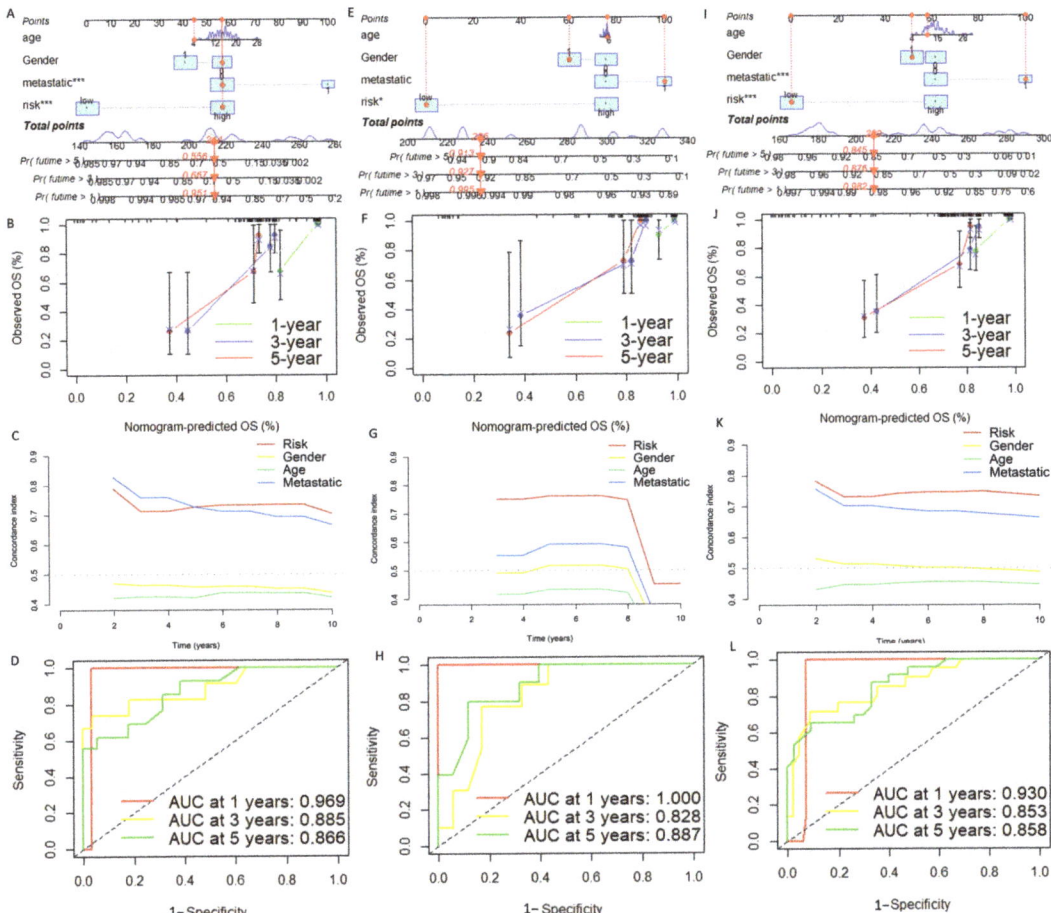

Figure 7. Construction and evaluation of a nomogram based on DGPS. Nomogram used to predict prognosis was constructed based on DGPS in the training set (**A**), test set (**E**), and entire cohort (**I**). Calibration curves of the nomogram in the training set (**B**), test set (**F**), and entire cohort (**J**). The C-index curves for assessing the discrimination ability of DGPS and other clinical characteristics at each time point in the training set (**C**), test set (**G**), and entire cohort (**K**). ROC curves of the nomograms at one, three, and five years in the training set (**D**), test set (**H**), and entire cohort (**L**). "*" represented "$p < 0.05$", "***" represented "$p < 0.001$".

3.8. Anticancer Drug Sensitivity Analysis

Targeted drug therapy is a crucial strategy in tumor therapy. We performed drug sensitivity analysis with 251 anticancer drugs using the R package "pRRophetic" (version 6). This was achieved by creating statistical models from gene expression and drug sensitivity data from cell lines in the Cancer Genome Project (CGP) and then applying these models to oncogene expression levels in tumor samples in order to generate in vivo drug sensitivity predictions. To determine the potential use of DGPS, we investigated the association between DGPS and drug IC50 in OS therapy by comparing the differences in anticancer drug sensitivity between the two different risk groups. The IC50 values of anticancer drugs were compared in the different risk subgroups. The IC50 values of four anticancer drugs were found to be statistically different between the different risk subgroups ($p < 0.05$), as can be seen in Figure 15. The IC50 values of MP470 and SB52334 were lower in the high-risk group, proving that the high-risk group had greater sensitivity to these drugs. In addition, the IC50 values of JNK Inhibitor VIII and TGX221 were lower in the low-risk group, indicating that the low-risk group had greater sensitivity to these drugs. This finding suggested that the new DGPS signal may be helpful in predicting the efficacy of chemotherapy in patients with osteosarcoma.

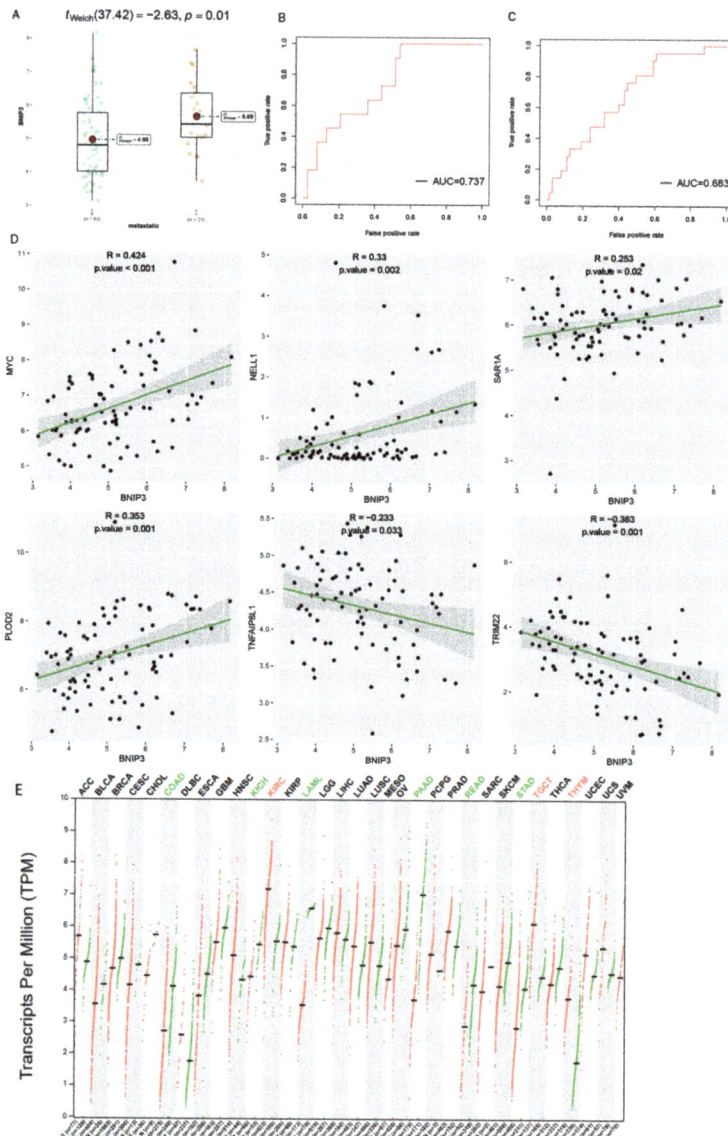

Figure 8. Cont.

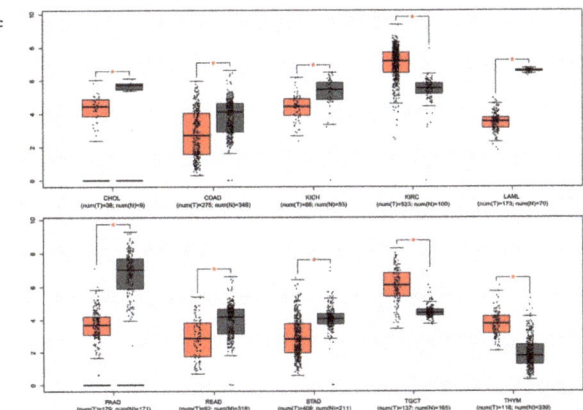

Figure 8. Exploration of the association of tumor metastasis with BNIP3. (**A**) Correlations between BNIP3 and osteosarcoma metastasis are displayed in box plots. ROC curve of diagnosis of osteosarcoma metastasis by BNIP3 in the training set (**B**) and in the entire cohort (**C**). (**D**) Relationship between the expression of BNIP3 and the expression of tumor metastasis-related genes MYC, NELL1, SAR1A, PLOD2, TNFAIP8L1, and TRIM22. (**E,F**) Expression of BNIP3 in different tumors. "*" represented "$p < 0.05$".

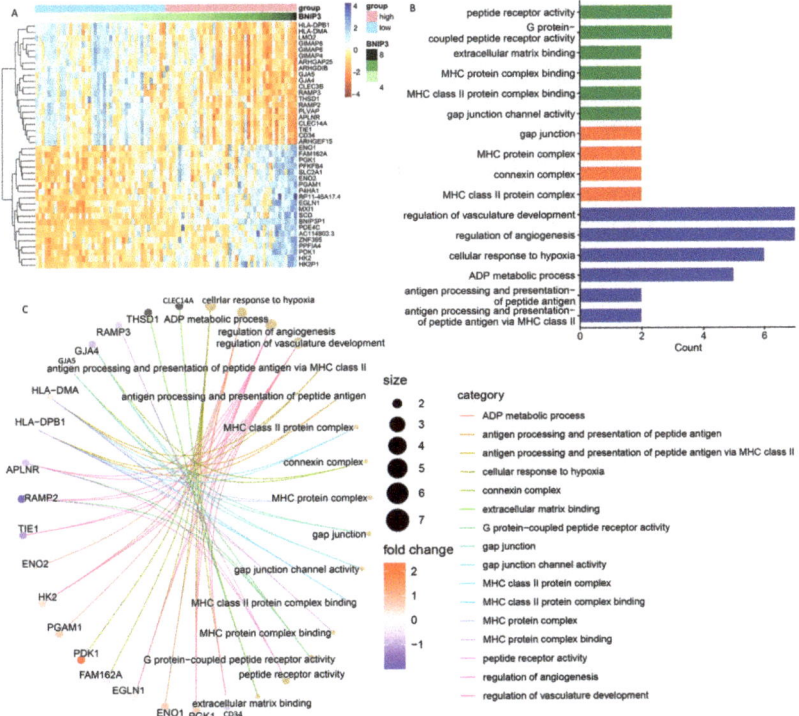

Figure 9. Pathway enrichment analysis of the genes most strongly associated with BNIP3. (**A**) Heatmap showing the 20 genes with the strongest positive or negative correlations with BNIP3 expression. (**B,C**) Pathway enrichment analysis showing the enrichment of genes in different pathways.

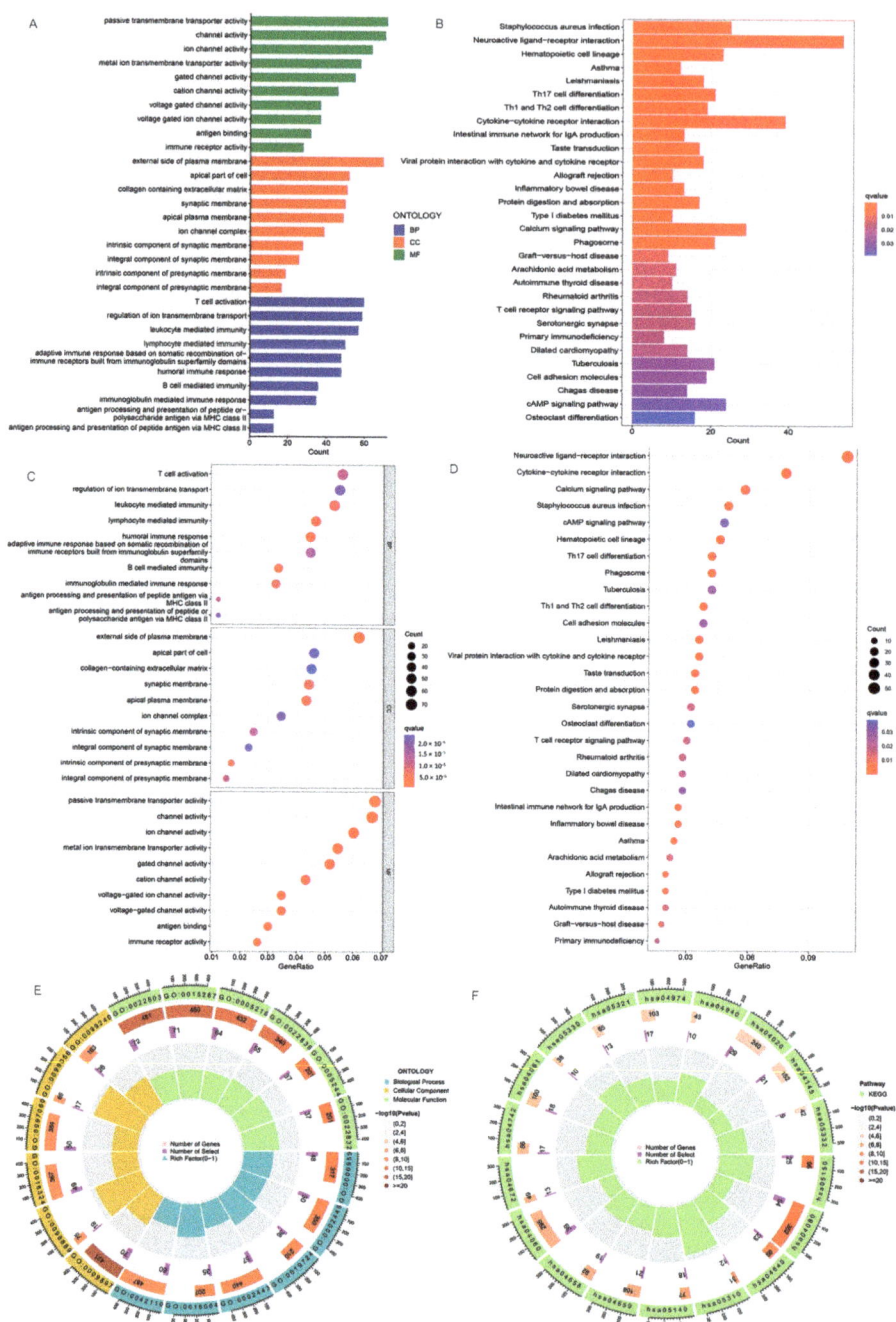

Figure 10. GO and KEGG pathway enrichment analyses. (**A**) Bar plot of the top 10 GO enrichment terms. (**B**) Bar plot of the top 30 KEGG enrichment terms. (**C**) Bubble chart of the top 10 GO enrichment terms. (**D**) Bubble chart of the top 30 KEGG enrichment terms. (**E**) Circle diagram of GO enrichment analysis. (**F**) Circle diagram of KEGG enrichment analysis. GO enrichment terms include biological process, cellular component, and molecular function.

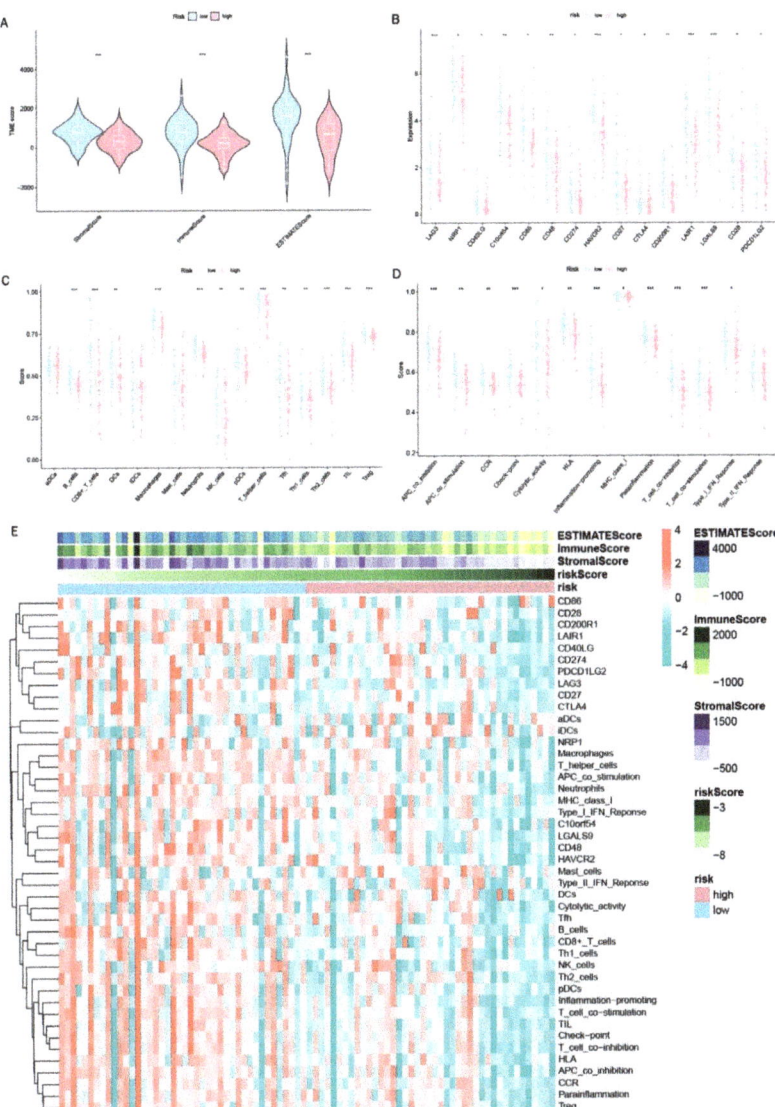

Figure 11. Immunoassay showing that DGPS is closely related to the immune system. (**A**) Analysis of TMB differences between high- and low-risk groups of patients with osteosarcoma. Box plots of the ssGSEA scores of 15 immune checkpoints (**B**), 13 immune cells (**C**), and 12 immune-related functions (**D**) between different risk groups. (**E**) Heatmap showing the landscape of immune characteristics and the tumor microenvironment in the TARGET cohort determined by the ssGSEA algorithm. "*"represented "$p < 0.05$","**"represented "$p < 0.01$","***"represented "$p < 0.001$".

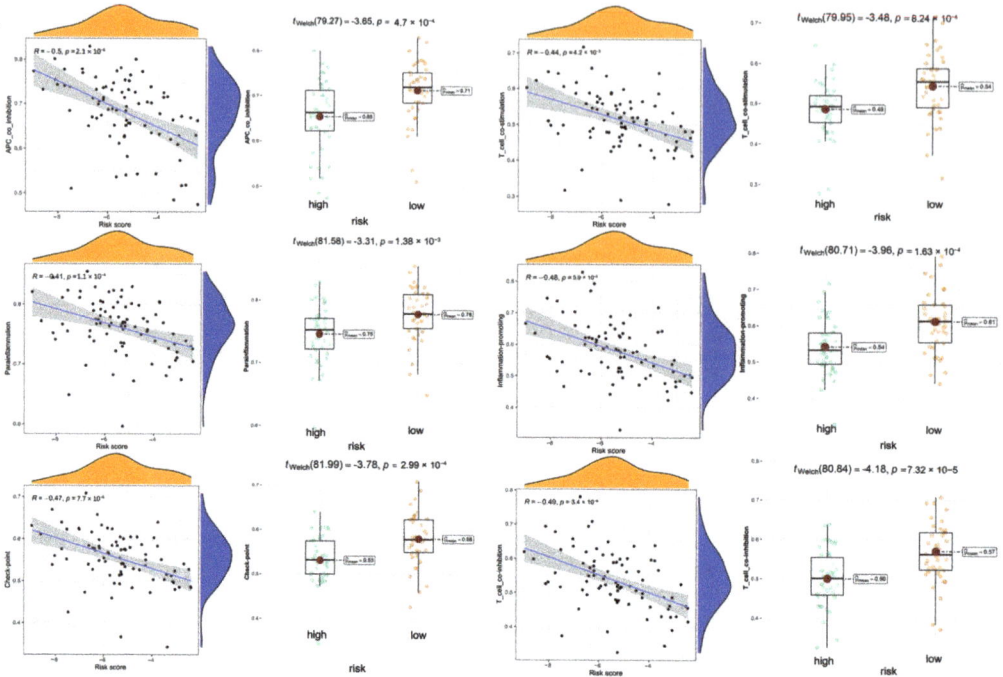

Figure 12. The association between immune functions and risk scores and immune function scores between different risk subgroups.

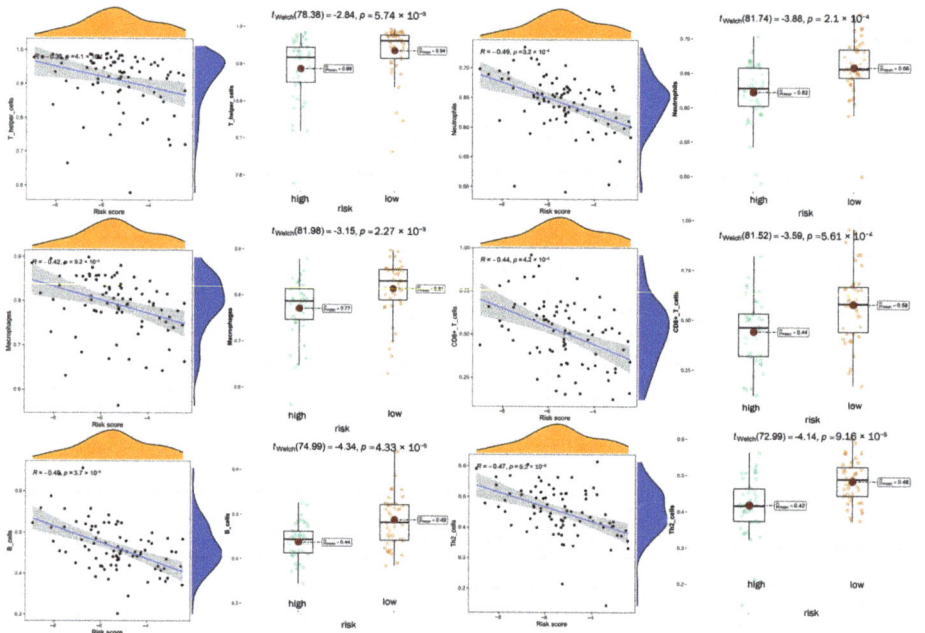

Figure 13. The association between immune cells and risk scores and immune cell scores between different risk subgroups.

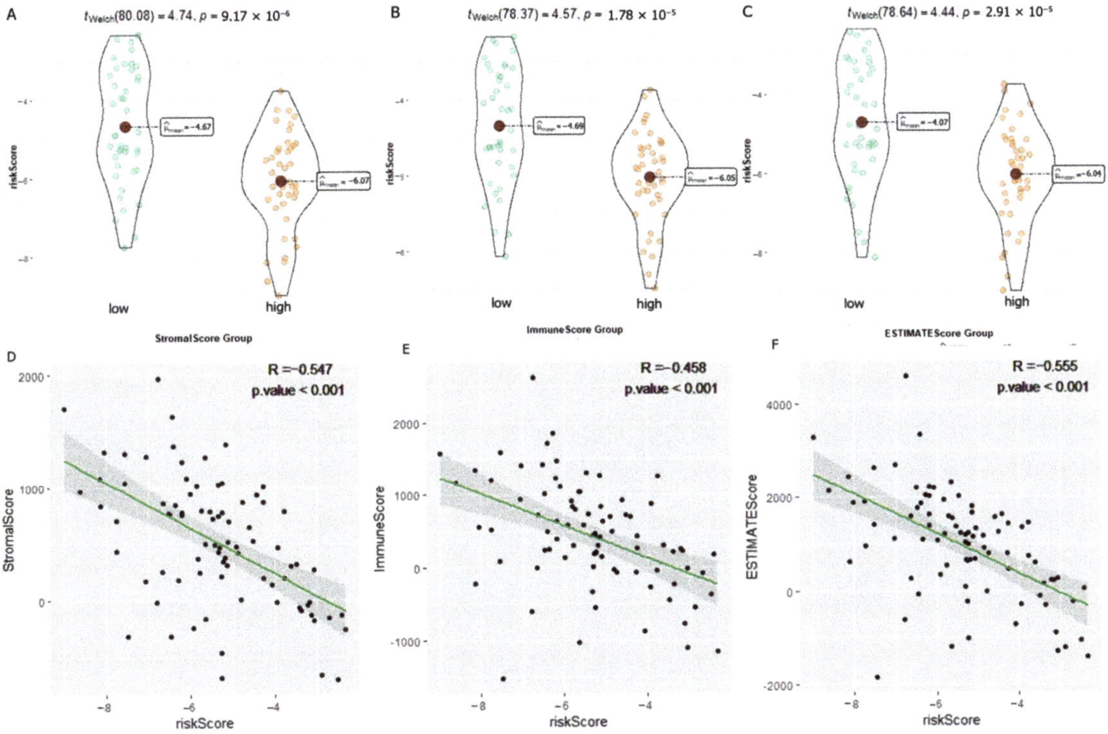

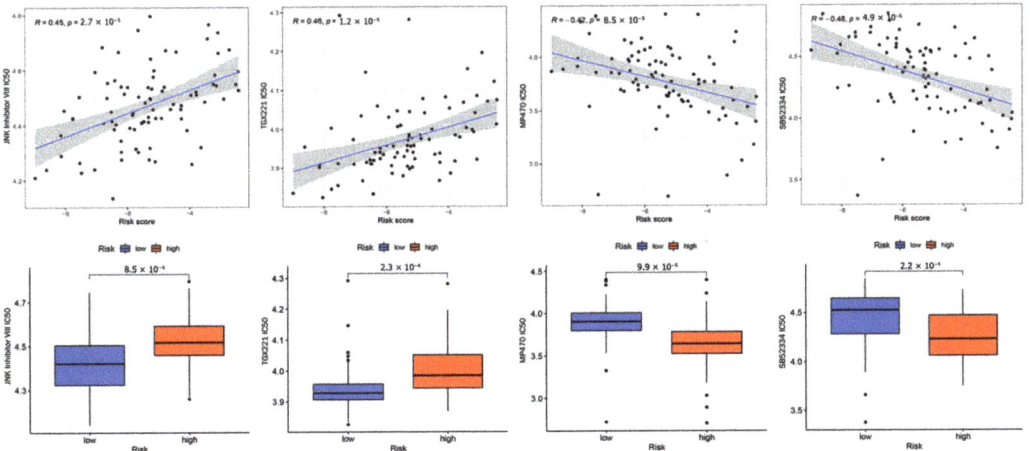

Figure 14. Correlation analysis of immune-related scores and risk scores. (**A**–**C**) Analysis of the variability of risk scores among different StromalScore (**A**), ImmuneScore (**B**), and ESTIMATEScore (**C**) subgroups. (**D**–**F**) Scatter plots of correlations between risk scores and StromalScore (**D**), ImmuneScore (**E**), and ESTIMATEScore (**F**).

Figure 15. Drug correlation and sensitivity analyses with JNK Inhibitor VIII, TGX221, MP470, and SB52334.

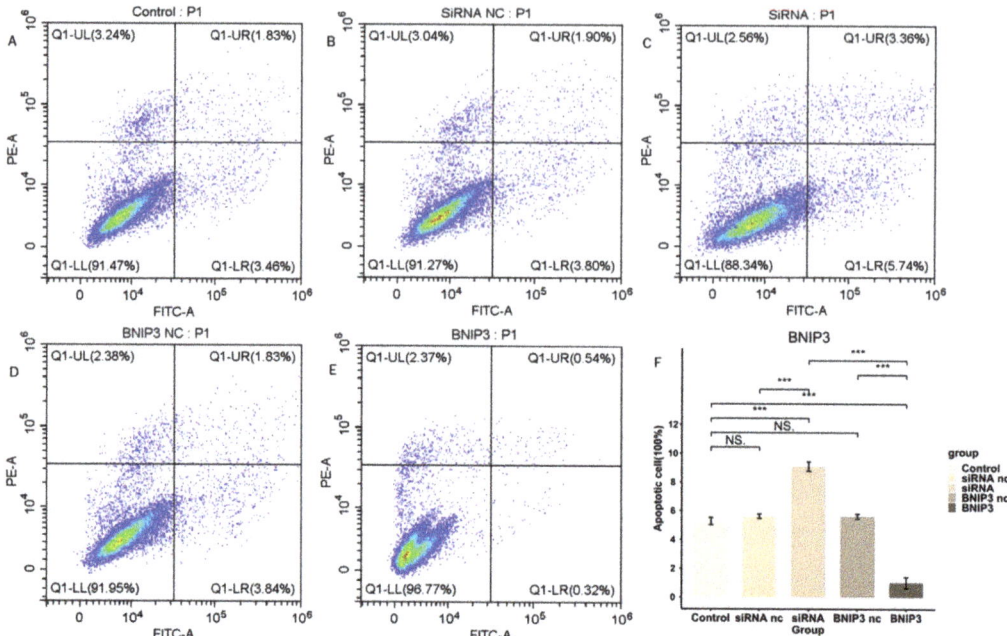

Figure 16. BNIP3 regulates the apoptosis of osteosarcoma cells. (**A–E**) Apoptosis of osteosarcoma cells after knockdown or overexpression of BNIP3. (**F**) Overexpression of BNIP3 inhibits apoptosis of osteosarcoma cells, while knockdown of BNIP3 promotes apoptosis of osteosarcoma cells. "NS" represented "No significant difference", "***" represented "$p < 0.001$".

3.9. BNIP3 Regulates Apoptosis in Osteosarcoma Cells

We investigated the regulation of apoptosis in osteosarcoma cell line 143B by BNIP3 expression levels. We knocked down BNIP3 expression in 143B cells by siRNA transfection and overexpressed BNIP3 in 143B cells by adenoviral transfection, and the apoptosis rate of cells was detected by flow cytometry (Figure 16). The results demonstrated that knockdown of BNIP3 significantly elevated the apoptosis rate of osteosarcoma cells, while overexpression of BNIP3 significantly decreased the apoptosis rate of osteosarcoma cells. In conclusion, the experimental results confirmed that the expression level of BNIP3 played an apoptosis-regulating role in osteosarcoma cell line 143B.

3.10. BNIP3 Promotes Osteosarcoma Progression

The proliferation of 143B cells was detected by EdU experiments. As shown in Figure 17, the proliferation of osteosarcoma cells was significantly inhibited after knockdown of BNIP3, while overexpression of BNIP3 significantly increased the proliferation of osteosarcoma cells. The wound healing assay was used to detect the migration ability of osteosarcoma cells, the results of which can be seen in Figure 18. Osteosarcoma cell migration significantly decreased following knockdown of BNIP3, while it was significantly enhanced following BNIP3 overexpression. These results confirmed the promoting effect of BNIP3 on osteosarcoma progression and metastasis.

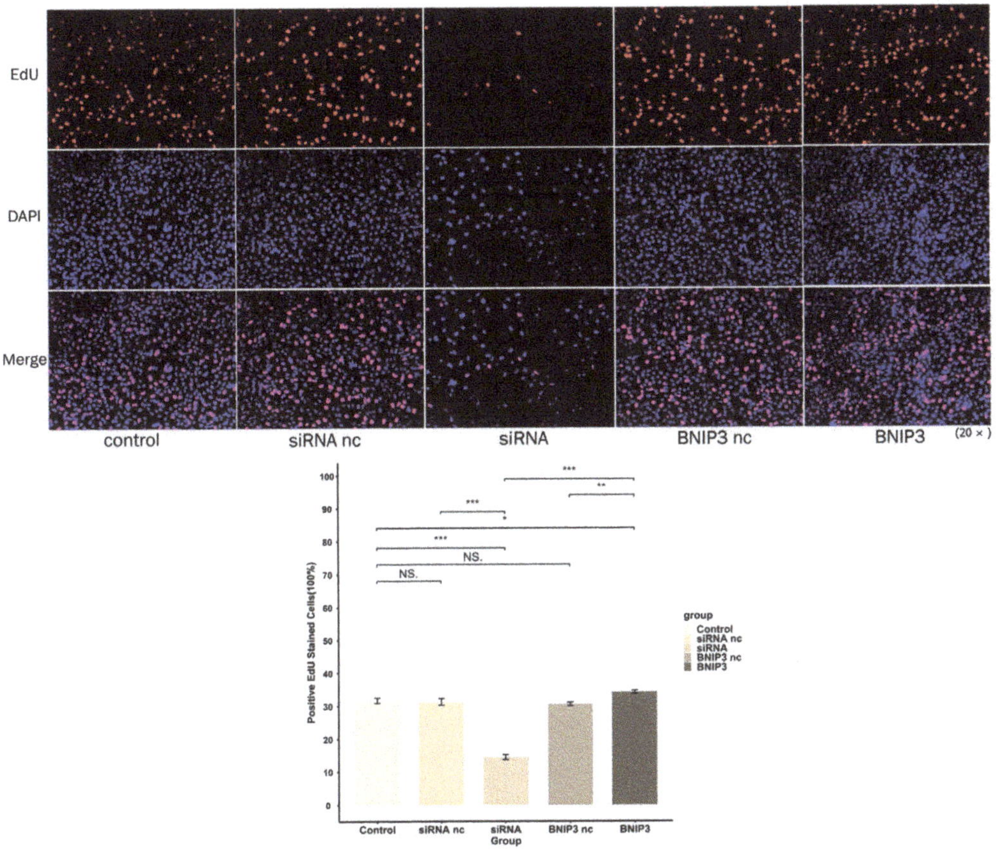

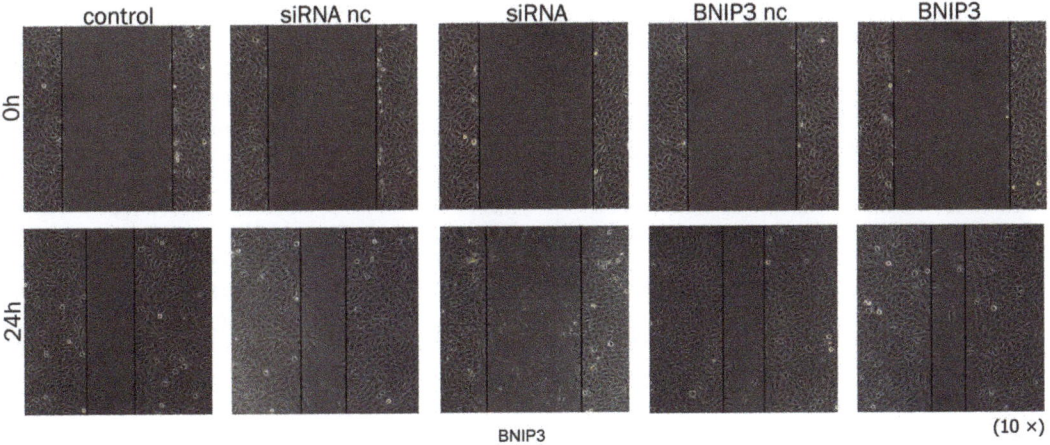

Figure 17. BNIP3 regulates the proliferation of osteosarcoma cells. Knockdown of BNIP3 inhibits the proliferation of osteosarcoma cells, while overexpression of BNIP3 promotes the proliferation of osteosarcoma cells. "NS" represented "No significant difference", "*" represented "$p < 0.05$", "**" represented "$p < 0.01$", "***" represented "$p < 0.001$".

Figure 18. *Cont.*

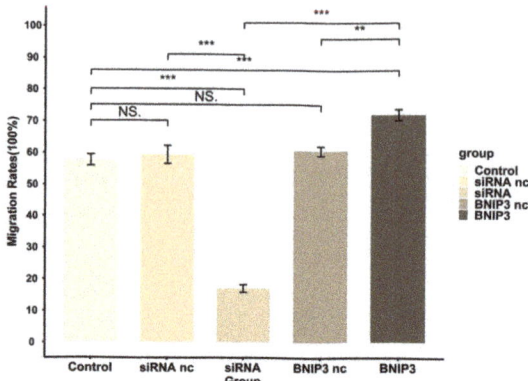

Figure 18. BNIP3 regulates the migration ability of osteosarcoma cells; knockdown of BNIP3 inhibits their migration ability, while overexpression of BNIP3 promotes the migration ability of osteosarcoma cells. "NS" represented "No significant difference", "**" represented "$p < 0.01$", "***" represented "$p < 0.001$".

4. Discussion

Tumor formation is a complex, multi-stage process in which human cells must break through multiple lines of defense before becoming tumor cells. Osteosarcoma is the most common primary malignant tumor of bone in children and young adults, which is characterized by easy recurrence, strong invasiveness, and early metastasis, and it is a tumor with a high degree of malignancy. Combination chemotherapy and complete surgical resection of osteosarcoma is key to a cure, but this only applies to localized osteosarcoma and primary metastatic osteosarcoma. Surgery requires removal of all known metastatic deposits [17], but osteosarcoma patients are prone to lung metastasis. The five-year survival rate for patients with metastatic osteosarcoma remains low, so predicting tumor metastasis and identifying new prognostic biomarkers are essential.

A potential relationship may exist between genes related to the defense response and tumor occurrence and development. In the process of tumor occurrence, the body initiates a series of defense responses, including cellular immune defense, humoral immune defense, and producing cytokines as a response to DNA damage events, all of which are important host defense responses [2,12]. The link between cancer and defense response genes has been identified by several previous studies, including key prognostic genes of osteosarcoma [4], pancreatic cancer [5] clear cell renal cell carcinoma [6], and breast cancer [7] that are significantly enriched in the defense response pathway. Defense response production helps the body to kill tumor cells while preventing their escape [8–10]. Therefore, defense response-related genes have a close relationship with osteosarcoma development and progression. Relatively few studies have been conducted on the role that defense response plays in osteosarcoma. This study established a signature composed of three genes for predicting osteosarcoma prognosis from a defense response perspective for the first time. The model was constructed using a GEO dataset and the TARGET database. It demonstrated good predictive performance for the overall survival of osteosarcoma patients and served as an independent prognosis predictor for osteosarcoma patients in both the training and test sets divided from the TARGET database. In addition, it exhibited excellent performance in distinguishing high- and low-risk groups. A new nomogram was produced for the purpose of guiding osteosarcoma treatment. Three key genes were studied to varying degrees, and BNIP3 was found to play an essential role in osteosarcoma metastasis and progression, verified by apoptosis, proliferation, and migration experiments. Apoptosis and EdU experiments confirmed that BNIP3 can inhibit osteosarcoma cell apoptosis and promote proliferation. Migration experiments confirmed that as a risk gene,

BNIP3 can enhance osteosarcoma cell invasiveness and promote metastasis. Box plots and ROC curves proved that BNIP3 had good performance in osteosarcoma metastasis prediction. Further correlation analysis found BNIP3 to have a significantly positive correlation with MYC, NELL1, SAR1A, PLOD2, and other genes proven to promote osteosarcoma metastasis [18–21]. However, a significantly negative correlation was found between TNFAIP8L1, TRIM22, and other genes proven to inhibit osteosarcoma metastasis [22,23]. In addition, pan-cancer analysis revealed that BNIP3 was also differentially expressed in different tumor tissues compared to that in normal tissues, including LAML, COAD, and KIRC, which was consistent with previous studies [24–27]. Enrichment analysis was conducted on the differentially expressed genes of the BNIP3 high–low expression group. The results indicated that the differentially expressed genes were significantly involved in antigen processing and the presentation of peptide antigen, the regulation of angiogenesis and cellular response to antigen hypoxia, gap junction channel activity, and other pathways, suggesting that BNIP3 may facilitate the regulation of osteosarcoma progression via these pathways, which needs to be explored in further experiments. All of these results suggested that BNIP3 has the potential to be a therapeutic target for osteosarcoma, with implications for clinical treatment and future research in osteosarcoma.

Among the three identified genes, BNIP3 has been reported to have an association with osteosarcoma, ovarian cancer, breast cancer, and melanoma prognosis [28–31], and BNIP3 is pro-apoptotic in most studies [32], although there are still some studies indicating that BNIP3 can inhibit apoptosis in tumor cells [33–35]. Burton et al. [35] reported that nuclear BNIP3 acts as a transcriptional repressor by binding to the promoter region of the AIF gene, thereby preventing apoptosis of glioma cells. Luo et al. [33] indicated that knockdown of BNIP3 significantly increased the apoptosis rate of lung cancer cells, and low expression levels of BNIP3 could increase the infiltration of immune cells and improve the prognosis of lung cancer patients. Moreover, the role of BNIP3 in various tumors is inconsistent. Vianello et al. [29] found that high levels of BNIP3 expression significantly reduced survival in ovarian cancer patients, and that BNIP3 affected tumor cell resistance by regulating mitochondrial autophagy and could also be a potential target for new therapeutic strategies. Niu et al. [30] discovered BNIP3 as a tumor suppressor by alleviating FTO-dependent breast tumor growth and metastasis. Hu et al. [36] found that BNIP3 could serve as a prognostic biomarker for breast cancer patients, and patients with breast cancer with high BNIP3 expression had poorer overall survival, disease-free survival (DFS, the measure of time after treatment during which no sign of cancer is found [37]), and disease-specific survival (DSS, the percentage of people who die from a specific disease in a defined period of time, i.e., patients who die from causes other than the disease being studied are not counted [38]). These studies have fully illustrated the diversity of BNIP3 modes of action and biological functions under different conditions.

ZYX has been reported to have an association with glioblastoma, colon cancer, and pancreatic cancer [39–42]. However, its role in various tumors is also not standardized, and studies on its role in osteosarcoma are lacking. Michiyo et al. [43] found that inhibition of ZYX expression could lead to tumor regression by affecting cell structure and motility in oral squamous cell carcinoma cells, while Aleksandra et al. [44] indicated that decreased expression of ZYX may promote the formation of non-small cell lung cancer. The role of PTGIS in osteosarcoma has not yet been reported, but some studies have demonstrated that PTGIS is associated with the prognosis of bladder and lung cancers [45–47]. Kai et al. [48] revealed that PTGIS promotes proliferation, migration, and invasion of lung squamous cell carcinoma (LUSC) and can be utilized as a therapeutic target for LUSC as well as a biomarker for prognosis and tumor immunity. Danian et al. [49] found that high expression of PTGIS promoted the infiltration of tumor-associated macrophages (TAMs) and Tregs in the tumor microenvironment and deteriorated the prognosis of patients with lung, ovarian, and gastric cancers.

Immunotherapy has been developed as a complementary treatment strategy to conventional chemotherapy. To find the application value of DGPS in the immunotherapy of osteosarcoma, we further explored the tumor microenvironment of osteosarcoma in our present study. We performed differential analysis of the tumor microenvironment in the high- and low-risk groups classified based on DGPS and found that immune infiltration was significantly higher in the low-risk group than in the high-risk group. The scores of most immune cells in the low-risk group in this study were found to be significantly higher than those of the high-risk group, such as B cells, macrophages, neutrophils, NK cells, CD8+ T cells, Th1 cells, and Th2 cells. Meanwhile, the enrichment analysis of DEGs in the different risk subgroups also revealed significant enrichment in KEGG enrichment pathways such as Th1 and Th2 cell differentiation and in GO enrichment pathways such as B cell-mediated immunity and T cell activation. The immune function scores of APC co-inhibition, CCR, checkpoint, cytolytic activity, and T cell co-stimulation were also found to be significantly higher in the low-risk group. This may serve as a basis for selecting appropriate therapeutic targets and chemotherapeutic agents. In addition, the low-risk group had higher stromal, immune, and ESTIMATE scores, which indicated lower tumor purity and better immunotherapy response among patients in the low-risk group [50,51]. Additionally, we also divided all samples into high and low ImmuneScore groups according to the median ImmuneScore for the difference analysis of DGPS risk scores, and the results indicated that the low ImmuneScore group had a significantly higher DGPS risk score than the high ImmuneScore group, with the same results validated for StromalScore and ESTIMATEScore. Correlation scatterplots indicated that DGPS risk scores were significantly and negatively correlated with ImmuneScore, StromalScore, and ESTIMATEScore. These results suggested that osteosarcoma in the high-risk group of DGPS can be classified as a cold tumor subgroup, i.e., with poorer immune infiltration and possibly poorer response to immunotherapy [52,53]. The expression of immune checkpoints LAG3, NRP1, CD40LG, C10orf54, CD86, CD48, CD274, HAVCR2, CD27, CTLA4, CD200R1, LAIR1, LGALS9, CD28, and PDCD1LG2 was significantly higher in the low-risk group than in the high-risk group, and it was previously confirmed in the literature that LAG3 [54], CD86 [55], HAVCR2 [56], CD27 [57], LAIR1 [58], and PDCD1LG2 [56] checkpoints play important roles in osteosarcoma cell therapy. These results suggested that these checkpoints could be potential targets for osteosarcoma therapy and that DGPS could provide a new criteria to guide osteosarcoma immunotherapy.

The sensitivity to chemotherapeutic drugs was represented by the half-maximal inhibitory concentration (IC50) of chemotherapeutic drugs. IC50 is a crucial indicator for assessing tumor response to therapy; a smaller IC50 value indicates higher sensitivity of tumor cells to this chemotherapeutic agent. IC50 values have been used by many researchers to predict drug sensitivity in order to explore personalized drug therapy guidance for different patients [59–64]. At the same time, high-risk patients in this study were found to have a greater sensitivity to MP479, SB52334, and other drugs, whereas low-risk patients were found to be more sensitive to JNK inhibitor VIII and TGX221. It was previously found that MP470 could be a potential therapeutic agent for osteosarcoma [65]. The results showed that DGPS has great potential for guiding clinical treatment strategies for osteosarcoma patients.

There were several limitations to this study. Firstly, the datasets were downloaded from the TARGET and GEO databases, and the sample quantities were limited. Secondly, external validation of the constructed model was not conducted to improve its applicability. Generally, the model had good prognostic value, and the role played by the BNIP3 gene in osteosarcoma occurrence and development was verified experimentally. At the same time, collecting more clinical samples is planned for further verification of this model.

From this study, it can be seen that the signature based on the defense response has good application value for the prediction of osteosarcoma prognosis, and it has strong potential for evaluation of the tumor immune microenvironment and personalized treatment guidance. In particular, the potential impact of BNIP3 in osteosarcoma was further explored. Additionally forward-looking evidence for assessing the signature's accuracy and applicability is required in the future.

5. Conclusions

This study elucidated the role and mechanism of BNIP3, PTGIS, and ZYX in OS progression and was well verified by the experimental results, enabling reliable prognostic means and treatment strategies to be proposed for OS patients.

This study established a signature (DGPS) composed of three genes for predicting osteosarcoma prognosis from a defense response perspective for the first time. DGPS had excellent performance in predicting one-, three-, and five-year survival rates and metastasis of osteosarcoma. It was also a strong predictor of survival in different clinical subgroups of osteosarcoma patients. The risk model DGPS we constructed taps into the relationship between osteosarcoma and the immune microenvironment; high-risk status classified by DGPS was associated with a reduction in immune infiltration. DGPS was also found to be instructive in the individualization of drug therapy for patients with osteosarcoma. BNIP3 was found to play an essential role in osteosarcoma metastasis and progression and was verified by apoptosis, proliferation, and migration experiments. Our findings have guiding significance in the clinical treatment and future research of osteosarcoma.

Author Contributions: Conceptualization, L.H. and F.S.; methodology, Z.L.; software, L.H. and J.C.; validation, W.J., Y.Z. and L.H.; formal analysis, C.Z.; investigation, L.H.; resources, W.L.; data curation, L.H.; writing—original draft preparation, F.S.; writing—review and editing, L.H.; visualization, Z.L.; supervision, H.P.; project administration, H.P.; funding acquisition, H.P. All authors have read and agreed to the published version of the manuscript.

Funding: This research was funded by the National Natural Science Foundation of China (grant number 81672154).

Institutional Review Board Statement: Not applicable.

Informed Consent Statement: Not applicable.

Data Availability Statement: These data were derived from the following resources available in the public domain: TARGET database (https://xena.ucsc.edu/, accessed on 6 April 2023), GEO database (https://www.ncbi.nlm.nih.gov/geo/, accessed on 6 April 2023).

Acknowledgments: We sincerely appreciated X. Wang for his advice on linguistic editing and manuscript writing.

Conflicts of Interest: The authors declare no conflict of interest.

References

1. Gupta, R.; Mehta, A.; Wajapeyee, N. Transcriptional determinants of cancer immunotherapy response and resistance. *Trends Cancer* **2022**, *8*, 404–415. [CrossRef] [PubMed]
2. Konno, H.; Yamauchi, S.; Berglund, A.; Putney, R.M.; Mulé, J.J.; Barber, G.N. Suppression of STING signaling through epigenetic silencing and missense mutation impedes DNA damage mediated cytokine production. *Oncogene* **2018**, *37*, 2037–2051. [CrossRef] [PubMed]
3. Riera-Domingo, C.; Audigé, A.; Granja, S.; Cheng, W.-C.; Ho, P.-C.; Baltazar, F.; Stockmann, C.; Mazzone, M. Immunity, Hypoxia, and Metabolism-the Ménage à Trois of Cancer: Implications for Immunotherapy. *Physiol. Rev.* **2020**, *100*, 1–102. [CrossRef] [PubMed]
4. Fan, H.; Lu, S.; Wang, S.; Zhang, S. Identification of critical genes associated with human osteosarcoma metastasis based on integrated gene expression profiling. *Mol. Med. Rep.* **2019**, *20*, 915–930. [CrossRef] [PubMed]
5. Tang, D.; Wu, Q.; Yuan, Z.; Xu, J.; Zhang, H.; Jin, Z.; Zhang, Q.; Xu, M.; Wang, Z.; Dai, Z.; et al. Identification of key pathways and gene changes in primary pancreatic stellate cells after cross-talk with pancreatic cancer cells (BXPC-3) using bioinformatics analysis. *Neoplasma* **2019**, *66*, 446–458. [CrossRef]
6. Li, S.; Xu, W. Mining TCGA database for screening and identification of hub genes in kidney renal clear cell carcinoma microenvironment. *J. Cell Biochem.* **2019**, *121*, 3952–3960. [CrossRef]
7. Wu, J.; Li, M.; Zhang, Y.; Cai, Y.; Zhao, G. Molecular mechanism of activated T cells in breast cancer. *Onco Targets Ther.* **2018**, *11*, 5015–5024. [CrossRef]
8. Kerneur, C.; Cano, C.E.; Olive, D. Major pathways involved in macrophage polarization in cancer. *Front. Immunol.* **2022**, *13*, 1026954. [CrossRef]

9. Nath, A.; Cosgrove, P.A.; Mirsafian, H.; Christie, E.L.; Pflieger, L.; Copeland, B.; Majumdar, S.; Cristea, M.C.; Han, E.S.; Lee, S.J.; et al. Evolution of core archetypal phenotypes in progressive high grade serous ovarian cancer. *Nat. Commun.* **2021**, *12*, 3039. [CrossRef]
10. Carenzo, A.; Serafini, M.S.; Roca, E.; Paderno, A.; Mattavelli, D.; Romani, C.; Saintigny, P.; Koljenović, S.; Licitra, L.; De Cecco, L.; et al. Gene Expression Clustering and Selected Head and Neck Cancer Gene Signatures Highlight Risk Probability Differences in Oral Premalignant Lesions. *Cells* **2020**, *9*, 1828. [CrossRef]
11. Gill, J.; Gorlick, R. Advancing therapy for osteosarcoma. *Nat. Rev. Clin. Oncol.* **2021**, *18*, 609–624. [CrossRef]
12. Chiesa, A.M.; Spinnato, P.; Miceli, M.; Facchini, G. Radiologic Assessment of Osteosarcoma Lung Metastases: State of the Art and Recent Advances. *Cells* **2021**, *10*, 553. [CrossRef]
13. Sasaki, R.; Osaki, M.; Okada, F. MicroRNA-Based Diagnosis and Treatment of Metastatic Human Osteosarcoma. *Cancers* **2019**, *11*, 553. [CrossRef]
14. Nørregaard, K.S.; Jürgensen, H.J.; Gårdsvoll, H.; Engelholm, L.H.; Behrendt, N.; Søe, K. Osteosarcoma and Metastasis Associated Bone Degradation-A Tale of Osteoclast and Malignant Cell Cooperativity. *Int. J. Mol. Sci.* **2021**, *22*, 6865. [CrossRef]
15. Geeleher, P.; Cox, N.; Huang, R.S. pRRophetic: An R package for prediction of clinical chemotherapeutic response from tumor gene expression levels. *PLoS ONE* **2014**, *9*, e107468. [CrossRef]
16. Lillo Osuna, M.A.; Garcia-Lopez, J.; El Ayachi, I.; Fatima, I.; Khalid, A.B.; Kumpati, J.; Slayden, A.V.; Seagroves, T.N.; Miranda-Carboni, G.A.; Krum, S.A. Activation of Estrogen Receptor Alpha by Decitabine Inhibits Osteosarcoma Growth and Metastasis. *Cancer Res.* **2019**, *79*, 1054–1068. [CrossRef]
17. Beird, H.C.; Bielack, S.S.; Flanagan, A.M.; Gill, J.; Heymann, D.; Janeway, K.A.; Livingston, J.A.; Roberts, R.D.; Strauss, S.J.; Gorlick, R. Osteosarcoma. *Nat. Rev. Dis. Prim.* **2022**, *8*, 77. [CrossRef]
18. Qin, Q.; Gomez-Salazar, M.; Tower, R.J.; Chang, L.; Morris, C.D.; McCarthy, E.F.; Ting, K.; Zhang, X.; James, A.W. NELL1 Regulates the Matrisome to Promote Osteosarcoma Progression. *Cancer Res.* **2022**, *82*, 2734–2747. [CrossRef]
19. Feng, W.; Dean, D.C.; Hornicek, F.J.; Spentzos, D.; Hoffman, R.M.; Shi, H.; Duan, Z. Myc is a prognostic biomarker and potential therapeutic target in osteosarcoma. *Ther. Adv. Med. Oncol.* **2020**, *12*, 1758835920922055. [CrossRef]
20. Zhan, F.; Deng, Q.; Chen, Z.; Xie, C.; Xiang, S.; Qiu, S.; Tian, L.; Wu, C.; Ou, Y.; Chen, J.; et al. SAR1A regulates the RhoA/YAP and autophagy signaling pathways to influence osteosarcoma invasion and metastasis. *Cancer Sci.* **2022**, *113*, 4104–4119. [CrossRef]
21. Wang, Z.; Fan, G.; Zhu, H.; Yu, L.; She, D.; Wei, Y.; Huang, J.; Li, T.; Zhan, S.; Zhou, S.; et al. PLOD2 high expression associates with immune infiltration and facilitates cancer progression in osteosarcoma. *Front. Oncol.* **2022**, *12*, 980390. [CrossRef] [PubMed]
22. Yang, M.; Zhang, Y.; Liu, G.; Zhao, Z.; Li, J.; Yang, L.; Liu, K.; Hu, W.; Lou, Y.; Jiang, J.; et al. TIPE1 inhibits osteosarcoma tumorigenesis and progression by regulating PRMT1 mediated STAT3 arginine methylation. *Cell Death Dis.* **2022**, *13*, 815. [CrossRef] [PubMed]
23. Liu, W.; Zhao, Y.; Wang, G.; Feng, S.; Ge, X.; Ye, W.; Wang, Z.; Zhu, Y.; Cai, W.; Bai, J.; et al. TRIM22 inhibits osteosarcoma progression through destabilizing NRF2 and thus activation of ROS/AMPK/mTOR/autophagy signaling. *Redox Biol.* **2022**, *53*, 102344. [CrossRef] [PubMed]
24. Sun, Y.; Wang, R.; Xie, S.; Wang, Y.; Liu, H. A Novel Identified Necroptosis-Related Risk Signature for Prognosis Prediction and Immune Infiltration Indication in Acute Myeloid Leukemia Patients. *Genes* **2022**, *13*, 1837. [CrossRef] [PubMed]
25. Ramirez, J.A.Z.; Romagnoli, G.G.; Falasco, B.F.; Gorgulho, C.M.; Fogolin, C.S.; dos Santos, D.C.; Junior, J.P.A.; Lotze, M.T.; Ureshino, R.P.; Kaneno, R. Blocking drug-induced autophagy with chloroquine in HCT-116 colon cancer cells enhances DC maturation and T cell responses induced by tumor cell lysate. *Int. Immunopharmacol.* **2020**, *84*, 106495. [CrossRef]
26. Wang, X.; Wu, F.; Deng, Y.; Chai, J.; Zhang, Y.; He, G.; Li, X. Increased expression of PSME2 is associated with clear cell renal cell carcinoma invasion by regulating BNIP3-mediated autophagy. *Int. J. Oncol.* **2021**, *59*, 5286. [CrossRef]
27. Deng, Q.; Li, X.; Fang, C.; Li, X.; Zhang, J.; Xi, Q.; Li, Y.; Zhang, R. Cordycepin enhances anti-tumor immunity in colon cancer by inhibiting phagocytosis immune checkpoint CD47 expression. *Int. Immunopharmacol.* **2022**, *107*, 108695. [CrossRef]
28. He, G.; Pan, X.; Liu, X.; Zhu, Y.; Ma, Y.; Du, C.; Liu, X.; Mao, C. HIF-1α-Mediated Mitophagy Determines ZnO Nanoparticle-Induced Human Osteosarcoma Cell Death both In Vitro and In Vivo. *ACS Appl. Mater. Interfaces* **2020**, *12*, 48296–48309. [CrossRef]
29. Vianello, C.; Cocetta, V.; Catanzaro, D.; Dorn, G.W.; De Milito, A.; Rizzolio, F.; Canzonieri, V.; Cecchin, E.; Roncato, R.; Toffoli, G.; et al. Cisplatin resistance can be curtailed by blunting BNIP3-mediated mitochondrial autophagy. *Cell Death Dis.* **2022**, *13*, 398. [CrossRef]
30. Niu, Y.; Lin, Z.; Wan, A.; Chen, H.; Liang, H.; Sun, L.; Wang, Y.; Li, X.; Xiong, X.-F.; Wei, B.; et al. RNA N6-methyladenosine demethylase FTO promotes breast tumor progression through inhibiting BNIP3. *Mol. Cancer* **2019**, *18*, 46. [CrossRef]
31. Vara-Pérez, M.; Rossi, M.; Van den Haute, C.; Maes, H.; Sassano, M.L.; Venkataramani, V.; Michalke, B.; Romano, E.; Rillaerts, K.; Garg, A.D.; et al. BNIP3 promotes HIF-1α-driven melanoma growth by curbing intracellular iron homeostasis. *EMBO J.* **2021**, *40*, e106214. [CrossRef]
32. Gorbunova, A.S.; Yapryntseva, M.A.; Denisenko, T.V.; Zhivotovsky, B. BNIP3 in Lung Cancer: To Kill or Rescue? *Cancers* **2020**, *12*, 3390. [CrossRef]
33. Luo, L.; Yao, X.; Xiang, J. Pyroptosis-Related Gene Model Predicts Prognosis and Immune Microenvironment for Non-Small-Cell Lung Cancer. *Oxid. Med. Cell Longev.* **2022**, *2022*, 1749111. [CrossRef]
34. Xu, S.; Zhou, Z.; Peng, X.; Tao, X.; Zhou, P.; Zhang, K.; Peng, J.; Li, D.; Shen, L.; Yang, L. EBV-LMP1 promotes radioresistance by inducing protective autophagy through BNIP3 in nasopharyngeal carcinoma. *Cell Death Dis.* **2021**, *12*, 344. [CrossRef]

35. Burton, T.R.; Eisenstat, D.D.; Gibson, S.B. BNIP3 (Bcl-2 19 kDa interacting protein) acts as transcriptional repressor of apoptosis-inducing factor expression preventing cell death in human malignant gliomas. *J. Neurosci.* **2009**, *29*, 4189–4199. [CrossRef]
36. Hu, T.; Zhao, X.; Zhao, Y.; Cheng, J.; Xiong, J.; Lu, C. Identification and Verification of Necroptosis-Related Gene Signature and Associated Regulatory Axis in Breast Cancer. *Front. Genet.* **2022**, *13*, 842218. [CrossRef]
37. Altorki, N.; Wang, X.; Kozono, D.; Watt, C.; Landrenau, R.; Wigle, D.; Port, J.; Jones, D.R.; Conti, M.; Ashrafi, A.S.; et al. Lobar or Sublobar Resection for Peripheral Stage IA Non-Small-Cell Lung Cancer. *N. Engl. J. Med.* **2023**, *388*, 489–498. [CrossRef]
38. Wang, T.S.; Sosa, J.A. Thyroid surgery for differentiated thyroid cancer—Recent advances and future directions. *Nat. Rev. Endocrinol.* **2018**, *14*, 670–683. [CrossRef]
39. De Semir, D.; Bezrookove, V.; Nosrati, M.; Scanlon, K.R.; Singer, E.; Judkins, J.; Rieken, C.; Wu, C.; Shen, J.; Schmudermayer, C.; et al. PHIP drives glioblastoma motility and invasion by regulating the focal adhesion complex. *Proc. Natl. Acad. Sci. USA* **2020**, *117*, 9064–9073. [CrossRef]
40. Zhou, J.; Zeng, Y.; Cui, L.; Chen, X.; Stauffer, S.; Wang, Z.; Yu, F.; Lele, S.M.; Talmon, G.A.; Black, A.R.; et al. Zyxin promotes colon cancer tumorigenesis in a mitotic phosphorylation-dependent manner and through CDK8-mediated YAP activation. *Proc. Natl. Acad. Sci. USA* **2018**, *115*, E6760–E6769. [CrossRef]
41. Zhu, Y.; Tian, J.; Peng, X.; Wang, X.; Yang, N.; Ying, P.; Wang, H.; Li, B.; Li, Y.; Zhang, M.; et al. A genetic variant conferred high expression of CAV2 promotes pancreatic cancer progression and associates with poor prognosis. *Eur. J. Cancer* **2021**, *151*, 94–105. [CrossRef] [PubMed]
42. Zhong, C.; Yu, J.; Li, D.; Jiang, K.; Tang, Y.; Yang, M.; Shen, H.; Fang, X.; Ding, K.; Zheng, S.; et al. Zyxin as a potential cancer prognostic marker promotes the proliferation and metastasis of colorectal cancer cells. *J. Cell Physiol.* **2019**, *234*, 15775–15789. [CrossRef] [PubMed]
43. Yamamura, M.; Noguchi, K.; Nakano, Y.; Segawa, E.; Zushi, Y.; Takaoka, K.; Kishimoto, H.; Hashimoto-Tamaoki, T.; Urade, M. Functional analysis of Zyxin in cell migration and invasive potential of oral squamous cell carcinoma cells. *Int. J. Oncol.* **2013**, *42*, 873–880. [CrossRef] [PubMed]
44. Partynska, A.; Gomulkiewicz, A.; Piotrowska, A.; Grzegrzolka, J.; Rzechonek, A.; Ratajczak-Wielgomas, K.; Podhorska-Okolow, M.; Dzięgiel, P. Expression of Zyxin in Non-Small Cell Lung Cancer-A Preliminary Study. *Biomolecules* **2022**, *12*, 827. [CrossRef]
45. Lu, M.; Ge, Q.; Wang, G.; Luo, Y.; Wang, X.; Jiang, W.; Liu, X.; Wu, C.-L.; Xiao, Y.; Wang, X. CIRBP is a novel oncogene in human bladder cancer inducing expression of HIF-1α. *Cell Death Dis.* **2018**, *9*, 1046. [CrossRef]
46. Fan, T.; Lu, Z.; Liu, Y.; Wang, L.; Tian, H.; Zheng, Y.; Zheng, B.; Xue, L.; Tan, F.; Xue, Q.; et al. A Novel Immune-Related Seventeen-Gene Signature for Predicting Early Stage Lung Squamous Cell Carcinoma Prognosis. *Front. Immunol.* **2021**, *12*, 665407. [CrossRef]
47. Liang, X.; Wang, J.; Liu, Y.; Wei, L.; Tian, F.; Sun, J.; Han, G.; Wang, Y.; Ding, C.; Guo, Z. Polymorphisms of COX/PEG2 pathway-related genes are associated with the risk of lung cancer: A case-control study in China. *Int. Immunopharmacol.* **2022**, *108*, 108763. [CrossRef]
48. Lei, J.; Liang, R.; Tan, B.; Li, L.; Lyu, Y.; Wang, K.; Wang, W.; Wang, K.; Hu, X.; Wu, D.; et al. Effects of Lipid Metabolism-Related Genes PTGIS and HRASLS on Phenotype, Prognosis, and Tumor Immunity in Lung Squamous Cell Carcinoma. *Oxid. Med. Cell Longev.* **2023**, *2023*, 6811625. [CrossRef]
49. Dai, D.; Chen, B.; Feng, Y.; Wang, W.; Jiang, Y.; Huang, H.; Liu, J. Prognostic value of prostaglandin I2 synthase and its correlation with tumor-infiltrating immune cells in lung cancer, ovarian cancer, and gastric cancer. *Aging* **2020**, *12*, 9658–9685. [CrossRef]
50. Zhao, F.; Li, Z.; Dong, Z.; Wang, Z.; Guo, P.; Zhang, D.; Li, S. Exploring the Potential of Exosome-Related LncRNA Pairs as Predictors for Immune Microenvironment, Survival Outcome, and Microbiotain Landscape in Esophageal Squamous Cell Carcinoma. *Front. Immunol.* **2022**, *13*, 918154. [CrossRef]
51. Zhou, Z.; Chen, M.-J.M.; Luo, Y.; Mojumdar, K.; Peng, X.; Chen, H.; Kumar, S.V.; Akbani, R.; Lu, Y.; Liang, H. Tumor-intrinsic SIRPA promotes sensitivity to checkpoint inhibition immunotherapy in melanoma. *Cancer Cell* **2022**, *40*, 1324–1340.e8. [CrossRef]
52. Chakravarthy, A.; Furness, A.; Joshi, K.; Ghorani, E.; Ford, K.; Ward, M.J.; King, E.V.; Lechner, M.; Marafioti, T.; Quezada, S.A.; et al. Pan-cancer deconvolution of tumour composition using DNA methylation. *Nat. Commun.* **2018**, *9*, 3220. [CrossRef]
53. Liu, J.; Geng, R.; Ni, S.; Cai, L.; Yang, S.; Shao, F.; Bai, J. Pyroptosis-related lncRNAs are potential biomarkers for predicting prognoses and immune responses in patients with UCEC. *Mol. Ther. Nucleic Acids* **2022**, *27*, 1036–1055. [CrossRef]
54. Yang, J.; Zhang, A.; Luo, H.; Ma, C. Construction and validation of a novel gene signature for predicting the prognosis of osteosarcoma. *Sci. Rep.* **2022**, *12*, 1279. [CrossRef]
55. Li, J.; Su, L.; Xiao, X.; Wu, F.; Du, G.; Guo, X.; Kong, F.; Yao, J.; Zhu, H. Development and Validation of Novel Prognostic Models for Immune-Related Genes in Osteosarcoma. *Front. Mol. Biosci.* **2022**, *9*, 828886. [CrossRef]
56. Song, Y.-J.; Xu, Y.; Deng, C.; Zhu, X.; Fu, J.; Chen, H.; Lu, J.; Xu, H.; Song, G.; Tang, Q.; et al. Gene Expression Classifier Reveals Prognostic Osteosarcoma Microenvironment Molecular Subtypes. *Front. Immunol.* **2021**, *12*, 623762. [CrossRef]
57. Pahl, J.H.; Santos, S.J.; Kuijjer, M.L.; Boerman, G.H.; Sand, L.G.; Szuhai, K.; Cleton-Jansen, A.; Egeler, R.M.; Boveé, J.V.; Schilham, M.W.; et al. Expression of the immune regulation antigen CD70 in osteosarcoma. *Cancer Cell Int.* **2015**, *15*, 31. [CrossRef]
58. Bu, X.; Liu, J.; Ding, R.; Li, Z. Prognostic Value of a Pyroptosis-Related Long Noncoding RNA Signature Associated with Osteosarcoma Microenvironment. *J. Oncol.* **2021**, *2021*, 2182761. [CrossRef]
59. Sethi, B.; Kumar, V.; Jayasinghe, T.D.; Dong, Y.; Ronning, D.R.; Zhong, H.A.; Coulter, D.W.; Mahato, R.I. Targeting BRD4 and PI3K signaling pathways for the treatment of medulloblastoma. *J. Control. Release* **2023**, *354*, 80–90. [CrossRef]

60. Abdelsalam, E.A.; Abd El-Hafeez, A.A.; Eldehna, W.M.; El Hassab, M.A.; Marzouk, H.M.M.; Elaasser, M.M.; Abou Taleb, N.A.; Amin, K.M.; Abdel-Aziz, H.A.; Ghosh, P.; et al. Discovery of novel thiazolyl-pyrazolines as dual EGFR and VEGFR-2 inhibitors endowed with in vitro antitumor activity towards non-small lung cancer. *J. Enzym. Inhib. Med. Chem.* **2022**, *37*, 2265–2282. [CrossRef]
61. Maurici, C.E.; Colenbier, R.; Wylleman, B.; Brancato, L.; van Zwol, E.; Van den Bossche, J.; Timmermans, J.-P.; Giovannetti, E.; Mori da Cunha, M.G.M.C.; Bogers, J. Hyperthermia Enhances Efficacy of Chemotherapeutic Agents in Pancreatic Cancer Cell Lines. *Biomolecules* **2022**, *12*, 651. [CrossRef] [PubMed]
62. Agena, R.; de Jesús Cortés-Sánchez, A.; Hernández-Sánchez, H.; Jaramillo-Flores, M.E. Pro-Apoptotic Activity of Bioactive Compounds from Seaweeds: Promising Sources for Developing Novel Anticancer Drugs. *Mar. Drugs* **2023**, *21*, 182. [CrossRef] [PubMed]
63. Kamali, M.; Webster, T.J.; Amani, A.; Hadjighassem, M.R.; Malekpour, M.R.; Tirgar, F.; Khosravani, M.; Adabi, M. Effect of folate-targeted Erlotinib loaded human serum albumin nanoparticles on tumor size and survival rate in a rat model of glioblastoma. *Life Sci.* **2023**, *313*, 121248. [CrossRef] [PubMed]
64. Mesas, C.; Garcés, V.; Martínez, R.; Ortiz, R.; Doello, K.; Dominguez-Vera, J.M.; Bermúdez, F.; Porres, J.M.; López-Jurado, M.; Melguizo, C.; et al. Colon cancer therapy with calcium phosphate nanoparticles loading bioactive compounds from Euphorbia lathyris: In vitro and in vivo assay. *Biomed. Pharmacother.* **2022**, *155*, 113723. [CrossRef]
65. Wang, X.; Xie, C.; Lin, L. Development and validation of a cuproptosis-related lncRNA model correlated to the cancer-associated fibroblasts enable the prediction prognosis of patients with osteosarcoma. *J. Bone Oncol.* **2023**, *38*, 100463. [CrossRef]

Disclaimer/Publisher's Note: The statements, opinions and data contained in all publications are solely those of the individual author(s) and contributor(s) and not of MDPI and/or the editor(s). MDPI and/or the editor(s) disclaim responsibility for any injury to people or property resulting from any ideas, methods, instructions or products referred to in the content.

Article

CD19 (+) B Cell Combined with Prognostic Nutritional Index Predicts the Clinical Outcomes of Patients with Gastric Cancer Who Underwent Surgery

Hao Sun [†], Huibo Wang [†], Hongming Pan, Yanjiao Zuo, Ruihu Zhao, Rong Huang, Yingwei Xue and Hongjiang Song *

Harbin Medical University Cancer Hospital, Harbin Medical University, 150 Haping Road, Nangang District, Harbin 150081, China; haosun@hrbmu.edu.cn (H.S.); 2021021826@hrbmu.edu.cn (H.W.)
* Correspondence: 600911@hrbmu.edu.cn
† These authors contributed equally to this work.

Simple Summary: Gastric cancer has a high degree of malignancy, and even with comprehensive surgical treatment, there is still a high probability of recurrence and metastasis. Finding accurate predictive biomarkers can screen high-risk patients and intervene in a timely manner, which is extremely important for prolonging patient survival. In addition, the value of lymphocyte subset detection in patients with gastric cancer who underwent surgery still needs further exploration. This study further explored the predictive ability of lymphocyte subsets on the prognosis of gastric cancer patients who underwent surgery on a larger sample size and explored the prognostic value of CD19 (+) B cell combined with the Prognostic Nutritional Index (PNI). The results showed that lymphocyte subsets were related to the clinical outcome, the combined index had a stronger prognostic predictive ability than single markers and other non-invasive biomarkers, and was a powerful predictive biomarker for gastric cancer patients who underwent surgery.

Abstract: (1) Background: The aim of this study was to explore the predictive ability of lymphocyte subsets for the prognosis of gastric cancer patients who underwent surgery and the prognostic value of CD19 (+) B cell combined with the Prognostic Nutritional Index (PNI). (2) Methods: This study involved 291 patients with gastric cancer who underwent surgery at our institution between January 2016 and December 2017. All patients had complete clinical data and peripheral lymphocyte subsets. Differences in clinical and pathological characteristics were examined using the Chi-square test or independent sample t-tests. The difference in survival was evaluated using Kaplan–Meier survival curves and the Log-rank test. Cox's regression analysis was performed to identify independent prognostic indicators, and nomograms were used to predict survival probabilities. (3) Results: Patients were categorized into three groups based on their CD19 (+) B cell and PNI levels, with 56 cases in group one, 190 cases in group two, and 45 cases in group three. Patients in group one had a shorter progression-free survival (PFS) (HR = 0.444, $p < 0.001$) and overall survival (OS) (HR = 0.435, $p < 0.001$). CD19 (+) B cell–PNI had the highest area under the curve (AUC) compared with other indicators, and it was also identified as an independent prognostic factor. Moreover, CD3 (+) T cell, CD3 (+) CD8 (+) T cell, and CD3 (+) CD16 (+) CD56 (+) NK T cell were all negatively correlated with the prognosis, while CD19 (+) B cell was positively associated with the prognosis. The C-index and 95% confidence interval (CI) of nomograms for PFS and OS were 0.772 (0.752–0.833) and 0.773 (0.752–0.835), respectively. (4) Conclusions: Lymphocyte subsets including CD3 (+) T cell, CD3 (+) CD8 (+) T cell, CD3 (+) CD16 (+) CD56 (+) NK T cell, and CD19 (+) B cell were related to the clinical outcomes of patients with gastric cancer who underwent surgery. Additionally, PNI combined with CD19 (+) B cell had higher prognostic value and could be used to identify patients with a high risk of metastasis and recurrence after surgery.

Keywords: gastric cancer; surgery; peripheral lymphocyte subsets; prognostic nutritional index; prognostic factor

1. Introduction

According to statistical data, gastric cancer continued to be the fifth most common type of cancer globally and was the third leading cause of cancer-related deaths, surpassed only by lung and liver cancers [1,2]. Currently, surgery is the primary treatment for gastric cancer. However, the recurrence and mortality rates for patients with gastric cancer remains high even after radical resection [3,4]. Thus, it is crucial to investigate effective non-invasive prognostic indicators.

The immune system is essential in preventing and resisting the occurrence and progression of tumors [5]. Normally, it can detect and eliminate abnormal cells in the body, including cancer cells [6]. When the immune system identifies abnormal cells, it triggers a complex cascade of cellular and molecular signals that activate immune cells to initiate an immune response and ultimately eliminate these abnormal cells [7–9]. Therefore, patients with a weakened immune status are more likely to experience tumor recurrence [10]. Detection techniques for lymphocyte subsets emerged many years ago. However, their limited reference values for surgery and high price have hindered their usage in gastric cancer patients receiving surgery. Unlike tumor-infiltrating lymphocytes, peripheral lymphocyte subsets are more easily detectable and can also serve as a reflection of a patient's immune function [11,12]. Previous studies have demonstrated that lymphocyte subsets are reliable biomarkers for cancer patients and are significantly associated with treatment outcomes and prognosis, but these studies were based on a small sample size, and the results need to be further validated [11,13–15]. The relationship between nutritional status and tumors is closely intertwined, with many cancer patients experiencing malnutrition due to metabolic changes, anorexia, nausea, vomiting, and other factors resulting from tumor growth and treatment. This is especially true for patients with gastric cancer [16–18]. Malnutrition can adversely affect the efficacy of tumor treatment and diminish the body's immune function, which, in turn, lowers its resistance to tumors and accelerates their growth [19,20]. The immune function of patients is closely linked to their nutritional status, meaning that proper nutrition is essential for maintaining optimal immune function.

The Prognostic Nutritional Index (PNI) can effectively indicate the nutritional and inflammatory status of patients, with numerous studies confirming its effectiveness in assessing gastric cancer [21,22]. By combining PNI, which indicates nutritional and inflammatory status, with lymphocyte subsets that reflect immune status, a more comprehensive evaluation of the condition of gastric cancer patients can be achieved.

2. Materials and Methods

2.1. Patients

We continuously collected data from 291 patients with gastric cancer who underwent surgery at our institution between January 2016 and December 2017. All patients underwent peripheral lymphocyte subset proportion testing and had complete clinical data. Clinical and pathological information were gathered using an electronic medical records system, and due to the retrospective nature of the study, the Ethics Committee of Harbin Medical University Cancer Hospital waived the need for informed consent (Ethics number: 2019-57-IIT). All analyses were conducted in accordance with the Helsinki Declaration and its amendments.

2.2. Data Collection

The study's endpoints were progression-free survival (PFS) and overall survival (OS), which were determined through centralized telephone follow-up conducted in December 2021. PFS was the period between the beginning of surgery and the progression of the disease, and evidence of disease progression was determined through imaging tests such as enhanced CT. For patients without evidence of disease progression, PFS also ended at the time of the last follow-up. OS was the period from the beginning of surgery to death or the last follow-up.

2.3. Peripheral Lymphocyte Subsets and PNI

The percentage of peripheral lymphocyte subsets were detected via flow cytometry and including CD3 (+) T cell, CD3 (+) CD4 (+) T cell, CD3 (+) CD8 (+) T cell, CD3 (+) CD4 (+) CD8 (+) T cell, CD19 (+) B cell, CD3 (−) CD16 (+) CD56 (+) NK cell, and CD3 (+) CD16 (+) CD56 (+) NK T cell. In addition, we also calculated the ratio of CD4 to CD8. The sum of their proportions was approximately equal to 100%. PNI was calculated as follows: PNI = albumin (g/L) + 5 × lymphocyte (10^9/L). The cut-off points for CD19 (+) B cell and PNI were obtained using the maximum Youden index [Sensitivity − (1 − Specificity)] calculated by the receiver operating characteristic (ROC) curve. The maximum Youden indexes for CD19 (+) B cell and PNI were 0.157 and 0.199, and their cut-off values were 15.40% and 45.82 (Figure 1C,G). Patients with CD19 (+) B cell levels < 15.40% and PNI < 45.82 were included in group 1, those with CD19 (+) B cell levels ≥ 15.40% and PNI ≥ 45.82 were placed in group 3, while the remaining cases were categorized under group 2.

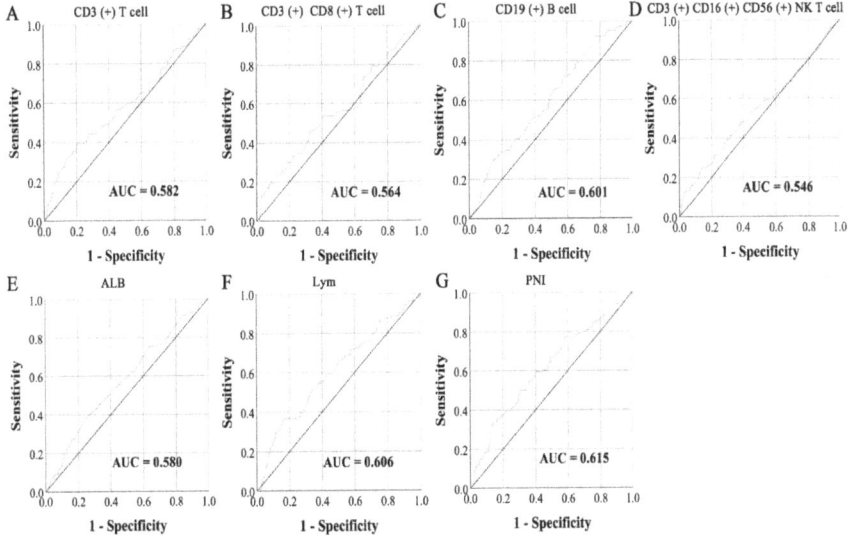

Figure 1. The ROC curve of (**A**) CD3 (+) T cell, (**B**) CD3 (+) CD8 (+) T cell, (**C**) CD19 (+) B cell, (**D**) CD3 (+) CD16 (+) CD56 (+) NK T cell, (**E**) ALB, (**F**) Lym, and (**G**) PNI.

2.4. Statistical Analysis

We performed all statistical analyses using R version 4.2.2 (https://www.r-project.org, accessed on 2 March 2023) and GraphPad Prism 8.0 (https://www.graphpad.com, accessed on 3 March 2023). Statistical significance was set at a two-sided p value of <0.05. Differences in clinical information were compared using Student's t-test, Chi-square test, or Fisher's exact test. Survival differences were evaluated using Kaplan–Meier survival curves and Log-rank test. Cox's regression analysis was conducted to identify prognostic markers, with relative risks estimated by the hazard ratio (HR) and 95% confidence interval (CI). Finally, we developed nomograms to predict the survival probability of patients and assessed their predictive performance using calibration curves.

3. Results

3.1. Patient Characteristics

This study enrolled a total of 291 cases, with 203 (69.8%) men and 88 (30.2%) women, and a mean age of 59.05 (10.45) years. All patients underwent surgery, with 274 patients (94.2%) receiving radical resection. Due to non-normal distribution of tumor markers, patients were categorized into two groups based on the median of tumor markers. Our results showed that CD19 (+) B cell–PNI was associated with age, body mass index (BMI), TNM stage, and CA724 (all $p < 0.05$) (Table 1).

Table 1. Patient characteristics.

	CD19 (+) B Cell–PNI Group			
	Group 1	Group 2	Group 3	p Value
Item	$n = 56$	$n = 190$	$n = 45$	
Age (years), mean (SD)	63.73 (10.56)	58.78 (9.80)	54.40 (10.85)	<0.001
Sex (%)				0.453
Male	41 (73.2)	134 (70.5)	28 (62.2)	
Female	15 (26.8)	56 (29.5)	17 (37.8)	
BMI (Kg/m^2), mean (SD)	21.68 (3.29)	22.91 (3.00)	24.13 (3.56)	0.001
Radical resection (%)				0.191
Yes	52 (92.9)	177 (93.2)	45 (100)	
No	4 (7.1)	13 (6.8)	0 (0.0)	
Primary tumor site (%)				0.610
Upper 1/3	1 (1.8)	8 (4.2)	2 (4.4)	
Middle 1/3	4 (7.1)	26 (13.7)	8 (17.8)	
Low 1/3	42 (75.0)	135 (71.1)	31 (68.9)	
Whole	9 (16.1)	21 (11.1)	4 (8.9)	
Borrmann type (%)				0.193
I	2 (3.6)	21 (11.1)	9 (20.0)	
II	15 (26.8)	59 (31.1)	13 (28.9)	
III	36 (64.3)	97 (51.1)	20 (44.4)	
IV	3 (5.4)	13 (6.8)	3 (6.7)	
LNP (%)				0.080
Yes	34 (60.7)	83 (43.7)	21 (46.7)	
No	22 (39.3)	107 (56.3)	24 (53.3)	
Tumor size (%)				<0.001
<20 mm	0 (0.0)	14 (7.4)	15 (33.3)	
20–50 mm	21 (37.5)	90 (47.4)	13 (28.9)	
>50 mm	35 (62.5)	86 (45.3)	17 (37.8)	
Differentiation (%)				0.116
Poor	21 (37.5)	64 (33.7)	16 (35.6)	
Moderately	31 (55.4)	100 (52.6)	18 (40.0)	
Well	2 (3.6)	15 (7.9)	9 (20.0)	
Unknown	2 (3.6)	11 (5.8)	2 (4.4)	
Lauren type (%)				0.989
Intestinal	27 (48.3)	93 (48.9)	23 (51.1)	
Diffuse	10 (17.9)	35 (18.4)	6 (13.3)	
Mixed	17 (30.4)	53 (27.9)	14 (31.1)	
Unknown	2 (3.6)	9 (4.7)	2 (4.4)	
TNM stage (%)				0.032
I	13 (23.2)	83 (43.7)	21 (46.7)	
II	13 (23.2)	48 (25.3)	10 (22.2)	
III	24 (42.9)	53 (27.9)	12 (26.7)	
IV	6 (10.7)	6 (3.2)	2 (4.4)	
CEA (%)				0.310
<1.97 ng/mL	32 (57.1)	88 (46.3)	24 (53.3)	
≥1.97 ng/mL	24 (42.9)	102 (53.7)	21 (46.7)	
CA199 (%)				0.141

Table 1. Cont.

	CD19 (+) B Cell–PNI Group			p Value
Item	Group 1 n = 56	Group 2 n = 190	Group 3 n = 45	
<10.19 U/L	24 (42.9)	93 (48.9)	28 (62.2)	
≥10.19 U/L	32 (57.1)	97 (51.1)	17 (37.8)	
CA724 (%)				0.001
<2.17 U/L	17 (30.4)	98 (51.6)	30 (66.7)	
≥2.17 U/L	39 (69.6)	92 (48.4)	15 (33.3)	
CA125II (%)				0.897
<10.21 U/L	28 (50.0)	96 (50.5)	21 (46.7)	
≥10.21 U/L	28 (50.0)	94 (49.5)	24 (53.3)	

BMI: body mass index; LNP: lymph node positive; CEA: carcinoembryonic antigen; CA199: carbohydrate antigen 199; CA724: carbohydrate antigen 724; CA125II: carbohydrate antigen 125II; PNI: Prognostic Nutritional Index.

Furthermore, Fisher's exact test revealed that patients in group one tended to have larger tumor sizes ($p < 0.001$). When analyzing blood parameters, we found that cases with low CD19 (+) B cell and PNI had lower γ-glutamyl transferase (γ-GGT), lower total bilirubin (TBIL), lower indirect bilirubin (IDBIL), lower total protein (TP), lower albumin (ALB), lower globulin (GLOB), lower prealbumin (PALB), lower lymphocyte (Lym), higher CD3 (+) T cell, higher CD3 (+) CD8 (+) T cell, lower CD19 (+) B cell, and higher CD3 (−) CD16 (+) CD56 (+) NK cell (all $p < 0.05$) (Table 2).

Table 2. Blood parameters.

	CD19 (+) B Cell–PNI Group			p Value
Item, Mean (SD)	Group 1 n = 56	Group 2 n = 190	Group 3 n = 45	
ALT (U/L)	19.32 (10.63)	21.27 (13.34)	23.52 (14.57)	0.277
AST (U/L)	21.98 (10.25)	21.81 (7.97)	22.38 (7.14)	0.918
γ-GGT (U/L)	15.65 (8.55)	26.14 (21.07)	22.96 (20.77)	0.002
TBIL (μmol/L)	10.78 (6.07)	13.46 (8.86)	11.21 (6.04)	0.042
DBIL (μmol/L)	4.11 (2.25)	4.31 (1.61)	3.99 (1.76)	0.503
IDBIL (μmol/L)	6.68 (4.25)	8.40 (3.46)	7.26 (4.58)	0.006
TP (g/L)	59.89 (6.29)	69.35 (5.42)	69.49 (4.57)	<0.001
ALB (g/L)	35.13 (3.53)	41.87 (3.46)	42.15 (3.17)	<0.001
GLOB (g/L)	25.16 (3.71)	27.42 (3.94)	27.34 (2.84)	<0.001
PALB (mg/L)	218.44 (72.14)	283.77 (72.60)	280.02 (73.89)	<0.001
Urea (mmol/L)	5.83 (1.51)	6.21 (5.02)	6.22 (1.84)	0.823
CREA (μmol/L)	80.25 (15.54)	87.52 (44.46)	78.38 (17.46)	0.206
UA (μmol/L)	265.27 (95.65)	304.58 (86.40)	311.42 (81.33)	0.007
Glu (mmol/L)	5.17 (1.04)	5.30 (1.22)	5.20 (1.00)	0.745
WBC (10^9/L)	6.34 (2.91)	6.79 (2.09)	7.04 (1.76)	0.257
NEU (10^9/L)	4.46 (2.95)	3.99 (1.92)	4.12 (1.55)	0.357
Lym (10^9/L)	1.29 (0.40)	2.11 (0.71)	2.21 (0.70)	<0.001
CD3 (+) (%)	82.63 (84.64)	68.60 (10.61)	66.08 (7.60)	0.036
CD3 (+) CD4 (+) (%)	41.89 (8.80)	40.41 (8.66)	41.19 (8.61)	0.507
CD3 (+) CD8 (+) (%)	24.26 (9.70)	23.86 (7.76)	20.50 (6.55)	0.029
CD4 (+)/CD8 (+)	2.10 (1.09)	1.96 (1.07)	2.34 (1.09)	0.094
CD3 (+) CD4 (+) CD8 (+) (%)	0.32 (0.36)	0.60 (1.47)	0.54 (0.69)	0.328
CD19 (+) (%)	9.58 (3.31)	10.01 (3.46)	19.02 (3.05)	<0.001
CD3 (−) CD16 (+) CD56 (+) (%)	15.70 (9.76)	18.27 (9.81)	11.45 (5.30)	<0.001
CD3 (+) CD16 (+) CD56 (+) (%)	3.51 (3.44)	3.04 (3.64)	3.02 (7.22)	0.761

ALT: alanine transaminase; AST: aspartate aminotransferase; γ-GGT: γ-glutamyl transferase; TBIL: total bilirubin; DBIL: direct bilirubin; IDBIL: indirect bilirubin; TP: total protein; ALB: albumin; GLOB: globulin; PALB: prealbumin; WBC: white blood cell; NEU: neutrophil; Lym: lymphocyte; PNI: Prognostic Nutritional Index.

3.2. Univariate and Multivariate Cox's Regression Analysis

We conducted Cox's regression analysis on the clinical and pathological information of patients. In addition, to explore the impact of lymphocyte subsets more accurately on prognosis, we have also included non-grouped lymphocyte subsets in the analysis. The results showed that age, BMI, CD3 (+) CD8 (+) T cell, CD19 (+) B cell, CD3 (+) CD16 (+) CD56 (+) NK T cell, ALB, Lym, PNI, CD19 (+)-B cell–PNI, radical resection, Borrmann type, lymph node positive (LNP), tumor size, and TNM stage (all $p < 0.05$) were significantly associated with both PFS and OS. Furthermore, CD3 (+) T cell was also identified as a prognostic factor for OS ($p = 0.028$). After incorporating meaningful indicators from univariate analysis into Cox's multivariate regression analysis, we found that age, CD19 (+) B cell–PNI, and TNM stage were identified as independent prognostic markers for both PFS and OS (all $p < 0.05$) (Tables 3 and 4).

Table 3. Univariate and multivariate analysis for PFS.

	PFS				
	Univariate Analysis			Multivariate Analysis	
Parameters	HR (95% CI)	p		HR (95% CI)	p
Age (years)	1.036 (1.015–1.057)	0.001		1.021 (1.000–1.042)	0.047
Sex					
Male	1 (Ref)				
Female	0.918 (0.601–1.401)	0.692			
BMI (Kg/m^2)	0.931 (0.877–0.988)	0.018			
CD3 (+) (%)	1.003 (1.000–1.005)	0.051			
CD3 (+) CD4 (+) (%)	0.998 (0.975–1.021)	0.854			
CD3 (+) CD8 (+) (%)	1.027 (1.003–1.051)	0.026			
CD4 (+)/CD8 (+)	0.934 (0.769–1.134)	0.493			
CD3 (+) CD4 (+) CD8 (+) (%)	0.909 (0.715–1.155)	0.435			
CD19 (+) (%)	0.934 (0.893–0.978)	0.003			
CD3 (−) CD16 (+) CD56 (+) (%)	0.994 (0.973–1.015)	0.581			
CD3 (+) CD16 (+) CD56 (+) (%)	1.031 (1.002–1.061)	0.039			
ALB (g/L)	0.949 (0.909–0.990)	0.016			
Lym (10^9/L)	0.690 (0.517–0.920)	0.012			
PNI	0.952 (0.924–0.982)	0.002			
CD19 (+) B cell–PNI					
Group 1	1 (Ref)			1 (Ref)	
Group 2	0.443 (0.293–0.670)	<0.001		0.763 (0.483–1.206)	0.248
Group 3	0.198 (0.088–0.447)	<0.001		0.352 (0.149–0.831)	0.017
Radical resection (%)					
Yes	1 (Ref)			1 (Ref)	
No	4.182 (2.335–7.492)	<0.001		1.411 (0.579–3.439)	0.448
Primary tumor site (%)					
Upper 1/3	1 (Ref)				
Middle 1/3	0.627 (0.196–2.000)	0.430			
Low 1/3	0.877 (0.320–2.401)	0.798			
Whole	2.084 (0.712–6.104)	0.180			
Borrmann type (%)					
I	1 (Ref)			1 (Ref)	
II	6.081 (1.448–25.533)	0.014		1.978 (0.400–9.783)	0.403
III	8.088 (1.977–33.091)	0.004		2.282 (0.476–10.928)	0.302
IV	28.997 (6.605–127.294)	<0.001		4.626 (0.877–24.383)	0.071
LNP (%)					
No	1 (Ref)			1 (Ref)	
Yes	3.537 (2.324–5.384)	<0.001		1.050 (0.511–2.158)	0.895
Tumor size (%)					
<20 mm	1 (Ref)			1 (Ref)	
20–50 mm	2.715 (0.831–8.870)	0.098		1.536 (0.402–5.871)	0.531
>50 mm	6.883 (2.165–21.878)	0.001		1.203 (0.576–1.431)	0.677

Table 3. Cont.

	PFS				
	Univariate Analysis			Multivariate Analysis	
Parameters	HR (95% CI)	p		HR (95% CI)	p
TNM stage (%)					
I	1 (Ref)			1 (Ref)	
II	3.875 (1.878–7.996)	<0.001		3.192 (1.388–7.340)	0.006
III	11.807 (6.187–22.533)	<0.001		8.472 (3.134–22.904)	<0.001
IV	45.844 (20.022–104.969)	<0.001		21.182 (6.246–71.836)	<0.001

HR: hazard ratio; BMI: body mass index; LNP: lymph node positive; PNI: Prognostic Nutritional Index; ALB: albumin; Lym: lymphocyte.

Table 4. Univariate and multivariate analysis for OS.

	OS				
	Univariate Analysis			Multivariate Analysis	
Items	HR (95% CI)	p		HR (95% CI)	p
Age (years)	1.037 (1.016–1.058)	<0.001		1.022 (1.001–1.043)	0.045
Sex					
Male	1 (Ref)				
Female	0.912 (0.597–1.392)	0.669			
BMI (Kg/m^2)	0.932 (0.879–0.989)	0.021			
CD3 (+) (%)	1.003 (1.000–1.003)	0.028			
CD3 (+) CD4 (+) (%)	0.998 (0.976–1.021)	0.885			
CD3 (+) CD8 (+) (%)	1.028 (1.004–1.052)	0.023			
CD4 (+)/CD8 (+)	0.935 (0.771–1.135)	0.496			
CD3 (+) CD4 (+) CD8 (+) (%)	0.913 (0.720–1.158)	0.454			
CD19 (+) (%)	0.933 (0.892–0.977)	0.003			
CD3 (−) CD16 (+) CD56 (+) (%)	0.994 (0.937–1.015)	0.549			
CD3 (+) CD16 (+) CD56 (+) (%)	1.032 (1.002–1.063)	0.035			
ALB (g/L)	0.947 (0.908–0.989)	0.013			
Lym (10^9/L)	0.684 (0.513–0.911)	0.009			
PNI	0.951 (0.922–0.980)	0.001			
CD19 (+) B cell–PNI					
Group 1	1 (Ref)			1 (Ref)	
Group 2	0.434 (0.287–0.656)	<0.001		0.721 (0.455–1.143)	0.164
Group 3	0.191 (0.085–0.430)	<0.001		0.319 (0.134–0.757)	0.010
Radical resection (%)					
Yes	1 (Ref)			1 (Ref)	
No	4.356 (2.431–7.807)	<0.001		1.769 (0.762–4.105)	0.184
Primary tumor site (%)					
Upper 1/3	1 (Ref)				
Middle 1/3	0.609 (0.191–1.944)	0.402			
Low 1/3	0.885 (0.323–2.423)	0.812			
Whole	2.056 (0.702–6.023)	0.189			
Borrmann type (%)					
I	1 (Ref)			1 (Ref)	
II	6.025 (1.435–25.300)	0.014		2.002 (0.405–9.909)	0.395
III	8.012 (1.958–32.780)	0.004		2.180 (0.454–10.467)	0.330
IV	27.087 (6.171–118.891)	<0.001		4.625 (0.876–24.410)	0.071
LNP (%)					
No	1 (Ref)			1 (Ref)	
Yes	3.445 (2.264–5.242)	<0.001		1.089 (0.532–2.232)	0.815
Tumor size (%)					
<20 mm	1 (Ref)			1 (Ref)	
20–50 mm	2.710 (0.829–8.858)	0.099		1.466 (0.386–5.568)	0.574
>50 mm	6.917 (2.176–21.988)	0.001		1.217 (0.546–1.355)	0.516

Table 4. *Cont.*

	OS				
	Univariate Analysis			Multivariate Analysis	
Items	HR (95% CI)	*p*		HR (95% CI)	*p*
TNM stage (%)					
I	1 (Ref)			1 (Ref)	
II	3.833 (1.858–7.910)	<0.001		3.282 (1.435–7.505)	0.005
III	11.441 (5.999–21.819)	<0.001		9.280 (3.441–25.029)	<0.001
IV	35.899 (15.895–81.079)	<0.001		15.617 (4.770–51.134)	<0.001

HR: hazard ratio; BMI: body mass index; LNP: lymph node positive; PNI: Prognostic Nutritional Index; ALB: albumin; Lym: lymphocyte.

In addition, we evaluated the predictive advantage of different parameters for prognosis using AUC calculated by ROC with death as the endpoint. At the same time, to highlight the prognostic value of combined indicators, we also included classic inflammation and nutritional markers in the analysis. Their calculation formulas are shown in Table 5. The results showed that CD19 (+) B cell had the highest area under curve (AUC) in lymphocyte subsets and PNI had the highest AUC in classic inflammatory and nutritional markers. The combined indicators, consisting of CD19 (+) B cell and PNI, demonstrated a significant advantage in predicting prognosis among non-invasive biomarkers (AUC = 0.648) (Table 6).

Table 5. The calculation formulas.

Items	Calculation Formulas
GNRI	$[1.519 \times$ albumin (g/L)$] + [41.7 \times$ (weight/Wlo)$]$
NRI	$[1.489 \times$ albumin (g/L)$] + [41.7 \times$ (weight/Wlo)$]$
SII	platelet (10^9/L) $\times$ neutrophil (10^9/L)/lymphocyte (10^9/L)
SIRI	Monocyte (10^9/L) $\times$ neutrophil (10^9/L)/lymphocyte (10^9/L)
ALI	BMI (Kg/m^2) $\times$ albumin (g/dL) $\times$ lymphocyte (10^9/L)/neutrophil (10^9/L)

GNRI, geriatric nutritional risk index; NRI, nutritional risk index; SII, systemic immune-inflammation index; SIRI, systemic inflammation response index; ALI, advanced lung cancer inflammation index; The Lorentz equations (Wlo) were as follows: male = Height − 100 − [(Height − 150)/4]; female = Height − 100 − [(Height − 150)/2.5].

Table 6. The AUC of different parameters.

Parameters	AUC	95% CI
CD19 (+) B cell–PNI	0.648	0.582–0.713
Age	0.621	0.555–0.687
BMI	0.584	0.517–0.651
Differentiation	0.562	0.494–0.629
TNM stage	0.817	0.766–0.868
Lauren type	0.537	0.469–0.605
Tumor size	0.668	0.605–0.731
Primary tumor site	0.571	0.502–0.640
Borrmann type	0.646	0.582–0.711
NRI	0.593	0.525–0.661
GNRI	0.591	0.523–0.598
PNI	0.615	0.547–0.683
SII	0.567	0.498–0.637
SIRI	0.561	0.491–0.631
ALI	0.536	0.466–0.607
ALT	0.533	0.465–0.602
AST	0.504	0.436–0.572
γ-GGT	0.533	0.465–0.601

Table 6. Cont.

Parameters	AUC	95% CI
TBIL	0.582	0.513–0.651
DBIL	0.547	0.478–0.615
IDBIL	0.586	0.518–0.655
TP	0.583	0.515–0.652
ALB	0.580	0.511–0.648
GLOB	0.542	0.473–0.611
A/G	0.533	0.464–0.601
PALB	0.640	0.599–0.727
Urea	0.516	0.446–0.586
CREA	0.537	0.467–0.607
UA	0.549	0.478–0.621
Glu	0.538	0.469–0.607
WBC	0.526	0.456–0.597
NEU	0.514	0.443–0.585
Lym	0.606	0.538–0.675
CEA	0.563	0.494–0.631
CA199	0.543	0.474–0.612
CA724	0.610	0.543–0.677
CA125II	0.588	0.520–0.655
CD3 (+)	0.582	0.511–0.652
CD3 (+) CD4 (+)	0.500	0.429–0.571
CD3 (+) CD8 (+)	0.564	0.494–0.632
CD4 (+)/CD8 (+)	0.533	0.462–0.603
CD3 (+) CD4 (+) CD8 (+)	0.511	0.442–0.579
CD19 (+)	0.601	0.534–0.668
CD3 (−) CD16 (+) CD56 (+)	0.536	0.466–0.607
CD3 (+) CD16 (+) CD56 (+)	0.546	0.475–0.617

AUC: area under curve; CI: confidence interval; PNI: Prognostic Nutritional Index; GNRI: geriatric nutritional risk index; NRI: nutritional risk index; SII: systemic immune-inflammation index; SIRI: systemic inflammation response index; ALI: advanced lung cancer inflammation index; ALT: alanine transaminase; AST: aspartate aminotransferase; γ-GGT: γ-glutamyl transferase; TBIL: total bilirubin; DBIL: direct bilirubin; IDBIL: indirect bilirubin; TP: total protein; ALB: albumin; GLOB: globulin; PALB: prealbumin; Urea: urea nitrogen; CREA: creatinine; UA: uric acid; Glu: glucose; WBC: white blood cell; NEU: neutrophil; Lym: lymphocyte; CEA: carcinoembryonic antigen; CA199: carbohydrate antigen 199; CA724: carbohydrate antigen 724; CA125II: carbohydrate antigen 125II.

3.3. Survival Analysis for Lymphocyte Subsets

As some of the lymphocyte subset indicators were found to be related to survival in Cox's regression analysis, the maximum Youden indexes for CD3 (+) T cell, CD3 (+) CD8 (+) T cell, and CD3 (+) CD16 (+) CD56 (+) NK T cell were 0.191, 0.138, and 0.110, and their cut-off values were 74.60%, 25.25%, and 4.85% (Figure 1A,B,D). There were 211 patients with CD3 (+) T cell < 74.60%, with 1-, 3-, and 5-year survival rates for PFS and OS of 90.5%, 75.2%, and 71.7%, and 91.0%, 77.7%, and 73.3%, respectively. There were 80 patients with CD3 (+) T cell ≥ 74.60%, with 1-, 3-, and 5-year survival rates for PFS and OS of 88.8%, 65.0%, and 51.2%, and 89.7%, 78.6%, and 75.2%, respectively. Patients with high CD3 (+) T cell levels had a shorter PFS (HR = 1.995, $p < 0.001$) and OS (HR = 2.051, $p < 0.001$) (Figure 2A,B).

After grouping, 182 cases were enrolled in the CD3 (+) CD8 (+) T cell < 25.25% group and 109 cases were enrolled in the CD3 (+) CD8 (+) T cell ≥ 25.25% group. The 1-, 3-, and 5-year survival rates for PFS in patients with CD3 (+) CD8 (+) T cell < 25.25% and CD3 (+) CD8 (+) T cell ≥ 25.25% were 90.8%, 75.6%, and 71.7% and 89.6%, 67.0%, and 56.5%, respectively. The corresponding survival rates for OS were 91.8%, 76.3%, and 71.8% and 90.1%, 71.6%, and 59.6%. Notably, patients with high CD3 (+) CD8 (+) T cell were associated with poorer PFS (HR = 1.513, $p = 0.030$) and OS (HR = 1.516, $p = 0.029$) (Figure 2C,D).

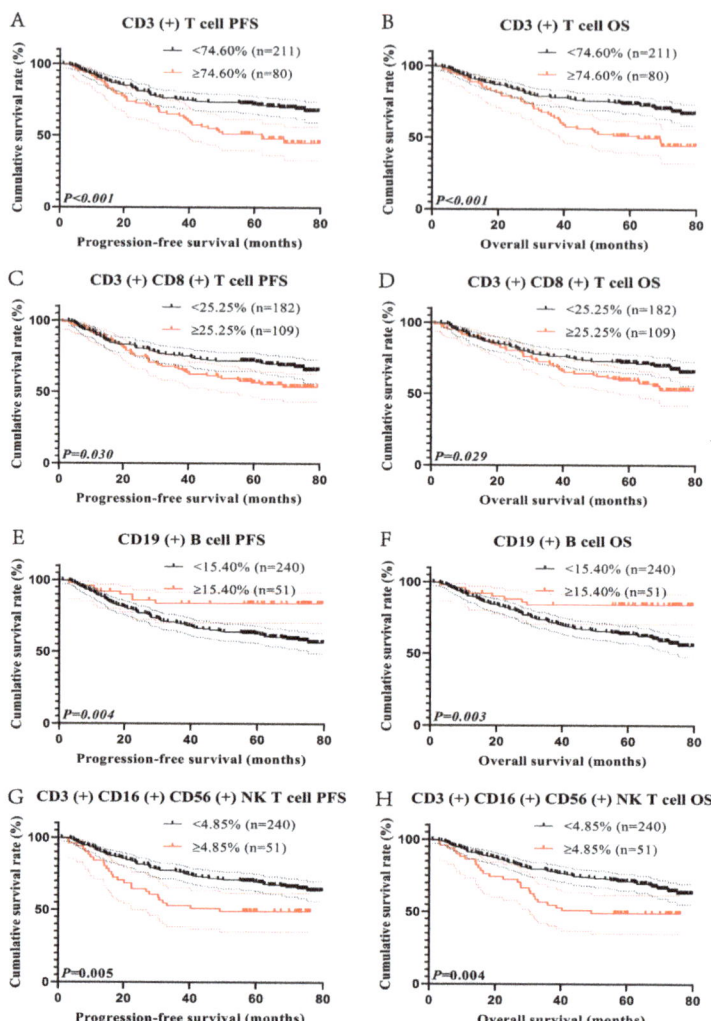

Figure 2. Survival curve for lymphocyte subset. CD3 (+)-related survival curve for (**A**) PFS and (**B**) OS; CD3 (+) CD8 (+)-related survival curve for (**C**) PFS and (**D**) OS; CD19 (+)-related survival curve for (**E**) PFS and (**F**) OS. CD3 (+) CD16 (+) CD56 (+)-related survival curve for (**G**) PFS and (**H**) OS.

There were 240 patients with CD19 (+) B cell < 15.40%, and their 1- and 3-year survival rates for PFS and OS were 89.6% and 90.0%, respectively, while there were 51 patients with CD19 (+) B cell ≥ 15.40%, and their 1- and 3-year survival rates for PFS and OS were 92.2% and 83.9% and 92.2% and 84.1%, respectively. Patients with low CD19 (+) B cell had shorter PFS (HR = 0.358, $p < 0.004$) and OS (HR = 0.351, $p < 0.003$) (Figure 2E,F).

There were then 240 cases with CD3 (+) CD16 (+) CD56 (+) NK T cell < 4.85% and 51 cases with CD3 (+) CD16 (+) CD56 (+) NK T cell ≥ 4.85%. Patients with CD3 (+) CD16 (+) CD56 (+) NK T cell < 4.85% had 1-, 3-, and 5-year survival rates for PFS and OS of 91.3%, 76.5%, and 69.6% and 91.3%, 78.3%, and 71.1%, respectively. In addition, patients with CD3 (+) CD16 (+) CD56 (+) NK T cell ≥ 4.85% had 1-, 3-, and 5-year survival rates for PFS and OS of 84.3%, 52.9%, and 49.0% and 86.3%, 56.9%, and 48.5%, respectively. Patients with high CD3 (+) CD16 (+) CD56 (+) NK T cell had significantly poorer PFS (HR = 1.865, $p = 0.005$) and OS (HR = 1.880, $p = 0.004$) (Figure 2G,H).

3.4. Survival Analysis for Prognostic Nutritional Index

In this study, we conducted a survival analysis for PNI because it has the highest ACU among classic inflammatory and nutritional markers. The maximum Youden indexes calculated by ROC for ALB and Lym were 0.140 and 0.200, and their cut-off values were 38.50 g/L and 1.43×10^9/L (Figure 1E,F). Of the total 291 patients, there were 84 cases with ALB < 38.50 g/L and 207 cases with ALB $\geq$ 38.50 g/L. The 1-, 3-, and 5-year survival rates for both PFS and OS in patients with ALB < 38.50 g/L were 89.3%, 65.2%, and 55.4% vs. 88.1%, 66.7%, and 57.1%, respectively. In addition, the corresponding survival rates in patients with ALB $\geq$ 38.50 g/L were 90.3%, 75.3%, and 70.2% vs. 91.3%, 77.7%, and 71.3%. Patients with low ALB levels had significantly shorter PFS and OS (HR = 0.600, $p = 0.013$ and HR = 0.583, $p = 0.009$, respectively) (Figure 3A,B).

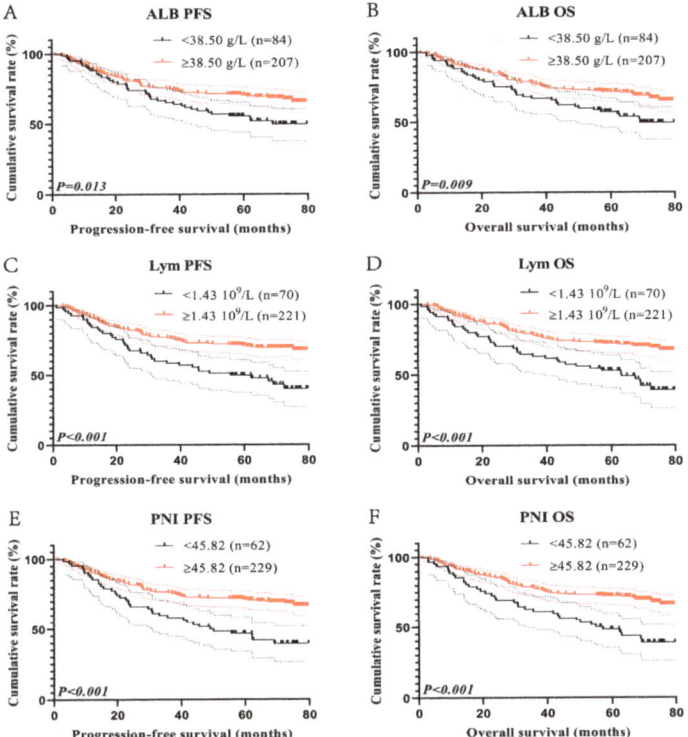

Figure 3. Survival curve for Prognostic Nutritional Index. ALB-related survival curve for (**A**) PFS and (**B**) OS; Lym-related survival curve for (**C**) PFS and (**D**) OS; PNI-related survival curve for (**E**) PFS and (**F**) OS.

There were 70 patients with Lym < 1.43×10^9/L and 221 patients with Lym $\geq 1.43 \times 10^9$/L. The 1-, 3-, and 5-year survival rates for PFS in patients with Lym < 1.43×10^9/L and Lym $\geq 1.43 \times 10^9$/L were 85.7%, 58.4%, and 49.6% and 91.4%, 76.8%, and 71.2%, respectively. Similarly, the corresponding survival rates for OS were 84.3%, 62.9%, and 52.8% and 92.3%, 78.2%, and 71.8%. Patients with low Lym had poorer PFS and OS (HR = 0.456, $p < 0.001$ and HR = 0.453, $p < 0.001$) (Figure 3C,D).

There were 62 patients with PNI < 45.82, with 1-, 3-, and 5-year survival rates for PFS and OS of 87.1%, 58.1%, and 46.6% and 85.5%, 61.3%, and 48.3%. Meanwhile, there were

229 patients with PNI $\geq$ 45.82, with 1-, 3-, and 5-year survival rates for PFS and OS of 90.8%, 76.3%, and 71.3% and 91.7%, 78.1%, and 72.3%. Patients with PNI < 45.82 also related to shorter PFS (HR = 0.441, p < 0.001) and OS (HR = 0.431, p < 0.001) (Figure 3E,F).

3.5. Survival Analysis for CD19 (+) B Cell–PNI

Due to the higher AUC of CD19 (+) B cell and PNI, we analyzed their relevant indicators and combined them for survival analysis. We also compared the ROC curves of grouped CD19 (+) B cell, PNI, and CD19 (+) B cell–PNI, and found that the AUC for PNI was 0.615, that for CD19 (+) B cell was 0.601, and that for CD19 (+) B cell–PNI was 0.648. The CD19 (+) B cell–PNI also had a higher AUC, indicating that it had a higher prognostic value compared with a single indicator (Figure 4).

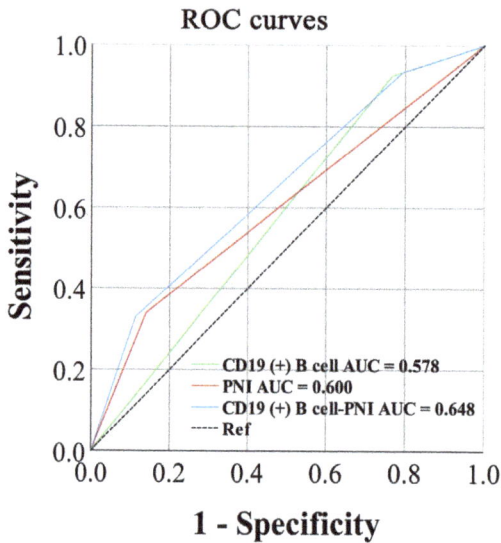

Figure 4. The ROC curve and AUC of grouped CD19 (+) B cell–PNI-related factors.

We grouped patients as follows: 56 cases in group one with 1-, 3-, and 5-year survival rates of 87.5%, 55.4%, and 42.7% for PFS and 85.7%, 58.9%, and 44.5% for OS; 190 cases in group two with 1-, 3-, and 5-year survival rates of 90.0%, 74.7%, and 68.9% for PFS and 91.1%, 76.8%, and 70.0% for OS; and 45 cases in group three with 1-, 3-, and 5-year survival rates of 93.3%, 83.9%, and 73.1% for PFS and 93.1%, 84.2%, and 73.3% for OS. Patients in group one had shorter PFS (HR = 0.444, p < 0.001) and OS (HR = 0.435, p < 0.001) (Figure 5A,B).

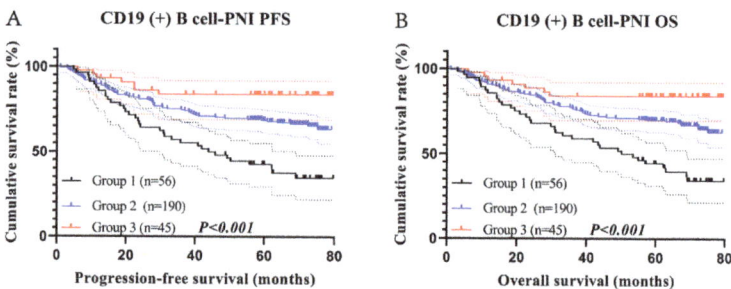

Figure 5. CD19 (+) B cell–PNI-related survival curve of (**A**) PFS and (**B**) OS.

3.6. Survival Analysis for CD19 (+) B Cell–PNI in Different TNM Stages

As the patients in this study were at different TNM stages, we explored the prognostic significance of combined indicators in different TNM stages. Additionally, due to the uneven distribution of CD19 (+) B cell–PNI in different TNM stages, we combined stages I and II, as well as stages III and IV for analysis. There were 188 cases with stage I and II, with 1-, 3-, and 5-year survival rates for PFS and OS of 97.9%, 87.7%, and 84.4% and 97.9%, 88.2%, and 85.6%. Meanwhile, there were 103 patients with stage III and IV, with 1-, 3-, and 5-year survival rates for PFS and OS of 75.7%, 44.0%, and 31.7% and 76.7%, 49.5%, and 33.7%. Patients with stage III and IV closely related to shorter PFS (HR = 6.723, $p < 0.001$) and OS (HR = 6.528, $p < 0.001$) (Figure 6A,B).

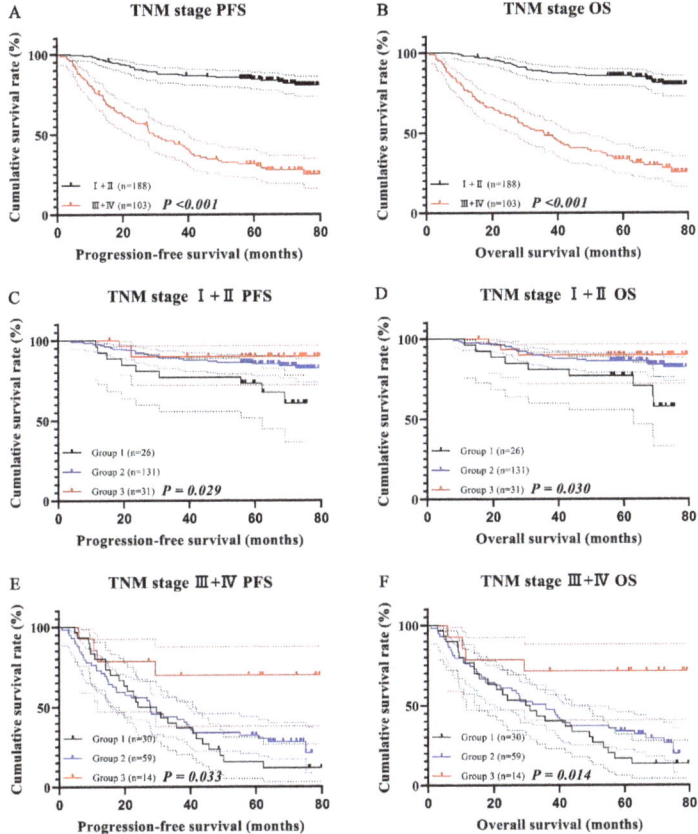

Figure 6. CD19 (+) B cell–PNI-related survival curves in different TNM stages. TNM-stage-related survival curve for PFS (**A**) and OS (**B**); CD19 (+) B cell–PNI-related survival curves in TNM stages I and II for PFS (**C**) and OS (**D**); CD19 (+) B cell–PNI-related survival curves in TNM stages III and IV for PFS (**E**) and OS (**F**).

In TNM stages I and II, there were 26 cases in group one with 1- and 3-year survival rates of 96.2% and 76.9% for PFS and 96.2% and 80.8% for OS. At the same time, there were 131 cases in group two with 1- and 3-year survival rates of 97.7% and 89.3% for PFS and 97.6% and 88.4% for OS. In addition, there were 31 cases in group three with 1- and 3-year survival rates of 99.9% and 90.0% for PFS and 100.0% and 91.1% for OS. Patients in group one had poorer PFS (HR = 0.466, $p = 0.029$) and OS (HR = 0.468, $p = 0.030$) (Figure 6C,D).

In TNM stages III and IV, there were 30 patients in group one with 1- and 3-year survival rates of 70.1% and 36.7% for PFS and 71.7% and 40.0% for OS. At the same time, there were 59 patients in group two with 1- and 3-year survival rates of 72.9% and 42.4% for PFS and 76.3% and 49.2% for OS. In addition, there were 14 patients in group three with 1- and 3-year survival rates of 78.6% and 69.8% for PFS and 78.6% and 71.4% for OS. Patients in group one also had shorter PFS (HR = 0.611, p = 0.033) and OS (HR = 0.570, p = 0.014) (Figure 6E,F).

3.7. Nomograms

To further verify the prognostic effectiveness of combined indicators, we constructed nomograms to predict the probability of PFS and OS based on age, CD19 (+) B cell–PNI, and TNM stage (Figure 7A,B). The C-index and 95% CI of the nomograms were 0.772 (0.752–0.833) for PFS and 0.773 (0.752–0.835) for OS. Furthermore, bootstrap correction showed good consistency of the nomograms (Figure 8A,B).

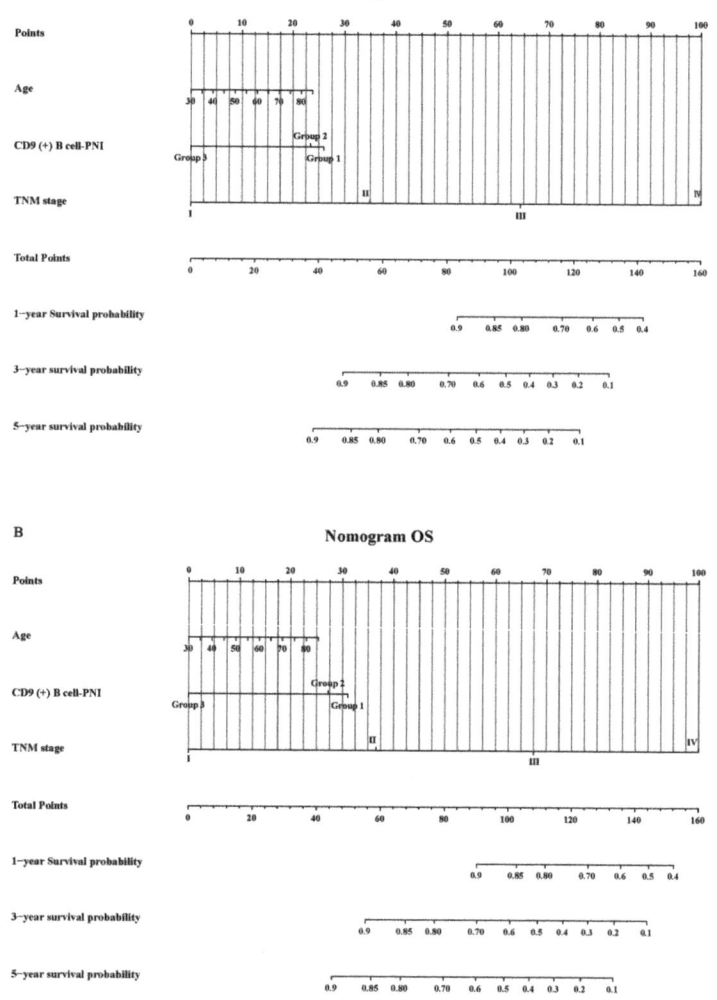

Figure 7. Nomograms of (**A**) PFS and (**B**) OS.

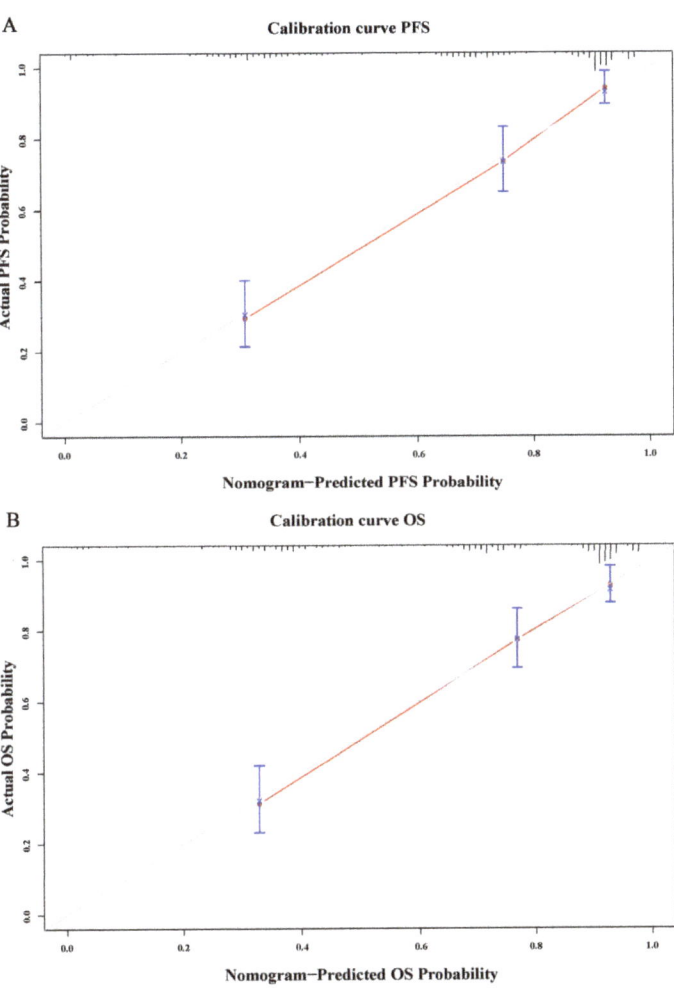

Figure 8. The calibration curves of the nomograms for (**A**) PFS and (**B**) OS.

4. Discussion

After the discovery that solid tumors can affect the composition and quantity of circulating lymphocyte subpopulations, the relationship between peripheral lymphocyte subpopulations and tumor prognosis has been extensively studied. Zhu and his colleagues gathered data from 220 patients with nasopharyngeal carcinoma who underwent concurrent chemoradiotherapy. They analyzed the patients' EBV status and peripheral lymphocyte subsets and found that higher levels of CD3 (+) CD8 (+) percentage and lower levels of CD3 (−) CD56 (+) percentage were linked to better OS [23]. In another study, Zhou and his colleagues also discovered the predictive value of certain subpopulations of peripheral lymphocytes. They collected data from 84 patients with stage III esophageal squamous cell carcinoma who had undergone neoadjuvant chemotherapy and analyzed their disease progression. Their analysis revealed that the percentage of NK cells was an independent predictor of pathological complete response [24]. In 2019, Yang and his colleagues studied the predictive ability of circulating lymphocyte subsets for clinical outcomes in metastatic breast cancer. Through survival analysis of 482 patients with metastatic breast cancer, they found that high levels of CD3 (+) T cell and CD3 (+) CD4 (+) T cell were associated with poor outcomes [25]. Peripheral lymphocyte subsets can also predict the prognosis of patients with gastric cancer. Gao et al. collected clinical information and peripheral lymphocyte subset data from 171 patients with gastric cancer who underwent radical resection. Survival analysis revealed that total T-cell count, B-cell count, and percentage of regulatory T-cells were independent predictors of recurrence-free survival [26]. Another study targeting gastric cancer also reached similar conclusions [27]. As a commonly used nutritional biomarker, PNI has been extensively studied and confirmed for its ability to predict the prognosis of gastric cancer [28–31].

This study further explored the relationship between lymphocyte subsets and prognosis in patients with gastric cancer who underwent surgery on a larger sample size. We performed Cox's regression analysis on all ungrouped peripheral lymphocyte subset indicators and found that patients with high percentages of CD3 (+) T cells, CD3 (+) CD8 (+) T cells, CD3 (+) CD16 (+) CD56 (+) NK T cells, and low percentages of CD19 (+) B cells had worse PFS and OS. After grouping based on ROC curves, the survival analysis still yielded the same results. This result seems different from previous studies which found that T lymphocyte subsets were positively correlated with the prognosis of cancer patients [23,32]. The possible reason was that the percentage of peripheral lymphocyte subsets could only reflect the changes in the composition of different lymphocyte populations but could not accurately reflect the quantity of a certain lymphocyte. In addition, many gastric cancer patients included in this study were at TNM stages I and II (64.6%). The weak ability of tumor tissue to suppress immune function allows the immune system to maintain a response to the tumor. The main type of tumor immunity is cellular immunity, and an increase in the proportion of T lymphocyte subsets may indicate a high tumor burden in patients [33–35].

Due to the close relationship between nutritional status and gastric cancer, we first combined lymphocyte subsets with PNI to determine the status of patients. In extensive analysis of the prognostic value of various parameters, we found that CD19 (+) B cell and PNI had the highest AUC among lymphocyte subsets and nutritional markers, respectively. Therefore, we mainly investigated the predictive ability of CD19 (+) B cell binding PNI on the disease progression and clinical outcomes of gastric cancer patients. Correlation analysis found that CD19 (+) B cell–PNI was related to age, BMI, TNM staging, CA724, tumor size, and a wide range of blood parameters. Survival analysis showed that CD19 (+) B cell–PNI was not only associated with the prognosis of gastric cancer patients who underwent surgery, but also an independent prognostic factor for them. The nomograms containing CD19 (+) B cell–PNI also showed a high consistency between the predicted survival probability and the actual survival probability. These results all confirm its predictive value in gastric cancer. In addition, due to the cautious attitudes of doctors and patients towards endoscopic submucosal dissection (ESD), as well as some early metastases that cannot be detected by imaging examinations, our study included patients with all TNM stages. Although the significant correlation between CD19 (+) B cell combined with PNI and TNM stage resulted in uneven distribution of patients in different groups, we could still find that it had prognostic value in different TNM stages.

Some possible mechanisms could explain how CD19 (+) B cell combined with PNI could accurately predict the prognosis of gastric cancer patients. CD19 was a molecule that was expressed on all B cell lineages except for plasma cells. Belonging to the immunoglobulin superfamily, it played a critical role in B cell development, activation, and proliferation [36,37]. An increase in CD19 (+) B cells reflected an enhancement of humoral immunity in patients and was important in anti-tumor immunity [38,39]. On the one hand, tumor tissues could produce tumor-associated antigens, and antibodies produced by B cells bind to these antigens to induce antibody-dependent cell-mediated cytotoxicity. On the other hand, B cells could bind to tumor-associated antigens, process and present the antigen to induce T cell immune response, or interact with macrophages and complement systems to eliminate tumor cells [40,41]. Albumin not only reflected the nutritional status of patients but also indicated liver function reserve and treatment tolerance [42,43]. Additionally, the decrease in serum albumin was related to systemic inflammatory status, as cytokines produced during inflammation could both inhibit liver synthesis of albumin and induce albumin denaturation, leading to a rapid decrease in serum albumin levels [19,44,45]. Prolonged inflammation could also inhibit the function of the immune system, leading to tumor progression. Lymphocytes were the main participants in immune response, and the decrease in lymphocyte levels resulted in a reduction in anti-tumor immune response, leading to a more rapid development of tumors [46]. Therefore, albumin combined with lymphocytes could predict the prognosis of tumor patients.

However, single indicators had certain limitations in predicting patient prognosis. Although ALB can accurately reflect the patient's status, it is influenced by various factors, including liver and kidney function, nutritional status, and inflammatory response. Changes in these factors can affect the level of ALB [47]. Additionally, patients with gastric cancer typically experience digestive symptoms, nausea, vomiting, and other issues, which may also impact their dietary intake and ALB levels [48]. Similarly, lymphocytes are influenced by factors such as infection, medication, nutritional status, and immune system diseases, leading to certain limitations [5]. CD19 (+) B cells reflect the immune function of a patient, but the immune function of cancer patients is also affected by various factors, such as inflammation and nutritional status, tumor activity, age, and psychological issues [49–51]. By combining PNI and CD19 (+) B cell measurements to predict patient prognosis, the limitations of using single indicators could be minimized, resulting in more accurate results. Overall, the combination of CD19 (+) B cells and PNI comprehensively assessed the patient's status from the perspective of immunity, nutrition, and inflammation, and could accurately predict the clinical outcome of gastric cancer patients.

In this study, we were unable to eliminate the potential bias in information brought about by a single-center retrospective study. In addition, this study only focused on gastric cancer patients who underwent surgery, and the application of CD19 (+) B cells combined with PNI in other types of cancer requires further exploration in subsequent studies. Another issue worth noting is that the differences of CD19 (+) B cells and PNI among different types of cancer patients made them still lack a recognized cut-off value. Finally, the conclusions of this study need to be further verified by a larger sample size prospective experiment.

5. Conclusions

The lymphocyte subsets including CD3 (+) T cell, CD3 (+) CD8 (+) T cell, CD3 (+) CD16 (+) CD56 (+) NK T cell, and CD19 (+) B cell were related to the clinical outcomes of patients with gastric cancer who underwent surgery. Additionally, PNI combined with CD19 (+) B cell as a new biomarker had higher prognostic value than single markers and other non-invasive biomarkers. This combination could be used to identify patients with a high risk of metastasis and recurrence after surgery.

Author Contributions: Writing—original draft and writing—review and editing: H.S. (Hao Sun) and H.W.; data curation and investigation: H.P. and Y.Z.; methodology and supervision: R.Z. and R.H.; resources, funding acquisition, and project administration: Y.X. and H.S. (Hongjiang Song). All authors have read and agreed to the published version of the manuscript.

Funding: This research was funded by Clinical Research Foundation of Wu Jieping Medical Foundation (No: 320.6750.2022-07-13).

Institutional Review Board Statement: This study was approved by the ethics committee of Harbin Medical University Cancer Hospital (Ethical approval number: 2019-57-IIT).

Informed Consent Statement: Due to the retrospective nature of this investigation, the Ethics Committee of Harbin Medical University Cancer Hospital decided to waive informed consent.

Data Availability Statement: The authors promise to provide the original data supporting this study without reservation.

Conflicts of Interest: The authors declare no conflict of interest.

References

1. Ajani, J.A.; D'Amico, T.A.; Bentrem, D.J.; Chao, J.; Cooke, D.; Corvera, C.; Das, P.; Enzinger, P.C.; Enzler, T.; Fanta, P.; et al. Gastric Cancer, Version 2.2022, NCCN Clinical Practice Guidelines in Oncology. *J. Natl. Compr. Cancer Netw.* **2022**, *20*, 167–192. [CrossRef]
2. Thrift, A.P.; El-Serag, H.B. Burden of Gastric Cancer. *Clin. Gastroenterol. Hepatol.* **2020**, *18*, 534–542. [CrossRef] [PubMed]
3. Pape, M.; Kuijper, S.C.; Vissers, P.A.J.; Ruurda, J.P.; Neelis, K.J.; van Laarhoven, H.W.M.; Verhoeven, R.H.A. Conditional relative survival in nonmetastatic esophagogastric cancer between 2006 and 2020: A population-based study. *Int. J. Cancer* **2023**, *152*, 2503–2511. [CrossRef] [PubMed]
4. Park, S.H.; Hyung, W.J.; Yang, H.K.; Park, Y.K.; Lee, H.J.; An, J.Y.; Kim, W.; Kim, H.I.; Kim, H.H.; Ryu, S.W.; et al. Standard follow-up after curative surgery for advanced gastric cancer: Secondary analysis of a multicentre randomized clinical trial (KLASS-02). *Br. J. Surg.* **2023**, *110*, 449–455. [CrossRef] [PubMed]
5. Gonzalez, H.; Hagerling, C.; Werb, Z. Roles of the immune system in cancer: From tumor initiation to metastatic progression. *Gene. Dev.* **2018**, *32*, 1267–1284. [CrossRef] [PubMed]
6. Abbott, M.; Ustoyev, Y. Cancer and the Immune System: The History and Background of Immunotherapy. *Semin. Oncol. Nurs.* **2019**, *35*, 150923. [CrossRef] [PubMed]
7. Janssen, L.M.E.; Ramsay, E.E.; Logsdon, C.D.; Overwijk, W.W. The immune system in cancer metastasis: Friend or foe? *J. Immunother. Cancer* **2017**, *5*, 79. [CrossRef]
8. Sattler, S. The Role of the Immune System Beyond the Fight Against Infection. *Adv. Exp. Med. Biol.* **2017**, *1003*, 3–14. [CrossRef]
9. Wu, Z.; Li, S.; Zhu, X. The Mechanism of Stimulating and Mobilizing the Immune System Enhancing the Anti-Tumor Immunity. *Front. Immunol.* **2021**, *12*, 682435. [CrossRef]
10. Pan, S.; Li, S.; Zhan, Y.; Chen, X.; Sun, M.; Liu, X.; Wu, B.; Li, Z.; Liu, B. Immune status for monitoring and treatment of bladder cancer. *Front Immunol.* **2022**, *13*, 963877. [CrossRef]
11. Miao, K.; Zhang, X.; Wang, H.; Si, X.; Ni, J.; Zhong, W.; Zhao, J.; Xu, Y.; Chen, M.; Pan, R.; et al. Peripheral Blood Lymphocyte Subsets Predict the Efficacy of Immune Checkpoint Inhibitors in Non-Small Cell Lung Cancer. *Front. Immunol.* **2022**, *13*, 912180. [CrossRef]
12. Wang, Q.; Li, S.; Qiao, S.; Zheng, Z.; Duan, X.; Zhu, X. Changes in T Lymphocyte Subsets in Different Tumors Before and After Radiotherapy: A Meta-analysis. *Front. Immunol.* **2021**, *12*, 648652. [CrossRef] [PubMed]
13. Wu, Y.; Ye, S.; Goswami, S.; Pei, X.; Xiang, L.; Zhang, X.; Yang, H. Clinical significance of peripheral blood and tumor tissue lymphocyte subsets in cervical cancer patients. *BMC Cancer* **2020**, *20*, 173. [CrossRef] [PubMed]
14. Li, P.; Qin, P.; Fu, X.; Zhang, G.; Yan, X.; Zhang, M.; Zhang, X.; Yang, J.; Wang, H.; Ma, Z. Associations between peripheral blood lymphocyte subsets and clinical outcomes in patients with lung cancer treated with immune checkpoint inhibitor. *Ann. Palliat. Med.* **2021**, *10*, 3039–3049. [CrossRef] [PubMed]
15. Mao, F.; Yang, C.; Luo, W.; Wang, Y.; Xie, J.; Wang, H. Peripheral blood lymphocyte subsets are associated with the clinical outcomes of prostate cancer patients. *Int. Immunopharmacol.* **2022**, *113 Pt A*, 109287. [CrossRef]
16. Bullock, A.F.; Greenley, S.L.; McKenzie, G.A.G.; Paton, L.W.; Johnson, M.J. Relationship between markers of malnutrition and clinical outcomes in older adults with cancer: Systematic review, narrative synthesis and meta-analysis. *Eur. J. Clin. Nutr.* **2020**, *74*, 1519–1535. [CrossRef]
17. Park, J.H.; Kim, E.; Seol, E.M.; Kong, S.H.; Park, D.J.; Yang, H.K.; Choi, J.H.; Park, S.H.; Choe, H.N.; Kweon, M.; et al. Prediction Model for Screening Patients at Risk of Malnutrition after Gastric Cancer Surgery. *Ann. Surg. Oncol.* **2021**, *28*, 4471–4481. [CrossRef]
18. Huang, D.D.; Wu, G.F.; Luo, X.; Song, H.N.; Wang, W.B.; Liu, N.X.; Yu, Z.; Dong, Q.T.; Chen, X.L.; Yan, J.Y. Value of muscle quality, strength and gait speed in supporting the predictive power of GLIM-defined malnutrition for postoperative outcomes in overweight patients with gastric cancer. *Clin. Nutr.* **2021**, *40*, 4201–4208. [CrossRef]
19. Alwarawrah, Y.; Kiernan, K.; MacIver, N.J. Changes in Nutritional Status Impact Immune Cell Metabolism and Function. *Front. Immunol.* **2018**, *9*, 1055. [CrossRef]
20. Zitvogel, L.; Pietrocola, F.; Kroemer, G. Nutrition, inflammation and cancer. *Nat. Immunol.* **2017**, *18*, 843–850. [CrossRef]
21. Sun, H.; Chen, L.; Huang, R.; Pan, H.; Zuo, Y.; Zhao, R.; Xue, Y.; Song, H. Prognostic nutritional index for predicting the clinical outcomes of patients with gastric cancer who received immune checkpoint inhibitors. *Front. Nutr.* **2022**, *9*, 1038118. [CrossRef]
22. Okadome, K.; Baba, Y.; Yagi, T.; Kiyozumi, Y.; Ishimoto, T.; Iwatsuki, M.; Miyamoto, Y.; Yoshida, N.; Watanabe, M.; Baba, H. Prognostic Nutritional Index, Tumor-infiltrating Lymphocytes, and Prognosis in Patients with Esophageal Cancer. *Ann. Surg.* **2020**, *271*, 693–700. [CrossRef] [PubMed]
23. Zhu, J.; Fang, R.; Pan, Z.; Qian, X. Circulating lymphocyte subsets are prognostic factors in patients with nasopharyngeal carcinoma. *BMC Cancer* **2022**, *22*, 716. [CrossRef] [PubMed]
24. Zhou, J.; Lin, H.P.; Xu, X.; Wang, X.H.; Rong, L.; Zhang, Y.; Shen, L.; Xu, L.; Qin, W.T.; Ye, Q.; et al. The predictive value of peripheral blood cells and lymphocyte subsets in oesophageal squamous cell cancer patients with neoadjuvant chemoradiotherapy. *Front. Immunol.* **2022**, *13*, 1041126. [CrossRef] [PubMed]
25. Yang, J.; Xu, J.; E, Y.; Sun, T. Predictive and prognostic value of circulating blood lymphocyte subsets in metastatic breast cancer. *Cancer Med.* **2019**, *8*, 492–500. [CrossRef] [PubMed]
26. Gao, C.; Tong, Y.X.; Zhu, L.; Dan Zeng, C.D.; Zhang, S. Short-term prognostic role of peripheral lymphocyte subsets in patients with gastric cancer. *Int. Immunopharmacol.* **2023**, *115*, 109641. [CrossRef]

27. Li, F.; Sun, Y.; Huang, J.; Xu, W.; Liu, J.; Yuan, Z. CD4/CD8 + T cells, DC subsets, Foxp3, and IDO expression are predictive indictors of gastric cancer prognosis. *Cancer Med.* **2019**, *8*, 7330–7344. [CrossRef]
28. Zhang, X.; Zhao, W.; Chen, X.; Zhao, M.; Qi, X.; Li, G.; Shen, A.; Yang, L. Combining the Fibrinogen-to-Pre-Albumin Ratio and Prognostic Nutritional Index (FPR-PNI) Predicts the Survival in Elderly Gastric Cancer Patients After Gastrectomy. *Onco Targets Ther.* **2020**, *13*, 8845–8859. [CrossRef]
29. Liu, J.Y.; Dong, H.M.; Wang, W.L.; Wang, G.; Pan, H.; Chen, W.W.; Wang, Q.; Wang, Z.J. The Effect of the Prognostic Nutritional Index on the Toxic Side Effects of Radiochemotherapy and Prognosis After Radical Surgery for Gastric Cancer. *Cancer Manag. Res.* **2021**, *13*, 3385–3392. [CrossRef]
30. Zhang, X.; Fang, H.; Zeng, Z.; Zhang, K.; Lin, Z.; Deng, G.; Deng, W.; Guan, L.; Wei, X.; Li, X.; et al. Preoperative Prognostic Nutrition Index as a Prognostic Indicator of Survival in Elderly Patients Undergoing Gastric Cancer Surgery. *Cancer Manag. Res.* **2021**, *13*, 5263–5273. [CrossRef]
31. Ding, P.; Yang, P.; Sun, C.; Tian, Y.; Guo, H.; Liu, Y.; Li, Y.; Zhao, Q. Predictive Effect of Systemic Immune-Inflammation Index Combined With Prognostic Nutrition Index Score on Efficacy and Prognosis of Neoadjuvant Intraperitoneal and Systemic Paclitaxel Combined With Apatinib Conversion Therapy in Gastric Cancer Patients With Positive Peritoneal Lavage Cytology: A Prospective Study. *Front. Oncol.* **2021**, *11*, 791912. [CrossRef]
32. Milasiene, V.; Stratilatovas, E.; Norkiene, V. The importance of T-lymphocyte subsets on overall survival of colorectal and gastric cancer patients. *Med. Lith.* **2007**, *43*, 548–554.
33. Baxter, D. Active and passive immunization for cancer. *Hum. Vacc Immunother.* **2014**, *10*, 2123–2129. [CrossRef]
34. Ostroumov, D.; Fekete-Drimusz, N.; Saborowski, M.; Kühnel, F.; Woller, N. CD4 and CD8 T lymphocyte interplay in controlling tumor growth. *Cell. Mol. Life Sci.* **2018**, *75*, 689–713. [CrossRef]
35. McGray, A.J.R.; Bramson, J. Adaptive Resistance to Cancer Immunotherapy. *Adv. Exp. Med. Biol.* **2017**, *1036*, 213–227. [CrossRef]
36. Li, X.; Ding, Y.; Zi, M.; Sun, L.; Zhang, W.; Chen, S.; Xu, Y. CD19, from bench to bedside. *Immunol. Lett.* **2017**, *183*, 86–95. [CrossRef]
37. Wang, Y.; Liu, J.; Burrows, P.D.; Wang, J.Y. B Cell Development and Maturation. *Adv. Exp. Med. Biol.* **2020**, *1254*, 1–22. [CrossRef] [PubMed]
38. Chen, V.E.; Greenberger, B.A.; Taylor, J.M.; Edelman, M.J.; Lu, B. The Underappreciated Role of the Humoral Immune System and B Cells in Tumorigenesis and Cancer Therapeutics: A Review. *Int. J. Radiat. Oncol.* **2020**, *108*, 38–45. [CrossRef] [PubMed]
39. Conejo-Garcia, J.R.; Biswas, S.; Chaurio, R. Humoral immune responses: Unsung heroes of the war on cancer. *Semin. Immunol.* **2020**, *49*, 101419. [CrossRef]
40. Zaenker, P.; Gray, E.S.; Ziman, M.R. Autoantibody Production in Cancer—The Humoral Immune Response toward Autologous Antigens in Cancer Patients. *Autoimmun. Rev.* **2016**, *15*, 477–483. [CrossRef] [PubMed]
41. Sato, Y.; Shimoda, M.; Sota, Y.; Miyake, T.; Tanei, T.; Kagara, N.; Naoi, Y.; Kim, S.J.; Noguchi, S.; Shimazu, K. Enhanced humoral immunity in breast cancer patients with high serum concentration of anti-HER2 autoantibody. *Cancer Med.* **2021**, *10*, 1418–1430. [CrossRef] [PubMed]
42. Oh, I.S.; Sinn, D.H.; Kang, T.W.; Lee, M.W.; Kang, W.; Gwak, G.Y.; Paik, Y.H.; Choi, M.S.; Lee, J.H.; Koh, K.C.; et al. Liver Function Assessment Using Albumin-Bilirubin Grade for Patients with Very Early-Stage Hepatocellular Carcinoma Treated with Radiofrequency Ablation. *Digest. Dis. Sci.* **2017**, *62*, 3235–3242. [CrossRef] [PubMed]
43. Zhang, Q.; Zhang, L.; Jin, Q.; He, Y.; Wu, M.; Peng, H.; Li, Y. The Prognostic Value of the GNRI in Patients with Stomach Cancer Undergoing Surgery. *J. Pers. Med.* **2023**, *13*, 155. [CrossRef] [PubMed]
44. Coffelt, S.B.; de Visser, K.E. Cancer: Inflammation lights the way to metastasis. *Nature* **2014**, *507*, 48–49. [CrossRef]
45. Bito, R.; Hino, S.; Baba, A.; Tanaka, M.; Watabe, H.; Kawabata, H. Degradation of oxidative stress-induced denatured albumin in rat liver endothelial cells. *Am. J. Physiol. Physiol.* **2005**, *289*, C531–C542. [CrossRef]
46. Gray, K.J.; Gibbs, J.E. Adaptive immunity, chronic inflammation and the clock. *Semin. Immunopathol.* **2022**, *44*, 209–224. [CrossRef]
47. Margarson, M.P.; Soni, N. Serum albumin: Touchstone or totem? *Anaesthesia* **1998**, *53*, 789–803. [CrossRef]
48. Zhang, Z.; Pereira, S.L.; Luo, M.; Matheson, E.M. Evaluation of Blood Biomarkers Associated with Risk of Malnutrition in Older Adults: A Systematic Review and Meta-Analysis. *Nutrients* **2017**, *9*, 829. [CrossRef]
49. Andersen, C.J. Lipid Metabolism in Inflammation and Immune Function. *Nutrients* **2022**, *14*, 1414. [CrossRef]
50. Lewis, E.D.; Wu, D.; Meydani, S.N. Age-associated alterations in immune function and inflammation. *Prog. Neuropsychopharmacol. Biol. Psychiatry.* **2022**, *118*, 110576. [CrossRef]
51. Antoni, M.H.; Dhabhar, F.S. The impact of psychosocial stress and stress management on immune responses in patients with cancer. *Cancer Am. Cancer Soc.* **2019**, *125*, 1417–1431. [CrossRef] [PubMed]

Disclaimer/Publisher's Note: The statements, opinions and data contained in all publications are solely those of the individual author(s) and contributor(s) and not of MDPI and/or the editor(s). MDPI and/or the editor(s) disclaim responsibility for any injury to people or property resulting from any ideas, methods, instructions or products referred to in the content.

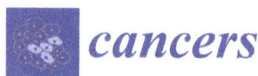 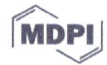

Article

The Membrane Protein Sortilin Is a Potential Biomarker and Target for Glioblastoma

Mark Marsland [1,2], Amiee Dowdell [1,2], Sam Faulkner [1,2], Craig Gedye [2,3,4], James Lynam [2,3,4], Cassandra P. Griffin [1,2,5], Joanne Marsland [1,2], Chen Chen Jiang [1,2,†] and Hubert Hondermarck [1,2,*,†]

1. School of Biomedical Sciences and Pharmacy, College of Health, Medicine and Wellbeing, University of Newcastle, Callaghan, NSW 2308, Australia; mark.marsland@uon.edu.au (M.M.); amiee.dowdell@uon.edu.au (A.D.); sam.faulkner@newcastle.edu.au (S.F.); cassandra.griffin@newcastle.edu.au (C.P.G.); joanne.marsland@uon.edu.au (J.M.); chenchen.jiang@newcastle.edu.au (C.C.J.)
2. Hunter Medical Research Institute, University of Newcastle, New Lambton Heights, NSW 2305, Australia; craig.gedye@calvarymater.org.au (C.G.); james.lynam@calvarymater.org.au (J.L.)
3. School of Medicine and Public Health, College of Health, Medicine and Wellbeing, University of Newcastle, Callaghan, NSW 2308, Australia
4. Department of Medical Oncology, Calvary Mater, Newcastle, NSW 2298, Australia
5. Hunter Cancer Biobank, NSW Regional Biospecimen and Research Services, University of Newcastle, Callaghan, NSW 2305, Australia
* Correspondence: hubert.hondermarck@newcastle.edu.au; Tel.: +61-2-49218830
† These authors contributed equally to this work.

Simple Summary: Glioblastoma (GBM) is the most lethal adult primary brain tumor, and has no cure. This study investigated the membrane protein sortilin as a prognosis biomarker for glioblastoma (GBM). We found that sortilin is overexpressed in GBM tumors and can be detected in the blood of GBM patients. In addition, in cell cultures, targeting sortilin resulted in the inhibition of GBM cell invasion. These data highlight the value of sortilin as a potential clinical biomarker and therapeutic target for GBM and warrant further translational investigation.

Abstract: Glioblastoma (GBM) is a devastating brain cancer with no effective treatment, and there is an urgent need for developing innovative biomarkers as well as therapeutic targets for better management of the disease. The membrane protein sortilin has recently been shown to participate in tumor cell invasiveness in several cancers, but its involvement and clinical relevance in GBM is unclear. In the present study, we explored the expression of sortilin and its potential as a clinical biomarker and therapeutic target for GBM. Sortilin expression was investigated by immunohistochemistry and digital quantification in a series of 71 clinical cases of invasive GBM vs. 20 non-invasive gliomas. Sortilin was overexpressed in GBM and, importantly, higher expression levels were associated with worse patient survival, pointing to sortilin tissue expression as a potential prognostic biomarker for GBM. Sortilin was also detectable in the plasma of GBM patients by enzyme-linked immunosorbent assay (ELISA), but no differences were observed between sortilin levels in the blood of GBM vs. glioma patients. In vitro, sortilin was detected in 11 brain-cancer-patient-derived cell lines at the anticipated molecular weight of 100 kDa. Interestingly, targeting sortilin with the orally bioavailable small molecule inhibitor AF38469 resulted in decreased GBM invasiveness, but cancer cell proliferation was not affected, showing that sortilin is targetable in GBM. Together, these data suggest the clinical relevance for sortilin in GBM and support further investigation of GBM as a clinical biomarker and therapeutic target.

Keywords: Glioblastoma; sortilin; cancer biomarkers; cancer therapeutic targets

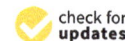

Citation: Marsland, M.; Dowdell, A.; Faulkner, S.; Gedye, C.; Lynam, J.; Griffin, C.P.; Marsland, J.; Jiang, C.C.; Hondermarck, H. The Membrane Protein Sortilin Is a Potential Biomarker and Target for Glioblastoma. *Cancers* **2023**, *15*, 2514. https://doi.org/10.3390/cancers15092514

Academic Editors: Daniel L. Pouliquen and Cristina Núñez González

Received: 28 March 2023
Revised: 24 April 2023
Accepted: 26 April 2023
Published: 27 April 2023

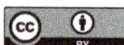

Copyright: © 2023 by the authors. Licensee MDPI, Basel, Switzerland. This article is an open access article distributed under the terms and conditions of the Creative Commons Attribution (CC BY) license (https://creativecommons.org/licenses/by/4.0/).

1. Introduction

Glioblastoma multiforme (GBM) is the most common and lethal malignant primary brain tumor in adults, accounting for 45% of brain cancer cases [1], with a median survival between 7 and 15 months [2]. This poor prognosis is due to the aggressive and invasive nature of GBM and the absence of effective targeted treatment [3]. The oral alkylating agent temozolomide (TMZ) is the standard first-line chemotherapy [4]. Unfortunately, resistance to TMZ and recurrence of GBM are inevitable, and this is particularly dramatic in the cases of GBM exhibiting unmethylated O6-methylguanine-DNA methyltransferase (MGMT); only 7% of GBM patients with this epigenetic silencing survive 5 years or longer [5]. Therefore, the identification of new therapeutic targets for GBM is necessary for the design of effective targeted treatment that could improve the currently limited efficacy of TMZ.

Sortilin (SORT1), also known as neurotensin receptor-3 (NTR3), is a membrane receptor that belongs to the VPS10P (vacuolar protein sorting 10 protein) family of receptors [6]. The biological roles of sortilin include sorting and transporting intracellular proteins. Sortilin has been associated with the progression and aggressiveness of several malignancies, including liver cancer [7,8], pancreatic cancer [9], breast cancer [10,11], metastatic melanoma [12], and colorectal cancer [13]. In GBM cells, sortilin promotes invasion and mesenchymal transition through a mechanism involving a GSK-3β/β-catenin/twist pathway [14] and presenilin1 [15], but the relevance of sortilin as a clinical biomarker or a therapeutic target is unclear.

In this study, we have explored the clinical relevance of sortilin in GBM. Using GBM patient samples and patient-derived cells, we have shown that sortilin expression is elevated in GBM compared to lower-grade glioma, and that sortilin was also detectable at varying concentrations in the blood of GBM and lower-grade glioma patients. In addition, sortilin inhibition was able to inhibit the invasion of GBM cells. These data point to sortilin as a potential biomarker and therapeutic target for GBM.

2. Materials and Methods

2.1. SORT1 (Sortilin) mRNA Data Mining

Gene Expression Profiling Interactive Analysis 2 (GEPIA2) (http://gepia.cancer-pku.cn (accessed on 1 December 2022)) was used to explore GBM data in TCGA [16] and normal brain tissue in Genotype-Tissue Expression (GTEx) [17] databases, using a standard processing pipeline [18]. SORT1 mRNA expressions in GBM, lower-grade glioma (LGG) and normal brain tissue were compared in terms of survival analysis in GBM and LGG comparing high (>median) vs. low (<median) gene expression of *SORT1*. One-way ANOVA was used for differential analysis of gene expression, using disease states (GBM, LGG or normal) as variables for the box plots. Log-rank tests for both disease-free survival and overall survival analyses were used.

2.2. Patient Samples

Patient cohort information included age, sex, tumor grade and primary tumor site (Table 1). Tumor samples were sourced from the Hunter Cancer Biobank (HCB, Newcastle, NSW, Australia) and then formalin-fixed paraffin-embedded (FFPE). All samples were graded by a clinical pathologist from the HCB using the clinically relevant histological features in the WHO guidelines used in clinical practice. The study was approved by the Human Research Ethics Committee of the University of Newcastle. Tumor samples included 71 cases of GBM, 12 cases of grade 3 glioma, 6 cases of grade 2 glioma, and 2 cases of grade 1 glioma. Matching plasma samples were obtained at the time of diagnosis and processed following standard clinical procedure for plasma, including centrifugation for 15 min at 1500 RPM, followed by 10 min at 2500 RPM. Samples were stored at −80 °C.

Table 1. Patient clinical information.

Characteristic	Subgroup	Total
Participants	n	91
Sex	Female	37 (40%)
	Male	55 (60%)
Age at diagnosis	Median (min, max)	63 (17, 82)
	Median (Q1, Q3)	63 (56.5, 72)
Grade	1	2 (2.2%)
	2	6 (6.6%)
	3	12 (13.2%)
	GBM	71 (78%)
Tumor site	Frontal	39 (42%)
	Temporal	30 (33%)
	Parietal	15 (16%)
	Other	8 (9%)

2.3. Immunohistochemical Detection and Quantification of Sortilin Expression

FFPE tissue sections of 4 μm were processed for sortilin immunohistochemical detection as previously described [19]. Sections were labelled with anti-sortilin (0.8 mg/mL, catalogue number ANT-009, Alomone labs, Jerusalem, Israel) followed by a secondary antibody (catalogue number MP-7401, Vector Laboratories, Newark, CA, USA). Following IHC, slides were digitized using the Aperio AT2 scanner (Leica Biosystems, Wetzlar, Germany) at 40× absolute resolution. Quantification of sortilin immunohistological staining intensities was performed using the HALOTM image analysis platform (version 3.3, Indica Labs, Albuquerque, NM, USA), as reported [19].

2.4. Sortilin Quantification in Patient Plasma Samples

Sortilin plasma concentration was determined by Enzyme-Linked ImmunoSorbent Assay (ELISA). The ELISA kit (catalogue number SK00472-01) was from Aviscera Bioscience (Santa Clara, CA, USA). The assays were performed as recommended by the manufacturer and as previously described [20]. The Wilcoxon Rank Sum or Kruskal–Wallis (for multiple comparisons) tests were used to study the distribution of concentrations. For the primary hypothesis (differential sortilin expression between pathological subtypes), a two-sided alpha of 0.05 was employed. Statistical analyses were performed on complete cases using Prism (version 8.2.0, GraphPad Software).

2.5. Cell lines and Culture Conditions

Glioblastoma cancer cell lines A172 (CRL-1620) and U87MG (HTB-14) were obtained from the American Type Culture Collection (ATCC, Manassas, VA, USA). Patient-derived GBM cell lines BAH1, MN1, WK1, RN1, RKI1, HW1, PB1, SB2b, and SJH1 were a generous gift from Dr Bryan Day (QIMR Berghofer Medical Research Institute, Brisbane, QLD, Australia). Human astrocytes (HA) were from ScienCell Research Laboratories (Wangara, WA, Australia (catalogue number 1800). GBM cell lines and patient-derived GBM cell lines, including their MGMT methylation status, have been described previously [21,22]. The cell culture conditions have been described previously [19].

2.6. Western Blotting

Conditions for protein extraction and Western blotting were as previously published [23] with an anti-sortilin antibody (catalogue number ANT-009, Alomone labs, Israel) used at a dilution of 1:300. Also, a β-actin antibody (catalogue number A1978, Sigma-Aldrich, St. Louis, MO, USA) was used for testing equal loading at a 1:5000 dilution.

2.7. Measurement of Cell Growth and Invasions

Cell growth assays were carried out using Cell Titer-Blue® (Promega, Hawthorne, VIC, Australia) according to the manufacturer's instructions and as previously reported [24]. Cells were treated with AF38469 (400 nM, catalogue number HY-12802, MedChemExpress, Monmouth Junction, NJ, USA), TMZ (50 µM, catalogue number S1237, Selleck Chem, Sapphire Bioscience, NSW, Australia), or AF38469 + TMZ for 72 h. Vehicle control was DMSO at the same concentration.

Invasion assays were carried out using the 6.5 mm Transwell® 8.0 µm Pore Polycarbonate Membrane Insert (Corning®, Sigma-Aldrich) as previously described [24]. Cells were treated with AF38469 (400 nM, catalogue number HY-12802, MedChemExpress, Monmouth Junction, NJ, USA). DMSO at the same concentration was used as vehicle control. For standard GBM cells U87MG and A172, cell invasion was quantified after 24 h, whereas the patient-derived cell lines (BAH1, RKI1, PB1) were quantified after 72 h.

2.8. Statistics

GraphPad Prism (La Jolla, CA, USA) was used. H-scores were analyzed as continuous variables, with summary statistics presented as group-level medians and interquartile ranges (IQR). Student's *t*-test with unpaired two-sided was used for single comparisons. One-way analysis of variance (ANOVA) or two-way analysis of variance with Dunnett's or Tukey's correction were used for multiple comparisons. When data was not normally distributed, the non-parametric Kruskal–Wallis test was performed. Pearson's correlation test was used to determine correlations. A p value less than 0.05 was deemed statistically significant. All experiments were performed at least in triplicate. All materials used and results generated were included for statistical analyses, with no exclusion of data points. All data are included in this publication and are presented as mean ± standard deviation (SD).

3. Results

3.1. SORT1 (Sortilin) mRNA Expression Is Not Increased in GBM Tissues

We first performed a data mining of sortilin gene (SORT1) expression using GEPIA2 [18] and accessing the GBM and Low-Grade Glioma (LGG) datasets of The Cancer Genome Atlas (TCGA) [16] database and GTEx [25]. While there was a wide range of SORT1 mRNA expression, there was no significant difference found between the GBM, LGG and normal groups (Figure 1A,B). Interestingly, there was significant differences in LGG patients' overall and disease-free survival comparing low and high SORT1 mRNA expression ($p = 0.0023$ and $p = 0.0004$ respectively): patients with low SORT1 expression survived longer (Figure 1C). However, this was not observed in GBM patients (Figure 1D).

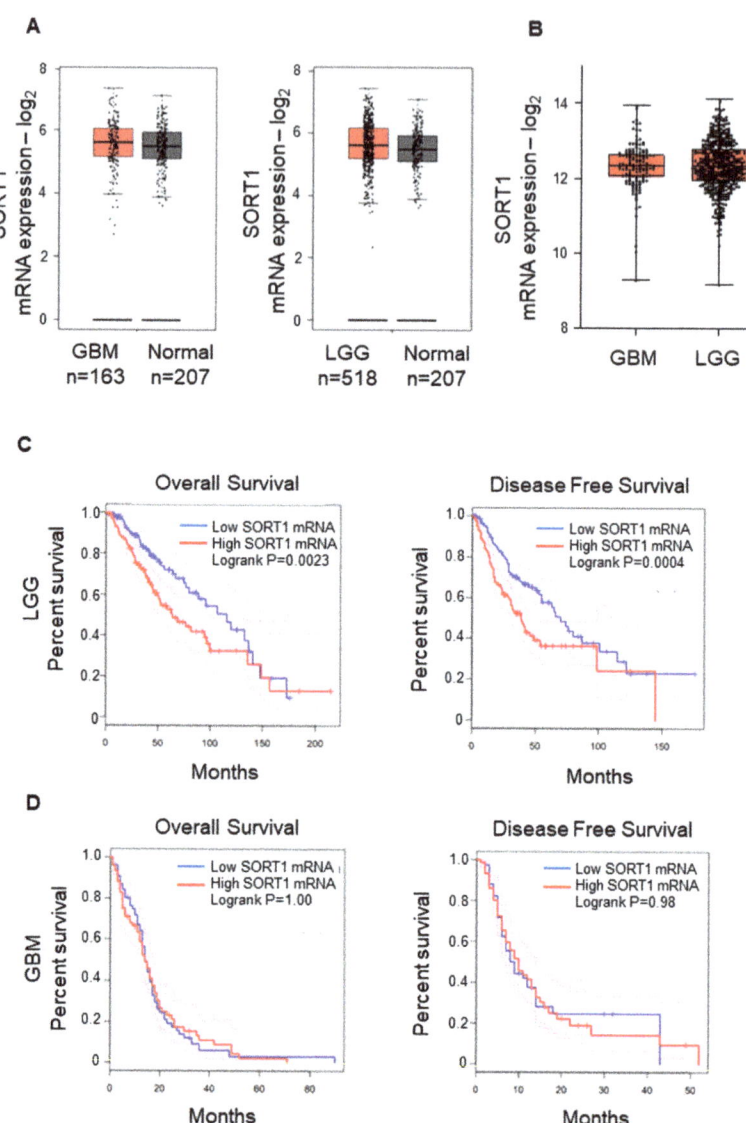

Figure 1. SORT1 (sortilin) mRNA expression in GBM and LGG vs. normal tissue. (**A**) The expression of SORT1 mRNA in GBM (left) and LGG (right) tissue was comparable to the expression in normal brain tissue. For normal brain tissue, GEPIA2 sourced the GTEx project (https://gtexportal.org/home/ (accessed on 1 December 2022)). (**B**) There was no observable difference between GBM and LGG SORT1 mRNA expression. (**C**) The overall survival (left) and disease-free survival (right) analysis for SORT1 mRNA in LGG revealed longer survival time for LGG patients with low SORT1 tumoral mRNA expression compared to those with high SORT1 mRNA expression ($p = 0.0023$ and $p = 0.0004$ respectively). (**D**) Analysis of overall survival (left) and disease-free survival (right) for SORT1 mRNA in GBM determined by GEPIA2.

3.2. Sortilin Protein Expression Is Increased in GBM Tissues Compared to Grade 1–3 Glioma

Immunohistochemical staining of sortilin was performed on all tissue samples obtained from GBM patients (71 cases) and lower-grade (1–3) glioma (20 cases); the results are presented in Figure 2 and Table 1. Sortilin staining intensity in grade 1–2 glioma was observed to be low in all cases (Figure 2A,B and Table 2), and ten out of twelve cases of grade 3 were observed to have low-intensity staining for sortilin (Figure 2C and Table 2). Sortilin protein expression was higher in GBM than in lower-grade glioma (Figure 2D). Visual observation was confirmed by digital quantification of sortilin staining intensity (Figure 2E), with high sortilin expression in GBM (median h-score = 22.19, IQR 11.52–36.01) compared to glioma grades 1–3 (median h-score = 4.87, IQR 2.24–13.66 p = 0.0016). The receiver operating characteristic (ROC) curve [26] indicated an area under the curve (AUC) of 0.81 (Figure 2F). Patient survival data on all glioma and GBM cases revealed that patients with low sortilin had longer survival, with a median survival of 18 months, compared to those with high sortilin, who had median survival of only 12 months (p = 0.0157) (Figure 2G). While the survival data for grade 1–3 (Figure S1) and GBM (Figure S2) show no significant difference, there was an observed trend of low sortilin levels associated with longer survival times (13 months and 1.5 months, respectively).

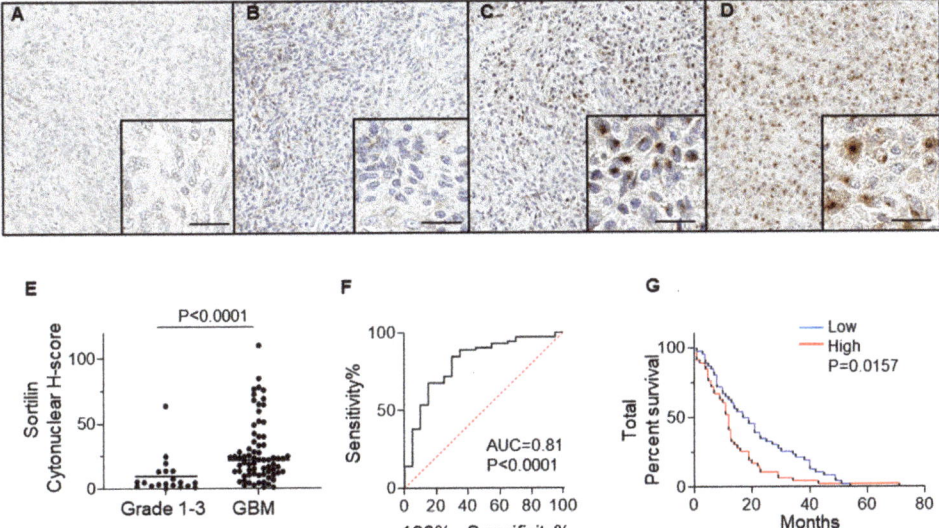

Figure 2. SORT1 Sortilin expression is increased in GBM vs. low grade gliomas. Representative pictures for the immunohistochemical detection of sortilin are shown for (**A**) grade 1, (**B**) grade 2, (**C**) grade 3, and (**D**) GBM. (**E**) Digital quantification of sortilin staining intensities according to grouped pathological subtypes: grade 1–3 (h-score = 4.87, IQR 2.24–13.66 p = 0.0016) and GBM (h-score = 22.19, IQR 11.52–36.01). Higher-magnification IHC staining pictures are shown in bottom right magnified insert; scale bar = 30 μm. Data are expressed as individual values with medians. Sortilin h-score median difference between grades 1–3 and GBM was analysed using Mann–Whitney statistical test. (**F**) ROC analysis for sortilin in GBM patient samples. (**G**) Kaplan–Meier survival analysis for patients with low staining (≤median h-score) and high staining (>median h-score). Cases with low sortilin h-score had longer median survival (18 months) compared to high sortilin h-score (12 months) (p = 0.0157). ROC: receiver operating characteristic.

Table 2. Association between sortilin expression and clinicopathological parameters in glioma.

Parameter	Sortilin Intensity		p-Value
	Low	High	
Sex			0.5219
Female	16 (44%)	20 (56%)	
Male	29 (53%)	26 (47%)	
Age			0.4043
≤63	25 (54%)	21 (46%)	
>63	20 (44%)	25 (56%)	
Grade			<0.0001
1–3	17 (85%)	3 (15%)	
GBM	28 (39%)	43 (61%)	
Tumor site			0.7241
Frontal	21 (54%)	18 (46%)	
Temporal	14 (48%)	15 (52%)	
Other	10 (43%)	13 (57%)	

The intensity of immunohistochemical staining was categorized as low-staining (≤median H-score) or high-staining (>median H-score). Statistical associations were investigated with Chi-squared test; p values of statistical significance (<0.05) are in bold.

3.3. Sortilin Is Detectable in the Plasma of GBM Patients

We measured the circulating concentration of sortilin in the plasma of GBM patients versus glioma grade 1–3 patients by ELISA; the results are reported in Figure 3 and Table 3. Sortilin was detected in all plasma samples at varying concentrations in both GBM and glioma grades 1–3 (Figure 3A). Grades 1–3 sortilin plasma concentrations (median = 0.163 ug/mL, IQR 0.063 ug/mL–5.136 ug/mL) were observed to be lower than GBM sortilin plasma concentrations (median = 0.377 ug/mL, IQR 0.057 ug/mL–2.91 ug/mL), but the difference was not statistically significant. We then wanted to see if circulating sortilin could be a potential biomarker for GBM. We observed a similar pattern to our findings in IHC sortilin-stained tissue samples, with low circulating sortilin concentrations corresponding to longer survival time (low sortilin = 13 months vs. high sortilin 10.5 months); however, this did not meet statistical significance (p = 0.2315) (Figure 3B). Interestingly, there was an association between sortilin tissue h-score and sortilin plasma concentration (Table 4); however, there was no significant correlation between tissue sortilin and sortilin plasma concentration (Figure S3A,B).

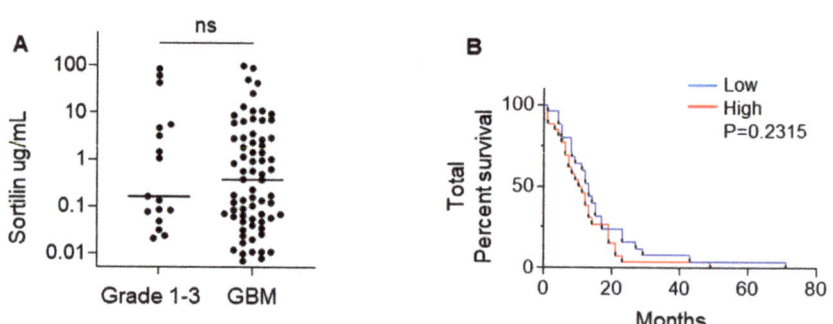

Figure 3. Sortilin plasma quantification in GBM vs. grade 1–3 gliomas. (**A**) Quantitation of circulating sortilin was obtained by ELISA in plasma from grade 1–3 vs. GBM patients. Sortilin plasma quantification is in µg/mL. The median sortilin concentration was 0.163 µg/mL (IQR 0.063 µg/mL–5.136 µg/mL) in combined grades 1–3 versus 0.377 ug/mL (IQR 0.057 µg/mL–2.907 µg/mL) in GBM. Mann–Whitney test was used to evaluate the sortilin concentration median difference between grades 1–3 and GBM. (**B**) Total patient survival based on low (≤median) and high (>median) sortilin concentration in plasma. Cases with low sortilin concentration had longer median survival (13 months) compared to cases with high sortilin concentration (10.5 months).

Table 3. Comparison of sortilin plasma concentration and clinicopathological parameters in glioma.

Parameter	Sortilin Conc.		p-Value
	Low	High	
Sex			>0.9999
Female	18 (51%)	17 (49%)	
Male	26 (50%)	26 (50%)	
Age			0.6700
≤63	23 (53%)	20 (47%)	
>63	21 (48%)	23 (52%)	
Grade			0.6927
1–3	8 (47%)	9 (53%)	
GBM	35 (50%)	35 (50%)	
Tumor site			0.6622
Frontal	20 (56%)	16 (44%)	
Temporal	14 (50%)	14 (50%)	
Other	10 (43%)	13 (57%)	

Sortilin was assayed by ELISA and categorized as low concentration (≤median µg/mL) vs. high concentration (>median µg/mL). Statistical associations were analysed using Chi-squared test; p values of statistical significance (<0.05).

Table 4. Association between sortilin concentration in plasma and IHC H-score.

Parameter	Sortilin Conc.		Total	p-Value
	Low	High		
Sortilin H-score				
Low	23 (55%)	19 (45%)	87	**<0.0001**
High	5 (11%)	40 (89%)		

Statistical associations were analysed using Chi-squared test; p values of statistical significance (<0.05) are in bold.

3.4. Sortilin Overexpression in Patient-Derived GBM Cell Lines

Western blot analysis (Figure 4A) was used to detect sortilin expression in human GBM cell lines. Sortilin was observed at the expected molecular weight of 100 kDa in all GBM and HA cell lines (Figure 4A). Densitometric analysis revealed that all GBM cell lines expressed higher levels of sortilin than the control HA cells (Figure 4B). Interestingly, two patient-derived GBM cell lines exhibiting the highest sortilin expression (SJH1 and PB1) were both MGMT-unmethylated and proneural subtype (Figure 4B). GBM cells with unmethylated MGMT seemed to express higher sortilin than GBM cells with methylated-MGMT status (Figure 4C); however, this did not meet statistical significance ($p = 0.0823$). Additionally, when we separated nine patient-derived GBM cell lines by their subtype [21,27], GBM cells with a proneural subtype had significant higher sortilin expression than the classical and mesenchymal subtype ($p = 0.0091$ and $p = 0.0131$, respectively) (Figure S4).

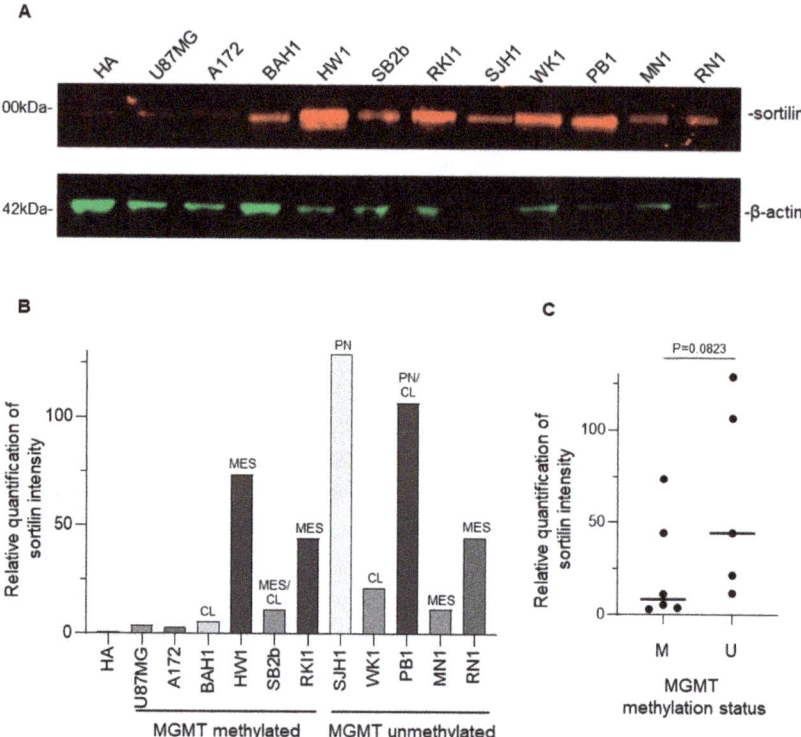

Figure 4. Western blot detection of sortilin in patient-derived GBM cell lines. (**A**) Sortilin was detected as a 100 kDa band (expected molecular mass) in every GBM cell line. The uncropped blots are shown in Figure S6. (**B**) Densitometry analysis of the Western blot. (**C**) Comparison of sortilin expression between GBM cell line, MGMT-methylated (M) and unmethylated (U) MGMT methylation status. Mann–Whitney test was used. Molecular subtypes: CL (classical), MES (mesenchymal), PN (proneural).

3.5. Targeting Sortilin with Small Molecule Inhibitor AF38469 Inhibits GBM Cell Invasion

We then wanted to test if targeting sortilin using the small molecular inhibitor AF38469 could reduce GBM cell viability and increase the sensitivity to TMZ treatment. Treatment with AF38469 alone did not reduce cell viability in any of the GBM cell lines (Figure 5A,B and Figure S5), suggesting that sortilin is not involved in cell proliferation. However, when combined with TMZ, AF38469 did reduce the cell viability in one of the patient-derived cell lines RKI1 ($p = 0.0039$) (Figure 5A) compared to treatment with TMZ alone. Whether GBM cell lines were MGMT-methylated (Figure 5A) or MGMT-unmethylated (Figure 5B) did not appear to affect AF38469 and TMZ interaction. To further investigate the effect of sortilin inhibition, Transwell invasion assays were performed. Crystal violet staining of invaded cells showed a decrease in the proportion of invaded cells after sortilin inhibition with AF38469 (Figure 6A). In the AF38469-treated GBM cell lines there was a 53% reduction of cell invasion in U87MG ($p = 0.0227$), 53% in A172 ($p = 0.0140$), 48% in BAH1, 38% in RKI1 ($p = 0.0150$), and 52% in PB1 ($p = 0.0005$) (Figure 6B). These results, based on the pharmacological inhibition of sortilin, show that sortilin is necessary for GBM cell invasion and targetable using AF38469.

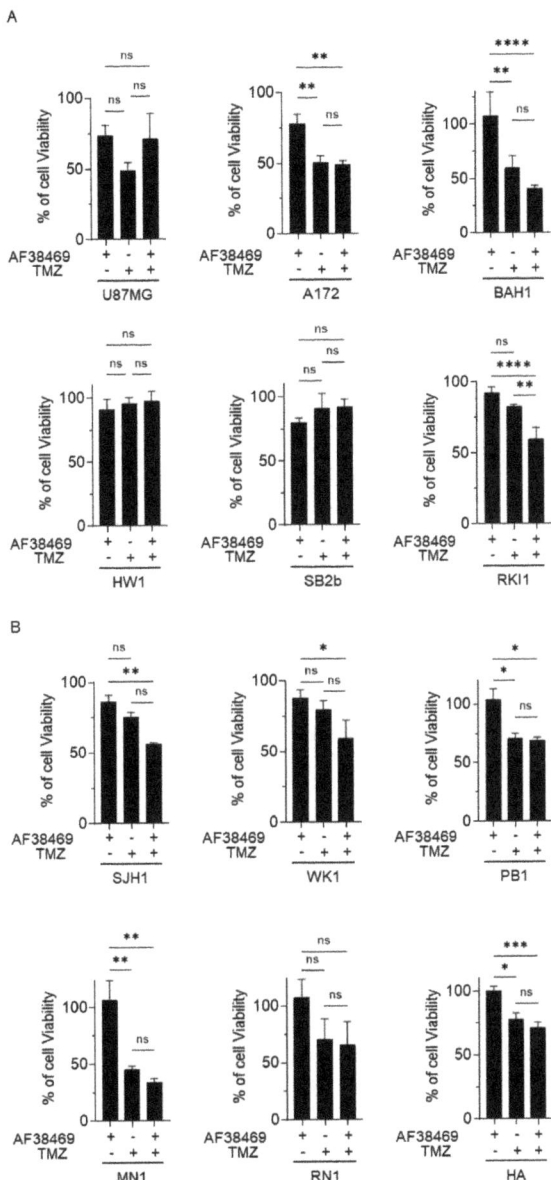

Figure 5. Sortilin targeting effect in GBM cell growth assay. Cell growth was investigated in GBM cells with methylated-MGMT status (**A**) and unmethylated-MGMT status (**B**). Human astrocytes (HA) were used as a control. Treatments were conducted with AF38469 (400 nM), a small molecule inhibitor of sortilin, TMZ (50 µM) and AF38469 in association with TMZ for a 72 h duration. Cell lines treated with TMZ and/or AF38469 were compared to vehicle control (DMSO) treated cells, with 100% viability being the viability of vehicle control (DMSO) treated cells. Data are represented as a mean +/− standard deviation (SD) of three independent experiments. For statistical significance, Student's t-test or ANOVA was used. * $p < 0.05$, ** $p < 0.01$, *** $p < 0.001$, **** $p < 0.0001$, ns: No Significance. TMZ: Temozolomide.

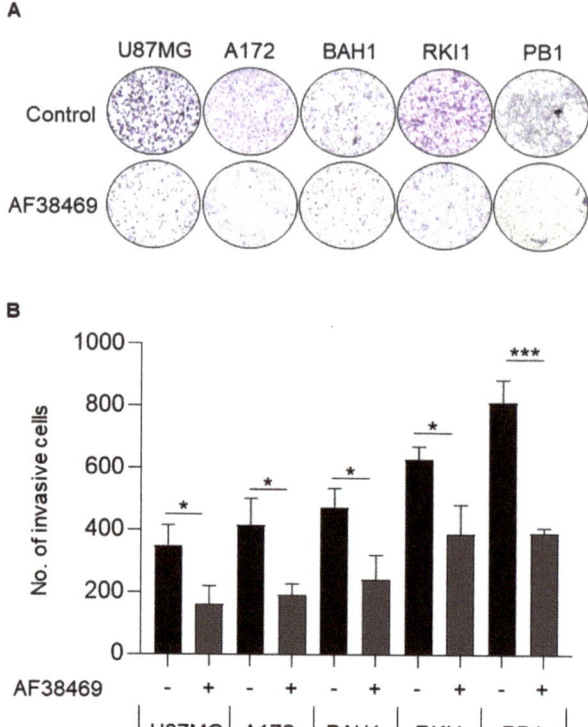

Figure 6. Inhibition of sortilin reduces GBM cell invasion. Cell invasion was investigated using Transwell assay. (A) Representative Transwell invasion assay images of untreated GBM cells (top) and GBM cells treated with AF38469 400 nM (bottom). The entire insert with invading cells was observed after crystal violet staining. (B) Average number of invading cells treated with AF34869 400 nM (+) compared to untreated (−). After AF38469 treatment there was a 53% reduction of cell invasion in U87MG ($p = 0.0227$), 53% in A172 ($p = 0.0140$), 48% in BAH1, 38% in RKI1 ($p = 0.0150$), and 52% in PB1 ($p = 0.0005$). Cell lines U87MG and A172 were treated for 24 h; BAH1, RKI1 and PB1 were treated for 72 h. Student's t-test was used and the data are the mean +/− standard deviation (SD) of three independent experiments. * $p < 0.05$, *** $p < 0.001$.

4. Discussion

The heterogeneity of GBM is complex and remains to be fully elucidated, not only to identify new effective targets for treatment, but also to identify noninvasive biomarkers that could enable accurate prognosis and help formulate appropriate treatments. The current study expands on previous observations of the expression and biological effects of sortilin in GBM [14,28] and further examines its potential as a clinical biomarker. The novelty of the present study is related to the following four points. First, we used a larger cohort of patient GBM cases compared to previous studies. Second, we used more recently obtained patient-derived cell lines, which are more clinically relevant. Third, we are the first to include the combined treatment of temozolomide and AF38469. And fourth, we report, for the first time, circulating sortilin in the blood of GBM patients.

In terms of gene expression, our data mining, using GEPIA2 to access the TCGA GBM and LGG datasets, contradicted other studies [14] and revealed no real difference between GBM, LGG and normal tissue expressing SORT1 mRNA. Interestingly, there was a significant difference in the survival outcome for LGG patients between those with high and low SORT1 mRNA expression. Patients with low SORT1 expression had longer survival (overall and disease-free) than patients with high SORT1 expression. However, it cannot be assumed that mRNA abundance equates to protein synthesis [9,29], and therefore it is essential to analyse the protein level directly.

The upregulation of sortilin protein has been reported in several cancers, including breast cancer [30], pancreatic cancer [9], and digestive cancers [6]. In the present study, we show higher sortilin protein expression in GBM compared to lower-grade glioma, and furthermore we show that a high sortilin protein level in tissue is associated with poor survival outcomes. Normal brain tissues were not included in this study, as it is not commonly excised during the surgical removal of the tumor to limit neurological complications in patients. Furthermore, due to the infiltrative nature of GBM, surrounding "normal" adjacent tissue could not be used as a proper control. Normal brain tissue samples could be obtained from cadavers, but we think such samples cannot be compared and are not appropriate controls for GBM biopsies. Therefore, we could not quantify sortilin in the adjacent normal or peritumoral region. In future studies, the peritumoral region would be an area worth exploring, as previous studies have reported that this region contains highly infiltrative cancer stem cells (CSC) [31].

Our study is the first to quantify soluble sortilin in the plasma of GBM patients. Outside GBM, soluble sortilin has already been reported and is presumably formed after proteolytic cleavage [32]. The ELISA used in this study to quantify sortilin was developed based on polyclonal antibodies raised against the extracellular domain (amino acids 78–765) of human sortilin. As such, the ELISA recognizes both the full-length and the cleaved sortilin, and does not discriminate between the two. The potential role of soluble sortilin remains to be elucidated, and while our study reported no significant difference in plasma sortilin concentrations between the glioma and GBM, there was a wide spread of sortilin plasma concentration. There was no correlation between plasma sortilin concentration and GBM tissue sortilin expression, but, interestingly, high concentrations of sortilin were significantly associated with high sortilin tissue expression, suggesting that a significant fraction of circulating sortilin originated from GBM. Other non-cancer studies have reported soluble sortilin as a potential biomarker for cardiac disease [33,34], and, interestingly, these non-cancer studies show a similar spread of concentrations to what we saw in this study, ranging from < 1 ug/mL to 100 ug/mL. The biological and clinical significance of circulating sortilin in GBM is unclear and warrants further investigations in normal and, in particular, GBM cell lines, and further analyses of larger clinical cohort are needed to clarify the clinical biomarker value of sortilin expression (both in tissue and plasma) in GBM.

Aside from tissue expression and plasma release of sortilin in GBM, an interesting finding of the present study was the inhibition of GBM cell invasion induced by sortilin targeting. Sortilin targeting by knockdown and inhibition with AF38469 has previously been shown to reduce cancer cell invasion in a few GBM cell lines. Here, we confirm that AF38469 not only reduces cell invasion in the traditional GBM cell lines (U87MG & A172), but, importantly, also reduces cell invasion in the more recently developed patient-derived cell lines (BAH1, RKI1 and PB1). In terms of GBM treatment, the use of a drug like AF38469 is more clinically relevant than a molecular knockdown, and AF38469 is the only blood-brain-barrier-crossing drug currently available to target sortilin. It is noteworthy to mention that the main issue with GBM recurrence is the invasive capacity of GBM cells, which can invade the brain tissue surrounding the tumor and thus escape surgery or radiotherapy. GBM rarely metastasises, and the main issue is the local invasion of GBM cells in the neural tissue. Interestingly, our data show that the pharmacological inhibition of sortilin, using the orally available blood-brain-barrier-crossing drug AF38469, resulted in the inhibition of patient-derived GBM cell lines. A statistically significant inhibition of GBM cell invasion by AF38469 was observed for tested patient-derived GBM cells, indicating that sortilin is a potential therapeutic target for inhibiting GBM invasiveness. In contrast, sortilin targeting with AF38469 was not found to have any effect on GBM cell survival, and was not found to potentiate the activity of TMZ. However, in one patient-derived cell line (RKI1), potentiation of the cytotoxic effect of TMZ by AF38469 was observed. It is unclear at this stage why RKI1 shows an increased sensitivity to TMZ in presence to AF38469, and this leaves open the possibility that in some GBM, sortilin inhibition could be a way to potentiate the efficacy of TMZ.

It is important to note that the mechanism of action for AF38469 is currently not clearly understood. The structural data published by Schrøder et al. [35] show that AF38469 can interfere with neurotensin binding, therefore preventing this ligand from engaging the sortilin receptor. While this interaction could partially explain the effect of AF38469 on the motility of GBM cell lines, the sortilin receptor has a plethora of additional functions that are independent of neurotensin binding. It is currently unclear whether (and to what degree) these functions are also impacted by AF38469. Furthermore, sortilin does not function as a primary receptor for neurotensin. This role is fulfilled by a different receptor (i.e., the high-affinity receptor for neurotensin or NTSR1), which is another molecule that is highly expressed in GBM [36]. More mechanistic studies are needed for a clear understanding of how sortilin and AF38469 work at the molecular level and how they mechanistically impact the motility of GBM cells. In any case, the finding reported here that sortilin targeting can decrease GBM cell invasion (and eventually proliferation in a limited fraction of GBM) warrants further in vivo investigation.

5. Conclusions

In conclusion, the present study points to sortilin as a new potential clinical biomarker for predicting GBM aggressiveness and patient survival. In addition, targeting sortilin seems to decrease GBM cell invasion, and could therefore be used in GBM therapy. Although further in vivo studies are needed, it should be noted that sortilin targeting in human cancers has recently entered a clinical trial phase. In breast [30], thyroid [37] and ovarian cancer [38], targeting sortilin has been shown to enhance the effect of existing chemotherapy by exploiting sortilin function as a receptor allowing targeted entry of a peptide conjugated to docetaxel (TH1902) [10,38–40]. There is currently a clinical trial underway targeting sortilin in patients with advanced solid tumors using TH1902 (NCT04706962). This phase 1 clinical trial will include patients with solid tumors in the breast, ovary, endometrium, skin, thyroid, lung, and prostate, and our findings suggest that GBM should be added to the list of cancers that could incorporate sortilin targeting as a therapeutic option.

Supplementary Materials: The following supporting information can be downloaded at https://www.mdpi.com/article/10.3390/cancers15092514/s1, Figure S1. (A) Grade 1–3 patient survival based on low staining (≤median h-score) and high staining (>median h-score). Cases with low sortilin h-score had longer median survival (36.5 months) compared to high sortilin h-score (23.5 months). (B) GBM patient survival based on low staining (≤median h-score) and high staining (>median h-score). Cases with low sortilin h-score had longer median survival (12.5 months) compared to high sortilin h-score (11 months); Figure S2. (A) Grade 1–3 patient survival based on low (≤median) and high (>median) sortilin concentration in plasma. Cases with low sortilin concentration had longer median survival (35 months) compared to high sortilin concentration (25 months). (B) GBM patient survival based on low (≤median) and high (>median) concentration in plasma. Cases with low sortilin concentration had longer median survival (12 months) compared to high sortilin concentration (10 months); Figure S3. (A) Correlation of sortilin in tissue cytonuclear h-score and soluble sortilin in plasma concentration. (B) Correlation of high sortilin expression in tissue cytonuclear h-score and high soluble sortilin concentration in plasma; Figure S4. Densitometric analysis of sortilin protein intensity by subgroups. CL = classic, MES = Mesenchymal, PN = Proneural. * $p < 0.05$, ** $p < 0.01$, Student's t-test or ANOVA; Figure S5. Viability assay Cell lines treated with AF38469 MGMT methylated v's MGMT unmethylated; Figure S6. The uncropped blots for Figure 4A.

Author Contributions: Conceptualization and methodology, H.H., S.F. and C.C.J.; formal analysis, H.H., C.C.J., C.G. and J.L.; biobanking, C.P.G.; experimental investigations, M.M., A.D. and J.M.; writing—original draft, H.H., C.C.J. and M.M.; writing—review and editing, H.H., S.F., C.G., M.M., A.D., J.L. and C.P.G. All authors have read and agreed to the published version of the manuscript.

Funding: This work was supported by the Mark Hughes Foundation (MHF), New South Wales, Australia.

Institutional Review Board Statement: The study was conducted in accordance with the Declaration of Helsinki and approved by the Human Research Ethics Committee of The University of Newcastle, Australia (X11-0023 and H-2012-0063).

Informed Consent Statement: Informed consent was obtained from all subjects involved in the study.

Data Availability Statement: The data presented in this study are available on request to the corresponding author.

Acknowledgments: We thank the Hunter Cancer Biobank (HCB) for providing tumor samples and assistance with pathology analysis. We also thank Kathryn Leaney for excellent Cancer Consumer Advice.

Conflicts of Interest: The authors declare no conflict of interest.

References

1. Ostrom, Q.T.; Gittleman, H.; Farah, P.; Ondracek, A.; Chen, Y.; Wolinsky, Y.; Stroup, N.E.; Kruchko, C.; Barnholtz-Sloan, J.S. CBTRUS statistical report: Primary brain and central nervous system tumors diagnosed in the United States in 2006–2010. *Neuro Oncol.* **2013**, *15* (Suppl. S2), ii1–ii56. [CrossRef] [PubMed]
2. Skaga, E.; Skretteberg, M.A.; Johannesen, T.B.; Brandal, P.; Vik-Mo, E.O.; Helseth, E.; Langmoen, I.A. Real-world validity of randomized controlled phase III trials in newly diagnosed glioblastoma: To whom do the results of the trials apply? *Neurooncol. Adv.* **2021**, *3*, vdab008. [CrossRef] [PubMed]
3. Iacob, G.; Dinca, E.B. Current data and strategy in glioblastoma multiforme. *J. Med. Life* **2009**, *2*, 386–393. [PubMed]
4. Stupp, R.; Mason, W.P.; van den Bent, M.J.; Weller, M.; Fisher, B.; Taphoorn, M.J.B.; Belanger, K.; Brandes, A.A.; Marosi, C.; Bogdahn, U.; et al. Radiotherapy plus Concomitant and Adjuvant Temozolomide for Glioblastoma. *N. Engl. J. Med.* **2005**, *352*, 987–996. [CrossRef]
5. Hegi, M.E.; Diserens, A.C.; Gorlia, T.; Hamou, M.F.; de Tribolet, N.; Weller, M.; Kros, J.M.; Hainfellner, J.A.; Mason, W.; Mariani, L.; et al. MGMT gene silencing and benefit from temozolomide in glioblastoma. *N. Engl. J. Med.* **2005**, *352*, 997–1003. [CrossRef]
6. Mazella, J. Deciphering Mechanisms of Action of Sortilin/Neurotensin Receptor-3 in the Proliferation Regulation of Colorectal and Other Cancers. *Int. J. Mol. Sci.* **2022**, *23*, 11888. [CrossRef]
7. Ye, S.; Wang, B.; Zhou, Y.; Sun, Q.; Yang, X. Sortilin 1 regulates hepatocellular carcinoma progression by activating the PI3K/AKT signaling. *Hum. Exp. Toxicol.* **2022**, *41*, 09603271221140111. [CrossRef]
8. Gao, Y.; Li, Y.; Song, Z.; Jin, Z.; Li, X.; Yuan, C. Sortilin 1 Promotes Hepatocellular Carcinoma Cell Proliferation and Migration by Regulating Immune Cell Infiltration. *J. Oncol.* **2022**, *2022*, 6509028. [CrossRef]
9. Gao, F.; Griffin, N.; Faulkner, S.; Li, X.; King, S.J.; Jobling, P.; Denham, J.W.; Jiang, C.C.; Hondermarck, H. The Membrane Protein Sortilin Can Be Targeted to Inhibit Pancreatic Cancer Cell Invasion. *Am. J. Pathol.* **2020**, *190*, 1931–1942. [CrossRef]
10. Demeule, M.; Charfi, C.; Currie, J.C.; Larocque, A.; Zgheib, A.; Kozelko, S.; Béliveau, R.; Marsolais, C.; Annabi, B. TH1902, a new docetaxel-peptide conjugate for the treatment of sortilin-positive triple-negative breast cancer. *Cancer Sci.* **2021**, *112*, 4317–4334. [CrossRef]
11. Rhost, S.; Hughes, É.; Harrison, H.; Rafnsdottir, S.; Jacobsson, H.; Gregersson, P.; Magnusson, Y.; Fitzpatrick, P.; Andersson, D.; Berger, K.; et al. Sortilin inhibition limits secretion-induced progranulin-dependent breast cancer progression and cancer stem cell expansion. *Breast Cancer Res.* **2018**, *20*, 137. [CrossRef]
12. Marsland, M.; Dowdell, A.; Jiang, C.C.; Wilmott, J.S.; Scolyer, R.A.; Zhang, X.D.; Hondermarck, H.; Faulkner, S. Expression of NGF/proNGF and Their Receptors TrkA, p75(NTR) and Sortilin in Melanoma. *Int. J. Mol. Sci.* **2022**, *23*, 4260. [CrossRef] [PubMed]
13. Blondy, S.; Talbot, H.; Saada, S.; Christou, N.; Battu, S.; Pannequin, J.; Jauberteau, M.O.; Lalloué, F.; Verdier, M.; Mathonnet, M.; et al. Overexpression of sortilin is associated with 5-FU resistance and poor prognosis in colorectal cancer. *J. Cell. Mol. Med.* **2021**, *25*, 47–60. [CrossRef] [PubMed]
14. Yang, W.; Wu, P.-f.; Ma, J.-x.; Liao, M.-j.; Wang, X.-h.; Xu, L.-s.; Xu, M.-h.; Yi, L. Sortilin promotes glioblastoma invasion and mesenchymal transition through GSK-3β/β-catenin/twist pathway. *Cell Death Dis.* **2019**, *10*, 208. [CrossRef] [PubMed]
15. Yang, W.; Xiang, Y.; Liao, M.-J.; Wu, P.-F.; Yang, L.; Huang, G.-H.; Shi, B.-Z.; Yi, L.; Lv, S.-Q. Presenilin1 inhibits glioblastoma cell invasiveness via promoting Sortilin cleavage. *Cell Commun. Signal.* **2021**, *19*, 112. [CrossRef]
16. Weinstein, J.N.; Collisson, E.A.; Mills, G.B.; Shaw, K.R.; Ozenberger, B.A.; Ellrott, K.; Shmulevich, I.; Sander, C.; Stuart, J.M. The Cancer Genome Atlas Pan-Cancer analysis project. *Nat. Genet.* **2013**, *45*, 1113–1120. [CrossRef]
17. Carithers, L.J.; Moore, H.M. The Genotype-Tissue Expression (GTEx) Project. *Biopreserv. Biobank* **2015**, *13*, 307–308. [CrossRef]
18. Tang, Z.; Kang, B.; Li, C.; Chen, T.; Zhang, Z. GEPIA2: An enhanced web server for large-scale expression profiling and interactive analysis. *Nucleic Acids Res.* **2019**, *47*, W556–W560. [CrossRef]
19. Marsland, M.; Dowdell, A.; Faulkner, S.; Jobling, P.; Rush, R.A.; Gedye, C.; Lynam, J.; Griffin, C.P.; Baker, M.; Marsland, J.; et al. ProNGF Expression and Targeting in Glioblastoma Multiforme. *Int. J. Mol. Sci.* **2023**, *24*, 1616. [CrossRef]

20. March, B.; Lockhart, K.R.; Faulkner, S.; Smolny, M.; Rush, R.; Hondermarck, H. ELISA-based quantification of neurotrophic growth factors in urine from prostate cancer patients. *FASEB Bioadv.* **2021**, *3*, 888–896. [CrossRef]
21. Stringer, B.W.; Day, B.W.; D'Souza, R.C.J.; Jamieson, P.R.; Ensbey, K.S.; Bruce, Z.C.; Lim, Y.C.; Goasdoué, K.; Offenhäuser, C.; Akgül, S.; et al. A reference collection of patient-derived cell line and xenograft models of proneural, classical and mesenchymal glioblastoma. *Sci. Rep.* **2019**, *9*, 4902. [CrossRef] [PubMed]
22. Festuccia, C.; Mancini, A.; Colapietro, A.; Gravina, G.L.; Vitale, F.; Marampon, F.; Delle Monache, S.; Pompili, S.; Cristiano, L.; Vetuschi, A.; et al. The first-in-class alkylating deacetylase inhibitor molecule tinostamustine shows antitumor effects and is synergistic with radiotherapy in preclinical models of glioblastoma. *J. Hematol. Oncol.* **2018**, *11*, 32. [CrossRef] [PubMed]
23. Pundavela, J.; Demont, Y.; Jobling, P.; Lincz, L.F.; Roselli, S.; Thorne, R.F.; Bond, D.; Bradshaw, R.A.; Walker, M.M.; Hondermarck, H. ProNGF correlates with Gleason score and is a potential driver of nerve infiltration in prostate cancer. *Am. J. Pathol.* **2014**, *184*, 3156–3162. [CrossRef] [PubMed]
24. Jiang, C.C.; Marsland, M.; Wang, Y.; Dowdell, A.; Eden, E.; Gao, F.; Faulkner, S.; Jobling, P.; Li, X.; Liu, L.; et al. Tumor innervation is triggered by endoplasmic reticulum stress. *Oncogene* **2022**, *41*, 586–599. [CrossRef]
25. Burgess, D.J. Reaching completion for GTEx. *Nat. Rev. Genet.* **2020**, *21*, 717. [CrossRef]
26. Søreide, K. Receiver-operating characteristic curve analysis in diagnostic, prognostic and predictive biomarker research. *J. Clin. Pathol.* **2009**, *62*, 1–5. [CrossRef]
27. Verhaak, R.G.; Hoadley, K.A.; Purdom, E.; Wang, V.; Qi, Y.; Wilkerson, M.D.; Miller, C.R.; Ding, L.; Golub, T.; Mesirov, J.P.; et al. Integrated genomic analysis identifies clinically relevant subtypes of glioblastoma characterized by abnormalities in PDGFRA, IDH1, EGFR, and NF1. *Cancer Cell* **2010**, *17*, 98–110. [CrossRef]
28. Xiong, J.; Zhou, L.; Yang, M.; Lim, Y.; Zhu, Y.H.; Fu, D.L.; Li, Z.W.; Zhong, J.H.; Xiao, Z.C.; Zhou, X.F. ProBDNF and its receptors are upregulated in glioma and inhibit the growth of glioma cells in vitro. *Neuro Oncol.* **2013**, *15*, 990–1007. [CrossRef]
29. Maier, T.; Güell, M.; Serrano, L. Correlation of mRNA and protein in complex biological samples. *FEBS Lett.* **2009**, *583*, 3966–3973. [CrossRef]
30. Roselli, S.; Pundavela, J.; Demont, Y.; Faulkner, S.; Keene, S.; Attia, J.; Jiang, C.C.; Zhang, X.D.; Walker, M.M.; Hondermarck, H. Sortilin is associated with breast cancer aggressiveness and contributes to tumor cell adhesion and invasion. *Oncotarget* **2015**, *6*, 10473–10486. [CrossRef]
31. Angelucci, C.; D'Alessio, A.; Lama, G.; Binda, E.; Mangiola, A.; Vescovi, A.L.; Proietti, G.; Masuelli, L.; Bei, R.; Fazi, B.; et al. Cancer stem cells from peritumoral tissue of glioblastoma multiforme: The possible missing link between tumor development and progression. *Oncotarget* **2018**, *9*, 28116–28130. [CrossRef] [PubMed]
32. Molgaard, S.; Demontis, D.; Nicholson, A.M.; Finch, N.A.; Petersen, R.C.; Petersen, C.M.; Rademakers, R.; Nykjaer, A.; Glerup, S. Soluble sortilin is present in excess and positively correlates with progranulin in CSF of aging individuals. *Exp. Gerontol.* **2016**, *84*, 96–100. [CrossRef] [PubMed]
33. Goettsch, C.; Iwata, H.; Hutcheson, J.D.; O'Donnell, C.J.; Chapurlat, R.; Cook, N.R.; Aikawa, M.; Szulc, P.; Aikawa, E. Serum Sortilin Associates With Aortic Calcification and Cardiovascular Risk in Men. *Arterioscler. Thromb. Vasc. Biol.* **2017**, *37*, 1005–1011. [CrossRef] [PubMed]
34. Jing, L.; Li, L.; Ren, X.; Sun, Z.; Bao, Z.; Yuan, G.; Cai, H.; Wang, L.; Shao, C.; Wang, Z. Role of Sortilin and Matrix Vesicles in Nε-Carboxymethyl-Lysine-Induced Diabetic Atherosclerotic Calcification. *Diabetes Metab. Syndr. Obes.* **2020**, *13*, 4141–4151. [CrossRef] [PubMed]
35. Schrøder, T.J.; Christensen, S.; Lindberg, S.; Langgård, M.; David, L.; Maltas, P.J.; Eskildsen, J.; Jacobsen, J.; Tagmose, L.; Simonsen, K.B.; et al. The identification of AF38469: An orally bioavailable inhibitor of the VPS10P family sorting receptor Sortilin. *Bioorg. Med. Chem. Lett.* **2014**, *24*, 177–180. [CrossRef]
36. Dong, Z.; Lei, Q.; Yang, R.; Zhu, S.; Ke, X.X.; Yang, L.; Cui, H.; Yi, L. Inhibition of neurotensin receptor 1 induces intrinsic apoptosis via let-7a-3p/Bcl-w axis in glioblastoma. *Br. J. Cancer* **2017**, *116*, 1572–1584. [CrossRef]
37. Faulkner, S.; Jobling, P.; Rowe, C.W.; Rodrigues Oliveira, S.M.; Roselli, S.; Thorne, R.F.; Oldmeadow, C.; Attia, J.; Jiang, C.C.; Zhang, X.D.; et al. Neurotrophin Receptors TrkA, p75(NTR), and Sortilin Are Increased and Targetable in Thyroid Cancer. *Am. J. Pathol.* **2018**, *188*, 229–241. [CrossRef]
38. Currie, J.C.; Demeule, M.; Charfi, C.; Zgheib, A.; Larocque, A.; Danalache, B.A.; Ouanouki, A.; Béliveau, R.; Marsolais, C.; Annabi, B. The Peptide-Drug Conjugate TH1902: A New Sortilin Receptor-Mediated Cancer Therapeutic against Ovarian and Endometrial Cancers. *Cancers* **2022**, *14*, 1877. [CrossRef]
39. Demeule, M.; Charfi, C.; Currie, J.C.; Zgheib, A.; Danalache, B.A.; Béliveau, R.; Marsolais, C.; Annabi, B. The TH1902 Docetaxel Peptide-Drug Conjugate Inhibits Xenografts Growth of Human SORT1-Positive Ovarian and Triple-Negative Breast Cancer Stem-like Cells. *Pharmaceutics* **2022**, *14*, 1910. [CrossRef]
40. Charfi, C.; Demeule, M.; Currie, J.C.; Larocque, A.; Zgheib, A.; Danalache, B.A.; Ouanouki, A.; Béliveau, R.; Marsolais, C.; Annabi, B. New Peptide-Drug Conjugates for Precise Targeting of SORT1-Mediated Vasculogenic Mimicry in the Tumor Microenvironment of TNBC-Derived MDA-MB-231 Breast and Ovarian ES-2 Clear Cell Carcinoma Cells. *Front. Oncol.* **2021**, *11*, 760787. [CrossRef]

Disclaimer/Publisher's Note: The statements, opinions and data contained in all publications are solely those of the individual author(s) and contributor(s) and not of MDPI and/or the editor(s). MDPI and/or the editor(s) disclaim responsibility for any injury to people or property resulting from any ideas, methods, instructions or products referred to in the content.

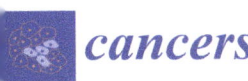

Article

The Indicative Value of Serum Tumor Markers for Metastasis and Stage of Non-Small Cell Lung Cancer

Chunyang Jiang [1,2,3,†], Mengyao Zhao [4,†], Shaohui Hou [3], Xiaoli Hu [5], Jinchao Huang [6], Hongci Wang [7], Changhao Ren [8], Xiaoying Pan [8], Ti Zhang [8], Shengnan Wu [8], Shun Zhang [4,*] and Bingsheng Sun [9,10,*]

1. Department of Thoracic Surgery, National Regional Medical Center, Binhai Campus of the First Affiliated Hospital, Fujian Medical University, Fuzhou 350212, China
2. Department of Thoracic Surgery, The First Affiliated Hospital, Fujian Medical University, 20 Chazhong Road, Fuzhou 350005, China
3. Department of Thoracic Surgery, Tianjin Union Medical Center, Nankai University, Tianjin 300121, China
4. Department of Occupational and Environmental Health, School of Public Health, Tongji Medical College, Huazhong University of Science and Technology, Wuhan 430030, China
5. Department of Respiratory, The Second People's Hospital of Linhai City, Linhai 317000, China
6. Department of Cancer Prevention, Tianjin Medical University Cancer Institute and Hospital, Tianjin 300181, China
7. Baodi District People's Hospital of Tianjin, Tianjin Baodi Hospital of Tianjin Medical University, Tianjin 301000, China
8. Medical College, Nankai University, Tianjin 300071, China
9. Department of Thoracic Surgery, Tianjin Medical University Cancer Institute and Hospital, Tianjin 300181, China
10. National Clinical Research Center for Cancer, Key Laboratory of Cancer Prevention and Therapy, Tianjin 300181, China
* Correspondence: shunzhang@hust.edu.cn (S.Z.); sbs129@163.com (B.S.)
† These authors contributed equally to this work.

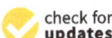

Citation: Jiang, C.; Zhao, M.; Hou, S.; Hu, X.; Huang, J.; Wang, H.; Ren, C.; Pan, X.; Zhang, T.; Wu, S.; et al. The Indicative Value of Serum Tumor Markers for Metastasis and Stage of Non-Small Cell Lung Cancer. Cancers 2022, 14, 5064. https://doi.org/10.3390/cancers14205064

Academic Editors: Daniel L. Pouliquen and Cristina Núñez González

Received: 27 September 2022
Accepted: 13 October 2022
Published: 16 October 2022

Publisher's Note: MDPI stays neutral with regard to jurisdictional claims in published maps and institutional affiliations.

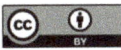

Copyright: © 2022 by the authors. Licensee MDPI, Basel, Switzerland. This article is an open access article distributed under the terms and conditions of the Creative Commons Attribution (CC BY) license (https://creativecommons.org/licenses/by/4.0/).

Simple Summary: This study recruited 3272 non-small cell lung cancer (NSCLC) cases to analyze the predictive abilities of serum tumor markers (CEA, SCC-Ag, CYFRA 21-1, NSE, ProGRP, TPSA and CA199) for metastasis and clinical stage, and found that tumor marker levels may be indicative of tumor metastasis (intrapulmonary, lymphatic and distant metastasis) and stage. Increased CEA and CA199 provided an accurate prediction of intrapulmonary and distant metastasis. Increased CEA, CYFRA 21-1 and CA199 provided an accurate prediction of lymphatic metastasis and higher tumor stage. Combined detection of serum tumor markers can indicate tumor metastasis and stage in NSCLC patients.

Abstract: Objective: This study aimed to explore the roles of serum tumor markers for metastasis and stage of non-small cell lung cancer (NSCLC). Methods: This study recruited 3272 NSCLC patients admitted to the Tianjin Union Medical Center and the Tianjin Medical University Cancer Institute and Hospital. The predictive abilities of some serum tumor markers (carcinoembryonic antigen (CEA), squamous cell carcinoma antigen (SCC-Ag), cytokeratin-19 fragment (CYFRA 21-1), neuron-specific enolase (NSE), pro-gastrin-releasing peptide (ProGRP), total prostate-specific antigen (TPSA) and carbohydrate antigen 199 (CA199)) for NSCLC metastasis (intrapulmonary, lymphatic and distant metastasis) and clinical stage were analyzed. Results: Tumor markers exhibited different numerical and proportional distributions in NSCLC patients. Elevated CEA, CYFRA 21-1 and CA199 levels were indicative of tumor metastasis and stage. Increased CEA and CA199 provided an accurate prediction of intrapulmonary and distant metastasis with the area under the receiver operator characteristic curve (AUC) of 0.69 both ($p < 0.001$); Increased CEA, CYFRA 21-1 and CA199 provided an accurate prediction of lymphatic metastasis with the AUC of 0.62 ($p < 0.001$). Conclusion: Combined detection of serum tumor markers can indicate tumor metastasis and stage in NSCLC patients.

Keywords: non-small cell lung cancer; serum tumor markers; tumor metastasis; tumor stage; prediction

1. Introduction

Lung cancer has been identified as one of the most common malignant tumors. In recent years, the incidence of lung cancer has gradually increased. Among different malignancies, lung cancer has the fastest-growing incidence and mortality, becoming the biggest threat to people's health and life [1,2]. Lung cancer is divided into two types: non-small cell lung cancer (NSCLC) and small cell lung cancer (SCLC). NSCLC accounts for about 80–85% of lung cancers, including squamous cell carcinoma, adenocarcinoma, and large cell carcinoma [3]. Compared with SCLC, NSCLC cells grow and divide slowly and metastasize relatively late [4]. The early clinical symptoms of lung cancer are not obvious; thus, lung cancer is usually diagnosed at an advanced stage, and optimal treatment and surgical opportunities are lost. Thus, improving the early detection rate of lung cancer is needed to immediately adopt positive treatment measures to reduce the harm of the disease.

Tumor markers reflect the presence of the tumor, and changes in the presence and level of markers indicate the nature of the tumor. Detecting tumor markers facilitates the early diagnosis and operation of tumor development. In recent years, more serum tumor markers have been identified for the early diagnosis of lung cancer. Due to the low sensitivity and specificity of single serum tumor markers, detecting multiple tumor markers has been used to improve the sensitivity and specificity of clinical diagnosis in lung cancer patients. Therefore, the application of single tumor markers has gradually progressed to the diagnostic use of multiple markers, thus improving the positive rate of diagnosis and monitoring the development of lung cancer [5,6]. Clinically significant serum tumor markers for lung cancer include carcinoembryonic antigen (CEA), cytokeratin-19 fragment (CYFRA 21-1), neuron-specific enolase (NSE), squamous cell carcinoma antigen (SCC-Ag), pro-gastrin-releasing peptide (ProGRP), total prostate-specific antigen (TPSA) and carbohydrate antigen 199 (CA199) [7–10]. Numerous studies have reported the application of these tumor markers in the diagnosis of lung cancer. Clinical studies have also focused on the use of these markers for monitoring treatment efficacy and prognosis; furthermore, progress has been made in the application of these markers [11–15]. High levels of tumor markers at baseline are correlated with worse survival in stage III-IV NSCLC patients [13]. Tumor markers such as CYFRA21-1, SCC-Ag, NSE, and CEA in the serum of lung cancer patients are significantly increased, and the degree of elevation are significantly correlated with tumor invasion, clinical stage and lymph node metastasis [16].

Serum tumor markers have been used for the early diagnosis of lung cancer and the clinical practice of tumor efficacy monitoring for more than 10 years. However, confirmative studies with large clinical sample size on the consistency of various tumor markers for determining the pathology and tumor progression of lung cancer remain lacking. Thus, the purpose of this study was to explore the effectiveness of serum markers in determining tumor metastasis and stage in lung cancer patients from two clinical centers with a large sample size.

2. Materials and Methods

2.1. Patients and Control Subjects

In total, 4690 lung cancer patients admitted to Tianjin Union Medical Center from September 2016 to September 2019 and 2700 lung cancer patients admitted to Tianjin Medical University Cancer Institute and Hospital from January 2018 to September 2019 were screened as study subjects. All patients were screened using case data, relevant laboratory examination data, imaging data, and pathological examination data. Patients were determined to be all Chinese from north China and northeast China. The inclusion criteria were complete information including age, sex, smoking history, and other basic data of the patients. Patients were excluded from the study if they had other tumors, inflammation in the lungs or areas other than the lungs, or a history of chronic gastritis or ulcer in the digestive system. A total of 3272 patients with NSCLC were included in this study.

Fasting blood samples were taken for determination of lung cancer-related serum tumor markers before surgery, chemotherapy, radiotherapy, or other special treatments at the first admission. The pathological diagnosis was based on lung cancer surgery, lung puncture biopsy or tracheoscopy. Pathological diagnoses of lung cancer included squamous cell carcinoma, adenocarcinoma, adenosquamous cell carcinoma, etc. Data entry for all patients included smoking index, intrapulmonary, lymphatic and distant metastasis, and tumor stage (according to the International Association for the Study of Lung Cancer, IASLC 2015 TNM stage for lung cancer).

2.2. Sample Collection and Measurement

All the patients had an empty stomach the morning after the first admission without any treatment. Venous blood (5 mL) was collected from each patient to detect lung cancer-related tumor markers. The whole blood was separated into serum and cellular fractions within 2 h by centrifugation at 4000 rpm for 10 min. Serum samples were obtained after separation, and serum concentrations of tumor markers were determined. CEA, SCC-Ag and CA199 were determined by chemiluminescent microparticle immunoassay (CMIA) using an Abbott ARCHITECT I2000SR automatic chemical microparticle immune analyzer and its supporting reagents. CYFRA 21-1, NSE, ProGRP, and TPSA were determined using a Roche Elecsys 2010 automatic electrochemiluminescence immune analyzer and its supporting reagents.

2.3. Statistical Analysis

All tumor markers had non-normal distribution, and markers were represented by the median (P25–P75). Nonparametric tests were used to compare the concentrations of tumor markers and the smoking index between the different groups. Chi-square tests were also used to determine the distribution differences of basic information (age, sex and smoking index) and tumor markers among different groups. The Bonferroni method was used for paired comparisons. Binary logistic analysis was used to analyze the influencing factors for lung tumor metastasis, lymphatic metastasis and distant metastasis, while ordinal logistic analysis was used in examining the influencing factors for tumor stage. The two logistic analyses were divided into two steps: (1) univariate factor analysis and logistic analysis for each potential influencing factor was conducted; (2) influencing factors of $p < 0.2$ [17] in univariate analysis were included in a multivariate logistic analysis. Finally, the prediction probabilities of tumor markers with $p < 0.05$ were reassessed by logistic analysis using multivariate analysis, and the receiver operating characteristic (ROC) curves were used for joint predictions. SPSS 24.0 (IBM, Chicago, IL, USA) was used for all analyses. For two-sided tests, a p value less than 0.05 was considered significant.

3. Results

3.1. Demographics and Clinical Characteristics

In total, 3272 NSCLC patients were analyzed in this study. Patient characteristics are described in Table 1. The correlations of age, sex, and smoking index with tumor metastasis, and the stage of patients with NSCLC, are presented in Table 2. The percentages of intrapulmonary and lymphatic metastases were higher in male patients than in female patients. Distribution ratios of tumor stage were statistically different; the proportions of patients with stages II–IV were lower than stage I; the proportions of patients with stages II and III were lower than stage IV.

The distribution of tumor stage, intrapulmonary and lymphatic metastases in patients ≤ 61 years old were statistically different from patients > 61 years. In patients > 61 years, the number of patients with stage II and III cancers was lower than stage I. Patients with lung tumor metastasis had a higher smoking index. Smoking indexes were statistically different for patients with different tumor stages.

Table 1. Basic information of the patients with NSCLC.

Patient Characteristics	Case or Median	%
Age		
median (P25–P75, year)	61 (55–67)	
Gender		
male	1812	55.4
female	1460	44.6
Smoking index		
median (P25–P75)	1.5 (0.00–600)	
non-smoking	1633	49.9
≤600 *	1009	31.2
>600	630	19.5
Intrapulmonary metastasis		
none	2656	83.8
yes	512	16.2
Lymphatic metastasis		
none	2147	67.6
yes	1031	32.4
Distant metastasis		
none	2607	81.7
yes	585	18.3
Histologic classification		
Squamous carcinoma	735	22.5
Adenocarcinoma	2354	72.0
Adenosquamous carcinoma	44	1.3
Others	139	4.2
Staging		
I	1997	61.3
II	503	15.4
III	175	5.4
IV	585	17.9

Note: * The P75 smoking index among smokers was 600.

Table 2. The correlation of age, sex, and smoking index with tumor metastasis, and stage of patients with NSCLC.

Variables	IM			LM			DM			Staging				
	None	Yes	p	None	Yes	p	None	Yes	p	I	II	III	IV	p
Gender (case)														
Male	1417	327	<0.001	1079	670	<0.001	1403	360	0.098	966	346	129	360	<0.001
Female	1239	185		1068	361		1204	225		1031	157 *	46 *	225 *#&	
Age (case)														
≤61 years	1377	221	<0.001	1111	494	0.047	1318	290	0.701	1064	206	77	290	<0.001
>61 years	1279	291		1036	537		1289	295		933	297 *	98 *	295	
Smoking index (case)														
non	1356	231	<0.001	1170	423	<0.001	1307	289	0.003	1112	178	52	289	<0.001
600	849	140		669	321		837	159		616	176	52	159	
>600	451	141		308	287		463	137		268	149 *	71 *#	137 *#&	

Note: DM, distant metastasis; IM, intrapulmonary metastasis; LM, lymphatic metastasis. Chi-square test was used to analyze. * Compared with staging I, adjustment $p < 0.05$; # compared with staging II, adjustment $p < 0.05$; & compared with staging III, adjustment $p < 0.05$.

3.2. Clinical Data and Risk Factor of Tumor Metastasis and Stage in NSCLC Patients

As shown in Tables 3 and 4, the levels of CEA, CYFRA 21-1 and NSE were significantly higher in patients with intrapulmonary, lymphatic and distant metastases when compared with those in non-metastatic patients. The levels of SCC-Ag, ProGRP and TPSA in patients with lymphatic metastasis were significantly higher than those in non-metastatic patients. The levels of CA199 in patients with lymphatic and distant metastases were significantly higher than those in non-metastatic patients. Moreover, the levels of the six tumor markers

CEA, SCC-Ag, CYFRA 21-1, NSE, TPSA and CA199 were significantly different in patients with different tumor stages.

Table 3. The difference in tumor metastasis for the tumor markers in the patients with NSCLC (CEA, SCC-Ag, CYFRA 21-1, NSE, ProGRP, TPSA and CA199).

Variables	IM			LM			DM		
	None	Yes	p	None	Yes	p	None	Yes	p
CEA	3.02 (1.78–5.86)	6.71 (3.18–34.55)	<0.001	2.71 (1.64–4.98)	5.67 (2.91–25.93)	<0.001	2.94 (1.73–5.47)	10.58 (3.43–58.54)	<0.001
SCC-Ag	0.9 (0.70–1.30)	0.9 (0.60–1.80)	0.129	0.9 (0.70–1.30)	1 (070–1.80)	<0.001	0.9 (0.70–1.40)	0.9 (0.60–1.70)	0.45
CYFRA 21-1	2.77 (1.92–4.56)	4.96 (2.63–10.13)	<0.001	2.59 (1.85–3.95)	4.6 (2.63–10.13)	<0.001	2.77 (1.92–4.47)	4.83 (2.58–12.57)	<0.001
NSE	13.32 (11.30–16.35)	16.5 (13.00–20.70)	<0.001	13.4 (11.30–16.00)	15.2 (12.33–20.70)	<0.001	13.36 (11.30–16.35)	16.09 (12.47–23.64)	<0.001
ProGRP	32.79 (26.23–40.64)	32.37 (26.04–38.82)	0.674	32.37 (26.06–40.28)	34.38 (27.90–42.08)	0.013	32.66 (26.16–40.66)	33.79 (27.48–39.34)	0.44
TPSA	45.73 (26.10–85.73)	50.12 (35.07–87.54)	0.17	44.46 (25.74–81.91)	56.28 (29.61–101.00)	<0.001	46.21 (26.20–85.83)	39.49 (25.27–80.74)	0.58
CA199	0.39 (0.26–0.63)	0.46 (0.26–1.03)	0.073	0.38 (0.25–0.61)	0.45 (0.31–0.87)	<0.001	0.39 (0.25–0.63)	0.48 (0.31–1.05)	<0.001

Note: DM, distant metastasis; IM, intrapulmonary metastasis; LM, lymphatic metastasis. Non-normal data are represented by median (P25–P75). Nonparametric test was used to analyze. Comparison of the concentrations of tumor markers between different groups was conducted by a nonparametric test.

Table 4. The difference in clinical stages for the tumor markers in the patients with NSCLC (CEA, SCC-Ag, CYFRA21-1, NSE, ProGRP, TPSA and CA199).

Variables	I	II	III	IV	p
CEA	2.59 (1.57–4.64)	4.10 (2.45–10.12) *	5.39 (3.26–15.75) *#	10.58 (3.43–58.54) *#&	<0.001
SCC-Ag	0.90 (0.70–1.20)	1.00 (0.70–2.10) *	1.10 (0.80–2.90) *#	0.90 (0.60–1.70) *#&	<0.001
CYFRA 21-1	2.50 (1.81–3.68)	4.21 (2.48–8.56) *	5.72 (3.62–14.22) *#	4.83 (2.58–12.57) *#&	<0.001
NSE	12.93 (11.07–15.60)	14.72 (12.20–18.59) *	17.45 (12.82–24.96) *#	16.09 (12.47–23.64) *#	<0.001
ProGRP	32.64 (26.15–40.76)	32.40 (26.01–39.19)	34.51 (29.14–41.78)	33.79 (27.48–39.34)	0.526
TPSA	44.37 (25.82–82.10)	56.94 (30.34–118.79) *	58.57 (45.11–128.41) *	39.49 (25.27–80.74) #&	<0.001
CA199	2.31 (1.35–5.60)	2.85 (1.36–7.35) *	3.01 (1.44–8.29) *#	3.25 (1.43–10.72) *	<0.001

Note: Non-normal data are represented by median (P25–P75). Nonparametric test was used to analyze. Comparison of the concentrations of tumor markers between different groups was conducted by a nonparametric test. * Compared with staging I, adjustment p < 0.05; # compared with staging II, adjustment p < 0.05; & compared with staging III, adjustment p < 0.05.

The results of the univariate analysis were summarized in Table 5. Single factors with p < 0.2 were included in the multivariate logistic analysis. The results of the collinearity analysis were presented in Table 6. The results of the multi-factor analysis were presented in Table 7. Binary logistic regression analysis showed that age, smoking index, CEA and CA199 were independent factors for intrapulmonary metastasis; age, CEA, CYFRA 21-1 and CA199 were independent factors for lymphatic metastasis; and age, CEA and CA199 were independent factors for distant metastasis. Ordinal logistic analysis showed that gender, age, adenocarcinoma (vs. squamous carcinoma), CEA, CYFRA 21-1, NSE and CA199 were independent factors for tumor stage.

Table 5. Univariate analysis of influencing factors for tumor metastasis and clinical stage in patients with NSCLC.

Variables	IM OR (95% CI)	p	LM OR (95% CI)	p	DM OR (95% CI)	p	Staging OR (95% CI)	p
Gender	0.64 (0.53–0.77)	<0.001	0.54 (0.47–0.63)	<0.001	0.73 (0.61–0.87)	<0.001	0.69 (0.64–0.76)	<0.001
Age	1.04 (1.03–1.05)	<0.001	1.02 (1.01–1.03)	<0.001	1.02 (1.01–1.03)	<0.001	1.01 (1.01–1.02)	<0.001
Smoking index								
non	Reference		Reference		Reference		Reference	
600	0.60 (0.48–0.75)	<0.001	0.82 (0.69–0.97)	0.019	0.60 (0.48–0.75)	<0.001	0.85 (0.78–0.94)	0.001
>600	2.00 (1.64–2.45)	<0.001	2.39 (2.00–2.86)	<0.001	1.55 (1.27–1.90)	<0.001	1.54 (1.39–1.71)	<0.001
Histologic classification								
Squamous carcinoma	Reference		Reference		Reference		Reference	
Adenocarcinoma	0.82 (0.66–1.03)	0.086	0.63 (0.74–1.62)	<0.001	0.98 (0.77–1.25)	0.873	0.63 (0.54–0.73)	<0.001
Adenosquamous carcinoma	1.33 (0.62–2.87)	0.469	1.80 (0.96–3.40)	0.068	1.55 (0.72–3.34)	0.259	1.31 (0.75–2.29)	0.338
Others	0.52 (0.29–0.93)	0.027	0.91 (0.62–1.34)	0.912	0.95 (0.55–1.64)	0.858	0.84 (0.60–1.19)	0.331
CEA	3.19 (2.66–3.82)	<0.001	3.60 (3.09–4.19)	<0.001	4.27 (3.57–5.11)	<0.001	2.40 (2.20–2.62)	<0.001
SCC-Ag	1.82 (1.49–2.22)	<0.001	2.02 (1.70–2.40)	<0.001	1.63 (1.34–2.00)	<0.001	1.52 (1.38–1.67)	<0.001
CYFRA 21-1	4.15 (3.38–5.08)	<0.001	4.28 (3.65–5.02)	<0.001	3.69 (3.04–4.47)	<0.001	2.63 (2.41–2.84)	<0.001
NSE	3.11 (2.59–3.74)	<0.001	2.59 (2.21–3.03)	<0.001	2.88 (2.41–3.44)	<0.001	1.95 (1.78–2.13)	<0.001
ProGRP	0.76 (0.18–3.17)	0.707	1.84 (1.07–3.16)	0.028	1.38 (0.55–3.51)	0.495	1.23 (0.89–1.69)	0.205
TPSA	0.92 (0.54–1.57)	0.760	1.61 (1.26–2.06)	<0.001	0.89 (0.57–1.40)	0.615	1.21 (1.05–1.39)	0.007
CA199	3.82 (2.23–6.54)	<0.001	0.32 (0.23–0.44)	<0.001	4.00 (2.53–6.31)	<0.001	2.08 (1.73–2.50)	<0.001

Note 1: DM, distant metastasis; IM, intrapulmonary metastasis; LM, lymphatic metastasis. Note 2: (1) The influencing factors of IM, LM and DM were analyzed by binary logistic analysis. Assignment of dependent variable: IM, LM and DM are all 0 = without and 1 = with. Independent variable assignment: gender (0 = male, 1 = female); age (0 = ≤61 years, 1 = >61 years); smoking index (0 = non, 1 = 1–600, 2 = ≥600); histologic classification (0 = Squamous carcinoma, 1 = Adenocarcinoma, 3 = Adenosquamous carcinoma, 4 = Others); CEA, SCC, CYFRA 21-1, NSE, ProGRP, TPSA, CA199 (0 = normal, 1 = high). (2) The influencing factors of tumor stage were analyzed by ordered logistics. Assignment of dependent variable: tumor stage (1–4 are stage I–IV, respectively); independent variable assignment: gender, age, smoking index, histologic classification and seven kinds of tumor markers are all the same as above.

Table 6. Collinearity examination of multifactor analysis for basic condition and tumor markers related with metastasis and stage of patients with NSCLC.

Variables	IM T	IM VIF	LM T	LM VIF	DM T	DM VIF	Staging T	Staging VIF
Gender	0.635	1.576	0.633	1.580	0.636	1.572	0.633	1.581
Age	0.937	1.067	0.937	1.067	0.936	1.068	0.937	1.067
Smoking index	0.629	1.589	0.628	1.591	0.629	1.589	0.628	1.592
Histologic classification	0.944	1.059	0.939	1.064	-	-	0.939	1.064

Table 6. Cont.

Variables	IM		LM		DM		Staging	
	T	VIF	T	VIF	T	VIF	T	VIF
CEA	0.891	1.122	0.892	1.122	0.895	1.118	0.891	1.122
SCC-Ag	0.900	1.111	0.896	1.116	0.911	1.097	0.896	1.116
CYFRA 21-1	0.863	1.159	0.737	1.356	0.872	1.147	0.737	1.357
NSE	0.975	1.025	0.976	1.025	0.980	1.020	0.976	1.025
TPSA	-	-	0.797	1.254	-	-	0.797	1.254
CA199	0.922	1.085	0.922	1.084	0.925	1.081	0.922	1.084

Note 1: DM, distant metastasis; IM, intrapulmonary metastasis; LM, lymphatic metastasis. Note 2: T, tolerance; VIF, variance inflation factor.

Table 7. Multivariate analysis of influencing factors for tumor metastasis and clinical stage in patients with NSCLC.

Variables	IM		LM		DM		Staging	
	OR (95% CI)	p	OR (95% CI)	p	OR (95% CI)	p	OR (95% CI)	p
Gender	0.52 (0.29–0.94)	0.031	0.85 (0.61–1.19)	0.335	0.66 (0.39–1.13)	0.117	0.68 (0.49–0.94)	0.021
Age	0.58 (0.34–0.99)	0.045	0.64 (0.48–0.83)	0.001	0.66 (0.42–1.03)	0.068	0.76 (0.59–0.98)	0.036
Smoking index								
non	Reference		Reference		Reference		Reference	
600	0.53 (0.27–1.03)	0.059	1.00 (0.70–1.42)	0.987	0.66 (0.37–1.15)	0.144	0.95 (0.67–1.34)	0.775
>600	0.28 (0.08–0.99)	0.048	1.22 (0.75–2.00)	0.413	0.45 (0.18–1.11)	0.082	1.03 (0.65–1.64)	0.889
Histologic classification								
Squamous carcinoma	Reference		Reference		Reference		Reference	
Adenocarcinoma	2.69 (0.78–9.31)	0.119	0.92 (0.62–1.38)	0.695	-	-	0.68 (0.47–0.97)	0.033
Adenosquamous carcinoma	-	-	1.58 (0.35–7.15)	0.553	-	-	1.05 (0.26–4.31)	0.948
Others	1.28 (0.20–8.12)	0.793	1.32 (0.72–2.43)	0.365	-	-	0.87 (0.49–1.54)	0.628
CEA	2.66 (1.53–4.63)	<0.001	3.08 (2.33–4.07)	<0.001	4.51 (2.86–7.12)	<0.001	2.85 (2.17–3.75)	<0.001
SCC-Ag	0.40 (0.14–1.18)	0.096	1.35 (0.95–1.93)	0.093	0.50 (0.24–1.03)	0.060	1.04 (0.74–1.45)	0.842
CYFRA 21-1	1.27 (0.73–2.22)	0.394	2.00 (1.48–2.69)	<0.001	1.06 (0.66–1.69)	0.822	2.56 (1.92–3.42)	<0.001
NSE	1.51 (0.86–2.66)	0.155	1.15 (0.84–1.57)	0.382	1.26 (0.77–2.08)	0.362	1.76 (1.33–2.34)	<0.001
TPSA	-	-	0.98 (0.72–1.32)	0.876	-	-	0.75 (0.56–1.01)	0.055
CA199	2.80 (1.49–5.17)	0.001	2.04 (1.41–2.96)	<0.001	2.20 (1.31–3.69)	0.003	2.20 (1.54–3.14)	<0.001

Notes are the same as in Table 5.

3.3. The Predictions of Single and Combined Factors for Tumor Metastasis and Stage in NSCLC Patients

Multivariate analysis of tumor markers with $p < 0.05$ was followed by a logistic analysis of prediction probability. For analysis of the influencing factors of tumor metastasis and clinical stage of NSCLC patients, the area under the ROC curve (AUC) for factors is shown in Table 8. ROC curves were used to predict lung cancer metastasis and stage, and the results were shown in Figure 1. CEA and CA199 provided an accurate prediction of intrapulmonary and distant metastasis with the AUC of 0.69 both ($p < 0.001$); CEA, CYFRA 21-1 and CA199 provided an accurate prediction of lymphatic metastasis with the AUC of 0.62 ($p < 0.001$).

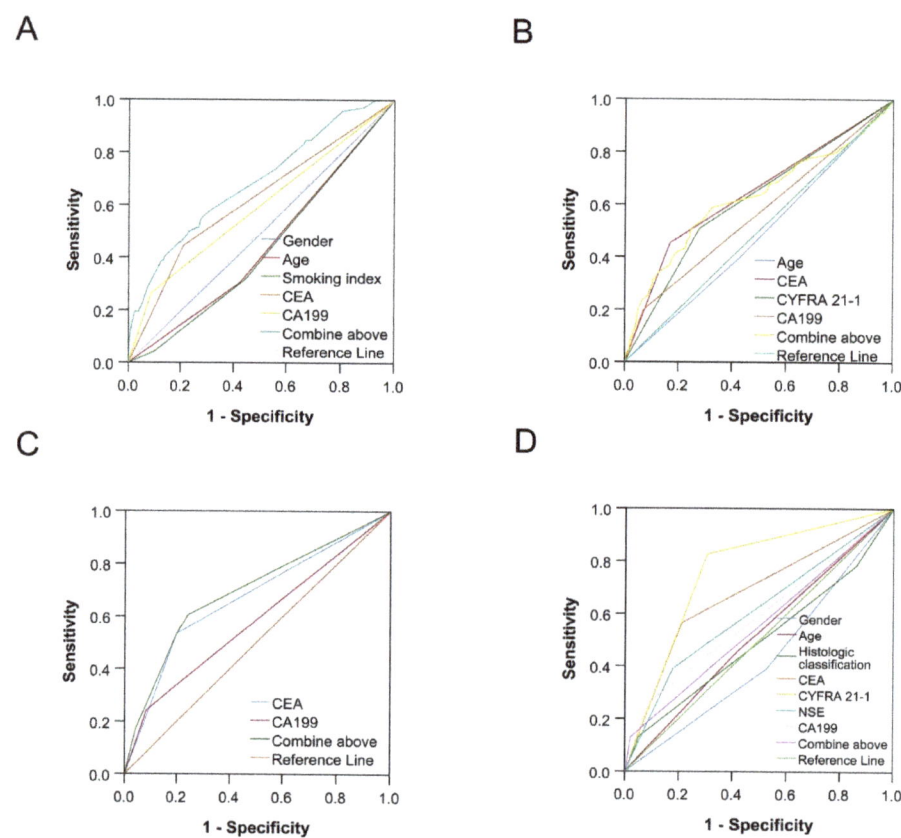

Figure 1. ROC curves of tumor markers for tumor metastasis and stage. (**A**) The ROC curve for gender, age, smoking index, CEA and CA199 in the diagnosis of intrapulmonary metastasis; (**B**) the ROC curve for age, CEA, CYFRA 21-1 and CA199 in the diagnosis of lymphatic metastasis. (**C**) the ROC curve for CEA and CA199 in the diagnosis of distant metastasis. (**D**) the ROC curve for gender, age, histologic classification, CEA, CYFRA 21-1, NSE and CA199 in the diagnosis of tumor stage.

Table 8. Receiver operating characteristic (ROC) curves of influencing factors for tumor metastasis and clinical stage in patients with NSCLC.

Variables	IM		LM		DM		Staging	
	AUC (95% CI)	p	AUC (95% CI)	p	AUC (95% CI)	p	AUC (95% CI)	p
Gender	0.49 (0.43–0.56)	0.862	-	-	-	-	0.43 (0.35–0.52)	0.116
Age	0.44 (0.38–0.51)	0.085	0.48 (0.45–0.52)	0.362	-	-	0.52 (0.43–0.60)	0.659
Smoking index	0.43 (0.37–0.49)	0.044	-	-	-	-	-	-

Table 8. *Cont.*

Variables	IM		LM		DM		Staging	
	AUC (95% CI)	p	AUC (95% CI)	p	AUC (95% CI)	p	AUC (95% CI)	p
Histologic classification	-	-	-	-	-	-	0.50 (0.40–0.59)	0.949
CEA	0.62 (0.55–0.69)	0.001	0.64 (0.61–0.68)	<0.001	0.67 (0.61–0.73)	<0.001	0.68 (0.59–0.76)	<0.001
CYFRA 21-1	-	-	0.62 (0.58–0.65)	<0.001	-	-	0.76 (0.70–0.83)	<0.001
NSE	-	-	-	-	-	-	0.61 (0.52–0.70)	0.013
CA199	0.59 (0.52–0.66)	0.011	0.56 (0.53–0.60)	<0.001	0.58 (0.52–0.64)	0.007	0.59 (0.49–0.68)	0.046
Combine	0.69 (0.62–0.75)	<0.001	0.62 (0.59–0.66)	<0.001	0.69 (0.63–0.75)	<0.001	0.55 (0.46–0.65)	0.205

Notes: DM, distant metastasis; IM, intrapulmonary metastasis; LM, lymphatic metastasis.

4. Discussion

Tumor markers have been widely used in the clinical diagnosis and treatment of malignant tumors as they serve as important indicators of disease outcome monitoring. At present, varied tumor markers, such as CEA, SCC-Ag, CYFRA 21-1, NSE, are applied in diagnosing lung cancer, which can also be used to monitor metastasis and recurrence of NSCLC [18]. Although tumor markers are widely used in clinical practice, the clinical analysis and validation of these markers using a large sample size remain lacking. In this study, a large sample of lung cancer patients from two medical centers was selected to verify the accuracy of tumor markers from multiple perspectives, including predicting tumor metastasis and clinical stage. Our results support the use of these markers in clinical practice.

CEA is widely found in adult cancer tissues and has been used in the auxiliary diagnosis, efficacy observation, prognostic judgment, and recurrence prediction of cancer [19,20]. CEA elevation is common in multisystem tumors, including lung cancer [21]. Due to the non-specificity of this indicator, CEA is often used in combination with other tumor markers in clinical practice [22,23]. SCC-Ag participates in the regulation of protein decomposition during malignant transformation, and it is the preferred tumor marker for cervical squamous cell carcinoma [24,25]. Additionally, this marker is observed to increase in lung squamous cell cancers [26]. CYFRA 21-1 is highly expressed in lung squamous cell carcinoma compared with adenocarcinoma and SCLC [27]. The use of increased serum levels of CYFRA 21-1 for predicting postoperative recurrence in lung cancer patients shows good sensitivity and specificity. CYFRA 21-1 is also a highly sensitive and specific biomarker for the prediction of post-chemotherapy progression [28].

A high concentration of serum NSE is a specific marker of neuroendocrine tumors [29,30]. SCLC regulates the secretion of a variety of related enzymes, active peptides, and hormones [31]. Thus, NSE is a preferred marker for SCLC. NSE is only significantly changed in middle and advanced SCLC. NSE has been found to be related to changes in tumor growth and can be combined with clinical observations and monitoring to predict metastasis and recurrence for NSCLC [32]. ProGRP is a marker of small cell lung cancer. Serum CA199 can be used for pancreatic cancer. Auxiliary diagnostic indicators for malignant tumors such as gallbladder cancer are mainly used as indicators for disease monitoring and predicting recurrence.

In this study, we have analyzed the differences in tumor markers among patients with different metastases and tumor stages. The results showed that the levels of SCC-Ag, ProGRP and CA199 in patients with lymphatic metastasis, and the levels of CEA, CYFRA 21-1 and NSE in patients with intrapulmonary, lymphatic, and distant metastasis, were significantly higher than those patients with non-metastasis. This data indicates that the increased tumor markers significantly correlate with NSCLC metastasis [13]. Lung cancer markers have been also associated with the clinical stage of lung cancer. Tumor markers related to NSCLC, such as CEA, SCC-Ag and CYFRA 21-1, show a clear relationship with tumor stage [12,33]. The results of this study showed that there were statistical differences in the numeric levels and proportion of six tumor markers, including SCC-Ag, CEA, CYFRA 21-1, NSE, CA199 and TPSA, among patients with different tumor stages of NSCLC.

The results of risk factors showed that the patients, with increased levels of CEA, CYFRA 21-1, NSE and CA199, tended to have higher tumor stages. The risk factors for intrapulmonary metastasis were smoking index > 600, and increased levels of CEA and CA199. The risk factors for lymphatic metastasis were higher levels of CEA, CYFRA 21-1 and CA199. The risk factors for distant metastasis were elevated CEA and CA199 levels.

Combined detection of certain serum tumor markers in lung cancer patients can significantly improve diagnostic sensitivity and the roles of monitoring tumor progression [34,35]. At last, joint predictions of combined lung cancer-related tumor markers for tumor metastasis have been performed by ROC curve analyses. The result showed that the combined elevations in CEA and CA199 were also useful for the diagnoses of lymphatic metastasis and distant metastasis, respectively. These results are in accordance with previous reports [36].

5. Conclusions

In summary, our results suggest that the levels of CEA, SCC-Ag, CYFRA 21-1, NSE and CA199 were positively related to tumor metastasis and stage. Elevated CEA and CA199 levels in NSCLC patients are indicative of intrapulmonary and distant metastases; elevated CEA, CYFRA 21-1 and CA199 levels in patients with NSCLC are indicative of lymphatic metastasis. These tumor markers could be useful in predicting tumor metastasis in patients with NSCLC.

Author Contributions: C.J. and S.Z. conceived and designed this study; C.J. and B.S. carried out the data collection; C.J., S.Z. and M.Z. mainly performed data statistical analysis; X.H. and S.H. mainly presented all tables; C.J., B.S., S.Z., M.Z. and X.H. participated in analyzing the analysis results and wrote the paper; all other authors participated in the data collection; C.J., B.S. and S.Z. supervised and directed the project. All authors have read and agreed to the published version of the manuscript.

Funding: This work was supported by the Natural Science Foundation of Tianjin-Municipal Science and Technology Commission (Grant Number: 20JCYBJC01030) and Social Development Science and Technology Project of TaiZhou City (Grant Number: 21ywb99).

Institutional Review Board Statement: This study was approved by the Medical Ethics Committees of Tianjin Union Medical Center (TUMCME20200228, approve date 28 February 2020) and Tianjin Medical University Cancer Institute and Hospital (20200115, approve date 15 January 2020).

Informed Consent Statement: All authors have approved the manuscript and consent for publication.

Data Availability Statement: Data are available upon request.

Conflicts of Interest: The authors declare no conflict of interest.

Abbreviations

CA199, carbohydrate antigens; CEA, carcinoembryonic antigen; CMIA, chemiluminescent microparticle immunoassay; CYFRA 21-1, cytokeratin-19 fragment; DM, Distant metastasis; IM, Intrapulmonary metastasis; LM, Lymphatic metastasis; NSCLC, non-small cell lung cancer; NSE, neuron-specific enolase; ProGRP, pro-gastrin-releasing peptide; ROC, receiver operating characteristic; SCC-Ag, squamous cell carcinoma antigen; SCLC, small cell lung cancer; TPSA, total prostate-specific antigen.

References

1. Elbeyli, L.; Sanli, M.; Kasap, M.; Gezici, S.; Ozaslan, M.; Akpinar, G. Comparative Proteomics and Bioinformatics Analysis of Tissue from Non-Small Cell Lung Cancer Patients. *Curr. Proteom.* **2017**, *14*, 58–77.
2. Siegel, R.L.; Miller, K.D.; Jemal, A. Cancer statistics, 2018. *CA Cancer J. Clin.* **2018**, *60*, 277–300. [CrossRef]
3. Zhan, M.; Wen, F.; Liu, L.; Chen, Z.; Wei, H.; Zhou, H. JMJD1A promotes tumorigenesis and forms a feedback loop with EZH2/let-7c in NSCLC cells. *Tumor Biol.* **2016**, *37*, 11237–11247. [CrossRef] [PubMed]
4. Funakoshi, T.; Tachibana, I.; Kimura, H.; Takeda, Y.; Kijima, T.; Hoshida, Y.; Nishino, K.; Goto, H.; Yoneda, T.; Kumagai, T.; et al. Expression of tetraspanins in human lung cancer cells: Frequent downregulation of CD9 and its contribution to cell motility in small cell lung cancer. *Oncogene* **2003**, *22*, 674–687. [CrossRef] [PubMed]
5. Wu, H.; Wang, Q.; Liu, Q.; Zhang, Q.; Huang, Q.; Yu, Z. The Serum Tumor Markers in Combination for Clinical Diagnosis of Lung Cancer. *Clin. Lab.* **2020**, *66*. [CrossRef] [PubMed]
6. Liu, L.; Teng, J.; Zhang, L.; Cong, P.; Yao, Y.; Sun, G.; Liu, Z.; Yu, T.; Liu, M. The Combination of the Tumor Markers Suggests the Histological Diagnosis of Lung Cancer. *Biomed. Res. Int.* **2017**, *2017*, 2013989. [CrossRef] [PubMed]
7. Molina, R.; Auge, J.M.; Escudero, J.M.; Marrades, R.; Viñolas, N.; Carcereny, E.; Ramirez, J.; Filella, X. Mucins CA 125, CA 19.9, CA 15.3 and TAG-72.3 as tumor markers in patients with lung cancer: Comparison with CYFRA 21-1, CEA, SCC and NSE. *Tumour Biol.* **2008**, *29*, 371–380. [CrossRef]
8. Hu, Q.; Xiao, P.; Li, J.; Yu, P. A retrospective analysis of serum tumor markers found in non-small cell lung cancer. *J. Cancer Res.* **2016**, *12*, 117–120.
9. Nisman, B.; Biran, H.; Ramu, N.; Heching, N.; Barak, V.; Peretz, T. The diagnostic and prognostic value of ProGRP in lung cancer. *Anticancer. Res.* **2009**, *29*, 4827–4832.
10. Wang, C.F.; Peng, S.J.; Liu, R.Q.; Yu, Y.J.; Ge, Q.M.; Liang, R.B.; Li, Q.Y.; Li, B.; Shao, Y. The Combination of CA125 and NSE Is Useful for Predicting Liver Metastasis of Lung Cancer. *Dis. Markers* **2020**, *2020*, 8850873. [CrossRef]
11. Wang, L.; Wang, D.; Zheng, G.; Yang, Y.; Du, L.; Dong, Z.; Zhang, X.; Wang, C. Clinical Evaluation and Therapeutic Monitoring Value of Serum Tumor Markers in Lung Cancer. *Int. J. Biol. Markers* **2016**, *31*, 80–87. [CrossRef] [PubMed]
12. Molina, R.; Filella, X.; Augé, J.M.; Fuentes, R.; Bover, I.; Rifa, J.; Moreno, V.; Canals, E.; Viñolas, N.; Marquez, A.; et al. Tumor Markers (CEA, CA 125, CYFRA 21-1, SCC and NSE) in Patients with Non-Small Cell Lung Cancer as an Aid in Histological Diagnosis and Prognosis. *Tumor Biol.* **2003**, *24*, 209–218. [CrossRef] [PubMed]
13. Cedrés, S.; Nuñez, I.; Longo, M.; Martinez, P.; Checa, E.; Torrejón, D.; Felip, E. Serum Tumor Markers CEA, CYFRA21-1, and CA-125 Are Associated with Worse Prognosis in Advanced Non–Small-Cell Lung Cancer (NSCLC). *Clin. Lung Cancer* **2011**, *12*, 172–179. [CrossRef] [PubMed]
14. Bello, M.G.D.; Filiberti, R.A.; Alama, A.; Orengo, A.M.; Mussap, M.; Coco, S.; Vanni, I.; Boccardo, S.; Rijavec, E.; Genova, C.; et al. The role of CEA, CYFRA21-1 and NSE in monitoring tumor response to Nivolumab in advanced non-small cell lung cancer (NSCLC) patients. *J. Transl. Med.* **2019**, *17*, 74. [CrossRef] [PubMed]
15. Shirasu, H.; Ono, A.; Omae, K.; Nakashima, K.; Omori, S.; Wakuda, K.; Kenmotsu, H.; Naito, T.; Murakami, H.; Endo, M.; et al. CYFRA 21-1 predicts the efficacy of nivolumab in patients with advanced lung adenocarcinoma. *Tumor Biol.* **2018**, *40*, 101042831876042. [CrossRef]
16. Li, Q.; Sang, S. Diagnostic Value and Clinical Significance of Combined Detection of Serum Markers CYFRA21-1, SCC Ag, NSE, CEA and ProGRP in Non-Small Cell Lung Carcinoma. *Clin. Lab.* **2020**, *66*, 11. [CrossRef]
17. Kang, S.J.; Cho, Y.R.; Park, G.M.; Ahn, J.M.; Han, S.B.; Lee, J.Y.; Kim, W.J.; Park, D.W.; Lee, S.W.; Kim, Y.H.; et al. Predictors for functionally significant in-stent restenosis: An integrated analysis using coronary angiography, IVUS, and myocardial perfusion imaging. *JACC Cardiovasc. Imaging* **2013**, *6*, 1183–1190. [CrossRef]
18. Vinolas, N.; Molina, R.; Fuentes, R.; Bover, I.; Rifa, J.; Moreno, V.; Canals, E.; Marquez, A.; Barreiro, E.; Borras, J.; et al. Tumor markers (CEA, CA 125, CYFRA 21.1, SCC and NSE) in non small cell lung cancer (NSCLC) patients as an aid in histological diagnosis and prognosis: Comparison with the main clinical and pathological prognostic factors. *Lung Cancer* **2000**, *29*, 195. [CrossRef]
19. Zamcheck, N. The present status of carcinoembryonic antigen (CEA) in diagnosis, detection of recurrence, prognosis and evaluation of therapy of colonic and pancreatic cancer. *Clin. Gastroenterol.* **1976**, *5*, 625–638. [CrossRef]
20. Grunnet, M.; Sorensen, J.B. Carcinoembryonic antigen (CEA) as tumor marker in lung cancer. *Lung Cancer* **2012**, *76*, 138–143. [CrossRef] [PubMed]
21. Kim, K.N.; Joo, N.S.; Je, S.Y.; Kim, K.M.; Kim, B.T.; Park, S.B.; Cho, D.Y.; Park, R.W.; Lee, D.J. Carcinoembryonic Antigen Level Can be Overestimated in Metabolic Syndrome. *J. Korean Med. Sci.* **2011**, *26*, 759–764. [CrossRef]
22. Hall, C.; Clarke, L.; Pal, A.; Buchwald, P.; Eglinton, T.; Wakeman, C.; Frizelle, F. A Review of the Role of Carcinoembryonic Antigen in Clinical Practice. *Ann. Coloproctol.* **2019**, *35*, 294–305. [CrossRef] [PubMed]
23. Hao, C.; Zhang, G.; Zhang, L. Serum CEA levels in 49 different types of cancer and noncancer diseases. *Prog. Mol. Biol. Transl. Sci.* **2019**, *162*, 213–227. [PubMed]
24. Suzuki, Y.; Nakano, T.; Ohno, T.; Abe, A.; Morita, S.; Tsujii, H. Serum CYFRA 21-1 in cervical cancer patients treated with radiation therapy. *J. Cancer Res. Clin. Oncol.* **2000**, *126*, 332–336. [CrossRef] [PubMed]

25. Holdenrieder, S.; Molina, R.; Qiu, L.; Zhi, X.; Rutz, S.; Engel, C.; Kasper-Sauer, P.; Dayyani, F.; Mkorse, C. Technical and clinical performance of a new assay to detect squamous cell carcinoma antigen levels for the differential diagnosis of cervical, lung, and head and neck cancer. *Tumour Biol.* **2018**, *40*, 1010428318772202. [CrossRef] [PubMed]
26. Schneider, J.; Velcovsky, H.G.; Morr, H.; Katz, N.; Neu, K.; Eigenbrodt, E. Comparison of the tumor markers tumor M2-PK, CEA, CYFRA 21-1, NSE and SCC in the diagnosis of lung cancer. *Anticancer. Res.* **2000**, *20*, 5053–5058.
27. Jiang, Z.F.; Wang, M.; Xu, J.L. Thymidine kinase 1 combined with CEA, CYFRA21-1 and NSE improved its diagnostic value for lung cancer. *Life Sci.* **2018**, *194*, 1–6. [CrossRef]
28. Zissimopoulos, A.; Stellos, K.; Permenopoulou, V.; Petrakis, G.; Theodorakopoulos, P.; Baziotis, N.; Thalassinos, N. The importance of the tumor marker CYFRA 21-1 in patients with lung cancer after surgery or chemotherapy. *Hell. J. Nucl. Med.* **2007**, *10*, 62–66.
29. Sandoval, J.A.; Malkas, L.H.; Hickey, R.J. Clinical significance of serum biomarkers in pediatric solid mediastinal and abdominal tumors. *Int. J. Mol. Sci.* **2012**, *13*, 1126–1153. [CrossRef]
30. Kamiya, N.; Suzuki, H.; Kawamura, K.; Imamoto, T.; Naya, Y.; Tochigi, N.; Kakuta, Y.; Yamaguchi, K.; Ishikura, H.; Ichikawa, T. Neuroendocrine differentiation in stage D2 prostate cancers. *Int. J. Urol.* **2008**, *15*, 423–428. [CrossRef]
31. Rosati, R.; Adil, M.R.; Ali, M.A.; Eliason, J.; Orosz, A.; Sebestyén, F.; Kalemkerian, G.P. Induction of apoptosis by a short-chain neuropeptide analog in small cell lung cancer. *Peptides* **1998**, *19*, 1519–1523. [CrossRef]
32. Tiseo, M.; Ardizzoni, A.; Cafferata, M.A.; Loprevite, M.; Chiaramondia, M.; Filiberti, R.; Marroniet, P.; Grossi, F.; Paganuzzi, M. Predictive and prognostic significance of neuron-specific enolase (NSE) in non-small cell lung cancer. *Anticancer. Res.* **2008**, *28*, 507–513. [PubMed]
33. Yang, Q.; Zhang, P.; Wu, R.; Lu, K.; Zhou, H. Identifying the Best Marker Combination in CEA, CA125, CY211, NSE, and SCC for Lung Cancer Screening by Combining ROC Curve and Logistic Regression Analyses: Is It Feasible? *Dis. Markers* **2018**, *2018*, 2082840. [CrossRef] [PubMed]
34. Wang, W.J.; Tao, Z.; Gu, W.; Sun, L.H. Clinical observations on the association between diagnosis of lung cancer and serum tumor markers in combination. *Asian Pac. J. Cancer Prev.* **2013**, *14*, 4369–4371. [CrossRef]
35. Chu, X.Y.; Hou, X.B.; Song, W.A.; Xue, Z.Q.; Wang, B.; Zhang, L.B. Diagnostic values of SCC, CEA, Cyfra21-1 and NSE for lung cancer in patients with suspicious pulmonary masses: A single center analysis. *Cancer Biol.* **2011**, *11*, 995–1000. [CrossRef]
36. Hatate, K.; Yamashita, K.; Hirai, K.; Kumamoto, H.; Sato, T.; Ozawa, H.; Nakamura, T.; Onozato, W.; Kokuba, Y.; Ihara, A.; et al. Liver metastasis of colorectal cancer by protein-tyrosine phosphatase type 4A, 3 (PRL-3) is mediated through lymph node metastasis and elevated serum tumor markers such as CEA and CA19-9. *Oncol Rep* **2008**, *20*, 737–743.

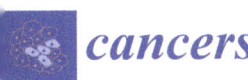

Article

Proteomic and Metabolomic Analysis of Bone Marrow and Plasma from Patients with Extramedullary Multiple Myeloma Identifies Distinct Protein and Metabolite Signatures

Katie Dunphy [1,*], Despina Bazou [2], Michael Henry [3], Paula Meleady [3], Juho J. Miettinen [4], Caroline A. Heckman [4], Paul Dowling [1,†] and Peter O'Gorman [2,†]

1. Department of Biology, Maynooth University, W23 F2K8 Kildare, Ireland; paul.dowlling@mu.ie
2. Department of Haematology, Mater Misericordiae University Hospital, D07 AX57 Dublin, Ireland; despina.bazou@ucd.ie (D.B.); pogorman@mirtireland.com (P.O.)
3. National Institute for Cellular Biotechnology, Dublin City University, D09 NR58 Dublin, Ireland; michael.henry@dcu.ie (M.H.); paula.meleady@dcu.ie (P.M.)
4. Institute for Molecular Medicine Finland-FIMM, HiLIFE–Helsinki Institute of Life Science, iCAN Digital Precision Cancer Medicine Flagship, University of Helsinki, 00290 Helsinki, Finland; juho.miettinen@helsinki.fi (J.J.M.); caroline.heckman@helsinki.fi (C.A.H.)
* Correspondence: katie.dunphy.2015@mumail.ie
† These authors contributed equally to this work.

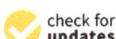

Citation: Dunphy, K.; Bazou, D.; Henry, M.; Meleady, P.; Miettinen, J.J.; Heckman, C.A.; Dowling, P.; O'Gorman, P. Proteomic and Metabolomic Analysis of Bone Marrow and Plasma from Patients with Extramedullary Multiple Myeloma Identifies Distinct Protein and Metabolite Signatures. *Cancers* **2023**, *15*, 3764. https://doi.org/10.3390/cancers15153764

Academic Editors: Daniel L. Pouliquen and Cristina Núñez González

Received: 5 July 2023
Revised: 19 July 2023
Accepted: 19 July 2023
Published: 25 July 2023

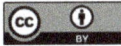

Copyright: © 2023 by the authors. Licensee MDPI, Basel, Switzerland. This article is an open access article distributed under the terms and conditions of the Creative Commons Attribution (CC BY) license (https://creativecommons.org/licenses/by/4.0/).

Simple Summary: Extramedullary multiple myeloma (EMM) is a rare and aggressive subtype of multiple myeloma which is associated with a poor prognosis. Here, we used mass spectrometry to illustrate that extramedullary multiple myeloma patients have a bone marrow and plasma protein signature that is distinct from multiple myeloma patients without extramedullary spread. We used bioinformatic tools to analyse differentially expressed proteins and verified the increased abundance of three proteins (VCAM1, HGFA, PEDF) in the plasma of patients with EMM. Considering the paucity of informative biomarkers and effective therapeutic approaches for the treatment of EMM, this study may provide direction for the discovery of novel diagnostic and therapeutic approaches and markers of extramedullary progression.

Abstract: Multiple myeloma (MM) is an incurable haematological malignancy of plasma cells in the bone marrow. In rare cases, an aggressive form of MM called extramedullary multiple myeloma (EMM) develops, where myeloma cells enter the bloodstream and colonise distal organs or soft tissues. This variant is associated with refractoriness to conventional therapies and a short overall survival. The molecular mechanisms associated with EMM are not yet fully understood. Here, we analysed the proteome of bone marrow mononuclear cells and blood plasma from eight patients (one serial sample) with EMM and eight patients without extramedullary spread. The patients with EMM had a significantly reduced overall survival with a median survival of 19 months. Label-free mass spectrometry revealed 225 proteins with a significant differential abundance between bone marrow mononuclear cells (BMNCs) isolated from patients with MM and EMM. This plasma proteomics analysis identified 22 proteins with a significant differential abundance. Three proteins, namely vascular cell adhesion molecule 1 (VCAM1), pigment epithelium derived factor (PEDF), and hepatocyte growth factor activator (HGFA), were verified as the promising markers of EMM, with the combined protein panel showing excellent accuracy in distinguishing EMM patients from MM patients. Metabolomic analysis revealed a distinct metabolite signature in EMM patient plasma compared to MM patient plasma. The results provide much needed insight into the phenotypic profile of EMM and in identifying promising plasma-derived markers of EMM that may inform novel drug development strategies.

Keywords: multiple myeloma; extramedullary multiple myeloma; extramedullary disease; proteomics; mass spectrometry; clinical proteomics; metabolomics

1. Introduction

Multiple myeloma (MM) is characterised by the uncontrolled proliferation of plasma cells in the bone marrow, resulting in the production of large amounts of non-functional monoclonal antibodies or paraproteins, which can be detected in the blood or urine [1]. MM is the second most common blood cancer and accounts for approximately 1% of all cancers [2]. The approval of various therapeutics, including proteasome inhibitors, immunomodulatory drugs, and monoclonal antibodies, have improved the overall survival of MM patients over the last two decades. However, despite the introduction of these novel therapeutics, MM remains an incurable disease due to the development of drug resistance and repeated relapses [3].

As outlined in the Revised International Staging System (RISS), multiple factors, including tumour burden, serum biomarker levels and the presence of high-risk cytogenetics, help define MM prognosis [4]. One poor prognostic factor is the presence of extramedullary multiple myeloma (EMM), an aggressive manifestation of MM where clonal plasma cells become independent of the bone marrow microenvironment (BME) and colonise distal organs and soft tissues outside of the bone marrow, such as the skin, liver and lungs [5]. EMM can be detected at diagnosis or relapse, both of which indicate poor prognosis. There is no consensus on the median survival of EMM patients; however, several studies have reported significantly reduced median survival in newly diagnosed and relapsed MM patients with extramedullary disease compared to those without plasmacytomas [6–8]. The reported incidence of EMM varies between studies, ranging from 0.5–4.8% in newly diagnosed MM and 3.4–14% in relapsed/refractory MM [8].

Treatment resistance is commonly associated with EMM [9,10]. When considering treatment options, EMM is treated aggressively, similarly to how high-risk MM is treated. MM is still treated empirically with conventional myeloma therapies, meaning there is a lack of targeted therapeutic options for MM variants, such as EMM. The low number of prospective studies specifically focusing on EMM impedes a clinician's ability to make strong treatment recommendations [8]. For this reason, several studies have advised future large MM-focused clinical trials to evaluate EMM patients as a defined subgroup to inform therapeutic decision making [8,11]. There is therefore a need for novel therapeutic targets and treatment strategies to improve the survival outcome for EMM patients.

Despite the aggressiveness of EMM, the molecular mechanisms that contribute to the escape of malignant plasma cells from the bone marrow and the colonization of distant tissues are poorly understood [5]. Several studies have reported high-risk genetic abnormalities, such as del(17p13), and dysregulated cell adhesion and migratory pathways, as contributing to extramedullary progression [12,13]. The increased expression of the chemokine receptor CXCR4 has been linked to the development of an epithelial-to-mesenchymal-like phenotype that is associated with medullary and extramedullary metastasis [14,15]. Furthermore, myeloma cells derived from extramedullary sites are often plasmablastic, a morphological trait associated with more aggressive disease [16,17]. Dissecting the key signalling pathways that facilitate the survival and proliferation of plasma cells outside of the bone marrow is crucial for identifying novel therapeutic targets in EMM. Furthermore, identifying clinically relevant non-invasive markers of EMM may facilitate the early detection of extramedullary lesions.

In this study, we performed a mass-spectrometry (MS)-based pilot proteomic analysis of matched bone marrow mononuclear cells (BMNCs) and blood plasma from MM patients with and without extramedullary spread ($n = 17$). A targeted metabolomic analysis of blood plasma was also performed to explore the metabolic signature of EMM plasma. Through these analyses, we aimed to (i) identify biological processes or signalling pathways associated with extramedullary transition, (ii) identify potential therapeutic targets and prognostic markers for further investigation and (iii) reveal plasma-based biomarkers for diagnostic and/or prognostic clinical use. Collectively, this study contributes to the current understanding of the molecular phenotype associated with EMM.

2. Materials and Methods

2.1. Patient Information and Sample Collection

Bone marrow mononuclear cells (BMNCs) and blood EDTA plasma samples from age- and gender-matched MM ($n = 8$) and EMM patients ($n = 9$, 1 serial sample) were obtained from the Finnish Hematology Registry and Clinical Biobank (FHRB). In this research paper, EMM refers to patients with soft tissue plasmacytomas outside of the bone marrow and not paraskeletal plasmacytomas [18]. Patient characteristics are summarised in Table 1. Cytogenetic information was also recorded (Figure S1). Sample collection, with informed consent, took place between 2013 and 2020 across several Finnish university hospitals and other haematology units. Median age was 65. Samples were obtained from 4 female and 12 male subjects. To analyse the association of the plasma-based markers of EMM with drug resistance, EDTA plasma was obtained from a second cohort of patients ($n = 44$) stratified based on ex vivo drug sensitivity resistance testing (DSRT) performed on CD138+ myeloma cells isolated from bone marrow aspirates. These plasma samples from 44 MM patients with corresponding DSRT data were also obtained from the FHRB. The FHRB is authorised and approved by the Finnish National Supervisory Authority for Welfare and Health (Valvira) and Finnish National Medical Ethics Committee, respectively. Samples were stored at $-80\ ^\circ$C.

Table 1. Clinical and demographic characteristics of patients involved in this study. Characteristics include diagnosis, status at diagnosis, sex, age and overall survival.

Sample ID	Diagnosis	Status	Sex	Age	OS (mo) from Diagnosis
D_EMM_2689	Myeloma, extramedullary	Diagnostic	Male	65	80
D_EMM_3497	Myeloma, extramedullary	Diagnostic	Male	65	87 *
D_EMM_3674	Myeloma, extramedullary	Diagnostic	Male	58	8
D_EMM_4296	Myeloma, extramedullary	Diagnostic	Male	65	22
D_EMM_1994	Myeloma, extramedullary	Diagnostic	Female	67	16
D_EMM_40725	Myeloma, extramedullary	Diagnostic	Male	49	2
PD_EMM_874	Myeloma, extramedullary	Progressive disease	Male	72	31
PD_EMM_1994 [†]	Myeloma, extramedullary	Progressive disease	Female	68	16
PD_EMM_40795	Myeloma, extramedullary	Progressive disease	Female	69	7
D_MM_5215	Myeloma, no extramedullary	Diagnostic	Male	65	61 *
D_MM_4314	Myeloma, no extramedullary	Diagnostic	Male	65	53
D_MM_5187	Myeloma, no extramedullary	Diagnostic	Male	59	62 *
D_MM_4317	Myeloma, no extramedullary	Diagnostic	Male	65	65
D_MM_40141	Myeloma, no extramedullary	Diagnostic	Male	49	43 *
PD_MM_899	Myeloma, no extramedullary	Progressive disease	Male	72	124
PD_MM_1579	Myeloma, no extramedullary	Progressive disease	Female	68	83
PD_MM_40301	Myeloma, no extramedullary	Progressive disease	Female	70	129 *

* Patient was alive at last follow-up. [†] D_EMM_1994 and PD_EMM_1994 were collected from the same patient. PD_EMM_1994 sample was collected approximately 1 year after D_EMM_1994.

2.2. Bone Marrow Mononuclear Cells Sample Preparation

Cryopreserved BMNCs were thawed in a 37 °C water bath. BMNCs were isolated and washed twice with phosphate-buffered saline (PBS). The supernatant was removed, and cell pellets were solubilised in 200 µL of lysis buffer (4% SDS, 100 mM Tris/HCl pH 7.6, 0.1 M DTT, protease inhibitors). Protein quantitation was performed using the Pierce™ 660 nm protein assay (Thermo Fisher Scientific, Waltham, MA, USA), as described by the manufacturer's guidelines. Filter-aided sample preparation (FASP) was applied for proteolytic digestion [19]. A total of 15 µg of protein from each sample was digested. Briefly, samples were subject to a series of centrifugal steps using 8 M urea and 50 mM iodoacetamide to facilitate detergent removal, buffer exchange and protein alkylation. Overnight trypsin digestion was carried out using a 1:25 enzyme-to-protein ratio in 50 mM ammonium bicarbonate digestion buffer. The tryptic peptides were acidified at a 1:10 ratio using 2% TFA and 20% ACN.

2.3. Label-Free Liquid Chromatography—Tandem Mass Spectrometry Analysis of BMNCs

Liquid chromatography tandem mass spectrometry (LC-MS/MS) was performed using the Thermo UltiMate 3000 nano system and directly coupled in-line with the Thermo Orbitrap Fusion Tribrid mass spectrometer. The maximum loading amount (~800 ng) was loaded for mass spectrometry analysis. PepMap100 (C18, 300 μm × 5 mm) and Acclaim PepMap 100 (75 μm × 50 cm, 3 μm bead diameter) columns were used as the trapping and analytical columns, respectively. Peptides were eluted over the following binary gradient: LC Solvent A and LC Solvent B using 2–32% Solvent B for 75 min, 32–90% Solvent B for 5 min and holding at 90% for 5 min at a flow rate of 300 nL/min. A data-dependent acquisition strategy was applied with full MS scans in the 380–1500 m/z range with a resolution of 120,000 at 200 m/z. A top-speed approach with a cycle time of 3 s was used for tandem MS analysis, with selected precursor ions isolated with an isolation width of 1.6 Da. The intensity threshold for fragmentation was set to 5000 and included peptides with charge states of 2+ to 7+. A higher energy collision dissociation (HCD) approach was applied with a normalised collision energy of 28% and tandem MS spectra were acquired in the linear ion trap with a fixed first m/z of 110, and a dynamic exclusion of 50 s was applied. A targeted automatic gain control (AGC) was set to 2×10^4 with a maximum injection time set at 35 ms.

2.4. Data Analysis of BMNCs Mass Spectrometry Results

The UniProtKB-SwissProt Homo Sapiens database with Proteome Discoverer 2.2 using Sequest HT (Thermo Fisher Scientific) and a percolator were used for the identification of peptides and proteins. Search parameters were set as follows: (i) MS/MS mass tolerance was set to 0.02 Da, (ii) peptide mass tolerance was set at 10 ppm, (iii) variable modifications included methionine oxidation, (iv) fixed modification settings for carbamido-methylation and (v) tolerance for up to two missed cleavages. Peptide probability was set to high confidence, and a minimum XCorr score of 1.5 for 1, 2.0 for 2, 2.25 for 3 and 2.5 for 4 charge states was applied for peptide filtering. The associated label-free quantitation software Progenesis QI for Proteomics (version 2.0; Nonlinear Dynamics, a Waters company, Newcastle upon Tyne, UK) was used for quantitative data analysis. Datasets were imported into Progenesis QI software. Protein identifications were deemed to be differentially expressed when specific criteria were met. Missing values were imputed using a width of 0.3 and down shift of 1.8 to enable statistical comparisons. The criteria were: ANOVA p-value of $\leq$0.05 between experimental groups, fold change $\geq$1.5 between experimental groups, proteins with $\geq$2 unique peptides contributing to the identification, and quantification data in >60% of samples. Pathway enrichment and gene ontology (GO) enrichment analysis was performed by submitting Uniprot accession IDs to the g:Profiler online bioinformatics tool (https://biit.cs.ut.ee/gprofiler/gost) (accessed on 24 November 2022) [20]. Term size was set to between 5 and 2000.

2.5. Gene Expression Analysis Using the CoMMpass Dataset

To determine the association of the most differentially abundant proteins with MM prognosis, we used the mRNA expression data from the MMRF CoMMpass study. The gene expression profiles and survival data of patients with MM (n = 784) were obtained and analysed using UCSC Xena (https://xena.ucsc.edu/) (accessed on 17 November 2022). Raw count values and clinical data were downloaded from the Xena website and normalised using the R package "deseq2". Survival analysis was performed using the "survival" and "RegParallel" packages and survival curves were illustrated using the Kaplan–Meier method. Proteins significantly changed between EMM BMNCs and MM BMNCs were analysed to identify the prognostic relevance of the gene expression of these proteins. Median expression values were used to binarise the genes. Gene expression results with log-rank p-values < 0.05 were considered significantly associated with MM survival.

2.6. Blood Plasma Sample Preparation

High abundant plasma proteins were depleted using the Proteome Purify 12 Human Serum Protein Immunodepletion Resin (R&D Systems, Minneapolis, MN, USA). Briefly, 10 µL of plasma was mixed with 1 mL of immunodepletion resin for 60 min. The mixture was transferred to Spin-X filter units and centrifuged. The protein concentration of the resulting eluate was determined using the Pierce™ 660 nm protein assay (Thermo Fisher Scientific). Protein digestion was performed using the FASP protocol, as described above. A total of 10 µg of protein was digested at a 1:25 enzyme-to-protein ratio. The tryptic digest was acidified at a 1:10 ratio using 2% TFA, 20% ACN.

2.7. Label-Free Liquid Chromatography-Tandem Mass Spectrometry Analysis of Plasma

LC-MS/MS was performed using the Ultimate 3000 NanoLC system (Dionex Corporation, Sunnyvale, CA, USA) coupled with a Q-Exactive mass spectrometer (Thermo Fisher Scientific). A total of 14 µL, containing ~1µg of digested protein was loaded. Samples were loaded onto a C18 trap column (C18 PepMap, 300 µm id × 5 mm, 5 µm particle size, 100 Å pore size; Thermo Fisher Scientific) and resolved on an analytical Biobasic C18 Picofrit column (C18 PepMap, 75 µm id × 50 cm, 2 µm particle size, 100 Å pore size; Dionex). Peptides generated were eluted over a 120 min gradient. The Q-Exactive was operated in positive, data-dependent acquisition (DDA) mode and externally calibrated. Full-scan spectra were collected at a fixed resolution of 140,000 and a mass range of 300–1700 m/z. Fragmentation spectra were acquired through the collision-induced dissociation (CID) of the fifteen most intense ions per scan, at a resolution of 17,500 and range of 200–2000 m/z. A dynamic exclusion window was applied within 30 s.

2.8. Data Analysis of Plasma Mass Spectrometry Results

Raw files from the mass spectrometry analysis were searched using the associated software, Proteome Discoverer 2.5 (Thermo Fisher Scientific). Protein identification and label-free quantitation (LFQ) was performed. The resulting dataset was imported into Perseus (1.6.14.0). Proteins with ≥ 2 peptides contributing to the identification and quantitative values in >70% samples were retained for downstream analysis. Missing values were imputed using a width of 0.3 and a down-shift of 1.8 to enable statistical comparisons. Statistically significant differentially abundant proteins were identified based on a false discovery rate (FDR)-adjusted p-value < 0.1 and fold change >1.5 between experimental groups.

2.9. Enzyme-Linked Immunosorbent Assays (ELISAs)

The concentrations of six proteins (vascular cell adhesion protein 1 (VCAM1), aminopeptidase N (CD13), butyrylcholinesterase (BCHE), hepatocyte growth factor activator (HGFA), alpha 2-macroglobulin (A2M) and pigment epithelium-derived factor (PEDF)) in blood plasma were measured by ELISA (DuoSet ELISA kits, R&D Systems). The following plasma dilutions were used: VCAM1 (1:1500), CD13 (1:75), BCHE (1:2000), HGFA (1:2000), A2M (1:100,000) and PEDF (1:8000). The plasma concentrations of VCAM1, PEDF and HGFA, at the same dilutions, were also analysed in the second MM patient cohort (n = 44).

2.10. Statistical Analysis

The statistical analysis of ELISA results, receiver-operating characteristic (ROC) curve analysis and correlation analyses were performed using Graphpad Prism (8.0.2.263) and MedCalc (version 20.118). Parametric t-tests were used to evaluate statistical significance. Outliers were removed using the ROUT method (Q = 1%). ROC curve analysis was used to determine the discriminatory performance of the verified statistically significant differentially abundant (SSDA) plasma proteins. The ROC curves evaluated the specificity (false positive fraction) and sensitivity (true positive fraction) of the potential protein biomarkers. Optimal cut-off points were selected using Youden's index. The area under the curve (AUC) was calculated to summarise the accuracy of the classification. Logistic regression analysis was performed using MedCalc.

2.11. Targeted Metabolomic Analysis

The targeted metabolomic analysis of medullary MM and EMM blood plasma samples was performed using the MxP® Quant 500 kit (Biocrates Life Sciences AG, Innsbruck, Austria) with a SCIEX QTRAP 6500plus mass spectrometer. The MxP® Quant 500 kit is capable of quantifying more than 600 metabolites from 26 compound classes. Quality control (QC) samples were employed to monitor the performance of the analysis with metabolite concentration in each sample normalised based on these QC samples. Isotopically labelled internal standards and seven-point calibration curves were used in the quantitation of amino acids and biogenic amines. The semi-quantitative analysis of other metabolites was performed using internal standards. Data quality was evaluated by checking the accuracy and reproducibility of QC samples. Metabolites were included only when the concentrations of the metabolites were above the limit of detection (LOD) in >75% of plasma samples. Data were imported into MetaboAnalyst 5.0 for further analysis. Feature filtering was performed based on relative standard deviation (RSD) and the resulting data were log-transformed and autoscaled. Metabolites of interest were identified based on p-value < 0.05 and fold-change >1.2 between experimental groups. Supervised statistical approaches were used to further interrogate the data.

3. Results

3.1. Clinical Information

Eight samples with MM but without extramedullary spread and nine samples with EMM were included in this study. Clinical data was obtained and summarised (Table 1, Figure S1). The median age was 65. Six males and two females were included in each group. Overall survival (OS) was statistically significantly decreased in patients with EMM compared to MM patients without extramedullary spread (Log-rank = 3.977, p = 0.046) (Figure S2). The median OS of patients with EMM and those without extramedullary spread was 19 months and 83 months, respectively.

3.2. Identification of Differentially Abundant Proteins in the Bone Marrow of MM Patients with and without Extramedullary Spread

To examine proteomic changes in the bone marrow of MM patients with and without EMM, BMNCs were isolated and proteolytically digested. Nine EMM samples—including one serial sample—and eight MM without extramedullary spread samples were analysed using LC-MS/MS. A total of 4589 proteins and 225 significantly differentially abundant proteins were identified based on ANOVA corrected p-value < 0.05 and fold change >1.5 (Figure 1, Table S1). Of these, 139 proteins were increased in abundance and 86 proteins were decreased in abundance in EMM BMNCs compared to MM BMNCs (Tables 2 and 3). The hierarchical clustering of protein abundance and principal component analysis (PCA) demonstrated a clear change in the proteomic profile of mononuclear cells from MM patients with extramedullary spread and those without (Figure 1A,B).

Table 2. Top 25 proteins with significantly increased abundance in EMM BMNCs compared to MM BMNCs as determined by label-free LC-MS/MS.

Uniprot ID	Description	Gene Name	Fold Change	FDR-Adjusted p-Value
P00918	Carbonic anhydrase 2	CA2	4.42	0.0001
Q8NBJ5	Procollagen galactosyltransferase 1	COLGALT1	1.77	0.0003
P09382	Galectin-1	LGALS1	1.94	0.0005
Q5JRX3	Presequence protease, mitochondrial	PITRM1	3.05	0.0006
P37802	Transgelin-2	TAGLN2	4.65	0.0006
P17301	Integrin alpha-2	ITGA2	34.90	0.0009
Q86WV6	Stimulator of interferon genes protein	TMEM173	3.02	0.0009
Q32MZ4	Leucine-rich repeat flightless-interacting protein 1	LRRFIP1	2.13	0.0009
Q15833	Syntaxin-binding protein 2	STXBP2	2.26	0.0011

Table 2. Cont.

Uniprot ID	Description	Gene Name	Fold Change	FDR-Adjusted p-Value
P62328	Thymosin beta-4	TMSB4X	8.64	0.0011
P08567	Pleckstrin	PLEK	5.45	0.0015
Q9UGT4	Sushi domain-containing protein 2	SUSD2	53.35	0.0017
O60610	Protein diaphanous homolog 1	DIAPH1	2.21	0.0018
P08758	Annexin A5	ANXA5	7.68	0.0018
P07951	Tropomyosin beta chain	TPM2	3.45	0.0019
Q7LDG7	RAS guanyl-releasing protein 2	RASGRP2	3.54	0.0019
Q14019	Coactosin-like protein	COTL1	2.38	0.0020
P18054	Polyunsaturated fatty acid lipoxygenase ALOX12	ALOX12	26.46	0.0020
Q9NYL9	Tropomodulin-3	TMOD3	2.90	0.0020
P63000	Ras-related C3 botulinum toxin substrate 1	RAC1	2.73	0.0025
P37840	Alpha-synuclein	SNCA	18.57	0.0025
Q9HBI1	Beta-parvin	PARVB	12.09	0.0026
P18206	Vinculin	VCL	5.78	0.0028
Q15942	Zyxin	ZYX	4.93	0.0029
P06753	Tropomyosin alpha-3 chain	TPM3	2.07	0.0030

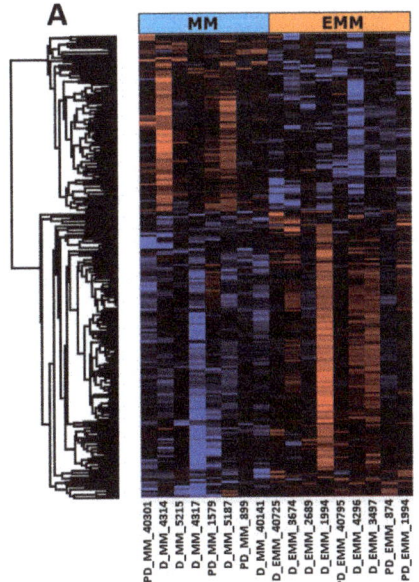
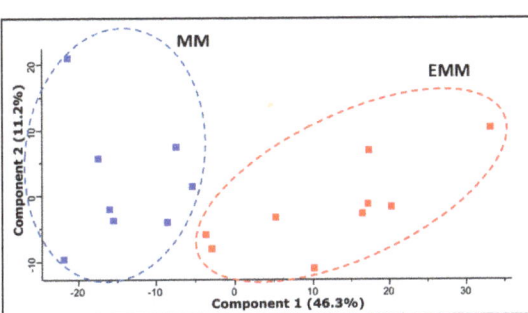

Figure 1. Proteomic profile of BMNCs from EMM patients and medullary MM patients. (A) Hierarchical clustering analysis of the statistically significant differentially abundant (SSDA) proteins between MM and EMM groups. The colours from blue to red represent the relative protein levels between the two groups. (B) Principal component analysis (PCA) illustrating a clear distinction between MM patients with EMM and those without. Each dot represents a patient sample with EMM samples highlighted in red and MM samples highlighted in blue.

Proteins found to be increased or decreased in abundance in EMM were characterised based on gene ontology enrichment and KEGG pathway enrichment (Figure 2). Proteins increased in abundance in EMM mononuclear cells were associated with migratory pathways, including focal adhesion, tight junction, Rap1 signalling pathway and leukocyte endothelial migration. Interestingly, proteins decreased in abundance in EMM BMNCs were associated with various metabolic pathways, including the tricarboxylic acid (TCA) cycle, suggesting a possible metabolic change in the cells of the bone marrow microenvironment during EMM transition [21].

Table 3. Top 25 proteins with significantly decreased abundance in EMM BMNCs compared to MM BMNCs as determined by label-free LC-MS/MS.

Uniprot ID	Description	Gene Name	Fold Change	FDR Adjusted p-Value
P22087	rRNA 2′-O-methyltransferase fibrillarin	FBL	1.65	0.0003
P16402	Histone H1.3	HIST1H1D	2.89	0.0007
Q8NBS9	Thioredoxin domain-containing protein 5	TXNDC5	4.33	0.0008
Q99798	Aconitate hydratase, mitochondrial	ACO2	1.61	0.0012
Q9NSE4	Isoleucine–tRNA ligase, mitochondrial	IARS2	2.22	0.0014
Q9Y320	Thioredoxin-related transmembrane protein 2	TMX2	5.92	0.0014
Q13263	Transcription intermediary factor 1-beta	TRIM28	2.19	0.0015
P30837	Aldehyde dehydrogenase X, mitochondrial	ALDH1B1	8.19	0.0015
Q9BY50	Signal peptidase complex catalytic subunit SEC11C	SEC11C	5.19	0.0016
Q13813	Spectrin alpha chain, non-erythrocytic 1	SPTAN1	2.10	0.0023
Q3SY69	Mitochondrial 10-formyltetrahydrofolate dehydrogenase	ALDH1L2	7.33	0.0033
P08240	Signal recognition particle receptor subunit alpha	SRPR	2.48	0.0035
P30044	Peroxiredoxin-5, mitochondrial	PRDX5	1.77	0.0037
Q7KZF4	Staphylococcal nuclease domain-containing protein 1	SND1	2.91	0.0042
P49257	Protein ERGIC-53	LMAN1	2.44	0.0043
Q9Y4P3	Transducin beta-like protein 2	TBL2	4.53	0.0045
P09874	Poly [ADP-ribose] polymerase 1	PARP1	2.67	0.0047
Q01105	Protein SET	SET	3.29	0.0054
Q92506	Estradiol 17-beta-dehydrogenase 8	HSD17B8	3.37	0.0054
P12235	ADP/ATP translocase 1	SLC25A4	4.43	0.0055
Q13310	Polyadenylate-binding protein 4	PABPC4	4.47	0.0056
P53992	Protein transport protein Sec24C	SEC24C	38.68	0.0057
Q16706	Alpha-mannosidase 2	MAN2A1	6.43	0.0058
Q01082	Spectrin beta chain, non-erythrocytic 1	SPTBN1	1.96	0.0060
P54886	Delta-1-pyrroline-5-carboxylate synthase	ALDH18A1	10.26	0.0072

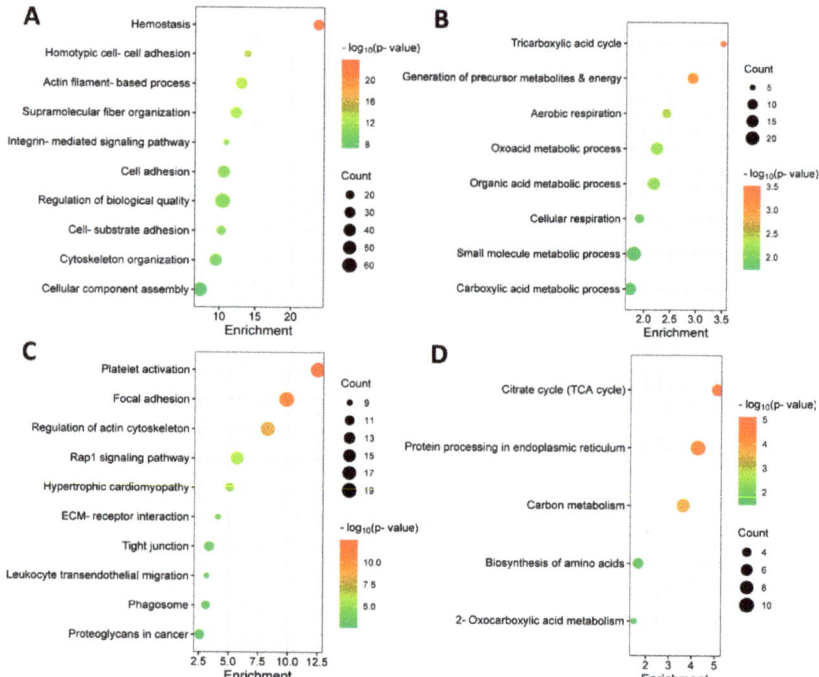

Figure 2. Gene ontology (GO) and Kyoto Encyclopedia of Genes and Genomes (KEGG) functional enrichment analysis of SSDA proteins. (A) Bubble plot of GO gene set enrichment analysis (biological processes) of proteins increased in abundance in EMM. (B) Bubble plot of GO gene set enrichment analysis (biological processes) of proteins decreased in abundance in EMM. (C) Bubble plot of KEGG pathway enrichment analysis of proteins increased in abundance in EMM. (D) Bubble plot of KEGG pathway enrichment analysis of proteins decreased in abundance in EMM. Enrichment value = $-\log_{10}(p\text{-value})$.

3.3. Association of Gene Expression with Prognosis Using the MMRF CoMMpass Study Data

To determine whether the proteins most significantly increased in abundance in EMM mononuclear cells were associated with a poor prognosis in MM, we performed a Kaplan–Meier gene expression analysis on the 25 proteins most significantly increased in abundance in EMM BMNCs using the MMRF CoMMpass dataset (Table 2). The increased expression of seven genes was associated with a significantly worse prognosis in MM. These included genes associated with focal adhesion and actin regulation, transgelin 2 (TAGLN2), integrin alpha 2 (ITGA2), tropomyosin beta chain (TPM2) and tropomyosin alpha-3 chain (TPM3), as well as carbonic anhydrase 2 (CA2), galectin-1 (LGALS1) and tropomodulin-3 (TMOD3) (Figure 3). For our cohort, we divided the samples into high and low expression groups for each of the seven biomarkers. Survival analysis revealed a trend towards decreased overall survival in those with the high expression of six (TAGLN2, CA2, ITGA2, LGALS1, TPM2, TMOD3) out of the seven proteins analysed. The high expression of TMOD3 was significantly associated with a poorer overall survival compared to those with a low expression of TMOD3 (Figure S3). Thus, the increased abundance of these proteins is associated with the aggressive EMM phenotype, as well as poorer overall survival in MM.

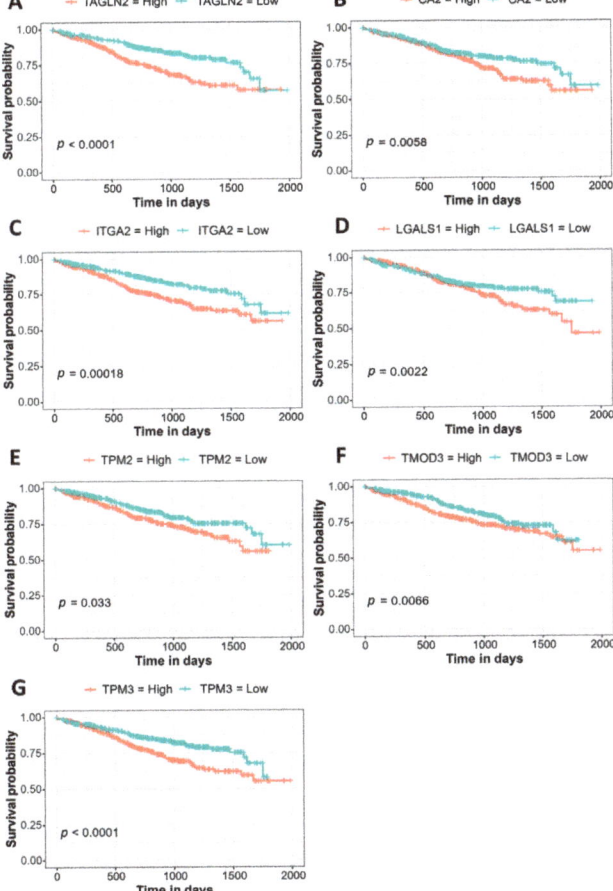

Figure 3. Kaplan–Meier curves illustrating genes whose expression (high/low) is significantly associated with survival in MM using the MMRF CoMMpass RNASeq dataset. (**A**) TAGLN2, (**B**) CA2, (**C**) ITGA2, (**D**) LGALS1, (**E**) TPM2, (**F**) TMOD3, (**G**) TPM3.

3.4. Identification of Significantly Differentially Abundant Proteins in the Plasma of MM Patients with and without Extramedullary Spread

Matched blood plasma samples from MM (n = 8) and EMM (n = 9, 1 serial sample) patients, taken on the same date as the BMNCs, were analysed through label-free LC-MS/MS to identify changes in the plasma proteome of patients with and without extramedullary lesions. A total of 524 proteins and 22 significantly differentially abundant proteins were identified based on FDR corrected p-value < 0.1 and fold change >1.5 (Figure 4, Table 4). All significant proteins were increased in abundance in EMM plasma samples compared to MM patient plasma without extramedullary spread. Only one protein, platelet glycoprotein Ib alpha chain (GP1BA), was differentially expressed in both BMNCs and blood plasma.

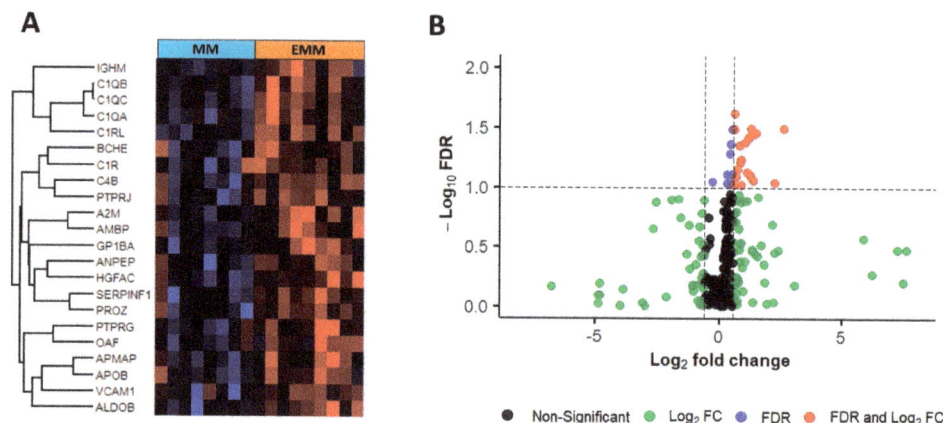

Figure 4. Heatmap and volcano plot of statistically significant differentially abundant (SSDA) proteins identified in the label-free mass spectrometry analysis of blood plasma. (**A**) Hierarchical clustering of SSDA proteins. The colours from blue to red represent the relative protein levels between the two groups. (**B**) Volcano plot of SSDA proteins. Red points represent proteins significantly increased in abundance in EMM plasma. Green points indicate proteins with a log2 fold change >1.5 but false discovery rate (FDR) p-value > 0.1. Blue points indicate proteins with an FDR p-value < 0.1 but log2 fold change <1.5. Black points indicate proteins with no significant difference.

Table 4. List of proteins significantly increased in abundance in the plasma of EMM patients compared to MM patients without extramedullary spread.

Uniprot ID	Description	Gene Name	Fold Change	FDR-Adjusted p-Value
Q9NZP8	Complement C1r subcomponent-like protein	C1RL	1.58	0.012
P02747	Complement C1q subcomponent subunit C	C1QC	2.45	0.030
P36955	Pigment epithelium-derived factor	SERPINF1	1.56	0.031
P23470	Receptor-type tyrosine-protein phosphatase gamma	PTPRG	2.87	0.035
P02745	Complement C1q subcomponent subunit A	C1QA	2.33	0.038
Q04756	Hepatocyte growth factor activator	HGFA	2.09	0.038
P05062	Fructose-bisphosphate aldolase B	ALDOB	2.31	0.039
P02746	Complement C1q subcomponent subunit B	C1QB	2.66	0.041
P22891	Vitamin K-dependent protein Z	PROZ	1.83	0.042
P06276	Cholinesterase	BCHE	1.88	0.056
Q9HDC9	Adipocyte plasma membrane-associated protein	APMAP	1.85	0.058
P02760	Protein AMBP	AMBP	1.69	0.062
P07359	Platelet glycoprotein Ib alpha chain	GP1BA	2.40	0.070
P19320	Vascular cell adhesion protein 1	VCAM1	2.23	0.078
P01023	Alpha-2-macroglobulin	A2M	2.50	0.079
P00736	Complement C1r subcomponent	C1R	1.63	0.079
P15144	Aminopeptidase N	ANPEP	2.65	0.081
P01871	Ig mu chain C region	IGHM	4.84	0.083
P04114	Apolipoprotein B-100	APOB	1.54	0.083
Q86UD1	Out at first protein homolog	OAF	2.24	0.085
P0C0L5	Complement C4-B	C4B	1.88	0.085
Q12913	Receptor-type tyrosine-protein phosphatase eta	PTPRJ	1.79	0.095

3.5. Verification of Differentially Expressed Plasma Proteins Identified by LC-MS/MS

Six proteins found to be increased in abundance in the blood plasma of EMM patients were verified via ELISA: ANPEP, VCAM1, BCHE, HGFA, PEDF and A2M. Three of the six proteins analysed (VCAM1, HGFA, PEDF) were verified as being significantly increased in abundance in EMM plasma (Figure 5). Although ANPEP, BCHE and A2M did not reach statistical significance, we observed trends towards increased abundance in EMM plasma, which would warrant further investigation in a larger cohort of samples. To explore the potential of the three verified proteins as biomarkers, we performed individual ROC curve analyses and a multivariate analysis of the biomarker combination. ROC curves were constructed and the area under the curve (AUC) values were calculated (Figure 6). VCAM1, HGFA and PEDF were found to have good prediction ability for EMM with AUC values of 0.806, 0.847 and 0.969, respectively. The combination of these biomarkers using a logistic regression analysis resulted in a larger AUC value of 1 and 95% confidence interval of 0.794–1.

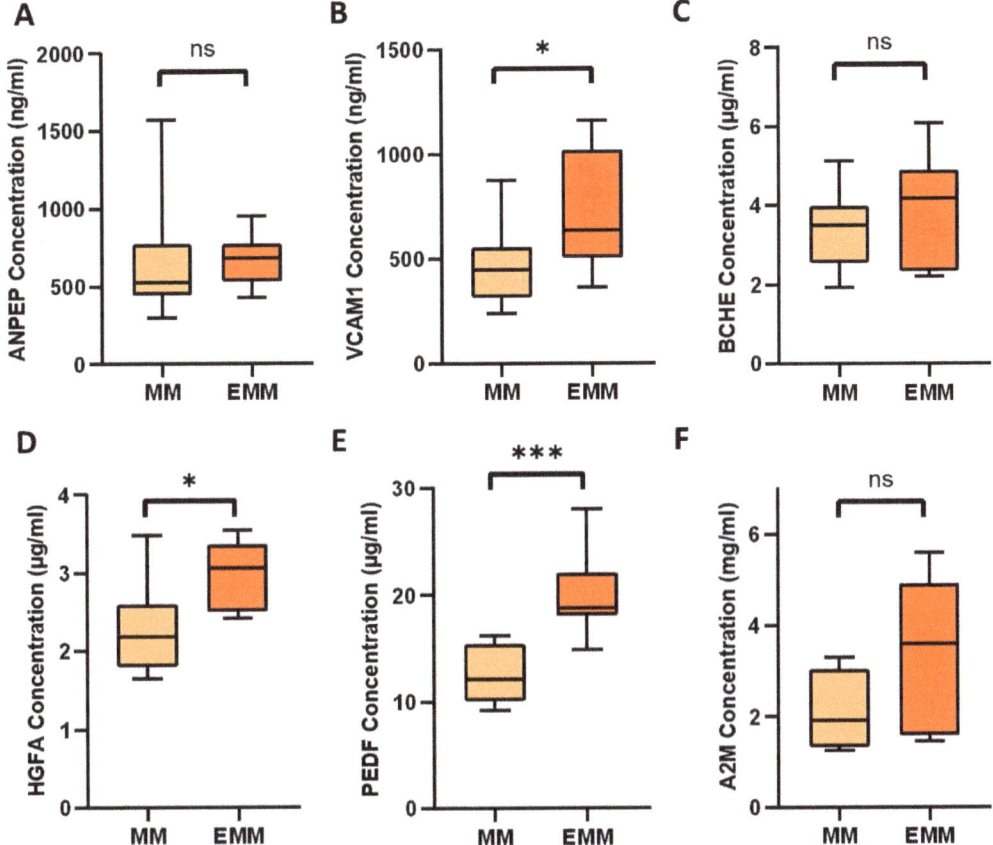

Figure 5. Plasma levels of SSDA proteins measured by ELISA. (**A**) ANPEP, (**B**) VCAM1, (**C**) BCHE, (**D**) HGFA, (**E**) PEDF and (**F**) A2M plasma levels in the EMM and medullary MM groups. Significance is marked as follows: ns 'not significant', $p \leq 0.05$ '*', $p \leq 0.001$ '***'.

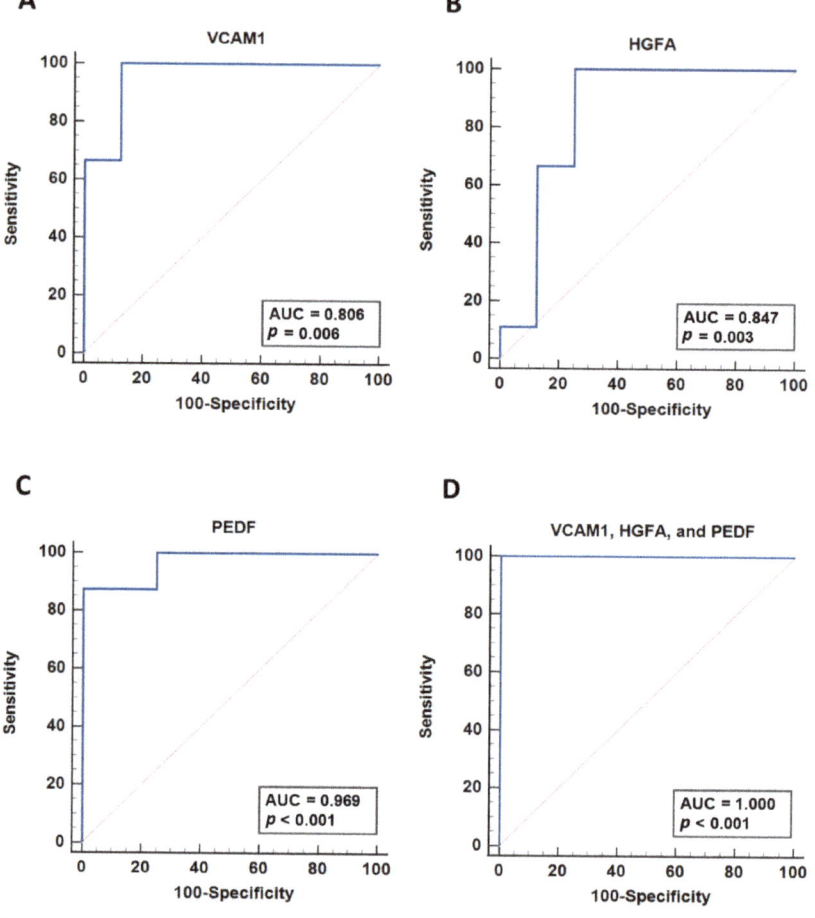

Figure 6. ROC curve analysis of three potential biomarkers. (**A**) VCAM1, (**B**) HGFA and (**C**) PEDF ROC curves. (**D**) Logistic regression analysis with a ROC curve illustrating the discriminatory power of combining VCAM1, HGFA and VCAM1.

3.6. VCAM1 Plasma Concentrations Are Increased in Patients Most Sensitive to the BCL-2 Inhibitors, Venetoclax and Navitoclax

As EMM is often associated with drug resistance, we tested the levels of VCAM1, HGFA and PEDF in the plasma of patients whose CD138+ myeloma cells had been evaluated by ex vivo drug sensitivity resistance testing (DSRT) ($n = 44$) [22,23]. VCAM1, HGFA, and PEDF plasma concentrations in this independent set of MM samples ($n = 43$, excluding 1 EMM sample) showed a similar pattern as observed in the MM group above. VCAM1 concentrations ranged from 150.9–488.2 ng/mL with a median and mean concentration of 289.7 ng/mL and 301 ng/mL, respectively. HGFA concentrations ranged from 1.039–3.372 µg/mL with a median and mean concentration of 2.155 µg/mL and 2.143 µg/mL, respectively. PEDF concentrations ranged from 8.901–19.22 µg/mL with a median and mean concentration of 12.97 µg/mL and 13.39 µg/mL, respectively. The median concentrations of VCAM1, HGFA and PEDF observed in this MM sample set were considerably lower than the median concentrations observed in the EMM group above (VCAM1 = 634.7 ng/mL, HGFA = 3.068 µg/mL, PEDF = 18.77 µg/mL) supporting our findings that these three proteins are increased in abundance in EMM patient plasma. We used Pearson's correlation analysis to evaluate whether plasma concentrations of VCAM1, HGFA and PEDF correlated with patient sensitivity to individual drugs based on the individual drug sensitivity scores (DSS). Based on the DSS, the samples were stratified into least sensitive and most sensitive groups to various drugs, including the BCL-2 inhibitors, venetoclax and navitoclax. The level of soluble VCAM1 (sVCAM1) was found to be significantly increased in patients considered most sensitive to venetoclax and navitoclax (Figure 7A,C). In addition, higher levels of sVCAM1 weakly correlated with increased sensitivity to venetoclax and navitoclax (Pearson's correlation coefficient r = 0.38 (p = 0.0116) and r = 0.44 (p = 0.0026), respectively) (Figure 7B,D). One patient from this cohort had EMM at the time of sampling and therefore had corresponding DSS values available. As expected, this patient was found to be resistant to many of the drugs tested (Figure 7E). Interestingly, this sample was highly sensitive to navitoclax and demonstrated some sensitivity to the other BCL-2 inhibitors tested, AT 101, venetoclax and obatoclax (Figure 7E).

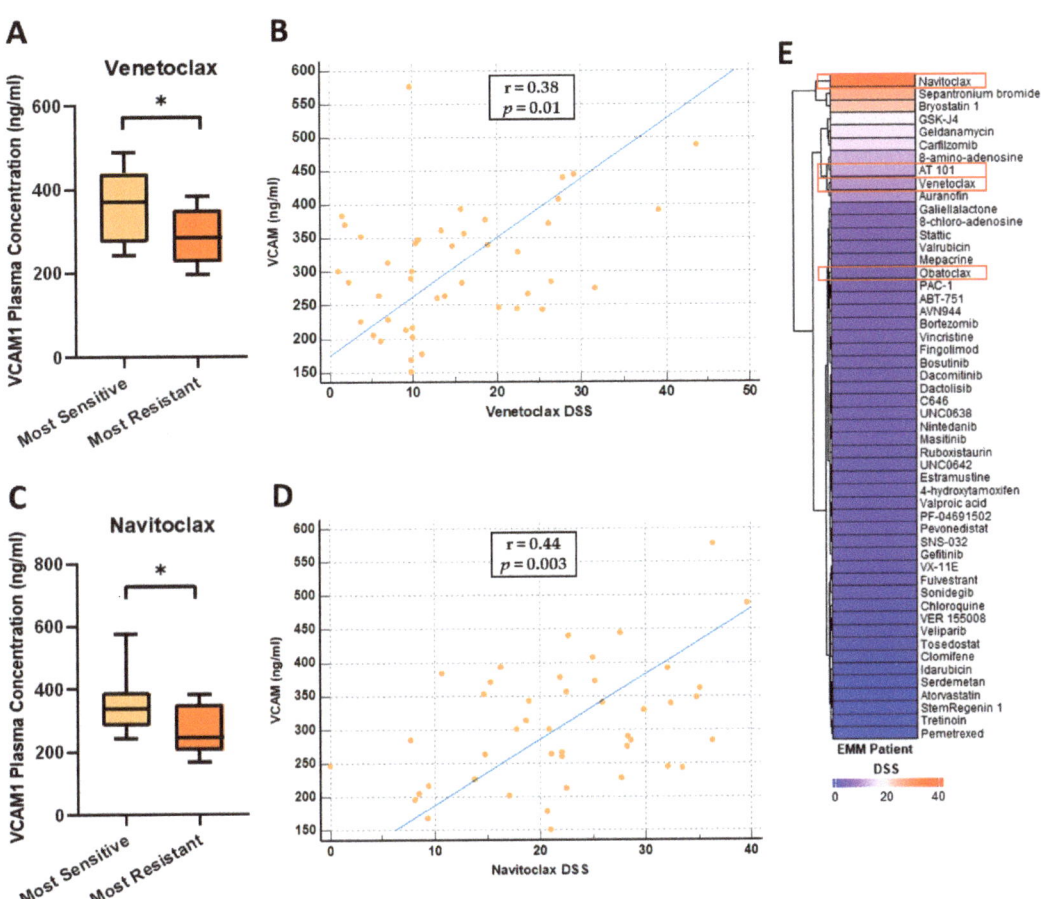

Figure 7. Plasma concentration of VCAM1 in patients most sensitive and most resistant to the BCL-2 inhibitors (**A**) venetoclax and (**C**) navitoclax. (**B**) Correlation between VCAM1 plasma concentration and venetoclax sensitivity. (**D**) Correlation between VCAM1 plasma concentration and navitoclax sensitivity. (**E**) Heatmap illustrating the varying DSS scores of an EMM patient. Drugs with DSS = 0 were removed from this figure. Drugs from the BCL2 inhibitor drug family are highlighted by the red boxes. Significance is marked as follows: $p \leq 0.05$ '*'.

3.7. Targeted Metabolomic Analysis of Blood Plasma from MM Patients with and without Extramedullary Spread

Using a targeted metabolomic/lipidomic technique, we compared the metabolic profile of MM and EMM patient plasma. We applied the unsupervised clustering approach and principal component analysis (PCA); however, no clear separation was observed between the EMM group and the medullary MM group (Figure 8A). A supervised clustering technique termed the orthogonal projection to latent structure discriminant analysis (OPLS-DA) was also used to determine separation between the two groups (Figure 8B). In the OPLS-DA model, R2 refers to the explained variance between the components, whereas Q2 is calculated by full cross validation to indicate the goodness of prediction. R2 and Q2 values closer to 1 indicate a better predictive model. Permutation analysis results (Q2 = 0.444, p = 0.042; R2Y = 0.99, p = 0.032) demonstrated that the model was not overfitted. In this analysis, the Q2 value of 0.444 indicated weak predictive power; however, due to the heterogeneity of human samples and the small sample size, a Q2 value of >0.4 is acceptable [24,25]. Discriminatory variables responsible for the group separation were identified using the OPLS-DA variable importance in the projection (VIP) score (Figure 8D).

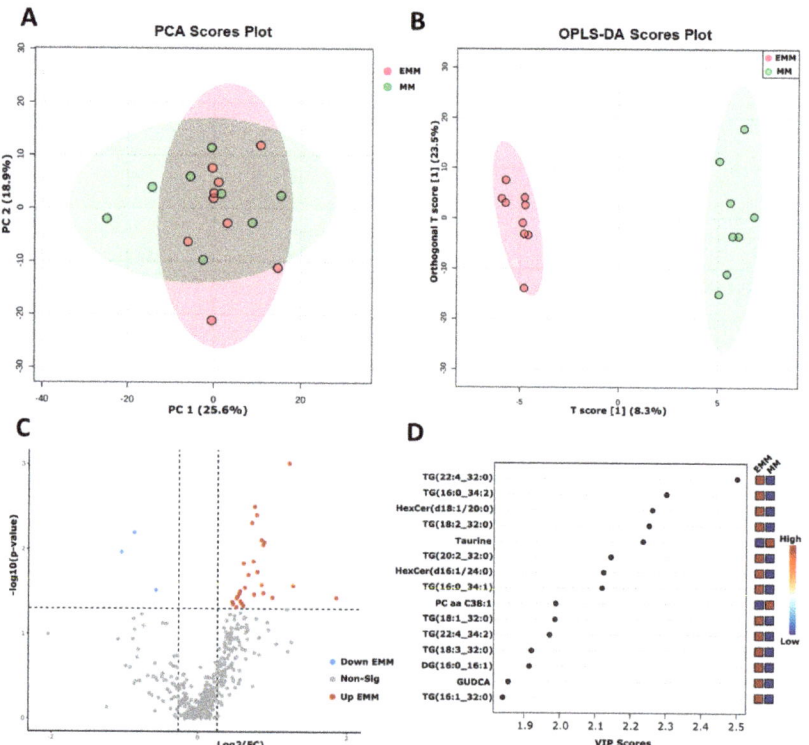

Figure 8. Targeted metabolomic analysis of EMM and MM plasma samples. (**A**) PCA score plot of EMM and MM samples. (**B**) Orthogonal projection to latent structure discriminant analysis (OPLS-DA) scores plot. Cumulative R2X = 0.555, R2Y = 0.99 and Q2 = 0.444. (**C**) Volcano plot identifying significantly altered metabolites in MM patients with and without extramedullary spread (p-value ≤ 0.05, FC > 1.2). (**D**) Variable importance in projection (VIP) scores plot depicting the 15 most significant metabolites contributing to the MM group separations observed in the model depicted in (**B**). Red squares indicate metabolites of high abundance in EMM plasma. Blue squares indicate metabolites of low abundance in EMM plasma.

Univariate analysis using a *t*-test identified 31 metabolites with significant differential abundance between the two groups (Figure 8C, Table S2). Of these, 28 metabolites were increased, and 3 metabolites were decreased in EMM plasma. A total of 26 of the 28 metabolites increased in EMM plasma were lipids. The total level of triglycerides was found to be higher in patients with EMM; however, this did not reach significance ($p = 0.099$) (Figure S3). The bile acid, glycoursodeoxycholic acid and the amino acid, tyrosine, were the only non-lipids found to be significantly increased in EMM plasma. We analysed the correlation between the metabolites/lipids and proteins identified in the plasma of EMM patients using Spearman's rank correlation (Figures S4 and S5). Taurine, phenylalanine betaine and phosphatidylcholine with a diacyl residue sum of C38:1 (PC aa C38:1) were negatively correlated with the proteins, whereas all other metabolites identified were positively correlated with the plasma proteins identified in our proteomics analysis.

4. Discussion

The introduction of novel therapeutics over the last 20 years has significantly improved survival rates of patients with MM. However, the presence of extramedullary lesions remains a poor prognostic indicator and an area of significant unmet need due to the lack of understanding of the history of this entity and the limited treatment options available. Historically, extramedullary spread was considered rare; however, the incidence has risen in recent years mainly due to improved sensitivity of imaging techniques and possible late emergence of EMM clones with the longer OS of MM patients [26]. Currently, EMM is diagnosed using imaging modalities. The International Myeloma Working Group (IMWG) recommends the use of fluorine 18 fluorodeoxyglucose (FDG) PET/CT to detect extramedullary lesions; however, the disadvantages of this imaging technique include the high cost, limited availability and lack of imaging standardization [9,27]. The underlying mechanisms that facilitate the spread and survival of malignant plasma cells outside of the bone marrow microenvironment are poorly understood [28].

This study aimed to characterise the proteome of the bone marrow microenvironment and blood plasma of MM patients with EMM to identify potential biomarkers that could serve as predictors of extramedullary development, prognostic biomarkers of MM and possibly contribute to the identification of novel therapeutic targets. Recent genomic and transcriptomic analyses have provided valuable insights into EMM; however, a quantitative proteomics analysis using mass spectrometry had not yet been applied for the study of EMM [29,30]. Examining changes at the protein level provides a comprehensive insight into the molecular events underlying EMM development. We used a label-free mass spectrometry approach to effectively quantify the proteomic changes that occur following extramedullary transition. This study has identified 225 SSDA proteins in BMNCs from MM patients with and without EMM. Furthermore, 22 SSDA proteins were detected in blood plasma with three of these proteins being verified as potential biomarkers for the detection of EMM.

Studies have implicated genetic factors, changes in the bone marrow microenvironment, the differential expression of adhesion molecules and immune evasion in the pathogenesis of EMM [29–32]. GO and KEGG analysis of proteins increased in abundance in EMM BMNCs revealed an enrichment of cell adhesion associated pathways and biological processes, including the integrin-mediated signalling pathway, cytoskeleton organization, focal adhesion, the Rap1 signalling pathway and, most interestingly, leukocyte transendothelial migration. Eight proteins involved in leukocyte transendothelial migration were increased in abundance in EMM (PECAM1, ITGB1, ACTB, ACTN1, VASP, VCL, RAP1B, RAC1, ROCK2) and may indicate a potential mechanism by which specific MM clones exit the bone marrow niche during extramedullary transition. The dynamic regulation of adhesion proteins during the intravasation of MM cells from the bone marrow has not been fully elucidated. One study reported that the loss of VLA4 (integrin α4 and integrin β1) increases extramedullary disease burden, whereas a recent transcriptomic analysis found that integrin α4 and integrin β1 are co-expressed on EMM cells [30,33]. PECAM1 (CD31) had previously been found to be expressed at higher levels in extramedullary plasmacytomas compared to primary MM cells [34].

Several proteins involved in the formation of focal adhesions, which are required to generate mechanical force during migration, were increased in EMM BMNCs [35]. An important component of focal adhesions is integrin linked kinase (ILK), which, when bound to LIM and senescent cell antigen-like-containing domain protein 1 (LIMS1/PINCH1) and β-Parvin, forms the ILK-PINCH-Parvin (IPP) complex [36]. ILK and the IPP complex promote metastasis by promoting a variety of cellular processes, including epithelial mesenchymal transition (EMT) and cell motility [37]. ILK, LIMS1, β-Parvin and another binding partner of LIMS1, Ras suppressor protein 1 (RSU1), were significantly increased in EMM BMNCs (Table S1). A recent study reported that ILK promotes lung adenocarcinoma progression and metastasis through the regulation of KRAS, the IPP complex and RSU1, with other studies also linking ILK to cancer metastasis [38–40]. Despite ILK being considered dispensable for myeloma cell survival, inhibiting ILK has previously been shown to reduce the invasive capabilities of myeloma cell lines [41,42]. This combined with the increased abundance of numerous components of the ILK signalling pathway in EMM BMNCs indicates a potential role of this signalling pathway in the migration of myeloma cells to extramedullary sites.

Proteins involved in the tricarboxylic acid (TCA) pathway were decreased in EMM BMNCs compared to MM BMNCs, indicating a potential metabolic change during extramedullary transition. Previous transcriptomic analysis reported the emergence of a metabolic cluster involving pyruvate kinase (PKM2) during extramedullary transition [30]. In this study, PKM2 levels were increased in EMM mononuclear cells. PKM2 has previously been linked to myeloma proliferation and adhesion, reporting that the silencing of PKM2 promoted cell adhesion in cell lines [43]. Interestingly, in lung cancer, secreted PKM2 was found to promote metastasis through interaction with integrin β1, which was also found to be increased in EMM BMNCs [44]. Further validation is required to fully elucidate the role of PKM2 and integrin β1 in the development of EMM.

EMM is frequently associated with an immature or plasmablastic morphology [11,45]. Interestingly, several of the cytoskeletal proteins increased in EMM BMNCs included proteins associated with a plasmablastic morphology (CNN2, PFN1, TMOD3, VASP, TLN1, TMSB4X, PLEK, ZYX) [6]. The hypoxic environment of the bone marrow promotes an immature phenotype in MM through the decreased expression of terminal differentiation markers such as syndecan 1 (CD138) [46]. The endoglycosidase, heparanase, has also been reported to promote myeloma stemness [47]. Our study found decreased levels of CD138 and increased levels of heparanase in the EMM mononuclear fraction. Heparanase promotes an invasive phenotype in MM through the cleavage of CD138 from the surface of MM cells. Shed CD138 subsequently binds to vascular endothelial cell growth factor receptor-2 (VEGFR2) to trigger the polarised migration of MM cells [48]. In EMM, the increased abundance of heparanase may contribute to the creation of a pro-migratory niche within the bone marrow. Further investigations should be performed to elucidate the roles of these proteins associated with the more aggressive, plasmablastic phenotype in extramedullary transition.

Proteomic analysis of EMM plasma identified VCAM1, PEDF and HGFA as potential markers of extramedullary myeloma. VCAM1, a member of the IgG immunoglobulin family, plays a well-known role in cancer development and progression [49]. In MM, the increased expression of VCAM1 and its receptor, VLA-4, correlates with disease progression, and increased levels of soluble VCAM1 (sVCAM1) in MM correlate with advanced disease and poor OS [50,51]. Soluble VCAM1 can be derived from endothelial cells, leukocytes and/or tumour cells via cleavage by metalloproteinases [52]. Interestingly, C-X-C chemokine receptor type 4 (CXCR4), a receptor widely reported to regulate extramedullary myeloma, was found to induce VCAM1 secretion in non-small cell lung cancer via the regulation of the metalloproteinase, ADAM17 [15,53]. The decreased expression of VCAM1 in the bone marrow microenvironment may induce the egress of B cells into circulation, while sVCAM1 has been widely reported to promote lymphocyte migration or stimulate lymphocyte chemotaxis [54–56]. The source of the increased concentration of VCAM1 in plasma is unknown and may derive from the shedding of VCAM1 from the surface of MM cells or from other cells known to express VCAM1, such as activated endothelial cells. Nonetheless, sVCAM1 represents a promising marker of EMM and warrants further investigation in a larger cohort of samples.

The increased levels of sVCAM1 correlated with increased sensitivity to the BCL-2 inhibitors, venetoclax and navitoclax, indicating a potential correlation with BCL-2 expression. VCAM1 and BCL2 are target genes of the nuclear factor kappa B (NF-κB) signalling pathway, a key pathway in MM pathogenesis [57]. Enhanced NF-κB activation may increase sVCAM1 and BCL2 levels, making sVCAM1 a potential surrogate plasma-based biomarker of response to BCL-2 inhibitors; however, further studies in a larger cohort of patients are required to further evaluate this link. The extrinsic activation of the NF-κB pathway via APRIL and BAFF provides survival signals in the early stages of MM, whereas during tumour progression, mutations in NF-κB pathway genes can result in autonomous NF-κB pathway activation and reduced dependence on the bone marrow microenvironment [58]. The link between EMM and the constitutive activation of the NF-κB has yet to be evaluated.

The monomeric glycoprotein, PEDF, was significantly increased in EMM plasma compared to the plasma of MM patients without extramedullary spread. PEDF has been widely reported as an anti-angiogenic and anti-tumorigenic protein in many cancers [59]. Literature focusing on PEDF in MM found that PEDF suppresses VEGF signalling and inhibits multiple myeloma through the inhibition of reactive oxygen species (ROS) generation [60,61]. In contrast, increased PEDF has been implicated in promoting metastasis and invasion in several cancers including hepatocellular carcinoma and oesophageal squamous cell carcinoma [62,63]. A recent study provides insight into the conflicting reports on PEDF as a metastatic biomarker and suggested a potential dual role depending on tissue type and stage of metastasis [64]. Therefore, an in-depth, focused investigation may determine the specific role of PEDF in the extramedullary transition of MM [65].

HGFA is a serine protease that catalyses the activation hepatocyte growth factor (HGF). MM cell lines and primary myeloma cells secrete HGFA which can then activate HGF [66]. Furthermore, HGFA has been reported to be present in high levels in the sera and bone marrow of MM patients [67]. HGF is a pleiotropic cytokine involved in the progression of the monoclonal gammopathy of undetermined significance (MGUS) to MM, myeloma cell proliferation and survival [68]. Interestingly, heparanase increases the expression and secretion of HGF in MM, and secreted HGF can form an active complex with cleaved CD138 which promotes c-Met signalling [69]. Combining HGFA, VCAM1 and PEDF into a three-marker panel for the detection of EMM using logistic regression analysis increased the discriminatory power when compared to the individual proteins. Further investigation on the use of this panel to detect EMM at an early stage is needed. The mechanisms driving the increase in circulating VCAM1, HGFA and PEDF in EMM plasma are currently unknown. Future mechanistic studies involving these proteins will provide more insight into the cellular processes that lead to increased levels of VCAM1, HGFA and PEDF in EMM plasma.

Targeted metabolomics/lipidomics analysis identified 26 lipids, tyrosine and GUDCA as increased in abundance in EMM plasma, and taurine, phenylalanine betaine and PC aa C38:1 as decreased in EMM plasma, indicating a distinct plasma metabolite profile in EMM compared to medullary MM. A trend towards an increase in triglyceride concentrations in the plasma of patients with EMM was also identified. Several EMM case studies have reported hyperlipidaemia, which is more predominant in patients with IgA myeloma [70–72]. MM patients with the IgA monoclonal protein type are also at higher risk of future EMM development [73]. Several studies have analysed triglyceride levels in healthy controls and MM patients, finding no change in triglyceride levels apart from one study which noted an increase in triglycerides during the active disease period [74]. The increased lipid levels observed in EMM plasma may indicate a link between dysregulated lipid metabolism and

EMM. A recent study found that targeting fatty acid binding proteins (FABPs), including FABP5, in MM reduced MYC signalling and induced apoptosis of myeloma cells, highlighting the association of aberrant lipid metabolism with MM [75]. The results of the cellular GO analysis in this study indicate a clear metabolic change, emphasised by the reduced abundance of TCA cycle proteins in EMM BMNCs. CD36, a fatty acid transporter that enhances fatty acid uptake into cells similarly to FABPs, was increased in abundance in EMM BMNCs and may contribute to abnormal lipid metabolism within the BME [76]. Statins are commonly used to lower lipid concentrations by targeting the mevalonate pathway. Statin use has been reported to reduce the risk of MM and improve MM survival rates, although the biological mechanisms have not been fully elucidated [77,78]. Recent evidence demonstrate that statins may act as metastasis inhibitors in various solid cancers, including colon cancer [79,80]. Statins may represent a promising approach to target lipid metabolism in EMM; however, further investigation is required to evaluate this. A strong anti-tumorigenic role of taurine has been reported; however, this has not been thoroughly analysed in MM [56].

The efficacy of current therapeutics in the treatment of EMM is limited, as exemplified by the known poor prognosis of patients who present with extramedullary lesions [81,82]. Despite developments in the treatment of MM through the introduction of immunotherapies, preliminary studies indicate that the long-term efficacy of these treatments is significantly worse in patients with EMM compared to MM patients without extramedullary spread [83,84]. Our study illustrates a clear phenotypic change in the bone marrow niche of EMM patients compared to MM patients without extramedullary spread, suggesting a need for novel drug combinations or drug targets for the treatment of EMM to improve patient prognosis and treatment response. The bone marrow microenvironment can influence the dissemination of myeloma cells. Targeting myeloma clones with capacity for extramedullary spread in the context of the bone marrow microenvironment may be a promising approach to limit extramedullary transition [21,85]. As increased levels of sVCAM1 were associated with EMM and correlated with sensitivity to BCL2 inhibitors, venetoclax and navitoclax may represent promising therapeutics for the treatment of EMM. Several proteins found to be increased in the bone marrow mononuclear fraction of EMM patients, such as heparanase and ROCK2, have specific inhibitors available that warrant investigation in the context of EMM progression (Table 5) [86,87]. Crucially, large multicentre studies are required to incorporate satisfactory sample sizes to comprehensively evaluate the molecular mechanisms associated with EMM and the efficacy of novel drug combinations in EMM.

Table 5. Potential targets/markers and associated therapeutics for the treatment of EMM patients based on the current literature. This table provides a rationale for future studies focusing on the detection of drug targets in EMM. BCL2, B-cell lymphoma 2; qPCR, quantitative polymerase chain reaction; BCL-XL, B-cell lymphoma—extra large; XPO1, exportin 1; MEK, mitogen-activated protein kinase kinase; BRAF, B-Raf.

Protein Target/Marker	Potential Therapeutic	Method of Target Detection	FDA Approval	References
Potential protein targets in extramedullary multiple myeloma (identified from the literature)				
BCL2	Venetoclax	Immunohistochemistry, qPCR, fl-w cytometry	Yes—Acute myeloid leukaemia, Chronic lymphocytic leukaemia	[88,89]
BCL2, BCL-XL	Navitoclax	Immunohistochemistry, qPCR, flow cytometry	No	[89,90]
XPO1	Selinexor	Immunohistochemistry	Yes—Multiple myeloma	[91,92]
Aminopeptidase expression (Correlates with Melflufen sensitivity)	Melflufen	RNA sequencing	No	[93,94]
MEK	Trametinib	Targeted sequencing for RAS mutations	Yes (in combination with dabrafenib)—Various metastatic solid tumours with BRAF V600 E mutation	[11,95]
CD44v	4SCAR-CD44v6	Immunohistochemistry, flow cytometry	No	[96,97]
BRAF V600E	Vemurafenib, encorafenib, binimetinib	Allele-specific PCR	Yes—Metastatic melanoma with BRAF V600 E mutation	[98,99]
Potential protein targets in extramedullary multiple myeloma (identified in this study)				
LGALS1	OTX008	Immunohistochemistry	No	[100–102]
HPSE	Roneparstat	Immunohistochemistry	No	[86]
ROCK2	Belumosudil	qPCR, immunohistochemistry	Yes—Chronic graft-versus-host disease	[103]
ILK	QLT0267, Compound 22	Immunohistochemistry	No	[104,105]
Lipids	Statins	Unknown	Yes	[78,79]

Our paper includes a small sample size and lacks cellular proteomic verification. This is due to the fact that EMM is a rare manifestation of multiple myeloma which limits the availability of clinical samples for initial analysis and subsequent validation. The use of the MMRF CoMMpass dataset to determine the prognostic value of the most significantly increased proteins in EMM BMNCs provides some insight into the association of these proteins with more aggressive disease; however, validation in an independent cohort of EMM patients would improve our confidence in the association of these proteins with EMM transition. Finally, BMNCs from EMM and MM patients were used for proteomic analysis, which means that proteomic changes seen between the two groups are not solely associated with myeloma cells and instead associated with changes in the mononuclear fraction. However, with the growing use of monoclonal and bispecific antibodies in the treatment of MM, analysing various cells from the bone marrow microenvironment is relevant.

Within these limitations, however, this study shows that the proteomic alterations in the bone marrow and plasma of patients with and without EMM is impactful. We assumed that the presence of extramedullary lesions is derived from changes in the bone marrow microenvironment, and we evaluated the change in the proteomic profile of the bone marrow and plasma in the context of EMM. The potential plasma biomarkers we identified may represent factors produced by myeloma cells from extramedullary lesions. Further molecular analyses and larger scaled studies are needed to explore and confirm the link between the proteins identified in this study and EMM more definitively.

5. Conclusions

To the best of our knowledge, this pilot study using label-free mass spectrometry to evaluate proteomic changes in MM patients with and without extramedullary spread is the first of its kind. Determining the underlying molecular processes involved in the development of EMM is crucial to advancing patient care. VCAM1, PEDF and HGFA warrant further investigation as markers of extramedullary transition in a larger cohort of patients. Ultimately, this study illustrates that extramedullary myeloma is phenotypically different to medullary myeloma and, as such, warrants a different therapeutic approach with novel drug targets and drug combinations to improve survival rates. We hope this proteomic study will inform future experimental designs and research in EMM.

Supplementary Materials: The following supporting information can be downloaded at: https://www.mdpi.com/article/10.3390/cancers15153764/s1: Figure S1: Cytogenetics of patient cohort; Figure S2: Survival graph illustrating the difference in OS between the EMM group ($n = 8$) and medullary MM group ($n = 8$); Figure S3: Survival graphs illustrating the difference in OS between patients with high expression and low expression of the seven proteins identified as potential prognostic biomarkers in the CoMMpass dataset. Samples were divided based on median expression levels. (A) TAGLN2, (B) CA2, (C) ITGA2, (D) LGALS1, (E) TPM2, (F) TMOD3, (G) TPM3; Figure S4: Targeted metabolomic analysis shows a trend towards increased triglycerides and lipids in the plasma of EMM patients (A) Total plasma triglyceride concentration in MM patients with and without extramedullary spread. (B) Total lipid concentration in MM patients with and without extramedullary spread; Figure S5: Spearman's correlation matrix between differential metabolites and proteins in plasma. Table S1: Full list of statistically significant differentially abundant (SSDA) proteins in EMM bone marrow mononuclear cells (BMNCs) and MM BMNCs; Table S2: Metabolites with significant differential abundance in the plasma of MM and EMM patients.

Author Contributions: Conceptualization, D.B., P.D. and P.O.; methodology, K.D., P.D. and J.J.M.; validation, K.D.; formal analysis, K.D.; investigation, K.D.; resources, P.M., M.H., C.A.H., J.J.M., P.D. and P.O.; data curation, K.D. and D.B.; writing—original draft preparation, K.D.; writing—review and editing, D.B., P.D., J.J.M., C.A.H. and P.O.; visualization, K.D.; supervision, P.D. and P.O.; project administration, D.B.; funding acquisition, P.D. and D.B. All authors have read and agreed to the published version of the manuscript.

Funding: This work was funded by the Kathleen Lonsdale Human Health Institute co-fund scholarship to K.D, UCD Seed Funding (SF20022) to D.B. and Mater Foundation Funding (MF092) to D.B.

Institutional Review Board Statement: The study was conducted in accordance with the Declaration of Helsinki. The Finnish Hematology Registry and Clinical Biobank (FHRB) is authorized by the Finnish National Supervisory Authority for Welfare and Health (Valvira) and has been approved by the Finnish National Medical Ethics Committee (decision number 3613/06.01.05.01.00/2014) (date of project approval 20 May 2021).

Informed Consent Statement: Informed consent to collect samples and publish data was obtained from all subjects involved in the study.

Data Availability Statement: The data presented in this study are available on request from the corresponding author. The data are not publicly available due to privacy and ethical limitations.

Acknowledgments: KD/PD acknowledge the Q-Exactive quantitative mass spectrometer at Maynooth University was funded by Science Foundation Ireland under the Research Infrastructure Call 2012 (SFI-12/RI/2346/3). We acknowledge the UCD Conway Metabolomics Facility where the targeted metabolomic analysis was performed.

Conflicts of Interest: The authors declare no conflict of interest.

References

1. Kumar, S.K.; Rajkumar, V.; Kyle, R.A.; van Duin, M.; Sonneveld, P.; Mateos, M.-V.; Gay, F.; Anderson, K.C. Multiple Myeloma. *Nat. Rev. Dis. Primers* **2017**, *3*, 17046. [CrossRef] [PubMed]
2. Pinto, V.; Bergantim, R.; Caires, H.R.; Seca, H.; Guimarães, J.E.; Vasconcelos, M.H. Multiple Myeloma: Available Therapies and Causes of Drug Resistance. *Cancers* **2020**, *12*, 407. [CrossRef] [PubMed]
3. van de Donk, N.W.C.J.; Pawlyn, C.; Yong, K.L. Multiple Myeloma. *Lancet* **2021**, *397*, 410–427. [CrossRef] [PubMed]
4. Rajkumar, S.V. Updated Diagnostic Criteria and Staging System for Multiple Myeloma. *Am. Soc. Clin. Oncol. Educ. Book* **2016**, *35*, e418–e423. [CrossRef]
5. Bhutani, M.; Foureau, D.M.; Atrash, S.; Voorhees, P.M.; Usmani, S.Z. Extramedullary Multiple Myeloma. *Leukemia* **2020**, *34*, 1–20. [CrossRef]
6. Gagelmann, N.; Eikema, D.-J.; Iacobelli, S.; Koster, L.; Nahi, H.; Stoppa, A.-M.; Masszi, T.; Caillot, D.; Lenhoff, S.; Udvardy, M.; et al. Impact of Extramedullary Disease in Patients with Newly Diagnosed Multiple Myeloma Undergoing Autologous Stem Cell Transplantation: A Study from the Chronic Malignancies Working Party of the EBMT. *Haematologica* **2018**, *103*, 890–897. [CrossRef]
7. Beksac, M.; Seval, G.C.; Kanellias, N.; Coriu, D.; Rosiñol, L.; Ozet, G.; Goranova-Marinova, V.; Unal, A.; Bila, J.; Ozsan, H.; et al. A Real World Multicenter Retrospective Study on Extramedullary Disease from Balkan Myeloma Study Group and Barcelona University: Analysis of Parameters That Improve Outcome. *Haematologica* **2020**, *105*, 201–208. [CrossRef]
8. Bladé, J.; Beksac, M.; Caers, J.; Jurczyszyn, A.; von Lilienfeld-Toal, M.; Moreau, P.; Rasche, L.; Rosiñol, L.; Usmani, S.Z.; Zamagni, E.; et al. Extramedullary Disease in Multiple Myeloma: A Systematic Literature Review. *Blood Cancer J.* **2022**, *12*, 45. [CrossRef]
9. Moreau, P.; Attal, M.; Caillot, D.; Macro, M.; Karlin, L.; Garderet, L.; Facon, T.; Benboubker, L.; Escoffre-Barbe, M.; Stoppa, A.-M.; et al. Prospective Evaluation of Magnetic Resonance Imaging and [18F]Fluorodeoxyglucose Positron Emission Tomography-Computed Tomography at Diagnosis and Before Maintenance Therapy in Symptomatic Patients with Multiple Myeloma Included in the IFM/DFCI 2009 Trial: Results of the IMAJEM Study. *J. Clin. Oncol.* **2017**, *35*, 2911–2918. [CrossRef]
10. Badar, T.; Srour, S.; Bashir, Q.; Shah, N.; Al-Atrash, G.; Hosing, C.; Popat, U.; Nieto, Y.; Orlowski, R.Z.; Champlin, R.; et al. Predictors of Inferior Clinical Outcome in Patients with Standard-Risk Multiple Myeloma. *Eur. J. Haematol.* **2017**, *98*, 263–268. [CrossRef]
11. Touzeau, C.; Moreau, P. How I Treat Extramedullary Myeloma. *Blood* **2016**, *127*, 971–976. [CrossRef] [PubMed]
12. Billecke, L.; Murga Penas, E.M.; May, A.M.; Engelhardt, M.; Nagler, A.; Leiba, M.; Schiby, G.; Kröger, N.; Zustin, J.; Marx, A.; et al. Cytogenetics of Extramedullary Manifestations in Multiple Myeloma. *Br. J. Haematol.* **2013**, *161*, 87–94. [CrossRef] [PubMed]
13. García-Ortiz, A.; Rodríguez-García, Y.; Encinas, J.; Maroto-Martín, E.; Castellano, E.; Teixidó, J.; Martínez-López, J. The Role of Tumor Microenvironment in Multiple Myeloma Development and Progression. *Cancers* **2021**, *13*, 217. [CrossRef]
14. Solimando, A.; Vià, M.D.; Croci, G.; Borrelli, P.; Tabares, P.; Brandl, A.; Munawar, U.; Steinbrunn, T.; Balduini, A.; Rauert-Wunderlich, H.; et al. OAB-041: Epithelial-Mesenchymal-Transition Regulated by Junctional Adhesion Molecule-A (JAM-A) Associates with Aggressive Extramedullary Multiple Myeloma Disease. *Clin. Lymphoma Myeloma Leuk.* **2021**, *21*, S26–S27. [CrossRef]
15. Roccaro, A.M.; Mishima, Y.; Sacco, A.; Moschetta, M.; Tai, Y.-T.; Shi, J.; Zhang, Y.; Reagan, M.R.; Huynh, D.; Kawano, Y.; et al. CXCR4 Regulates Extra-Medullary Myeloma through Epithelial-Mesenchymal-Transition-like Transcriptional Activation. *Cell Rep.* **2015**, *12*, 622–635. [CrossRef] [PubMed]

16. Greipp, P.R.; Leong, T.; Bennett, J.M.; Gaillard, J.P.; Klein, B.; Stewart, J.A.; Oken, M.M.; Kay, N.E.; Van Ness, B.; Kyle, R.A. Plasmablastic Morphology—An Independent Prognostic Factor with Clinical and Laboratory Correlates: Eastern Cooperative Oncology Group (ECOG) Myeloma Trial E9486 Report by the ECOG Myeloma Laboratory Group. *Blood* **1998**, *91*, 2501–2507. [CrossRef] [PubMed]
17. Liu, Y.; Jelloul, F.; Zhang, Y.; Bhavsar, T.; Ho, C.; Rao, M.; Lewis, N.E.; Cimera, R.; Baik, J.; Sigler, A.; et al. Genetic Basis of Extramedullary Plasmablastic Transformation of Multiple Myeloma. *Am. J. Surg. Pathol.* **2020**, *44*, 838–848. [CrossRef]
18. Weinstock, M.; Ghobrial, I.M. Extramedullary Multiple Myeloma. *Leuk. Lymphoma* **2013**, *54*, 1135–1141. [CrossRef]
19. Wiśniewski, J.R.; Zougman, A.; Nagaraj, N.; Mann, M. Universal Sample Preparation Method for Proteome Analysis. *Nat. Methods* **2009**, *6*, 359–362. [CrossRef]
20. Raudvere, U.; Kolberg, L.; Kuzmin, I.; Arak, T.; Adler, P.; Peterson, H.; Vilo, J. G:Profiler: A Web Server for Functional Enrichment Analysis and Conversions of Gene Lists (2019 Update). *Nucleic Acids Res.* **2019**, *47*, W191–W198. [CrossRef]
21. Forster, S.; Radpour, R. Molecular Impact of the Tumor Microenvironment on Multiple Myeloma Dissemination and Extramedullary Disease. *Front. Oncol.* **2022**, *12*, 941437. [CrossRef] [PubMed]
22. Majumder, M.M.; Silvennoinen, R.; Anttila, P.; Tamborero, D.; Eldfors, S.; Yadav, B.; Karjalainen, R.; Kuusanmäki, H.; Lievonen, J.; Parsons, A.; et al. Identification of Precision Treatment Strategies for Relapsed/Refractory Multiple Myeloma by Functional Drug Sensitivity Testing. *Oncotarget* **2017**, *8*, 56338–56350. [CrossRef] [PubMed]
23. Tierney, C.; Bazou, D.; Majumder, M.M.; Anttila, P.; Silvennoinen, R.; Heckman, C.A.; Dowling, P.; O'Gorman, P. Next Generation Proteomics with Drug Sensitivity Screening Identifies Sub-Clones Informing Therapeutic and Drug Development Strategies for Multiple Myeloma Patients. *Sci. Rep.* **2021**, *11*, 12866. [CrossRef]
24. Godzien, J.; Ciborowski, M.; Angulo, S.; Barbas, C. From Numbers to a Biological Sense: How the Strategy Chosen for Metabolomics Data Treatment May Affect Final Results. A Practical Example Based on Urine Fingerprints Obtained by LC-MS. *Electrophoresis* **2013**, *34*, 2812–2826. [CrossRef]
25. An, R.; Yu, H.; Wang, Y.; Lu, J.; Gao, Y.; Xie, X.; Zhang, J. Integrative Analysis of Plasma Metabolomics and Proteomics Reveals the Metabolic Landscape of Breast Cancer. *Cancer Metab.* **2022**, *10*, 13. [CrossRef] [PubMed]
26. Sevcikova, S.; Minarik, J.; Stork, M.; Jelinek, T.; Pour, L.; Hajek, R. Extramedullary Disease in Multiple Myeloma—Controversies and Future Directions. *Blood Rev.* **2019**, *36*, 32–39. [CrossRef]
27. Ormond Filho, A.G.; Carneiro, B.C.; Pastore, D.; Silva, I.P.; Yamashita, S.R.; Consolo, F.D.; Hungria, V.T.M.; Sandes, A.F.; Rizzatti, E.G.; Nico, M.A.C. Whole-Body Imaging of Multiple Myeloma: Diagnostic Criteria. *RadioGraphics* **2019**, *39*, 1077–1097. [CrossRef] [PubMed]
28. Gozzetti, A.; Kok, C.H.; Li, C.-F. Editorial: Molecular Mechanisms of Multiple Myeloma. *Front. Oncol.* **2022**, *12*, 870123. [CrossRef] [PubMed]
29. Kriegova, E.; Fillerova, R.; Minarik, J.; Savara, J.; Manakova, J.; Petrackova, A.; Dihel, M.; Balcarkova, J.; Krhovska, P.; Pika, T.; et al. Whole-Genome Optical Mapping of Bone-Marrow Myeloma Cells Reveals Association of Extramedullary Multiple Myeloma with Chromosome 1 Abnormalities. *Sci. Rep.* **2021**, *11*, 14671. [CrossRef]
30. Ryu, D.; Kim, S.J.; Hong, Y.; Jo, A.; Kim, N.; Kim, H.-J.; Lee, H.-O.; Kim, K.; Park, W.-Y. Alterations in the Transcriptional Programs of Myeloma Cells and the Microenvironment during Extramedullary Progression Affect Proliferation and Immune Evasion. *Clin. Cancer Res.* **2020**, *26*, 935–944. [CrossRef]
31. Gregorova, J.; Vychytilova-Faltejskova, P.; Kramarova, T.; Knechtova, Z.; Almasi, M.; Stork, M.; Pour, L.; Kohoutek, J.; Sevcikova, S. Proteomic Analysis of the Bone Marrow Microenvironment in Extramedullary Multiple Myeloma Patients. *Neoplasma* **2022**, *69*, 412–424. [CrossRef]
32. Bou Zerdan, M.; Nasr, L.; Kassab, J.; Saba, L.; Ghossein, M.; Yaghi, M.; Dominguez, B.; Chaulagain, C.P. Adhesion Molecules in Multiple Myeloma Oncogenesis and Targeted Therapy. *Int. J. Hematol. Oncol.* **2022**, *11*, IJH39. [CrossRef] [PubMed]
33. Hathi, D.; Chanswangphuwana, C.; Cho, N.; Fontana, F.; Maji, D.; Ritchey, J.; O'Neal, J.; Ghai, A.; Duncan, K.; Akers, W.J.; et al. Ablation of VLA4 in Multiple Myeloma Cells Redirects Tumor Spread and Prolongs Survival. *Sci. Rep.* **2022**, *12*, 30. [CrossRef] [PubMed]
34. Hedvat, C.V.; Comenzo, R.L.; Teruya-Feldstein, J.; Olshen, A.B.; Ely, S.A.; Osman, K.; Zhang, Y.; Kalakonda, N.; Nimer, S.D. Insights into Extramedullary Tumour Cell Growth Revealed by Expression Profiling of Human Plasmacytomas and Multiple Myeloma. *Br. J. Haematol.* **2003**, *122*, 728–744. [CrossRef] [PubMed]
35. Nagano, M.; Hoshino, D.; Koshikawa, N.; Akizawa, T.; Seiki, M. Turnover of Focal Adhesions and Cancer Cell Migration. *Int. J. Cell Biol.* **2012**, *2012*, e310616. [CrossRef]
36. Górska, A.; Mazur, A.J. Integrin-Linked Kinase (ILK): The Known vs. the Unknown and Perspectives. *Cell. Mol. Life Sci.* **2022**, *79*, 100. [CrossRef]
37. McDonald, P.C.; Dedhar, S. New Perspectives on the Role of Integrin-Linked Kinase (ILK) Signaling in Cancer Metastasis. *Cancers* **2022**, *14*, 3209. [CrossRef]
38. Nikou, S.; Arbi, M.; Dimitrakopoulos, F.-I.D.; Sirinian, C.; Chadla, P.; Pappa, I.; Ntaliarda, G.; Stathopoulos, G.T.; Papadaki, H.; Zolota, V.; et al. Integrin-Linked Kinase (ILK) Regulates KRAS, IPP Complex and Ras Suppressor-1 (RSU1) Promoting Lung Adenocarcinoma Progression and Poor Survival. *J. Mol. Hist.* **2020**, *51*, 385–400. [CrossRef]

39. Tsoumas, D.; Nikou, S.; Giannopoulou, E.; Tsaniras, S.C.; Sirinian, C.; Maroulis, I.; Taraviras, S.; Zolota, V.; Kalofonos, H.P.; Bravou, V. ILK Expression in Colorectal Cancer Is Associated with EMT, Cancer Stem Cell Markers and Chemoresistance. *Cancer Genom. Proteom.* 2018, 15, 127–141.
40. Chen, D.; Zhang, Y.; Zhang, X.; Li, J.; Han, B.; Liu, S.; Wang, L.; Ling, Y.; Mao, S.; Wang, X. Overexpression of Integrin-Linked Kinase Correlates with Malignant Phenotype in Non-Small Cell Lung Cancer and Promotes Lung Cancer Cell Invasion and Migration via Regulating Epithelial–Mesenchymal Transition (EMT)-Related Genes. *Acta Histochem.* 2013, 115, 128–136. [CrossRef]
41. Wang, X.; Zhang, Z.; Yao, C. Targeting Integrin-Linked Kinase Increases Apoptosis and Decreases Invasion of Myeloma Cell Lines and Inhibits IL-6 and VEGF Secretion from BMSCs. *Med. Oncol.* 2011, 28, 1596–1600. [CrossRef] [PubMed]
42. Steinbrunn, T.; Siegmund, D.; Andrulis, M.; Grella, E.; Kortüm, M.; Einsele, H.; Wajant, H.; Bargou, R.C.; Stühmer, T. Integrin-Linked Kinase Is Dispensable for Multiple Myeloma Cell Survival. *Leuk. Res.* 2012, 36, 1165–1171. [CrossRef] [PubMed]
43. He, Y.; Wang, Y.; Liu, H.; Xu, X.; He, S.; Tang, J.; Huang, Y.; Miao, X.; Wu, Y.; Wang, Q.; et al. Pyruvate Kinase Isoform M2 (PKM2) Participates in Multiple Myeloma Cell Proliferation, Adhesion and Chemoresistance. *Leuk. Res.* 2015, 39, 1428–1436. [CrossRef]
44. Wang, C.; Zhang, S.; Liu, J.; Tian, Y.; Ma, B.; Xu, S.; Fu, Y.; Luo, Y. Secreted Pyruvate Kinase M2 Promotes Lung Cancer Metastasis through Activating the Integrin Beta1/FAK Signaling Pathway. *Cell Rep.* 2020, 30, 1780–1797.e6. [CrossRef] [PubMed]
45. Dah, K.; Lavezo, J.L.; Dihowm, F. Aggressive Plasmablastic Myeloma with Extramedullary Cord Compression and Hyperammonemic Encephalopathy: Case Report and Literature Review. *Anticancer Res.* 2021, 41, 5839–5845. [CrossRef] [PubMed]
46. Muz, B.; de la Puente, P.; Azab, F.; Luderer, M.; Azab, A.K. Hypoxia Promotes Stem Cell-like Phenotype in Multiple Myeloma Cells. *Blood Cancer J.* 2014, 4, e262. [CrossRef] [PubMed]
47. Tripathi, K.; Ramani, V.C.; Bandari, S.K.; Amin, R.; Brown, E.E.; Ritchie, J.P.; Stewart, M.D.; Sanderson, R.D. Heparanase Promotes Myeloma Stemness and in Vivo Tumorigenesis. *Matrix Biol.* 2020, 88, 53–68. [CrossRef] [PubMed]
48. Jung, O.; Trapp-Stamborski, V.; Purushothaman, A.; Jin, H.; Wang, H.; Sanderson, R.D.; Rapraeger, A.C. Heparanase-Induced Shedding of Syndecan-1/CD138 in Myeloma and Endothelial Cells Activates VEGFR2 and an Invasive Phenotype: Prevention by Novel Synstatins. *Oncogenesis* 2016, 5, e202. [CrossRef]
49. Zhang, D.; Bi, J.; Liang, Q.; Wang, S.; Zhang, L.; Han, F.; Li, S.; Qiu, B.; Fan, X.; Chen, W.; et al. VCAM1 Promotes Tumor Cell Invasion and Metastasis by Inducing EMT and Transendothelial Migration in Colorectal Cancer. *Front. Oncol.* 2020, 10, 1066. [CrossRef]
50. Hao, P.; Zhang, C.; Wang, R.; Yan, P.; Peng, R. Expression and Pathogenesis of VCAM-1 and VLA-4 Cytokines in Multiple Myeloma. *Saudi J. Biol. Sci.* 2020, 27, 1674–1678. [CrossRef]
51. Terpos, E.; Migkou, M.; Christoulas, D.; Gavriatopoulou, M.; Eleutherakis-Papaiakovou, E.; Kanellias, N.; Iakovaki, M.; Panagiotidis, I.; Ziogas, D.C.; Fotiou, D.; et al. Increased Circulating VCAM-1 Correlates with Advanced Disease and Poor Survival in Patients with Multiple Myeloma: Reduction by Post-Bortezomib and Lenalidomide Treatment. *Blood Cancer J.* 2016, 6, e428. [CrossRef]
52. Okugawa, Y.; Miki, C.; Toiyama, Y.; Koike, Y.; Yokoe, T.; Saigusa, S.; Tanaka, K.; Inoue, Y.; Kusunoki, M. Soluble VCAM-1 and Its Relation to Disease Progression in Colorectal Carcinoma. *Exp. Ther. Med.* 2010, 1, 463–469. [CrossRef]
53. Liao, T.; Chen, W.; Sun, J.; Zhang, Y.; Hu, X.; Yang, S.; Qiu, H.; Li, S.; Chu, T. CXCR4 Accelerates Osteoclastogenesis Induced by Non-Small Cell Lung Carcinoma Cells Through Self-Potentiation and VCAM1 Secretion. *CPB* 2018, 50, 1084–1099. [CrossRef] [PubMed]
54. Alexiou, D.; Karayiannakis, A.J.; Syrigos, K.N.; Zbar, A.; Kremmyda, A.; Bramis, I.; Tsigris, C. Serum Levels of E-Selectin, ICAM-1 and VCAM-1 in Colorectal Cancer Patients: Correlations with Clinicopathological Features, Patient Survival and Tumour Surgery. *Eur. J. Cancer* 2001, 37, 2392–2397. [CrossRef] [PubMed]
55. Ding, Y.-B.; Chen, G.-Y.; Xia, J.-G.; Zang, X.-W.; Yang, H.-Y.; Yang, L. Association of VCAM-1 Overexpression with Oncogenesis, Tumor Angiogenesis and Metastasis of Gastric Carcinoma. *World J. Gastroenterol.* 2003, 9, 1409–1414. [CrossRef]
56. Kitani, A.; Nakashima, N.; Izumihara, T.; Inagaki, M.; Baoui, X.; Yu, S.; Matsuda, T.; Matsuyama, T. Soluble VCAM-1 Induces Chemotaxis of Jurkat and Synovial Fluid T Cells Bearing High Affinity Very Late Antigen-4. *J. Immunol.* 1998, 161, 4931–4938. [CrossRef]
57. Roy, P.; Sarkar, U.A.; Basak, S. The NF-κB Activating Pathways in Multiple Myeloma. *Biomedicines* 2018, 6, 59. [CrossRef]
58. Demchenko, Y.N.; Glebov, O.K.; Zingone, A.; Keats, J.J.; Bergsagel, P.L.; Kuehl, W.M. Classical and/or Alternative NF-κB Pathway Activation in Multiple Myeloma. *Blood* 2010, 115, 3541–3552. [CrossRef] [PubMed]
59. Becerra, S.P.; Notario, V. The Effects of PEDF on Cancer Biology: Mechanisms of Action and Therapeutic Potential. *Nat. Rev. Cancer* 2013, 13, 258–271. [CrossRef]
60. Seki, R.; Yoshida, T.; Nakamura, K.; Yamagishi, S.; Imaizumi, T.; Okamura, T.; Sata, M. Pigment Epithelium-Derived Factor (PEDF) Inhibits Multiple Myeloma through Suppressing NADPH Oxidase ROS Generation. *Blood* 2005, 106, 3389. [CrossRef]
61. Seki, R.; Yamagishi, S.; Matsui, T.; Yoshida, T.; Torimura, T.; Ueno, T.; Sata, M.; Okamura, T. Pigment Epithelium-Derived Factor (PEDF) Inhibits Survival and Proliferation of VEGF-Exposed Multiple Myeloma Cells through Its Anti-Oxidative Properties. *Biochem. Biophys. Res. Commun.* 2013, 431, 693–697. [CrossRef]
62. Chen, Z.; Che, D.; Gu, X.; Lin, J.; Deng, J.; Jiang, P.; Xu, K.; Xu, B.; Zhang, T. Upregulation of PEDF Predicts a Poor Prognosis and Promotes Esophageal Squamous Cell Carcinoma Progression by Modulating the MAPK/ERK Signaling Pathway. *Front. Oncol.* 2021, 11, 625612. [CrossRef] [PubMed]

63. Hou, J.; Ge, C.; Cui, M.; Liu, T.; Liu, X.; Tian, H.; Zhao, F.; Chen, T.; Cui, Y.; Yao, M.; et al. Pigment Epithelium-Derived Factor Promotes Tumor Metastasis through an Interaction with Laminin Receptor in Hepatocellular Carcinomas. *Cell Death Dis.* **2017**, *8*, e2969. [CrossRef] [PubMed]
64. Abooshahab, R.; Al-Salami, H.; Dass, C.R. The Increasing Role of Pigment Epithelium-Derived Factor in Metastasis: From Biological Importance to a Promising Target. *Biochem. Pharmacol.* **2021**, *193*, 114787. [CrossRef] [PubMed]
65. Kuriyama, S.; Tanaka, G.; Takagane, K.; Itoh, G.; Tanaka, M. Pigment Epithelium Derived Factor Is Involved in the Late Phase of Osteosarcoma Metastasis by Increasing Extravasation and Cell-Cell Adhesion. *Front. Oncol.* **2022**, *12*, 818182. [CrossRef]
66. Tjin, E.P.M.; Derksen, P.W.B.; Kataoka, H.; Spaargaren, M.; Pals, S.T. Multiple Myeloma Cells Catalyze Hepatocyte Growth Factor (HGF) Activation by Secreting the Serine Protease HGF-Activator. *Blood* **2004**, *104*, 2172–2175. [CrossRef]
67. Wader, K.F.; Fagerli, U.M.; Holt, R.U.; Stordal, B.; Børset, M.; Sundan, A.; Waage, A. Elevated Serum Concentrations of Activated Hepatocyte Growth Factor Activator in Patients with Multiple Myeloma. *Eur. J. Haematol.* **2008**, *81*, 380–383. [CrossRef]
68. Giannoni, P.; de Totero, D. The HGF/c-MET Axis as a Potential Target to Overcome Survival Signals and Improve Therapeutic Efficacy in Multiple Myeloma. *Cancer Drug Resist.* **2021**, *4*, 923–933. [CrossRef]
69. Ramani, V.C.; Yang, Y.; Ren, Y.; Nan, L.; Sanderson, R.D. Heparanase Plays a Dual Role in Driving Hepatocyte Growth Factor (HGF) Signaling by Enhancing HGF Expression and Activity. *J. Biol. Chem.* **2011**, *286*, 6490–6499. [CrossRef]
70. Misselwitz, B.; Goede, J.S.; Pestalozzi, B.C.; Schanz, U.; Seebach, J.D. Hyperlipidemic Myeloma: Review of 53 Cases. *Ann. Hematol.* **2010**, *89*, 569–577. [CrossRef]
71. Ilyas, U.; Umar, Z.; Pansuriya, A.M.; Mahmood, A.; Lopez, R. Multiple Myeloma with Retroperitoneal Extramedullary Plasmacytoma Causing Renal Failure and Obstructive Shock From Inferior Vena Cava Compression: A Case Report. *Cureus* **2022**, *14*, e31056. [CrossRef]
72. Shimokihara, K.; Kawahara, T.; Chiba, S.; Takamoto, D.; Yao, M.; Uemura, H. Extramedullary Plasmacytoma of the Testis: A Case Report. *Urol. Case Rep.* **2018**, *16*, 101–103. [CrossRef]
73. Stork, M.; Sevcikova, S.; Minarik, J.; Krhovska, P.; Radocha, J.; Pospisilova, L.; Brozova, L.; Jarkovsky, J.; Spicka, I.; Straub, J.; et al. Identification of Patients at High Risk of Secondary Extramedullary Multiple Myeloma Development. *Br. J. Haematol.* **2022**, *196*, 954–962. [CrossRef] [PubMed]
74. Lazaris, V.; Hatziri, A.; Symeonidis, A.; Kypreos, K.E. The Lipoprotein Transport System in the Pathogenesis of Multiple Myeloma: Advances and Challenges. *Front. Oncol.* **2021**, *11*, 638288. [CrossRef] [PubMed]
75. Farrell, M.; Fairfield, H.; Karam, M.; D'Amico, A.; Murphy, C.S.; Falank, C.; Pistofidi, R.S.; Cao, A.; Marinac, C.R.; Dragon, J.A.; et al. Targeting the Fatty Acid Binding Proteins Disrupts Multiple Myeloma Cell Cycle Progression and MYC Signaling. *eLife* **2023**, *12*, e81184. [CrossRef] [PubMed]
76. Kobari, L.; Auclair, M.; Piau, O.; Ferrand, N.; Zaoui, M.; Delhommeau, F.; Fève, B.; Sabbah, M.; Garderet, L. Circulating Cytokines Present in Multiple Myeloma Patients Inhibit the Osteoblastic Differentiation of Adipose Stem Cells. *Leukemia* **2022**, *36*, 540–548. [CrossRef]
77. Ponvilawan, B.; Charoenngam, N.; Rittiphairoj, T.; Ungprasert, P. Receipt of Statins Is Associated with Lower Risk of Multiple Myeloma: Systematic Review and Meta-Analysis. *Clin. Lymphoma Myeloma Leuk.* **2020**, *20*, e399–e413. [CrossRef] [PubMed]
78. Brånvall, E.; Ekberg, S.; Eloranta, S.; Wästerlid, T.; Birmann, B.M.; Smedby, K.E. Statin Use Is Associated with Improved Survival in Multiple Myeloma: A Swedish Population-Based Study of 4315 Patients. *Am. J. Hematol.* **2020**, *95*, 652–661. [CrossRef]
79. Gohlke, B.; Zincke, F.; Eckert, A.; Kobelt, D.; Preissner, S.; Liebeskind, J.M.; Gunkel, N.; Putzker, K.; Lewis, J.; Preissner, S.; et al. Real-world Evidence for Preventive Effects of Statins on Cancer Incidence: A Trans-Atlantic Analysis. *Clin. Transl. Med.* **2022**, *12*, e726. [CrossRef]
80. Juneja, M.; Kobelt, D.; Walther, W.; Voss, C.; Smith, J.; Specker, E.; Neuenschwander, M.; Gohlke, B.-O.; Dahlmann, M.; Radetzki, S.; et al. Statin and Rottlerin Small-Molecule Inhibitors Restrict Colon Cancer Progression and Metastasis via MACC1. *PLoS Biol.* **2017**, *15*, e2000784. [CrossRef]
81. Lonial, S.; Lee, H.C.; Badros, A.; Trudel, S.; Nooka, A.K.; Chari, A.; Abdallah, A.; Callander, N.; Sborov, D.; Suvannasankha, A.; et al. Longer Term Outcomes with Single-agent Belantamab Mafodotin in Patients with Relapsed or Refractory Multiple Myeloma: 13-month Follow-up from the Pivotal DREAMM-2 Study. *Cancer* **2021**, *127*, 4198–4212. [CrossRef]
82. Rosiñol, L.; Beksac, M.; Zamagni, E.; Van de Donk, N.W.C.J.; Anderson, K.C.; Badros, A.; Caers, J.; Cavo, M.; Dimopoulos, M.-A.; Dispenzieri, A.; et al. Expert Review on Soft-Tissue Plasmacytomas in Multiple Myeloma: Definition, Disease Assessment and Treatment Considerations. *Br. J. Haematol.* **2021**, *194*, 496–507. [CrossRef]
83. Jelinek, T.; Sevcikova, T.; Zihala, D.; Popkova, T.; Kapustova, V.; Broskevicova, L.; Capkova, L.; Rihova, L.; Bezdekova, R.; Sevcikova, S.; et al. Limited Efficacy of Daratumumab in Multiple Myeloma with Extramedullary Disease. *Leukemia* **2022**, *36*, 288–291. [CrossRef]
84. Li, W.; Liu, M.; Yuan, T.; Yan, L.; Cui, R.; Deng, Q. Efficacy and Follow-up of Humanized Anti-BCMA CAR-T Cell Therapy in Relapsed/Refractory Multiple Myeloma Patients with Extramedullary-Extraosseous, Extramedullary-Bone Related, and without Extramedullary Disease. *Hematol. Oncol.* **2022**, *40*, 223–232. [CrossRef] [PubMed]
85. Ho, M.; Xiao, A.; Yi, D.; Zanwar, S.; Bianchi, G. Treating Multiple Myeloma in the Context of the Bone Marrow Microenvironment. *Curr. Oncol.* **2022**, *29*, 8975–9005. [CrossRef] [PubMed]
86. Galli, M.; Chatterjee, M.; Grasso, M.; Specchia, G.; Magen, H.; Einsele, H.; Celeghini, I.; Barbieri, P.; Paoletti, D.; Pace, S.; et al. Phase I Study of the Heparanase Inhibitor Roneparstat: An Innovative Approach for Ultiple Myeloma Therapy. *Haematologica* **2018**, *103*, e469–e472. [CrossRef]

87. Federico, C.; Alhallak, K.; Sun, J.; Duncan, K.; Azab, F.; Sudlow, G.P.; de la Puente, P.; Muz, B.; Kapoor, V.; Zhang, L.; et al. Tumor Microenvironment-Targeted Nanoparticles Loaded with Bortezomib and ROCK Inhibitor Improve Efficacy in Multiple Myeloma. *Nat. Commun.* **2020**, *11*, 6037. [CrossRef]
88. Sidiqi, M.H.; Al Saleh, A.S.; Kumar, S.K.; Leung, N.; Jevremovic, D.; Muchtar, E.; Gonsalves, W.I.; Kourelis, T.V.; Warsame, R.; Buadi, F.K.; et al. Venetoclax for the Treatment of Multiple Myeloma: Outcomes Outside of Clinical Trials. *Am. J. Hematol.* **2021**, *96*, 1131–1136. [CrossRef] [PubMed]
89. Ludwig, L.M.; Maxcy, K.L.; LaBelle, J.L. Flow Cytometry-Based Detection and Analysis of BCL-2 Family Proteins and Mitochondrial Outer Membrane Permeabilization (MOMP). *Methods Mol. Biol.* **2019**, *1877*, 77–91. [CrossRef] [PubMed]
90. Ackler, S.; Mitten, M.J.; Foster, K.; Oleksijew, A.; Refici, M.; Tahir, S.K.; Xiao, Y.; Tse, C.; Frost, D.J.; Fesik, S.W.; et al. The Bcl-2 Inhibitor ABT-263 Enhances the Response of Multiple Chemotherapeutic Regimens in Hematologic Tumors in Vivo. *Cancer Chemother. Pharmacol.* **2010**, *66*, 869–880. [CrossRef]
91. Yee, A.J.; Huff, C.A.; Chari, A.; Vogl, D.T.; Gavriatopoulou, M.; Nooka, A.K.; Moreau, P.; Dingli, D.; Cole, C.E.; Lonial, S.; et al. Response to Therapy and the Effectiveness of Treatment with Selinexor and Dexamethasone in Patients with Penta-Exposed Triple-Class Refractory Myeloma Who Had Plasmacytomas. *Blood* **2019**, *134*, 3140. [CrossRef]
92. Bahlis, N.J.; Sutherland, H.; White, D.; Sebag, M.; Lentzsch, S.; Kotb, R.; Venner, C.P.; Gasparetto, C.; Del Col, A.; Neri, P.; et al. Selinexor plus Low-Dose Bortezomib and Dexamethasone for Patients with Relapsed or Refractory Multiple Myeloma. *Blood* **2018**, *132*, 2546–2554. [CrossRef] [PubMed]
93. Richardson, P.G.; Oriol, A.; Larocca, A.; Bladé, J.; Cavo, M.; Rodriguez-Otero, P.; Leleu, X.; Nadeem, O.; Hiemenz, J.W.; Hassoun, H.; et al. Melflufen and Dexamethasone in Heavily Pretreated Relapsed and Refractory Multiple Myeloma. *J. Clin. Oncol.* **2021**, *39*, 757–767. [CrossRef] [PubMed]
94. Miettinen, J.J.; Kumari, R.; Traustadottir, G.A.; Huppunen, M.-E.; Sergeev, P.; Majumder, M.M.; Schepsky, A.; Gudjonsson, T.; Lievonen, J.; Bazou, D.; et al. Aminopeptidase Expression in Multiple Myeloma Associates with Disease Progression and Sensitivity to Melflufen. *Cancers* **2021**, *13*, 1527. [CrossRef]
95. Sriskandarajah, P.; De Haven Brandon, A.; MacLeod, K.; Carragher, N.O.; Kirkin, V.; Kaiser, M.; Whittaker, S.R. Combined Targeting of MEK and the Glucocorticoid Receptor for the Treatment of RAS-Mutant Multiple Myeloma. *BMC Cancer* **2020**, *20*, 269. [CrossRef] [PubMed]
96. Gupta, S.; Master, S.; Graham, C. Extramedullary Multiple Myeloma: A Patient-Focused Review of the Pathogenesis of Bone Marrow Escape. *World J. Oncol.* **2022**, *13*, 311–319. [CrossRef]
97. Dahl, I.M.S.; Rasmussen, T.; Kauric, G.; Husebekk, A. Differential Expression of CD56 and CD44 in the Evolution of Extramedullary Myeloma. *Br. J. Haematol.* **2002**, *116*, 273–277. [CrossRef]
98. Mey, U.J.M.; Renner, C.; von Moos, R. Vemurafenib in Combination with Cobimetinib in Relapsed and Refractory Extramedullary Multiple Myeloma Harboring the BRAF V600E Mutation. *Hematol. Oncol.* **2017**, *35*, 890–893. [CrossRef] [PubMed]
99. Giesen, N.; Chatterjee, M.; Scheid, C.; Poos, A.M.; Besemer, B.; Miah, K.; Benner, A.; Becker, N.; Moehler, T.; Metzler, I.; et al. A Phase 2 Clinical Trial of Combined BRAF/MEK Inhibition for BRAFV600E-Mutated Multiple Myeloma. *Blood* **2023**, *141*, 1685–1690. [CrossRef] [PubMed]
100. Mariño, K.V.; Cagnoni, A.J.; Croci, D.O.; Rabinovich, G.A. Targeting Galectin-Driven Regulatory Circuits in Cancer and Fibrosis. *Nat. Rev. Drug Discov.* **2023**, *22*, 295–316. [CrossRef]
101. Storti, P.; Marchica, V.; Giuliani, N. Role of Galectins in Multiple Myeloma. *Int. J. Mol. Sci.* **2017**, *18*, 2740. [CrossRef] [PubMed]
102. Storti, P.; Marchica, V.; Airoldi, I.; Donofrio, G.; Fiorini, E.; Ferri, V.; Guasco, D.; Todoerti, K.; Silbermann, R.; Anderson, J.L.; et al. Galectin-1 Suppression Delineates a New Strategy to Inhibit Myeloma-Induced Angiogenesis and Tumoral Growth in Vivo. *Leukemia* **2016**, *30*, 2351–2363. [CrossRef] [PubMed]
103. Cutler, C.; Lee, S.J.; Arai, S.; Rotta, M.; Zoghi, B.; Lazaryan, A.; Ramakrishnan, A.; DeFilipp, Z.; Salhotra, A.; Chai-Ho, W.; et al. Belumosudil for Chronic Graft-versus-Host Disease after 2 or More Prior Lines of Therapy: The ROCKstar Study. *Blood* **2021**, *138*, 2278–2289. [CrossRef] [PubMed]
104. Kalra, J.; Warburton, C.; Fang, K.; Edwards, L.; Daynard, T.; Waterhouse, D.; Dragowska, W.; Sutherland, B.W.; Dedhar, S.; Gelmon, K.; et al. QLT0267, a Small Molecule Inhibitor Targeting Integrin-Linked Kinase (ILK), and Docetaxel Can Combine to Produce Synergistic Interactions Linked to Enhanced Cytotoxicity, Reductions in P-AKT Levels, Altered F-Actin Architecture and Improved Treatment Outcomes in an Orthotopic Breast Cancer Model. *Breast Cancer Res.* **2009**, *11*, R25. [CrossRef] [PubMed]
105. García-Marín, J.; Rodríguez-Puyol, D.; Vaquero, J.J. Insight into the Mechanism of Molecular Recognition between Human Integrin-Linked Kinase and Cpd22 and Its Implication at Atomic Level. *J. Comput. Aided Mol. Des.* **2022**, *36*, 575–589. [CrossRef] [PubMed]

Disclaimer/Publisher's Note: The statements, opinions and data contained in all publications are solely those of the individual author(s) and contributor(s) and not of MDPI and/or the editor(s). MDPI and/or the editor(s) disclaim responsibility for any injury to people or property resulting from any ideas, methods, instructions or products referred to in the content.

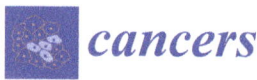

Article

Exosome-Mediated Activation of the Prostasin-Matriptase Serine Protease Cascade in B Lymphoma Cells

Li-Mei Chen * and Karl X. Chai *

Burnett School of Biomedical Sciences, College of Medicine, University of Central Florida, Orlando, FL 32816, USA
* Correspondence: limei.chen@ucf.edu (L.-M.C.); karl.chai@ucf.edu (K.X.C.)

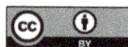

Citation: Chen, L.-M.; Chai, K.X. Exosome-Mediated Activation of the Prostasin-Matriptase Serine Protease Cascade in B Lymphoma Cells. Cancers 2023, 15, 3848. https://doi.org/10.3390/cancers15153848

Academic Editors: Daniel L. Pouliquen and Cristina Núñez González

Received: 25 June 2023
Revised: 25 July 2023
Accepted: 26 July 2023
Published: 28 July 2023

Copyright: © 2023 by the authors. Licensee MDPI, Basel, Switzerland. This article is an open access article distributed under the terms and conditions of the Creative Commons Attribution (CC BY) license (https://creativecommons.org/licenses/by/4.0/).

Simple Summary: Prostasin and matriptase are serine proteases co-expressed on the cell membrane in almost all epithelial cells. They reciprocally activate each other to maintain epithelial integrity. In cancers, matriptase is an oncoprotein with key roles in tumor initiation and progression, whereas prostasin acts in the opposite way. A subgroup of Burkitt lymphoma ectopically over-express matriptase without co-expressing prostasin. Reducing the matriptase expression level via small interfering RNAs in the lymphoma cells reduced tumor growth in vitro and in vivo. We hypothesized that an endowment of prostasin in the lymphoma cells can regulate the expression and function of matriptase. We show that prostasin can be introduced to the cancer cells via exosomes to initiate the prostasin–matriptase protease activation cascade and remove matriptase. The method of assembling this protease cascade in B cells via exosomes could be further exploited in animal models for developing alternative treatments for lymphoma.

Abstract: Prostasin and matriptase are extracellular membrane serine proteases with opposing effects in solid epithelial tumors. Matriptase is an oncoprotein that promotes tumor initiation and progression, and prostasin is a tumor suppressor that reduces tumor invasion and metastasis. Previous studies have shown that a subgroup of Burkitt lymphoma have high levels of ectopic matriptase expression but no prostasin. Reducing the matriptase level via small interfering RNAs in B lymphoma cells impeded tumor xenograft growth in mice. Here, we report a novel approach to matriptase regulation in B cancer cells by prostasin via exosomes to initiate a prostasin–matriptase protease activation cascade. The activation and shedding of matriptase were monitored by measuring its quantity and trypsin-like serine protease activity in conditioned media. Sustained activation of the protease cascade in the cells was achieved by the stable expression of prostasin. The B cancer cells with prostasin expression presented phenotypes consistent with its tumor suppressor role, such as reduced growth and increased apoptosis. Prostasin exosomes could be developed as an agent to initiate the prostasin–matriptase cascade for treating B lymphoma with further studies in animal models.

Keywords: exosomes; prostasin; matriptase; protease activation cascade; gelatinase activity; lymphoma

1. Introduction

Many physiological and pathophysiological functions are performed by serine proteases, e.g., blood coagulation and fibrinolysis, food digestion, cell apoptosis, and tumor metastasis [1]. These proteolytic enzymes use the hydroxyl group of an active-site serine residue to carry out a nucleophilic attack on the carbonyl group of the scissile peptide bond in their substrates. The results of the substrate cleavage can range from the activation of growth factors or zymogens to protein turnover and tissue remodeling. Most serine proteases, such as the quintessential pancreatic trypsin, are synthesized as precursors (zymogens) and secreted into extracellular spaces or bodily fluids. The secreted zymogens are activated by various factors and mechanisms for various functions. In the past 30 years, several membrane-bound extracellular serine proteases have been discovered, such as hepsin [2], prostasin [3,4], and matriptase [5,6], with specifically defined functions at this cellular localization. The activation and regulation of these enzymes can and also must occur at the membrane, as well.

Prostasin is entirely extracellular, anchored to the membrane via a glycosylphosphatidylinositol (GPI) moiety [7], whereas matriptase is a type-II transmembrane protein with a long carboxyl terminal portion outside the cell, including its serine protease domain [5,6]. Both prostasin and matriptase have been implicated in functional involvements in the initiation and progression of human cancers, but they seem to act in opposite manners. Prostasin is a tumor suppressor, which reduces cancer cell migration, invasion, and metastasis, and its expression level is usually downregulated in cancers [8,9]. Matriptase, on the other hand, is an oncoprotein, and its expression level is usually upregulated in cancers [10].

A co-expression of prostasin and matriptase has been observed in almost all normal epithelial cells, in which the pair reciprocally activate each other and maintain the epithelium integrity in a dynamic state [11–17]. The matriptase zymogen can be activated by prostasin. Subsequently, the activated matriptase can auto-activate additional matriptase zymogen, resulting in matriptase shedding from the cell surface [18–20]. Regulation of the prostasin–matriptase proteolytic activation cascade can be achieved via two Kunitz-type transmembrane serine protease inhibitors, hepatocyte growth factor activator inhibitor-1 and -2 (HAI-1 and HAI-2) [19,21–24]. The active prostasin is presented on the cell surface, whereas the active matriptase is hardly seen and almost always in a complex with HAI-1 on the cell surface or in the extracellular space [7,25,26]. HAI-1 is considered a bona fide inhibitor for matriptase, as its location is on the plasma membrane, bound to the activated matriptase [23]. HAI-2 normally shows an intracellular localization [27,28], with less chance to control the activity of matriptase on the plasma membrane.

Lymphoma is a cancer of the lymphatic system, presenting in two main types, Hodgkin lymphoma and non-Hodgkin lymphoma (NHL). The latter accounts for about 88% of all lymphoma cases and is one of the most common cancers in the United States. There will be 80,550 estimated new cases and 20,180 estimated deaths due to NHL in the United States in 2023 according to the American Cancer Society cancer facts and figures. Lymphoma is also common in children and teens, accounting for about 12% of all childhood cancers. NHL can be subdivided into more than 60 types, including Burkitt lymphoma, which is one of the fastest growing and a very aggressive tumor in humans. Treatment options for NHL are chemotherapy, radiation, and immunotherapy. For recurrent NHL patients or those refractory to the first-line therapy, there is no standard treatment, and the survival rate is rather low (10–30%), presenting an unmet challenge.

A subgroup of Burkitt lymphoma ectopically over-express matriptase [29,30] without the co-expression of prostasin (this study) typically observed in a normal epithelium. In addition, the two cognate inhibitors of matriptase, HAI-1 and HAI-2, are lacking or expressed at very low levels. An extensive survey was performed on 945 human cancer cell lines for the expression of matriptase and HAI-1 and HAI-2 [31]. Almost all epithelial cancer cell lines expressed both HAI-1 and HAI-2 (98%, 382 out of 391 cell lines), but only 20% of the hematological cancer cell lines (10 out of 51) expressed both HAI-1 and HAI-2 in the same cell line. In hematological cancer cell lines, the levels of HAI-1 and HAI-2 were relatively low. HAI-2 was more frequently co-expressed with matriptase (in 25 out of 51 cell lines, 49%) in the absence of HAI-1. Further, Burkitt lymphoma B cells expressed the highest levels of the matriptase protein and moderate levels of HAI-2 but almost no HAI-1.

It was hypothesized that the ectopic over-expression of matriptase in blood cancer cells promotes cancer progression. In two Burkitt lymphoma cell lines, Namalwa and Raji, silencing or downregulation of matriptase expression reduced the tumor cell invasion in vitro, reduced tumor growth, and increased apoptosis of xenografts in vivo in SCID mice [29,30].

The ectopic over-expression of matriptase in B cell lymphoma is an anomaly in two senses. First, it is a non-epithelial tissue in which matriptase is not normally expressed. Second, it is expressed rather independently from the familiar network of prostasin and HAIs in epithelial tissue, a feature that most likely underscores its tumor-promoting phenotype in B cell lymphoma. Intuitively, these observations invite the question of what would happen if a prostasin co-expression is introduced in the B cells over-expressing matriptase.

As a GPI-anchored protein, prostasin is known to be released into bodily fluids or in tissue culture media in the exosomes [7,32]. Exosomes are small membrane vesicles (30–150 nm in diameter) produced and released by most eukaryotic cells [33]. They contain specific membrane and cellular proteins and nucleic acids depending on the cell origin. Exosomes are capable of merging with other cells via specific receptor–ligand binding, followed by membrane fusion or endocytosis.

In recent years, prostasin exosomes in circulation or bodily fluids have been studied as potential diagnostic biomarkers in various diseases or conditions, e.g., in the urine of patients with primary aldosteronism, essential hypertension, or albuminuria [34–37]; in the blood of patients with severe coronavirus disease-2019 (COVID-19) [38]; and in the saliva of patients with oral squamous cell carcinomas [39]. Importantly, prostasin in the exosomes retains its serine protease activity [40,41].

In this study, we explore the utility of prostasin exosomes in matriptase activation in B lymphoma cells. Several B lymphoma cell lines over-expressing matriptase were chosen and were co-cultured with prostasin exosomes. Both the prostasin and matriptase serine proteases have a functional domain located outside the plasma membrane, enabling the interaction between the prostasin in the exosomes and the matriptase in the cells. Upon co-culturing, the matriptase content in the cells and in the conditioned media was determined. The activation of the prostasin–matriptase cascade was monitored by measuring the serine protease activity in the conditioned media. The migration and invasion abilities of the B lymphoma cells were examined during the prostasin–matriptase cascade activation.

2. Materials and Methods

2.1. Cell Culture

The human Burkitt lymphoma cell lines Daudi (ATCC® CCL-213™), Namalwa (ATCC® CRL-1432™), Ramos (RA 1) (ATCC® CRL-1596™), Raji (ATCC® CCL-86™), the JeKo-1 (ATCC® CRL-3006™) human mantle cell lymphoma cell line, and the RS4;11 (ATCC® CRL-1432™) human acute lymphoblastic leukemia cell line were purchased from the ATCC (American Type Culture Collection, Manassas, VA, USA). All cells were maintained according to the ATCC instructions in an incubator at 37 °C with a humidified atmosphere of 5% CO_2 in air. Tissue culture flasks and dishes were purchased from Sarstedt, Inc. (Newton, NC, USA). Heat-inactivated fetal bovine serum (FBS) was purchased from Sigma-Aldrich (St. Louis, MO, USA). Other cell culture media and reagents were purchased from Thermo Fisher Scientific (Waltham, MA, USA).

2.2. Establishment of an HEK293T Subline Over-Expressing Prostasin for Exosome Production

The HEK293T-Pro and HEK293T-Vec sublines expressing human prostasin or carrying empty pLVX-Puro vector (Clontech laboratories, Inc., Mountain View, CA, USA) were produced from the HEK293T (ATCC® CRL-3216™) human embryonic kidney cells using lentiviruses and procedures described previously [42]. The human prostasin protein was confirmed to be located on the cell-surface membrane of nearly 100% of the prostasin-expressing cells, as determined by flow cytometry.

We also established a tetracycline-regulated prostasin expression in the Namalwa cells (NamalwaTR-Pro, or NamalwaTR-ProM, a serine active-site mutant) using a previously described method [43]. Cells with the vector alone were used as the control (NamalwaTR-Vec).

2.3. Exosome Isolation and Cell Treatment

The HEK293T subline cells were cultured to confluence, and the conditioned media were collected. The conditioned media were centrifuged to remove cell debris and large vesicles and subjected to the PEG method of exosome isolation, as described in [41]. The exosome pellets were resuspended in phosphate-buffered saline (PBS) and further purified by ultracentrifugation at $100,000 \times g$ for 90 min to remove soluble protein carryovers from the culture medium. The exosome total protein concentration was determined using the Pierce™ BCA Protein Assay Kit (Thermo Fisher Scientific, Waltham, MA, USA). Calu-3 (ATCC® HTB-55™) human lung adenocarcinoma cells and derivative cells expressing various forms of prostasin, or having the prostasin gene knocked-out, were cultured as described previously [41]. B cancer cells were collected and resuspended in an assay buffer (2%FBS in RPMI medium). The amount of exosomes from 1 mL of the culture medium was defined as 1 unit. For cell–exosome co-cultures, the isolated exosomes were added at a ratio of 1 unit per 1×10^6 cells, with the final exosome concentration by total protein at 25–30 µg/mL. The cell–exosome mixture was incubated at 37 °C overnight.

2.4. Reverse Transcription and Real-Time Quantitative Polymerase Chain Reaction (RT-qPCR)

The procedures were carried out as described previously [41]. One microgram of total RNA from each sample was used for reverse transcription using the iScript reagent kit (Bio-Rad, Hercules, CA, USA), and one-fifth of the iScript product was used for each gene-specific qPCR. For quantitative comparison between samples, the relative expression levels were compared using the glyceraldehyde 3-phosphate dehydrogenase (GAPDH) copy number as the reference.

2.5. SDS-Polyacrylamide Gel Electrophoresis (PAGE), Western Blot Analysis, Gelatin-Gel Zymography

SDS-PAGE and western blot analysis were performed as described previously [41]. The original western blot figures could be found in File S1. All samples were mixed with the Laemmli sample buffer, including reducing agents, and boiled before electrophoresis. For western blot analysis, the following antibodies were used: prostasin [7]; matriptase (sc-365482, monoclonal, Santa Cruz Biotechnology, Inc., Dallas, TX, USA, or A300-221A, polyclonal, Bethyl Laboratories, Montgomery, TX, USA, or AF3946, polyclonal, R&D Systems, Inc., Minneapolis, MN, USA); HAI-2 (AF1106, R&D Systems, Inc.); and GAPDH (Santa Cruz Biotechnology). The western blot images were captured using a ChemiDoc MP Imager and analyzed with Image Lab software 6.1 (Bio-Rad).

Gelatin zymography was carried out as described previously [44]. Briefly, gelatin (Sigma) at a final concentration of 0.1% was incorporated into SDS-polyacrylamide gel (7.5–10%). Cell lysate and conditioned media were incubated with non-reducing Laemmli sample buffer at room temperature for 15 min and were resolved on the gelatin gel. After electrophoresis, the samples in the gel were renatured in a 2% Triton® X-100 (Thermo Fisher) solution with agitation for 1 h with one solution change. The gel was then incubated overnight in a buffer of 50 mM Tris at pH 8.0, containing 137 mM NaCl and 5 mM $CaCl_2$. The gel was stained with 0.25% Coomassie blue for 30–60 min, destained, and imaged using the ChemiDoc MP Imager.

2.6. Protease Activity Assay

Trypsin-like serine protease activity was measured using a synthetic tripeptide substrate Gln-Ala-Arg (QAR) with the fluorogenic leaving group AMC (Boc-QAR-AMC, R&D Systems). The conditioned media were collected by centrifugation at 24 h of co-culturing. In a 96-well plate, 10 µL of each medium sample were mixed with 90 µL of 0.1 M Tris at pH 8.5, containing 100 mM NaCl and 20 µM of the QAR substrate. The mixtures were read immediately using a SpectraMax i3x Multi-Mode Microplate Reader (Molecular Devices, San Jose, CA, USA) in the kinetic mode at 380 nm/480 nm excitation/emission for 2 h, with intervals of 2 min between readings.

2.7. Flow Cytometry

Flow cytometry was performed as described previously [41] with some modifications. A human Fc receptor-binding inhibitor polyclonal antibody (50-112-9053, Fisher Scientific) was used as a blocking agent prior to adding the primary antibodies in all B cell surface-labeling experiments. Rabbit anti-human prostasin sera or pre-immune rabbit sera [7] and the matriptase antibody (A6135, ABclonal Technology, Woburn, MA, USA) were used as the primary antibodies at 1:100 dilution. A goat anti-rabbit IgG-cyanine-Cy™3 (Jackson ImmunoResearch Laboratories, Inc., West Grove, PA, USA) was used as the secondary antibody at 1:200 dilution. The labeled cells (10,000) were analyzed using a CytoFLEX S flow cytometer with the laser configuration of V2B2Y3R2, operated by CytExpert software v2.3 (Beckman Coulter, Brea, CA, USA). The data were analyzed with FlowJo™ software v10.8.1.

2.8. Migration and Invasion

Transwell® inserts for migration and invasion were purchased from Corning Inc. (Corning, NY, USA). Human chemokines SDF-1 and CXCL 13 (BCA-1) were purchased from ProSpec (Rehovot, Israel). Chemoattractant-induced cell migration assays were performed according to procedures described previously [45] with modifications, using 5 μm Transwell cartridges (Corning, cat. No. 3421). Cells were washed with RPMI medium and incubated with exosomes at a ratio of 1 unit per 1 million cells in 100 μL of RPMI medium. The cell–exosome mixture was incubated for 2–3 h at 37 °C before seeding into the Transwells (3×10^5/100 μL per Transwell). The bottom well contained the growth medium with BCA-1 and SDF-1, at 10 ng/mL and 50 ng/mL, respectively. After 24 h of incubation, the cells in the bottom chamber were counted using the CytoFLEX S flow cytometer. The data were analyzed with FlowJo software v10.8.1. The invasion assay was performed the same way as the migration assay, with 50 μL of Matrigel® Matrix (Corning, Corning, NY, USA) added in the Transwell cartridge and gelled at 37 °C for 2 h before seeding the cells on top of the gelled matrix.

2.9. Statistical Analysis

Data were analyzed in GraphPad Prism 9 or Excel and were expressed as mean ± standard errors (SE). A student's t test was used to compare the means between two groups, in which a p value less than 0.05 was considered statistically significant. One-way analysis of variance (ANOVA) coupled with the Tukey post hoc test was used to determine statistical significance when comparing three or more independent groups, in which a p value less than 0.05 was considered statistically significant.

3. Results

3.1. Expression of Matriptase and Hepatocyte Growth Factor Activator Inhibitors (HAIs) in B Lymphoma Cell Lines

Six cell lines, including four Burkitt lymphoma cell lines, Daudi, Namalwa, Ramos, Raji, a mantle cell lymphoma cell line JeKo-1, and an acute lymphoblastic leukemia cell line RS4;11 (referred to as RS4 hereon), were evaluated for the expression of matriptase, prostasin, and HAIs at the mRNA level. As shown in Figure 1a, all four Burkitt lymphoma cell lines and the JeKo-1 cells express the matriptase (Mat) and HAI-2 mRNAs, but not the HAI-1 or the prostasin mRNA. The RS4 cells do not express matriptase or prostasin but have detectable amounts of HAI-1 and HAI-2 mRNAs. The quantitative ratio of HAI-2 to matriptase (HAI-2/Mat) differed over a wide range (Figure 1b): 0.04 in the Daudi, 2.69 in the Namalwa, 1.31 in the Ramos, 1.45 in the Raji, and 1.37 in the JeKo-1 cells.

The matriptase protein levels were analyzed in the Daudi, Namalwa, and Ramos cells, and the ratios of HAI-2 to matriptase were 0.002 in the Daudi, 0.27 in the Namalwa, and 0.07 in the Ramos cells (Figure 1c–e). The matriptase protein expression pattern is similar to that at the mRNA level. The matriptase protein levels are relatively high in the Daudi and the Ramos but low in the Namalwa cells. The HAI-2 level is high in the Ramos but hardly detectable in the Daudi cells. The proteolytic activity of matriptase may be better controlled by HAI-2 in the Namalwa cells than in the Ramos cells, but it is not well-controlled in the Daudi cells. These results are in agreement with previous studies [30,31].

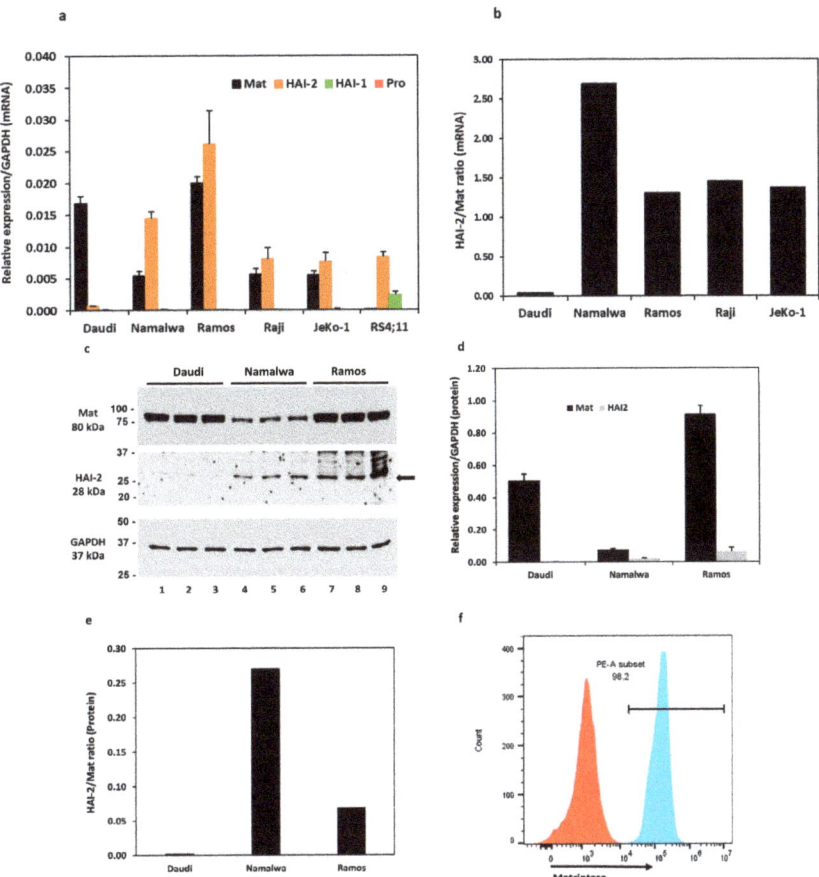

Figure 1. Expression analysis of matriptase, HAI-1, HAI-2, and prostasin in B cancer cells by reverse-transcription/qPCR (**a**,**b**), western blotting (**c**–**e**), and flow cytometry (**f**). (**a**) Bar graph of relative mRNA expression levels of matriptase (Mat), HAI-1, HAI-2, prostasin (Pro) in Daudi ($n = 4$), Namalwa ($n = 5$), Ramos ($n = 3$), Raji ($n = 3$), JeKo-1 ($n = 3$), and RS4;11 cells ($n = 2$) using GAPDH as the reference. The prostasin bars do not appear in the bar graph, as the actual qPCR readouts were registered as "N/A" by the instrument. (**b**) Bar graph of mRNA quantity ratio of HAI-2 to matriptase after normalization with the GAPDH level in each cell line in (**a**). (**c**) Western blotting images of matriptase (Ab: A300-221A), HAI-2, and GAPDH. Twenty micrograms of total protein from the cell lysate of each individual culture (including 2 repeats) were analyzed. Daudi, lanes 1–3; Namalwa, lanes 4–6; Ramos, lanes 7–9. Top panel, matriptase (Mat); middle panel, HAI-2; bottom panel, GAPDH. (**d**) Densitometry bar graph of relative protein quantities of matriptase and HAI-2 using GAPDH as the reference. (**e**) The quantitative ratio of HAI-2 to matriptase in each cell line. (**f**) Flow cytometry histogram of matriptase expression evaluation in Ramos cells. The Ramos cells (4×10^5) were labeled with the matriptase antibody as described in the Materials and Methods section. The matriptase-positive cells are shown in the PE-A subset (blue peak). Cells without the matriptase antibody labeling (red peak) were not detected in the PE-A subset and were used as the gating control.

We further showed by flow cytometry that the matriptase protein is localized on the cell surface of Ramos cells. The Ramos cells were fixed without permeabilization and labeled with a polyclonal matriptase antibody, followed by the secondary antibody conjugated with the fluorophore Cy3 (Figure 1f, PE-A subset/blue peak). Matriptase was localized on the cell surface in 98.2% of the live singlet Ramos cells. The cells that went through the labeling procedures without the matriptase antibody were used as the gating control (Figure 1f, red peak). The matriptase protein in these B lymphoma cells is transported to the cell surface and has an opportunity to interact with its substrates, e.g., prostasin, or inhibitors, e.g., the HAIs.

3.2. Prostasin Exosomes Reduce the Matriptase Protein Level in B Lymphoma Cells

We have previously shown in Calu-3 human lung adenocarcinoma cells that the prostasin protein can be released into the culturing medium, retaining its serine protease activity in the lipid bilayer of exosomes [41]. Prostasin has been reported to activate matriptase [40,42,46–48]. Here, we show that adding prostasin exosomes in the Daudi cell culture activated matriptase and released matriptase into the culturing medium (Figure 2). Prostasin-enriched exosomes were isolated from the conditioned medium of Calu-3 cells over-expressing prostasin (Pro), whereas prostasin-depleted exosomes were isolated from Calu-3 cells lacking prostasin expression as a result of CRISPR/Cas9 mediated gene knock-out (KO) [41]. As shown in Figure 2a (top panel), upon incubation with the prostasin exosomes (Pro, lanes 2, 4, 6, 8), the quantity of matriptase in the Daudi cells was greatly reduced to about 22% of that in the cells incubated with the exosomes without prostasin (KO, lanes 1, 3, 5, 7). Conversely, the amount of matriptase released into the medium of cells incubated with the prostasin KO exosomes was only about 4% of that in the medium of cells incubated with the prostasin exosomes. The amounts of matriptase in the cell lysate and media are inversely correlated (Figure 2c,d). This result indicated that prostasin can devolve matriptase from the cell surface into the medium. The GAPDH protein was detected in all cell lysate samples but barely detectable in the media (Figure 2b).

Similarly, as shown in Figure 2e, the prostasin-enriched exosomes (Pexo) isolated from the HEK293T cells over-expressing prostasin greatly reduced the matriptase amount in the Daudi (lane 3), the Namalwa (lane 6), and the Ramos (lane 9) cells, in comparison to the cells treated with the vector control exosomes (Vexo) isolated from the HEK293T cells harboring the empty lentiviral vector (lanes 2, 5, 8). Cells treated with the Vexo exosomes appeared to have a lower matriptase level than cells without the exosome treatment (None, lanes 1, 4, 7), but the difference was not statically significant ($p > 0.05$). The HEK293T exosomes were validated using exosome markers, and the exosomal prostasin was shown to be active using an established protease nexin-1 binding assay [7] (Figure S1).

These results suggest that matriptase ectopically expressed in B cancer cells was activated by the prostasin exosomes and shed from the cells, similar to observations described for epithelial cells [18–20]. The event of matriptase activation and shedding from the cells is accompanied by the release of a low-molecular-weight (LMW) fragment (28–30 kDa) in the medium. As shown in Figure 2g, this LMW matriptase fragment was detected more prominently in the conditioned media of cells treated with the prostasin exosomes (Pexo, lanes 4, 6, 8), in comparison to that of cells treated with the vector control exosomes (Vexo, lanes 3, 5, 7). The matriptase profile, including the matriptase complexes, in the conditioned media is very similar to that reported previously for these B lymphoma cell lines upon acid activation of matriptase [31].

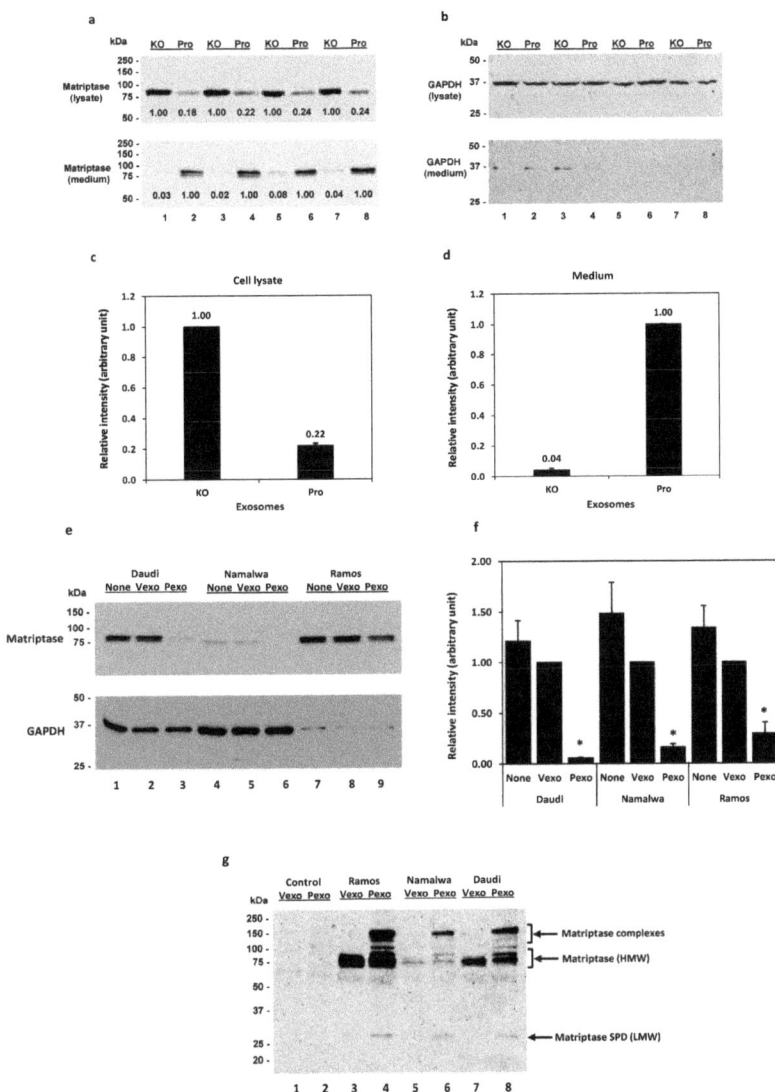

Figure 2. Prostasin exosomes reduce matriptase quantity in B cancer cells. (**a**) Western blot images of matriptase (Ab: A300-221A) in samples from the cell lysate (top panel) and the conditioned media (bottom panel) after incubation with prostasin exosomes (Pro) or exosomes without prostasin (KO). The Daudi cells (2×10^5 cells each) were incubated with the exosomes in 50 µL of OPTI-MEM I/2%FBS (lanes 1–4) or RPMI medium (lanes 5–8) overnight. One-half of each cell lysate or 40 µL of each media supernatant were analyzed. (**b**) Western blot images of GAPDH from (**a**). (**c**) Densitometry of relative intensities of matriptase in the cell lysate or media (**d**). Data presented are the average intensity of lanes 1, 3, 5, 7 versus that of lanes 2, 4, 6, 8 after normalization with GAPDH in (**b**). (**e**) Western blot images of matriptase (top panel; Ab: sc-365482) in the Daudi, Namalwa, and Ramos cells treated with exosomes isolated from the HEK293T cells. Cells (2.5×10^5) were co-cultured with prostasin exosomes (Pexo, lanes 3, 6, 9) or vector exosomes (Vexo, lanes 2, 5, 8) in 100 µL of OPTI-MEM I/2%FBS. Cells without exosomes (None, lanes 1, 4, 7) were cultured in the same conditions. Bottom, GAPDH western blot image. (**f**) Bar graph of (**e**) expressed as the relative intensities of matriptase

in cells treated with vector exosomes (Vexo), prostasin exosomes (Pexo), or no exosomes (None) using GAPDH as the reference. * denotes $p < 0.05$ between Vexo and Pexo. (**g**) Western blot image of matriptase (Ab: AF3946) in conditioned media (20 µL each) of samples in (**e**) treated with exosomes. The AF3946 human matriptase/ST14 catalytic domain antibody recognized a 28–30 kDa band in the Pexo-treated sample media. This antibody also recognized the high-molecular-weight (HMW) matriptase at 80-kDa as well as unknown/uncharacterized matriptase complexes in the Pexo-treated sample media. The Vexo and Pexo samples alone were included in the blot as controls, in which no specific proteins were recognized by this antibody.

3.3. The GPI Anchor and the Serine Active Site of Prostasin Play Roles in the Reduction of Matriptase Quantity in B Lymphoma Cells

Exosomes carrying over-expressed prostasin variants were isolated from a series of Calu-3 sublines as previously described [41] and incubated with the Daudi, Ramos, and Namalwa cells. The amount of cell-associated matriptase was analyzed by SDS-PAGE/western blotting and quantified by densitometry using GAPDH as the reference. The amount of matriptase was much less in the Daudi, Ramos, and Namalwa cells treated with exosomes carrying the GPI-anchored active prostasin (P) than in the cells treated with exosomes carrying a prostasin active-site mutant (M) or exosomes from cells expressing a GPI-anchor-free prostasin (G). The GPI-anchor-free prostasin is secreted and not expected to be present on the exosomes. Exosomes isolated from other Calu-3 sublines, including the prostasin-knockout (KO) and its control (CC), and the control subline (V) for the over-expression lines (P, M, G) did not significantly reduce the matriptase level in the B lymphoma cells (Figure 3a,b). The wild-type prostasin with both the membrane anchorage and the serine active site provided the most robust matriptase removal power (Figure 3c).

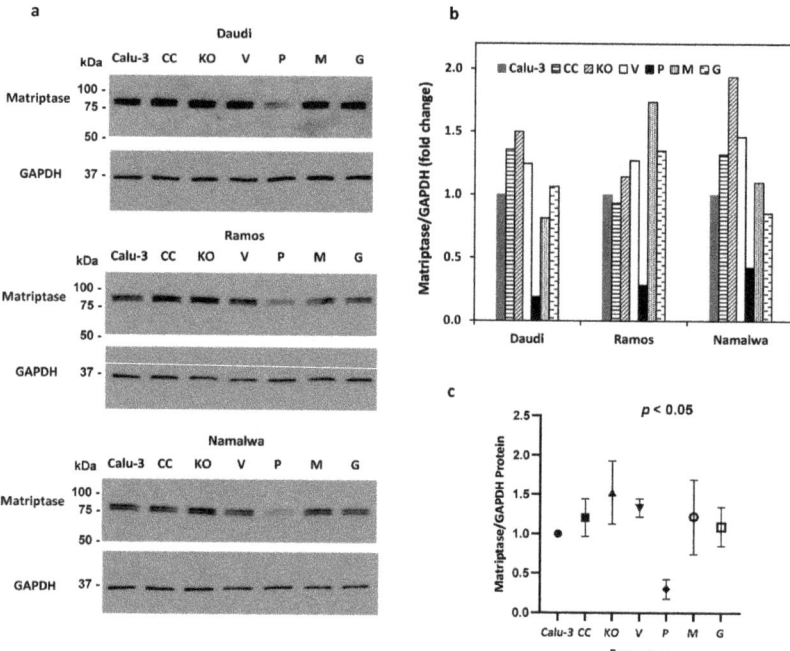

Figure 3. B cell matriptase quantity reduction by wild-type prostasin. (**a**) Western blot images of matriptase (Ab: sc-365482) and GAPDH in the Daudi (top two panels), Ramos (middle two panels), and Namalwa (bottom two panels) cells treated with exosomes isolated from the Calu-3 cells and sublines with over-expressed prostasin or variants. Calu-3, parent cells; KO, subline with prostasin

gene knockout; P, subline with the wild-type prostasin; M, subline with a serine active-site mutant prostasin; G, subline with an active prostasin without the GPI anchor; CC and V are control sublines for KO and P,M,G, respectively. The intensity of each band was quantified using Image Lab 6.1 software (Bio-Rad), normalized against the corresponding GAPDH signal, and is shown in the bar graph (**b**). (**c**) Effects of various prostasin exosomes on matriptase quantity reduction in B cancer cells. Data from (**b**) were combined and analyzed in GraphPad Prism 9 and are shown in the dot plot. ANOVA $p < 0.05$.

3.4. Trypsin-like Serine Protease Activity Is Increased in the Conditioned Media of Cells Treated with Prostasin Exosomes

The Daudi, Namalwa, Ramos, Raji, Jeko, and RS4 cells were co-cultured overnight with prostasin exosomes (Pexo) or the vector control exosomes (Vexo) prepared from the HEK293T-Pro or Vec cells, respectively. Cells without any addition of exosomes were also cultured in the same conditions. As shown in Figure 4a,c, the conditioned media from the cells treated with the prostasin exosomes (Pexo) had a higher trypsin-like serine protease activity than that of cells treated with the vector exosomes (Vexo). The highest activity was detected in the Pexo media of the Daudi cells, coinciding with the high matriptase expression level in these cells (Figure 1a). The lowest activity was in the Pexo media of the Jeko-1 cells, coinciding with a lower matriptase expression level (Figure 1a). The media of cells with the Vexo or no exosome (RPMI) have similar and low levels of protease activity (Figure 4a). The Vexo or Pexo sample with the exosomes alone also has measurable serine protease activity (Figure 4b) but at much lower levels. The activity of Pexo measures at ~2.3% of that in the Daudi conditioned media or ~9% of that in the Jeko-1 conditioned media from co-culturing with Pexo. This low level of protease activity is attributed to the intrinsic serine protease activity of the exosomes, especially in Pexo [7,41].

In duplicate experiments, we showed that upon prostasin exosome treatment, the elevated trypsin-like serine protease activity remained high for at least 10 days (Figure 4d). This phenomenon was only seen for the matriptase-expressing cells, but not the RS4 cells, which do not express matriptase. These results suggest that the increased trypsin-like serine protease activity may be attributed to the increased amount of matriptase released into the conditioned media after the prostasin exosome treatment.

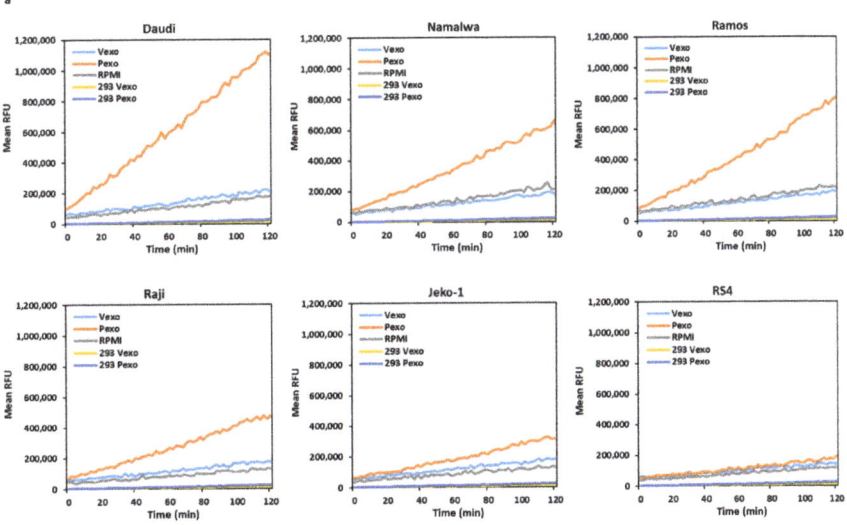

Figure 4. *Cont.*

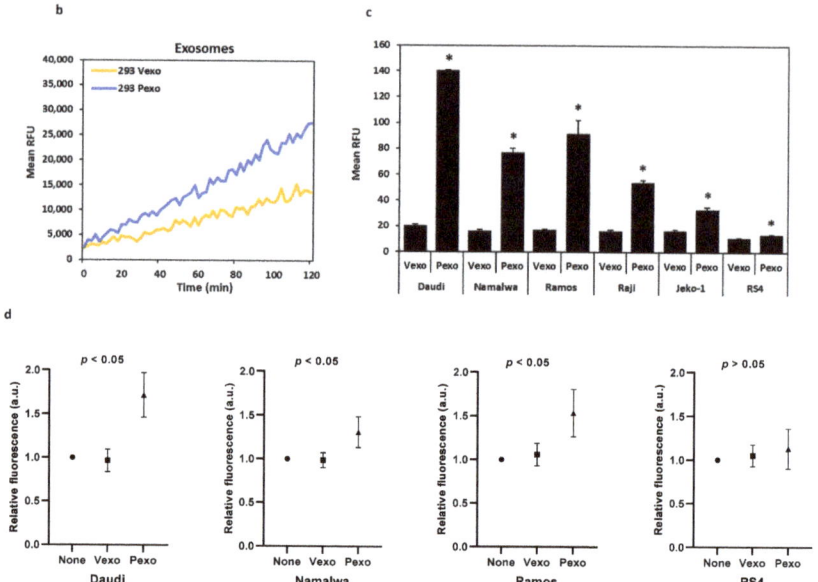

Figure 4. Trypsin-like serine protease activity measurement. (**a**) Line graphs of trypsin-like serine protease activity expressed as relative fluorescent units (RFU). After mixing 2×10^6 cells with exosomes (Vexo or Pexo) or with RPMI medium alone in a total volume of 500 µL for 24 h, the activity in the conditioned medium was measured continually for 120 min. (**b**) Activity graph of Vexo or Pexo exosomes from the HEK293T-Vec or Pro cells in RPMI medium without cells, used as background controls. (**c**) Bar graph of data from (**a**) after subtracting the background controls of (**b**). * denotes $p < 0.05$. (**d**) Dot plots of trypsin-like serine protease activity in media collected 10 days after cell–exosome co-culturing. a.u., arbitrary units. Data were analyzed in GraphPad Prism 9. ANOVA, $p < 0.05$ for Daudi, Namalwa, and Ramos, $p > 0.05$ for RS4.

3.5. Over-Expression of Prostasin Reduces Matriptase Quantity in B Cells

The Daudi, Namalwa, and Ramos cells were transduced with a lentivirus harboring the human prostasin cDNA for over-expression [42]. The cells were collected 24 h post-infection, lysed, and subjected to SDS-PAGE/western blot analysis using antibodies against matriptase, prostasin, or GAPDH, respectively. In cells with prostasin over-expression (Figure 5a, middle panel, lanes 2, 4, 6), the matriptase expression was almost abolished, in comparison to the cells without prostasin (Figure 5a, top panel, lanes 1, 3, 5). The GAPDH contents were used as the loading controls (Figure 5a, bottom panel).

In the NamalwaTR sublines, upon tetracycline induction, the NamalwaTR-Pro cells expressed a great amount of prostasin at the cell surface with the GPI anchor (Figure 5b, green peak), whereas the NamalwaTR-Vec cells did not express prostasin (Figure 5b, orange peak). At least 95.4% of the NamalwaTR cells were shown by flow cytometry to express prostasin after the tetracycline induction, as indicated by the right-shifted peak (PE-A subset/green peak), representing the cells labeled with a polyclonal prostasin antibody and the fluorophore-conjugated secondary antibody. The tetracycline-treated NamalwaTR-Vec (red peak) and NamalwaTR-Pro (sky-blue peak) cells without the prostasin antibody incubation that went through the same labeling procedures were negative for prostasin staining. Their representative peaks appear to the far left on the x-axis. The ectopically expressed prostasin protein in the B cells was correctly transported on the B cell surface.

In the long-term culture of tet-regulated NamalwaTR sublines, a sustained presence of the wild-type prostasin abolished the cellular matriptase presence (Figure 5c, lane 2), but the serine active-site mutant prostasin did not elicit such an effect (Figure 5c, lane 3). The cells cultured without tetracycline were analyzed and run as controls, wherein the cellular matriptase level appeared similar across the sublines (Figure 5c, lanes 4, 5, 6). The wild-type prostasin expressed in the NamalwaTR-Pro cells appeared in two bands, indicating a sustained activation. The conditioned media of these sublines in the long-term tet-induced culture also reproduced the shed-off matriptase profile (Figure 5d). The NamalwaTR-Pro cell medium had a much higher quantity of LMW matriptase, in comparison to that of the NamalwaTR-Vec or ProM cells.

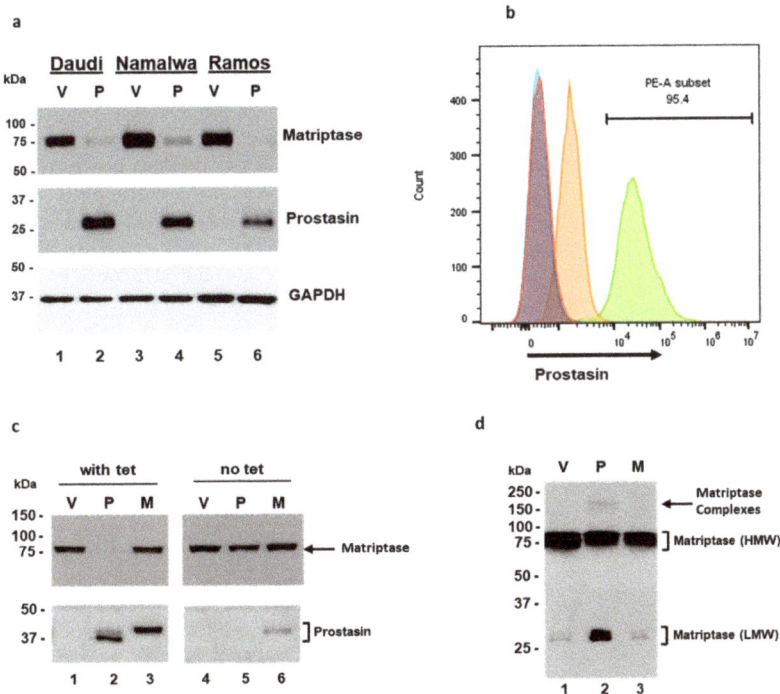

Figure 5. Ectopic expression of prostasin in B cancer cells. (a) Western blot analysis of transient expression of prostasin (P) or vector alone (V) in the Daudi, Namalwa, and Ramos cells. The lysate from 2×10^5 cells of each type was analyzed. Top panel, matriptase (Ab: sc-365482); middle panel, prostasin; bottom panel, GAPDH. (b) Flow cytometry analysis of Namalwa sublines with tetracycline-induced prostasin expression or vector alone. Red peak (vector-alone cells) and sky-blue peak (prostasin-expressing cells) are samples without the prostasin antibody incubation. Orange peak (vector-alone cells) and green peak (prostasin-expressing cells) are samples incubated with the prostasin antibody. All samples were incubated with a secondary antibody conjugated with the fluorophore Cy3, and 10,000 cells of each sample were analyzed in a CytoFLEX S flow cytometer. The data were analyzed with FlowJo™ software v10.8.1 and are presented in the histogram. (c) Western blot analysis of NamalwaTR sublines. One hundred thousand cells of each sample were analyzed. Lanes 1 and 4 or V, samples of the vector control subline; lanes 2 and 5 or P, samples of the subline with the wild-type prostasin; lanes 3 and 6 or M, samples of the subline with a serine active-site mutant prostasin. Left panel, cells were grown in OPTI-MEM I/2%FBS with 1 µg/mL tetracycline (with tet); right panel, cells were grown without tetracycline (no tet) for 8 days. Top two panels, matriptase antibody (sc-365482); bottom two panels, prostasin antibody. (d) Western blot analysis of tet-conditioned media from (c). Two hundred milliliters of the conditioned media were precipitated with trichloroacetic acid (TCA) (final 16.7%) at 4 °C overnight. The pellet was collected via centrifugation and analyzed. The membrane was blotted with the AF3946 human matriptase/ST14 catalytic domain antibody.

3.6. Proliferation, Migration, Invasion, and Gelatinase Activity Changes Associated with Prostasin

We have shown in Figures 2, 3 and 5 that prostasin reduced the matriptase level in B cancer cells, similar to the observations in epithelial cells in which prostasin over-expression reduced cellular matriptase levels [42,47]. We set out experiments to determine whether the prostasin-exosome-mediated reduction in the matriptase level impacts the growth, migration, and invasion properties of the B cancer cells.

3.6.1. Proliferation and Apoptosis

The Namalwa, Ramos, Raji, and Jeko-1 cells were cultured with prostasin exosomes (Pexo) or the control vector exosomes (Vexo) in a serum-reduced medium at a ratio of 1 unit of exosomes per 1×10^6 cells in 500 μL. The number of cells in each sample was monitored by flow cytometry. Cell numbers were not significantly different in two days of the co-culture between the samples treated with prostasin exosomes and vector exosomes, except for the Namalwa cells. There was a slight decrease (by 9%) in cell number in the samples treated with prostasin exosomes in 24 h, in comparison to that treated with the vector exosomes (Figure 6a). When the NamalwaTR-Pro cells at a concentration of 2.5×10^5 cells per milliliter were induced to over-express prostasin (Pro) with tetracycline (1 μg/mL), the growth rate of these cells decreased significantly on Day 4, with lower cell numbers in comparison to the tetracycline-treated NamalwaTR-Vec control cells (Vec) (Figure 6b, left graph). The cells were then diluted to a density of 5×10^5 cells per milliliter and re-cultured for another five days in the serum-reduced medium. The growth rate of the NamalwaTR-Pro cells continued to decline, in comparison to the NamalwaTR-Vec cells in the same culturing condition (Figure 6b, right graph).

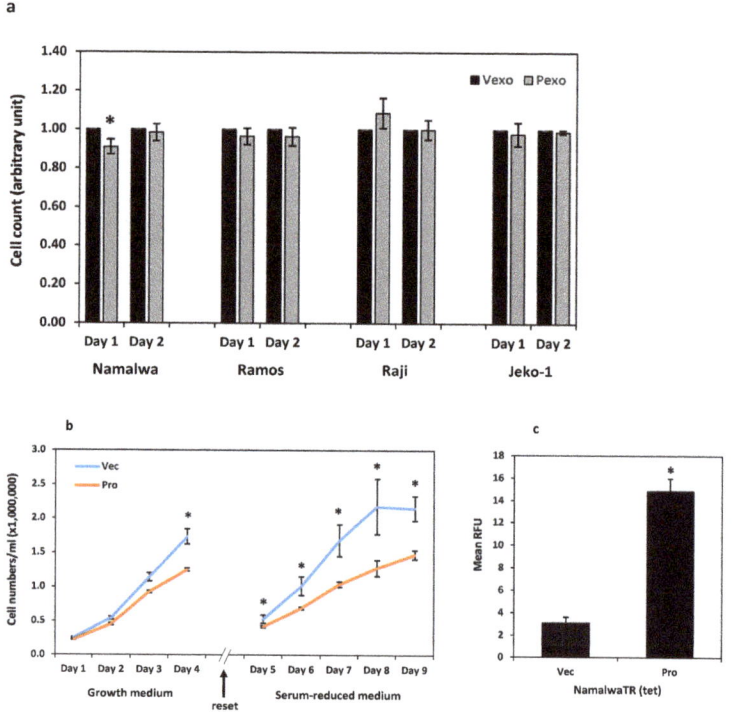

Figure 6. *Cont.*

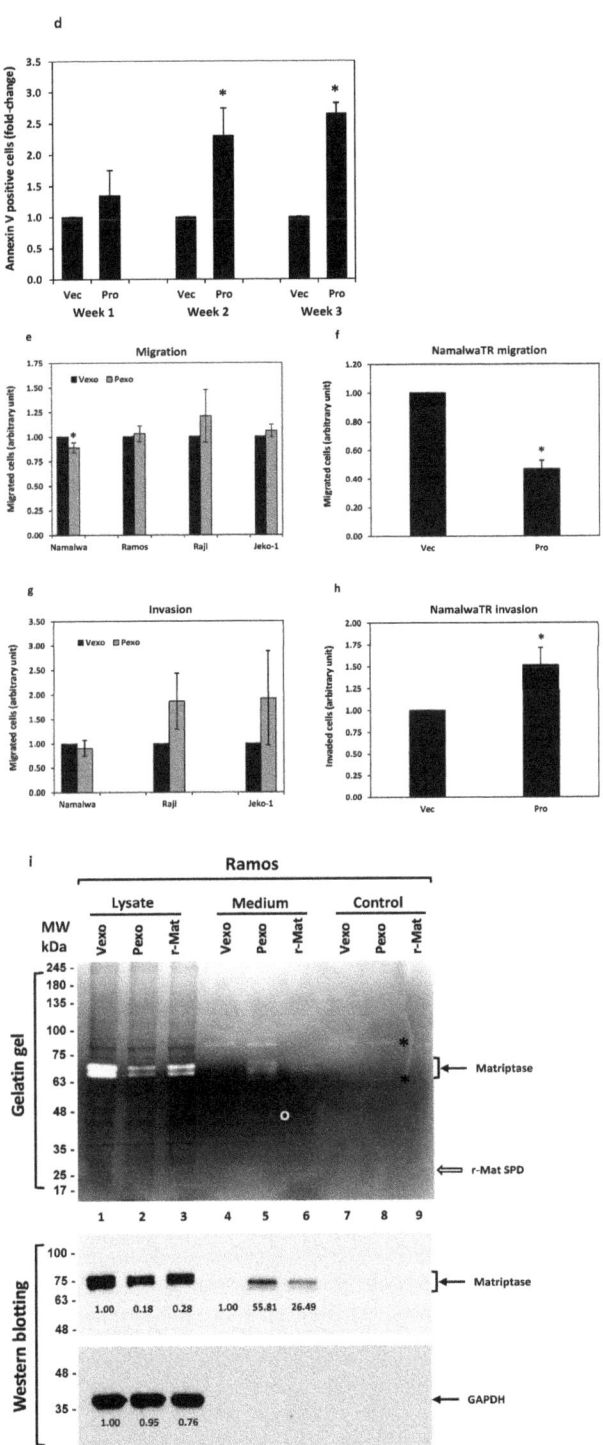

Figure 6. Cont.

j

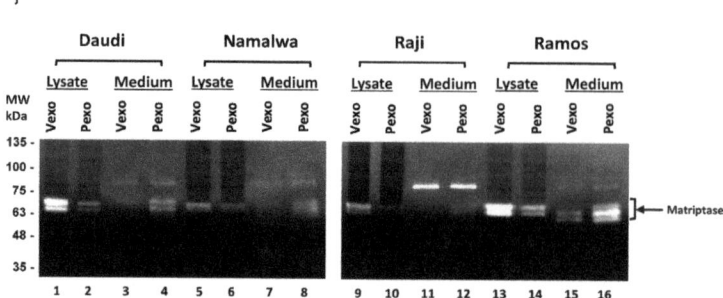

Figure 6. Impact of prostasin–matriptase cascade activation on B cancer cells. (**a**) Bar graph of cell count for two consecutive days of B cells treated with exosomes. Namalwa, $n = 7$; Ramos, $n = 6$; Raji, $n = 5$; Jeko-1, $n = 6$. * denotes $p < 0.05$. (**b**) Growth curves of NamalwaTR-Vec and NamalwaTR-Pro cells under tetracycline induction. Left graph, cells were set at 2.5×10^5/mL on day 0 and cultured in the growth medium containing 10%FBS for 4 days. Right graph, on day 4 (reset, indicated by the arrow), the cells were diluted in OPTI-MEM I/2%FBS to 5×10^5/mL and cultured for another 5 days. Tetracycline at 1 µg/mL was added into the culture on day 0 and maintained through culturing. $n = 4$ for each cell line, and * denotes $p < 0.05$. (**c**) Trypsin-like serine protease activity in the conditioned media of NamalwaTR-Vec and NamalwaTR-Pro cells ($n = 4$). Data were analyzed in Excel with student's t test. * denotes $p < 0.05$ between the two sample groups. (**d**) Bar graph of annexin-V-positive cells analyzed by flow cytometry. Cells under tetracycline induction were cultured for various times (week 1, $n = 3$; week 2, $n = 4$; week 3, $n = 3$) and subjected to direct labeling of annexin V conjugated with fluorophore allophycocyanin (APC). Ten thousand cells for each sample were analyzed on the CytoFLEX S flow cytometer. Propidium iodide staining and FSC/SSC discrimination were used for gating the live singlets, which were further analyzed for annexin V staining. (**e**) Bar graph of migrated cells treated with exosomes for 24 h. * denotes $p < 0.05$. (**f**) Bar graph of migrated Namalwa sublines with the induction of prostasin expression for 2–4 days and reconditioned in RPMI medium for 1 day before seeding in Transwells for migration ($n = 7$). * denotes $p < 0.05$. (**g**) Bar graph of invaded cells treated with exosomes for 24 h. (**h**) Bar graph of invaded Namalwa sublines ($n = 5$) treated as in (**f**). * denotes $p < 0.05$. (**i**) Gelatin zymography and western blot analysis. Top panel, the Ramos cells (2×10^6) in 500 µL of RPMI/0.1%BSA were treated with vector exosomes (Vexo), prostasin exosomes (Pexo), or a purified recombinant human matriptase serine protease domain (r-Mat SPD) overnight. One-fifth of the cell lysate (lanes 1–3) or 20 µL of the conditioned medium (lanes 4–6) were analyzed. The Vexo or Pexo exosomes or the r-Mat SPD alone were incubated in RPMI/0.1%BSA and used as controls (lanes 7–9). The clear bands at ~70 kDa marked by a filled arrow are matriptase. These were recognized by matriptase antibodies (middle panel). Unidentified bands with gelatinase activity marked at * locations in lanes 4, 5, 7, 8 are inherited from the exosomes, as shown in the samples with the exosomes alone (lanes 7 and 8). The band marked by the white circle is unknown. Bands at ~28 kDa marked by an unfilled arrow are r-Mat SPD. Bottom panel is GAPDH, which is detected only in the cell lysate, not in media samples or the controls without cells. (**j**) Gelatin zymography of B cancer cells treated as described in (**i**). The matriptase gelatinase activity is decreased in the cell lysate (lanes 2, 6, 10, 14) but increased in the corresponding media samples (lanes 4, 8, 12, 16) upon Pexo treatment in comparison to that of the Vexo-treated samples (in lysate, lanes 1, 5, 9, 13; in media, lanes 3, 7, 11, 15), correspondingly.

The prolonged presence of prostasin in B cancer cells reduced cell growth, a phenotype possibly associated with a sustained activation of the prostasin-matriptase cascade. Indeed, the conditioned media of the cells over-expressing prostasin (Pro) had higher trypsin-like serine protease activity than that of the cells with the empty vector (Vec) (Figure 6c). This result is also consistent with the data presented in Figure 4, in which the conditioned media of the cells treated with prostasin exosomes have higher trypsin-like serine protease activity than that of the cells treated with the vector exosomes.

The active matriptase is toxic to cells [10,23,48–50] when its inhibitors, i.e., the HAIs are absent in the cells. Such is the case in most hematological cancer cell lines [31]. The annexin V protein is an established cellular marker for apoptotic cells with its high binding affinity to the anionic phospholipid phosphatidylserine (PS), which is localized to the outer leaflet of the plasma membrane in apoptotic cells [51,52]. We show in Figure 6d that the amount of cell-surface annexin V in the NamalwaTR-Pro cells increased during longer culturing times, in comparison to that in the NamalwaTR-Vec cells. The increased apoptosis of the NamalwaTR-Pro cells might have contributed at least partially to the reduced growth of these cells (Figure 6b).

3.6.2. Migration and Invasion

Physiologically, B cells migrate from one tissue to another, with chemotaxis following an increasing chemokine concentration gradient. We assessed the chemotactic migration ability of B cancer cells during the activation of the prostasin-matriptase cascade. Upon treatment with either prostasin exosomes or vector exosomes, the Ramos, Raji, and Jeko-1 cells did not have a significant change in migration through the membrane with a 5 μm pore size (Figure 6e). The Namalwa cells in the same setting had a slightly reduced migration (by ~11%). The Daudi cells did not migrate or invade under the same experimental conditions, and the RS4 cells did not express matriptase. Both cells were excluded here. For the NamalwaTR-Pro cells induced to over-express prostasin (Pro), a significant reduction in migration (by over 50%) was observed (Figure 6f) in comparison to the NamalwaTR-Vec cells.

When the Matrigel matrix was constructed in the Transwell to assess the invasion properties of the B cancer cells under the influence of prostasin exosomes, there were no significant changes in invasion (Figure 6g). The Ramos cells did not invade efficiently through the Matrigel matrix under the same conditions. The NamalwaTR-Pro cells over-expressing prostasin showed a significant increase in invasion (by over 50%) through the Matrigel matrix (Figure 6h). A sustained prostasin–matriptase cascade activation appeared to decrease migration but increase invasion for the Namalwa cells in the presence of chemokines.

3.6.3. Gelatinase Activity

Matriptase was reported to have gelatinase activity [44,53], which offers a direct method to visually monitor the matriptase expression and function regulation phenotypes associated with prostasin endowment in B cancer cells. We evaluated the matriptase gelatinase activity in gelatin gels following electrophoresis. As shown in Figure 6i (top panel, lane 1), matriptase in the Ramos cells treated with vector exosomes (Vexo) cleaved the gelatin in the gel, producing clear doublet bands after staining with Coomassie blue dye. The bands correspond to the matriptase protein, recognized by the matriptase antibody (Figure 6i, middle panel, lane 1). Due to the different conditions used for the gelatin gel, i.e., non-reducing and without sample boiling, the matriptase protein appeared at the ~70 kDa position in the gelatin gel, as opposed to the ~80 kDa position in the SDS-APGE/western blot. The prostasin exosome (Pexo) treatment reduced the matriptase level in the Ramos cells (Figure 6i, middle panel, lane 2) and correspondingly reduced the associated gelatinase activity (Figure 6i, top panel, lane 2). A purified recombinant human matriptase serine protease domain (r-Mat SPD, R&D Systems), when added (0.2 nM) in the Ramos cell culture, also reduced the quantity of the endogenous matriptase (Figure 6i, middle panel, lane 3) and the gelatinase activity of the endogenously expressed matriptase (Figure 6i, top panel, lane 3), suggesting that the soluble active matriptase can further activate more cellular matriptase zymogen.

Prostasin exosomes mediated a reduction in the matriptase level in B cancer cells but an increase in the amount of matriptase in the culturing medium, with correspondingly increased gelatinase activity (Figure 6i, top panel, lane 5). The shed matriptase was recognized by the matriptase antibody (Figure 6i, middle panel, lane 5). Cells treated with the vector exosomes did not show very much matriptase released into the medium (Figure 6i, top and middle panels, lane 4). Cells treated with the r-Mat SPD released the endogenously expressed matriptase into the medium as well (Figure 6i, top and middle panels, lane 6). There was no detectable matriptase protein or gelatinase activity in samples with exosomes alone (lanes 7 and 8). The gelatinase activity of the r-Mat SPD was detected in samples either alone or in the Ramos cell culture medium (Figure 6i, top panel, lanes 9 and 6).

The gelatinase activity of matriptase was also examined in the Daudi, Namalwa, and Raji cells, as shown in Figure 6j. Consistent with the results from the Ramos cells, the gelatinase activity of matriptase was low in the cells but high in the media after the prostasin exosome treatment in comparison to that of the cells treated with vector exosomes. The RS4 cells do not express matriptase and do not have matriptase-associated gelatinase activity (Figure S2). These results suggest that prostasin exosomes mediated the shedding of matriptase from the cell surface into the extracellular medium, whereas the shed-off matriptase retained its gelatinase activity, which could be involved in extracellular matrix modification.

4. Discussion

Therapies targeting B-cell-specific markers have been developed in recent years for treating B cell diseases such as B cell lymphoma [54]. Rituximab is a monoclonal antibody developed to target CD20 on the B cell surface to remove aberrant B cells. MEDI-551, another monoclonal antibody, was developed to target CD19 on B cells to induce cytotoxicity. The required dose of MEDI-551 is lower than that of rituximab, and MEDI-551 depletes different subsets of plasma cells due to differential expression patterns of CD20 and CD19 on B cells. The monoclonal antibody epratuzumab targets CD22 to trigger signaling pathways in B cells and interfere with B cell proliferation. Other therapeutic strategies targeting B cell survival factors and mediators involved in intercellular and intracellular B cell functions are also in progress.

The prominent ectopic over-expression of matriptase, an otherwise epithelial-specific extracellular membrane serine protease in B cancer cells, presents a logical cell-surface molecule for targeting. In epithelial cells in which prostasin and matriptase are co-expressed, prostasin over-expression downregulates the matriptase level, and an insufficient prostasin expression level results in an upregulation of the matriptase level [42,47]. Upon zymogen activation, matriptase is shed from the cells, with an accumulation of the shed-off active matriptase in the culturing medium [20]. In most cases, the activated matriptase is almost immediately complexed with its inhibitor HAI-1, preventing further unwarranted matriptase activation and subsequent cytotoxicity. However, in hematological cancer cell lines, only 20% express both HAI-1 and HAI-2 in the same cells. In a subgroup of Burkitt lymphoma, HAI-1 is not expressed, with HAI-2 expressed at a very low quantity.

Such a molecular landscape would suggest that the over-expressed matriptase in the B cancer cells is in the inactive zymogen form. If matriptase is activated in these B cells, it could initiate an untamed matriptase auto-activation cascade with a subsequent cytotoxicity triggered by a stressed Gogi-endoplasmic reticulum apparatus [23]. Given the peculiarity of matriptase over-expression in B cancer cells in the absence of prostasin, and absence or scarcity of HAIs, we hypothesized that an endowment of prostasin expression could initiate the proteolytic activation cascade. We aimed to use prostasin exosomes to achieve this, with a long-term consideration of developing a clinically feasible approach for alternative treatment of B cell lymphoma, based on the burgeoning momentum of exosomes on this front.

Our attempt at directing a prostasin action onto the B cancer cell surface via the exosomes appeared to have been successful, with a very clear phenotype of matriptase quantity and functional changes. This was achieved with prostasin exosomes prepared from a cell type with a full complement of relevant proteins, Calu-3 human lung cancer cells, expressing endogenous prostasin, HAI-1, and HAI-2; or HEK293T cells, with null or minimal expression levels of all three. The cellular matriptase content was greatly reduced, with a corresponding increase in the shed-off soluble enzyme in the culture medium. Along with the molecular changes, tumor cell behaviors were also modified, with phenotypes consistent with the tumor suppressor role of prostasin, such as reduced growth and increased apoptosis. It is not surprising that not all cell lines manifested a uniform phenotypic response to prostasin, given the nature of cancer cells.

Using the various control conditions and prostasin variants as described, the action is more robust with GPI-anchored membrane-bound serine protease-active prostasin. It remains technically challenging to ascertain an actual molecular transfer of the exosome prostasin cargo onto the recipient B cells. But a prostasin-specific effect was supported by the lentiviral-transduced prostasin expression in the B cells, recapitulating the exosome delivery phenotypes. The lentiviral-transduced prostasin expression also allowed us to tease out a long-term phenotype associated with prostasin expression in B cancer cells, i.e., growth inhibition (Figure 6b).

The introduction of prostasin to the B cancer cells clearly resulted in the release of matriptase into the culture medium (Figure 2a), which had a corresponding gain of trypsin-like serine protease activity, as measured by the cleavage of the synthetic substrate QAR-AMC (Figure 4a). The QAR (P3-P1) is a highly selective matriptase and prostasin substrate that has been routinely used to demonstrate proteolysis by these specific serine proteases in complex sample contexts, such as cell lysate or living cells [25]. The B lymphoma cell lines used in this study were all validated for QAR selectivity toward matriptase in the conditioned media upon acid activation by a previous study [31]. The conditioned media tested for QAR cleavage would not have very appreciable amounts of prostasin, which would be even across the different cell types if there were residual amounts from the exosome treatment. The QAR-cleaving activities in the conditioned media at different levels across the cell types may thus be attributed to the shed-off active matriptase. The cellular matriptase in the B cancer cells was considered to be in the zymogen form, but in the gelatin zymography experiment, it showed gelatinase activity in the cell lysate (Figure 6i). The gelatin-degrading matriptase in the gel in situ underwent SDS denaturation during electrophoresis and renaturation for zymography. This process may very well have resulted in the activation of the enzyme in situ. Such a phenomenon was documented for the zymogen of trypsin (trypsinogen), showing a strong activity in gelatin zymography performed under conditions similar to those used here [55].

A question that arises and also remains concerns the fate and function of the shed-off soluble active matriptase upon the introduction of prostasin in the B cancer cells. We were able to induce a similar response with the use of a soluble recombinant human matriptase protease domain (Figure 6i). Thus, we may speculate that the shed-off soluble active matriptase would be able to do the same. We may also expect that newly synthesized matriptase zymogen would be perpetually subjected to a cycle of proteolytic activation and shedding, independent of the initial prostasin trigger. The data presented in Figure 4c with a sustained high trypsin-like serine protease activity in the culture medium over 10 days past the exosome treatment would be supportive of this.

We should be cautious when interpreting the results of the in vitro experiments. The active matriptase is a well-known tumor progression promoter by activating growth factors for cell migration. However, in our study, the advent of matriptase activation triggered by prostasin promotes invasion, but it also inhibits migration and induces apoptosis. The prostasin-mediated matriptase activation in B cancer cells may have different outcomes in an in vivo context. In solid tumors of B cell lymphoma, the active matriptase may be accumulated in situ, playing roles in the tumor microenvironment. The sustained matriptase activation could modify the extracellular matrix by degrading matrix proteins, such as collagen IV, or acting on its substrates, such as the urokinase plasminogen activator (uPA) and hepatocyte growth factor (HGF) in the neighboring cells, especially the fibroblasts [56,57]. On the other hand, the accumulation of active matriptase in the tumor microenvironment may also induce cell apoptosis, as the active matriptase is toxic to the cells [10,23,48–50].

In this study, prostasin exosomes could activate matriptase in all B cells tested here, as evidenced by the reduced cellular matriptase, increased trypsin-like serine protease activity in the conditioned media, and the accumulation of soluble matriptase therein. The matriptase in the JeKo-1 cells was reported as not being able to go through auto-activation induced by acid [31], but it could apparently be activated by the prostasin exosomes, as we have shown (Figure 4). This may suggest that different activation mechanisms were involved in the two experimental conditions.

Our study focused on a limited selection of four Burkett lymphoma cell lines with high levels of matriptase protein expression in the absence of its physiological inhibitor HAI-1 [31], which is also an inhibitor of prostasin. In future studies, we may consider testing the prostasin exosome activation of matriptase in cell lines representing the most common subtype of NHL, i.e., diffuse large B-cell lymphoma (DLBCL), such as OCI-LY3 and OCI-LY10. These have different molecular genetic and gene expression backgrounds than the Burkett cell lines we investigated, especially with regard to the expression of HAI-1 [31]. This would be very informative as to the potential role of HAI-1 in the prostasin-exosome-induced matriptase activation in these cell lines, with an abundance of the HAI-1 protein in the OCI-LY10 cells but an absence in the OCI-LY3 cells.

5. Conclusions

Our study began with the question as to what would happen if we imposed prostasin expression in B cancer cells ectopically expressing the otherwise epithelial-specific matriptase. The hypothesis was that matriptase would be activated by prostasin, shed from the cells, and reduced in quantity, recapitulating the phenotypes previously reported with matriptase expression silencing using siRNA. Our results supported this hypothesis. Prostasin-exosome-mediated matriptase removal from B cancer cells is an attractive and novel idea, shown to be efficient in the in vitro setting in this study. The use of an exosome-mediated proteolytic cascade to kill cancer cells could be exploited as an alternative approach to treat B cell lymphoma, but this requires validation in vivo, e.g., in xenografted tumors using animal models.

Supplementary Materials: The following supporting information can be downloaded at: https://www.mdpi.com/article/10.3390/cancers15153848/s1, File S1: The original western blots; Figure S1: Western blot analysis of exosomes. The vector control exosomes (Vexo, 10 µg) and prostasin exosomes (Pexo, 10 µg) prepared from the HEK293T cells were tested with four different exosome markers using antibodies against CD63, HSP70, Tsg101, and Alix (all from Santa Cruz Biotechnology). Lanes 1 & 2, CD63; lanes 3 & 4, HSP70; lanes 5 & 6, Tsg101; lanes 7 & 8, Alix. The panel of HSP70 membrane was stripped and re-blotted with the prostasin antibody (lanes 9 & 10). In a different experiment (right panel, lanes 11–14), the exosomes were incubated with 0.5 µg of purified mouse protease nexin 1 (PN-1) for 2 h at 37 °C before SDS-PAGE/western blotting; Figure S2. Gelatin zymography and western blot analysis of B lymphoma cell lines. Lysate from 2×10^5 cells of each line was analyzed in gelatin gel (left panel), western blotting with matriptase antibody (AF3946, middle panel) and western blotting with GAPDH antibody (right panel). Lanes 1, RS4; lanes 2, Daudi; lanes 3 Namalwa; lanes 4, Raji; lanes 5, Ramos; lanes 6, Jeko. RS4 cells do not express matriptase (middle panel, lane 1) and do not have matriptase-associated gelatinase activity (left panel, lane 1).

Author Contributions: L.-M.C. and K.X.C. contributed to the conceptualization, investigation, formal analysis, writing of the manuscript, and funding acquisition. All authors have read and agreed to the published version of the manuscript.

Funding: This work was partially supported by the Florida Department of Health Live Like Bella Pediatric Cancer Research Initiative, Public Health Research, Biomedical Research Program [grant number 20L06]; and by University of Central Florida College of Medicine internal funds to L.-M.C. and K.X.C. The funders had no role in the design of the study; in the collection, analyses, or interpretation of data; in the writing of the manuscript; or in the decision to publish the results.

Institutional Review Board Statement: Not applicable.

Informed Consent Statement: Not applicable.

Data Availability Statement: The data presented in this study are available in this article.

Acknowledgments: The instruments used in this study were supported by the BMS Core Facility of the Burnett School of Biomedical Sciences, University of Central Florida College of Medicine.

Conflicts of Interest: The authors declare no conflict of interest.

References

1. Barrett, A.J.; Rawlings, N.D.; Salvesen, G.; Woessner, J.F. Introduction. In *Handbook of Proteolytic Enzymes*, 3rd ed.; Rawlings, N.D., Salvesen, G., Eds.; Academic Press: Cambridge, MA, USA; Elsevier: London, UK, 2013; Volume 1, pp. li–liv. [CrossRef]
2. Leytus, S.P.; Loeb, K.R.; Hagen, F.S.; Kurachi, K.; Davie, E.W. A novel trypsin-like serine protease (hepsin) with a putative transmembrane domain expressed by human liver and hepatoma cells. *Biochemistry* **1988**, *27*, 1067–1074. [CrossRef]
3. Yu, J.X.; Chao, L.; Chao, J. Prostasin is a novel human serine proteinase from seminal fluid. Purification, tissue distribution, and localization in prostate gland. *J. Biol. Chem.* **1994**, *269*, 18843–18848. [CrossRef] [PubMed]
4. Yu, J.X.; Chao, L.; Chao, J. Molecular Cloning, Tissue-specific Expression, and Cellular Localization of Human Prostasin mRNA. *J. Biol. Chem.* **1995**, *270*, 13483–13489. [CrossRef] [PubMed]
5. Lin, C.-Y.; Anders, J.; Johnson, M.; Sang, Q.A.; Dickson, R.B. Molecular Cloning of cDNA for Matriptase, a Matrix-degrading Serine Protease with Trypsin-like Activity. *J. Biol. Chem.* **1999**, *274*, 18231–18236. [CrossRef] [PubMed]
6. Takeuchi, T.; Shuman, M.A.; Craik, C.S. Reverse biochemistry: Use of macromolecular protease inhibitors to dissect complex biological processes and identify a membrane-type serine protease in epithelial cancer and normal tissue. *Proc. Natl. Acad. Sci. USA* **1999**, *96*, 11054–11061. [CrossRef]
7. Chen, L.M.; Skinner, M.L.; Kauffman, S.W.; Chao, J.; Chao, L.; Thaler, C.D.; Chai, K.X. Prostasin is a glycosylphosphati-dylinositol-anchored active serine protease. *J. Biol. Chem.* **2001**, *276*, 21434–21442. [CrossRef]
8. Chen, L.M.; Chai, K.X. PRSS8 (protease, serine, 8). *Atlas Genet. Cytogenet. Oncol. Haematol.* **2012**, *16*, 658–664. [CrossRef]
9. Bao, Y.; Guo, Y.; Yang, Y.; Wei, X.; Zhang, S.; Zhang, Y.; Li, K.; Yuan, M.; Guo, D.; Macias, V.; et al. PRSS8 suppresses colorectal carcinogenesis and metastasis. *Oncogene* **2019**, *38*, 497–517; Erratum in *Oncogene* **2021**, *40*, 1922–1924. [CrossRef]
10. List, K.; Szabo, R.; Molinolo, A.; Sriuranpong, V.; Redeye, V.; Murdock, T.; Burke, B.; Nielsen, B.S.; Gutkind, J.S.; Bugge, T.H. Deregulated matriptase causes *ras*-independent multistage carcinogenesis and promotes *ras*-mediated malignant transformation. *Genes Dev.* **2005**, *19*, 1934–1950. [CrossRef]
11. Netzel-Arnett, S.; Currie, B.M.; Szabo, R.; Lin, C.-Y.; Chen, L.-M.; Chai, K.X.; Antalis, T.M.; Bugge, T.H.; List, K. Evidence for a Matriptase-Prostasin Proteolytic Cascade Regulating Terminal Epidermal Differentiation. *J. Biol. Chem.* **2006**, *281*, 32941–32945. [CrossRef]
12. List, K.; Hobson, J.P.; Molinolo, A.; Bugge, T.H. Co-localization of the channel activating protease prostasin/(CAP1/PRSS8) with its candidate activator, matriptase. *J. Cell Physiol.* **2007**, *213*, 237–245. [CrossRef]
13. Chen, M.; Chen, L.-M.; Lin, C.-Y.; Chai, K.X. The epidermal growth factor receptor (EGFR) is proteolytically modified by the Matriptase–Prostasin serine protease cascade in cultured epithelial cells. *Biochim. Biophys. Acta (BBA)-Mol. Cell Res.* **2008**, *1783*, 896–903. [CrossRef]
14. Chen, Y.-W.; Wang, J.-K.; Chou, F.-P.; Chen, C.-Y.; Rorke, E.A.; Chen, L.-M.; Chai, K.X.; Eckert, R.L.; Johnson, M.D.; Lin, C.-Y. Regulation of the Matriptase-Prostasin Cell Surface Proteolytic Cascade by Hepatocyte Growth Factor Activator Inhibitor-1 during Epidermal Differentiation. *J. Biol. Chem.* **2010**, *285*, 31755–31762. [CrossRef] [PubMed]
15. Xu, Z.; Chen, Y.-W.; Battu, A.; Wilder, P.; Weber, D.; Yu, W.; MacKerell, A.D.; Chen, L.-M.; Chai, K.X.; Johnson, M.D.; et al. Targeting Zymogen Activation to Control the Matriptase-Prostasin Proteolytic Cascade. *J. Med. Chem.* **2011**, *54*, 7567–7578. [CrossRef] [PubMed]
16. Miller, G.S.; List, K. The matriptase-prostasin proteolytic cascade in epithelial development and pathology. *Cell Tissue Res.* **2012**, *351*, 245–253. [CrossRef] [PubMed]
17. Friis, S.; Sales, K.U.; Godiksen, S.; Peters, D.E.; Lin, C.-Y.; Vogel, L.K.; Bugge, T.H. A Matriptase-Prostasin Reciprocal Zymogen Activation Complex with Unique Features: Prostasin as a non-enzymatic co-factor for matriptase activation. *J. Biol. Chem.* **2013**, *288*, 19028–19039. [CrossRef]
18. Oberst, M.D.; Williams, C.A.; Dickson, R.B.; Johnson, M.D.; Lin, C.-Y. The Activation of Matriptase Requires Its Noncatalytic Domains, Serine Protease Domain, and Its Cognate Inhibitor. *J. Biol. Chem.* **2003**, *278*, 26773–26779. [CrossRef]
19. Friis, S.; Sales, K.U.; Schafer, J.M.; Vogel, L.K.; Kataoka, H.; Bugge, T.H. The Protease Inhibitor HAI-2, but Not HAI-1, Regulates Matriptase Activation and Shedding through Prostasin. *J. Biol. Chem.* **2014**, *289*, 22319–22332. [CrossRef]
20. Tseng, C.-C.; Jia, B.; Barndt, R.; Gu, Y.; Chen, C.-Y.; Tseng, I.-C.; Su, S.-F.; Wang, J.-K.; Johnson, M.D.; Lin, C.-Y. Matriptase shedding is closely coupled with matriptase zymogen activation and requires de novo proteolytic cleavage likely involving its own activity. *PLoS ONE* **2017**, *12*, e0183507. [CrossRef]
21. Shimomura, T.; Denda, K.; Kitamura, A.; Kawaguchi, T.; Kito, M.; Kondo, J.; Kagaya, S.; Qin, L.; Takata, H.; Miyazawa, K.; et al. Hepatocyte Growth Factor Activator Inhibitor, a Novel Kunitz-type Serine Protease Inhibitor. *J. Biol. Chem.* **1997**, *272*, 6370–6376. [CrossRef]
22. Marlor, C.W.; Delaria, K.A.; Davis, G.; Muller, D.K.; Greve, J.M.; Tamburini, P.P. Identification and Cloning of Human Placental Bikunin, a Novel Serine Protease Inhibitor Containing Two Kunitz Domains. *J. Biol. Chem.* **1997**, *272*, 12202–12208. [CrossRef]

23. Oberst, M.D.; Chen, L.-Y.L.; Kiyomiya, K.-I.; Williams, C.A.; Lee, M.-S.; Johnson, M.D.; Dickson, R.B.; Lin, C.-Y. HAI-1 regulates activation and expression of matriptase, a membrane-bound serine protease. *Am. J. Physiol. Physiol.* **2005**, *289*, C462–C470. [CrossRef] [PubMed]
24. Szabo, R.; Sales, K.U.; Kosa, P.; Shylo, N.A.; Godiksen, S.; Hansen, K.K.; Friis, S.; Gutkind, J.S.; Vogel, L.K.; Hummler, E.; et al. Reduced Prostasin (CAP1/PRSS8) Activity Eliminates HAI-1 and HAI-2 Deficiency–Associated Developmental Defects by Preventing Matriptase Activation. *PLOS Genet.* **2012**, *8*, e1002937. [CrossRef] [PubMed]
25. Nimishakavi, S.; Besprozvannaya, M.; Raymond, W.W.; Craik, C.S.; Gruenert, D.C.; Caughey, G.H.; Menou, A.; Duitman, J.; Flajolet, P.; Sallenave, J.-M.; et al. Activity and inhibition of prostasin and matriptase on apical and basolateral surfaces of human airway epithelial cells. *Am. J. Physiol. Cell Mol. Physiol.* **2012**, *303*, L97–L106. [CrossRef] [PubMed]
26. Chang, H.-H.D.; Xu, Y.; Lai, H.; Yang, X.; Tseng, C.-C.; Lai, Y.-J.J.; Pan, Y.; Zhou, E.; Johnson, M.D.; Wang, J.-K.; et al. Differential Subcellular Localization Renders HAI-2 a Matriptase Inhibitor in Breast Cancer Cells but Not in Mammary Epithelial Cells. *PLoS ONE* **2015**, *10*, e0120489. [CrossRef]
27. Larsen, B.R.; Steffensen, S.D.; Nielsen, N.V.; Friis, S.; Godiksen, S.; Bornholdt, J.; Soendergaard, C.; Nonboe, A.W.; Andersen, M.N.; Poulsen, S.S.; et al. Hepatocyte growth factor activator inhibitor-2 prevents shedding of matriptase. *Exp. Cell Res.* **2013**, *319*, 918–929. [CrossRef]
28. Lee, S.-P.; Kao, C.-Y.; Chang, S.-C.; Chiu, Y.-L.; Chen, Y.-J.; Chen, M.-H.G.; Chang, C.-C.; Lin, Y.-W.; Chiang, C.-P.; Wang, J.-K.; et al. Tissue distribution and subcellular localizations determine in vivo functional relationship among prostasin, matriptase, HAI-1, and HAI-2 in human skin. *PLoS ONE* **2018**, *13*, e0192632. [CrossRef]
29. Gao, L.; Liu, M.; Dong, N.; Jiang, Y.; Lin, C.-Y.; Huang, M.; Wu, D.; Wu, Q. Matriptase is highly upregulated in chronic lymphocytic leukemia and promotes cancer cell invasion. *Leukemia* **2013**, *27*, 1191–1194. [CrossRef]
30. Chou, F.-P.; Chen, Y.-W.; Zhao, X.F.; Xu-Monette, Z.Y.; Young, K.H.; Gartenhaus, R.B.; Wang, J.-K.; Kataoka, H.; Zuo, A.H.; Barndt, R.J.; et al. Imbalanced Matriptase Pericellular Proteolysis Contributes to the Pathogenesis of Malignant B-Cell Lymphomas. *Am. J. Pathol.* **2013**, *183*, 1306–1317. [CrossRef]
31. Chiu, Y.-L.; Wu, Y.-Y.; Barndt, R.B.; Yeo, Y.H.; Lin, Y.-W.; Sytwo, H.-P.; Liu, H.-C.; Xu, Y.; Jia, B.; Wang, J.-K.; et al. Aberrant regulation favours matriptase proteolysis in neoplastic B-cells that co-express HAI-2. *J. Enzym. Inhib. Med. Chem.* **2019**, *34*, 692–702. [CrossRef]
32. Chatterjee, S.; Smith, E.R.; Hanada, K.; Stevens, V.L.; Mayor, S. GPI anchoring leads to sphingolipid-dependent retention of endocytosed proteins in the recycling endosomal compartment. *EMBO J.* **2001**, *20*, 1583–1592. [CrossRef] [PubMed]
33. Doyle, L.; Wang, M. Overview of Extracellular Vesicles, Their Origin, Composition, Purpose, and Methods for Exosome Isolation and Analysis. *Cells* **2019**, *8*, 727. [CrossRef] [PubMed]
34. van der Lubbe, N.; Jansen, P.M.; Salih, M.; Fenton, R.A.; van den Meiracker, A.H.; Danser, A.H.; Zietse, R.; Hoorn, E.J. The Phosphorylated Sodium Chloride Cotransporter in Urinary Exosomes Is Superior to Prostasin as a Marker for Aldosteronism. *Hypertension* **2012**, *60*, 741–748. [CrossRef]
35. Olivieri, O.; Chiecchi, L.; Pizzolo, F.; Castagna, A.; Raffaelli, R.; Gunasekaran, M.; Guarini, P.; Consoli, L.; Salvagno, G.; Kitamura, K. Urinary prostasin in normotensive individuals: Correlation with the aldosterone to renin ratio and urinary sodium. *Hypertens. Res.* **2013**, *36*, 528–533. [CrossRef] [PubMed]
36. Qi, Y.; Wang, X.; Rose, K.L.; MacDonald, W.H.; Zhang, B.; Schey, K.L.; Luther, J.M. Activation of the Endogenous Renin-Angiotensin-Aldosterone System or Aldosterone Administration Increases Urinary Exosomal Sodium Channel Excretion. *J. Am. Soc. Nephrol.* **2016**, *27*, 646–656. [CrossRef]
37. Zachar, R.; Jensen, B.L.; Svenningsen, P.; Takeda, R.; Stickford, A.S.; Best, S.A.; Yoo, J.-K.; Hissen, S.L.; Liu, Y.-L.; Fu, Q. Dietary Na$^+$intake in healthy humans changes the urine extracellular vesicle prostasin abundance while the vesicle excretion rate, NCC, and ENaC are not altered. *Am. J. Physiol. Physiol.* **2019**, *317*, F1612–F1622. [CrossRef]
38. Krishnamachary, B.; Cook, C.; Spikes, L.; Chalise, P.; Dhillon, N.K. The Potential Role of Extracellular Vesicles in COVID-19 Asso-ciated Endothelial injury and Pro-inflammation. *medRxiv* **2020**. [CrossRef]
39. Fontana, S.; Mauceri, R.; Novara, M.E.; Alessandro, R.; Campisi, G. Protein Cargo of Salivary Small Extracellular Vesicles as Potential Functional Signature of Oral Squamous Cell Carcinoma. *Int. J. Mol. Sci.* **2021**, *22*, 11160. [CrossRef]
40. Chen, L.M. *Prostasin in Human Health and Disease*; World Scientific Publishing Co. Pte. Ltd.: Singapore, 2023; ISBN 978-981-126-814-4.
41. Chen, L.-M.; Chai, J.C.; Liu, B.; Strutt, T.M.; McKinstry, K.K.; Chai, K.X. Prostasin regulates PD-L1 expression in human lung cancer cells. *Biosci. Rep.* **2021**, *41*, BSR20211370. [CrossRef]
42. Chai, A.C.; Robinson, A.L.; Chai, K.X.; Chen, L.-M. Ibuprofen regulates the expression and function of membrane-associated serine proteases prostasin and matriptase. *BMC Cancer* **2015**, *15*, 1025. [CrossRef]
43. Fu, Y.-Y.; Gao, W.-L.; Chen, M.; Chai, K.X.; Wang, Y.-L.; Chen, L.-M. Prostasin regulates human placental trophoblast cell proliferation via the epidermal growth factor receptor signaling pathway. *Hum. Reprod.* **2010**, *25*, 623–632. [CrossRef]
44. Shi, Y.E.; Torri, J.; Yieh, L.; Wellstein, A.; Lippman, M.E.; Dickson, R.B. Identification and characterization of a novel ma-trix-degrading protease from hormone-dependent human breast cancer cells. *Cancer Res.* **1993**, *53*, 1409–1415. [PubMed]
45. Trentin, L.; Cabrelle, A.; Facco, M.; Carollo, D.; Miorin, M.; Tosoni, A.; Pizzo, P.; Binotto, G.; Nicolardi, L.; Zambello, R.; et al. Homeostatic chemokines drive migration of malignant B cells in patients with non-Hodgkin lymphomas. *Blood* **2004**, *104*, 502–508. [CrossRef] [PubMed]

46. Camerer, E.; Barker, A.; Duong, D.N.; Ganesan, R.; Kataoka, H.; Cornelissen, I.; Darragh, M.R.; Hussain, A.; Zheng, Y.-W.; Srinivasan, Y.; et al. Local Protease Signaling Contributes to Neural Tube Closure in the Mouse Embryo. *Dev. Cell* **2010**, *18*, 25–38. [CrossRef]
47. Buzza, M.S.; Martin, E.W.; Driesbaugh, K.H.; Désilets, A.; Leduc, R.; Antalis, T.M. Prostasin Is Required for Matriptase Activation in Intestinal Epithelial Cells to Regulate Closure of the Paracellular Pathway. *J. Biol. Chem.* **2013**, *288*, 10328–10337. [CrossRef]
48. List, K.; Bugge, T.H.; Szabo, R. Matriptase: Potent Proteolysis on the Cell Surface. *Mol. Med.* **2006**, *12*, 1–7. [CrossRef] [PubMed]
49. Ma, J.; Scott, C.A.; Ho, Y.N.; Mahabaleshwar, H.; Marsay, K.S.; Zhang, C.; Teow, C.K.; Ng, S.S.; Zhang, W.; Tergaonkar, V.; et al. Matriptase activation of Gq drives epithelial disruption and inflammation via RSK and DUOX. *eLife* **2021**, *10*, e66596. [CrossRef]
50. Gaymon, D.O.; Barndt, R.; Stires, H.; Riggins, R.B.; Johnson, M.D. ROS is a master regulator of in vitro matriptase activation. *PLoS ONE* **2023**, *18*, e0267492. [CrossRef]
51. Balasubramanian, K.; Schroit, A.J. Aminophospholipid Asymmetry: A Matter of Life and Death. *Annu. Rev. Physiol.* **2003**, *65*, 701–734. [CrossRef]
52. Demchenko, A.P. Beyond annexin V: Fluorescence response of cellular membranes to apoptosis. *Cytotechnology* **2012**, *65*, 157–172. [CrossRef]
53. Lin, C.-Y.; Wang, J.-K.; Torri, J.; Dou, L.; Sang, Q.A.; Dickson, R.B. Characterization of a Novel, Membrane-bound, 80-kDa Matrix-degrading Protease from Human Breast Cancer Cells. Monoclonal antibody production, isolation, and localization. *J. Biol. Chem.* **1997**, *272*, 9147–9152. [CrossRef] [PubMed]
54. Blüml, S.; McKeever, K.; Ettinger, R.; Smolen, J.; Herbst, R. B-cell targeted therapeutics in clinical development. *Arthritis Res. Ther.* **2013**, *15* (Suppl. S1), S4. [CrossRef] [PubMed]
55. Paju, A.; Sorsa, T.; Tervahartiala, T.; Koivunen, E.; Haglund, C.; Leminen, A.; Wahlström, T.; Salo, T.; Stenman, U.-H. The levels of trypsinogen isoenzymes in ovarian tumour cyst fluids are associated with promatrix metalloproteinase-9 but not promatrix metalloproteinase-2 activation. *Br. J. Cancer* **2001**, *84*, 1363–1371. [CrossRef] [PubMed]
56. Matsuoka, H.; Sisson, T.H.; Nishiuma, T.; Simon, R.H. Plasminogen-Mediated Activation and Release of Hepatocyte Growth Factor from Extracellular Matrix. *Am. J. Respir. Cell Mol. Biol.* **2006**, *35*, 705–713. [CrossRef]
57. Jedeszko, C.; Victor, B.C.; Podgorski, I.; Sloane, B.F. Fibroblast Hepatocyte Growth Factor Promotes Invasion of Human Mammary Ductal Carcinoma in situ. *Cancer Res.* **2009**, *69*, 9148–9155. [CrossRef]

Disclaimer/Publisher's Note: The statements, opinions and data contained in all publications are solely those of the individual author(s) and contributor(s) and not of MDPI and/or the editor(s). MDPI and/or the editor(s) disclaim responsibility for any injury to people or property resulting from any ideas, methods, instructions or products referred to in the content.

Review

A Disintegrin and Metalloproteinase (ADAM) Family—Novel Biomarkers of Selected Gastrointestinal (GI) Malignancies?

Marta Łukaszewicz-Zając [1,*], Sara Pączek [2] and Barbara Mroczko [1,3]

1. Department of Biochemical Diagnostics, Medical University of Bialystok, 15-269 Bialystok, Poland; barbara.mroczko@umb.edu.pl
2. Department of Biochemical Diagnostics, University Hospital of Bialystok, 15-269 Bialystok, Poland; sara.paczek@umb.edu.pl
3. Department of Neurodegeneration Diagnostics, Medical University, 15-269 Bialystok, Poland
* Correspondence: marta.lukaszewicz-zajac@umb.edu.pl

Simple Summary: A disintegrin and metalloproteinase (ADAM) proteins are proteolytic enzymes that are responsible for destroying the extracellular matrix, but they also have adhesive properties. Recent investigations have demonstrated that the expression of several ADAMs is upregulated in gastrointestinal (GI) tumour cells and have linked the secretion of these proteins to pathogenesis of GI malignancies. Therefore, the aim of this review is to establish the involvement of selected ADAMs in the progression of GI malignancies as well as their prognostic significance. It was found that selected ADAMs might stimulate the proliferation and invasion of malignant cells and may be associated with unfavourable survival of patients with GI tumours. In conclusion, this review confirms the significance of selected ADAMs in the pathogenesis of the most common GI cancers and indicates their promising significance as potential prognostic biomarkers as well as therapeutic targets for GI malignancies.

Abstract: The global burden of gastrointestinal (GI) cancers is expected to increase. Therefore, it is vital that novel biomarkers useful for the early diagnosis of these malignancies are established. A growing body of data has linked secretion of proteolytic enzymes, such as metalloproteinases (MMPs), which destroy the extracellular matrix, to pathogenesis of GI tumours. A disintegrin and metalloproteinase (ADAM) proteins belong to the MMP family but have been proven to be unique due to both proteolytic and adhesive properties. Recent investigations have demonstrated that the expression of several ADAMs is upregulated in GI cancer cells. Thus, the objective of this review is to present current findings concerning the role of ADAMs in the pathogenesis of GI cancers, particularly their involvement in the development and progression of colorectal, pancreatic and gastric cancer. Furthermore, the prognostic significance of selected ADAMs in patients with GI tumours is also presented. It has been proven that ADAM8, 9, 10, 12, 15, 17 and 28 might stimulate the proliferation and invasion of GI malignancies and may be associated with unfavourable survival. In conclusion, this review confirms the role of selected ADAMs in the pathogenesis of the most common GI cancers and indicates their promising significance as potential prognostic biomarkers as well as therapeutic targets for GI malignancies. However, due to their non-specific nature, future research on ADAM biology should be performed to elucidate new strategies for the diagnosis of these common and deadly malignancies and treatment of patients with these diseases.

Keywords: ADAM; biomarker; gastrointestinal tumours

1. Gastrointestinal Cancers—General Characteristics

According to estimates from the American Cancer Society, in 2018 there were approximately 1.7 million new cancer cases and 610,000 cancer deaths [1]. Gastrointestinal (GI) cancers are defined as a group of malignancies that includes cancers of the liver, oesophagus, gallbladder, pancreas, stomach, large and small intestine and anus [2–4]. Neoplasms originating from the GI tract, including colorectal cancer (CRC) and gastric cancer (GC), are among the five most common malignancies in both men and women worldwide. It is estimated that CRC is one of the most frequently diagnosed cancers and the second most common cause of cancer-related deaths worldwide. Gastric cancer is the fourth most common cancer and accounts for 8.8% of all cancer-related deaths [2–4].

The incidence of GI cancers shows significant geographical variation. CRC incidence is higher in Western Europe and North America, while the incidence of GC and liver cancer (LC) is elevated in Asia and Africa. The main risk factors for GI cancers include tobacco and alcohol intake, genetic factors, viruses such as Papillomaviruses, Epstein–Barr virus (EBV) or hepatitis B and C. Other risk indicators that may cause tumour development are bacterial infections and microbiome imbalance, *Helicobacter pylori* infection, as well as an unhealthy diet and obesity. It was suggested that *Fusobacterium nucleatum* plays a role in CRC development via promotion of tumour progression include generating a proinflammatory tumour-promoting microenvironment [5–7]. Moreover, the study of Yoshimura revealed that *Helicobacter pylori* stimulated temporal changes in the levels of proteolytic enzymes such as ADAM10 and ADAM17 transcripts in gastric epithelial cells, while chronic infection with *Helicobacter pylori* may result in persistent mucosal increases in members of the ADAM family [8]. Some epidemiological studies have shown an increased risk of GI cancers in overweight and obese individuals, while substantial evidence has linked reduced physical activity with an increased risk of colon cancer. Moreover, it has been proven that a high salt intake is associated with enhanced prevalence of GC, whereas a diet high in red and processed meats has been linked to an increased risk of GC, EC, PC and CRC [2–9]. Furthermore, changes in lifestyle, the growing population and environmental factors as well as advances in medicine may also affect the epidemiology of GI cancers [2].

Clinical symptoms of GI cancers depend on the type of malignancy and tumour stage as well as the development of systemic symptoms such as early satiety nausea, anorexia, changes in the sense of smell, stress or dysgeusia [10]. It has been revealed that fatigue is a major sign followed by pain, anxiety, poor well-being, sleep disturbances, poor appetite, depression, drowsiness, dyspnoea and nausea [10,11]. Moreover, in EC, GC and PC, signs of disease may occur early. However, symptoms are directly related to the cancer or release of inflammatory cytokines [10,11]. Neoplasms of the alimentary tract are characterized by rapid progression and a very unfavourable prognosis. The diagnostic process of GI cancers includes endoscopic evaluation as an important tool in diagnosis and staging. Diagnosis is confirmed with an upper gastrointestinal endoscopy and biopsy. Other imaging tests useful in diagnosis of GI tumours include computed tomography (CT), positron emission tomography–CT (PET–CT) and endoscopic ultrasound (EUS) [12]. It is also recommended that apart from imaging tests, diagnosis of GI tumours should include laboratory tests. Measurements of the well-investigated classical tumour markers for GI malignancies such as carcinoembryonic antigen (CEA), cancer antigen 19-9 (CA 19.9), cancer antigen 50 (CA 50) or cancer antigen 72.4 (CA 72.4) are not useful in the early detection of these malignancies due to their low diagnostic sensitivity and specificity. A number of candidates for novel biochemical markers for GI malignancies such as matrix metalloproteinases and their tissue inhibitors, cytokines and chemokines as well as specific proteins such as C-reactive protein or interleukin-6 have been evaluated by scientists in the last decade. However, no studies have confirmed their significance in early diagnosis of GI malignancies [13–23]. Therefore, future research should focus on the search for new, non-invasive and easily accessible biomarkers characterized by high diagnostic sensitivity and specificity, which would be useful in the early detection and tumour staging as well as improve treatment implementation.

Remodelling of the extracellular matrix (ECM) plays an important role in tumour progression, including growth, proliferation and angiogenesis. Moreover, many authors link these proteases to tumour invasiveness, particularly metastasis [13]. Therefore, in our previous studies we assessed the usefulness of selected MMPs and their tissue inhibitors in the diagnosis and progression of GI malignancies such as CRC, PC, EC and GC. In addition, selected MMPs, such as MMP-14, are able to regulate a variety of signalling pathways and cell functions, including apoptosis. It has been proven that the proteolytic activity of MMPs is physiologically inhibited by tissue inhibitors of metalloproteinases (TIMPs). TIMP-2 regulates several cell functions including migration, proliferation and apoptosis through MMP-dependent and -independent mechanisms, e.g., via inhibition of FGF-2-induced endothelial cell proliferation, suppression of the mitogenic activity of epidermal growth factor (EGF) or inhibition of angiogenic factor-induced endothelial cell proliferation and angiogenesis [24]. Our previous results indicated that selected MMPs, especially MMP9, might be used as potential biomarkers in the diagnosis and progression of several GI malignancies [14–19]. Based on the most recent literature reports, we believe that another member of the MMP family—ADAM (A disintegrin and metalloproteinase)—might be considered a potential candidate for a biochemical marker involved in GI carcinogenesis because of both proteolytic and adhesive activities. Thus, the goal of our review is to summarize the current knowledge concerning the significance of selected ADAMs in the pathogenesis of GI cancers and their potential utility in diagnosis and prognosis of patients with these malignancies.

2. A Disintegrin and Metalloproteinase (ADAM)—General Information

A disintegrin and metalloproteinases (ADAMs) belong to the family of zinc-dependent proteases, such as metalloproteinases, which consist of 21 members, 13 of which have proteolytic activity [25,26]. They are also known as metalloproteinase, disintegrin, cysteine-rich (MDC) proteins. ADAMs regulate the shedding of membrane-bound proteins, cytokines, growth factors as well as ligands and receptors. It has been demonstrated that the structure of most of these proteins consists of a prodomain, a metalloprotease region, a disintegrin domain for adhesion, a cysteine-rich region, epidermal-growth-factor (EGF) repeats, a transmembrane module as well as a cytoplasmic tail [27,28].

It has been observed that among other cell-surface proteins, ADAMs are unique because of both adhesive and proteolytic activities. Moreover, it has been indicated that EGF repeats and the cysteine-rich region mediate cell fusion or the interaction of these proteins with other molecules [29–32]. ADAMs are mostly transmembrane proteins, but selected ADAMs, such as ADAM11, 12, 17 and 28 may generate a soluble, secreted protein. About 50% of the ADAM family consists of a metalloproteinase domain with a catalytic site consensus sequence that allows for protein–protein interactions [27,28]. The structures of both transmembrane and soluble ADAMs are presented in Figure 1 [30–32].

Several ADAM genes initiate more than one protein due to differential splicing of mRNA, a post-transcriptional modification in which a single gene can code for multiple proteins. This promotes the synthesis of a secreted ADAM structure, in addition to membrane-anchored forms, or variation in the length of the cytoplasmic tail of ADAM proteins. According to differences in the active site sequence of the metalloproteinase domain, 60% of the members are non-proteolytic ADAM molecules. By contrast, active sites in the metalloproteinase domain of the proteinase-type ADAM molecules (ADAM8, 9, 10, 12, 15, 17, 19–21, 28, 30 and 33) contain a common HEXGHXXGXXHD sequence with a 'Met-turn' which is also present in the catalytic metalloproteinase domain of MMP members [33]. ADAM10 and ADAM17 have a similar structure and are characterized by a membrane-proximal domain in the extracellular region in place of the EGF-like, cysteine-rich domain that provides substrate recognition [34,35]. A distinct subfamily of ADAMs is a disintegrin and metalloproteinase with thrombospondin motifs (ADAMTS), which consists of a pro-domain and a disintegrin, metalloproteinase, and cysteine-rich domain. In addition, ADAMTS have a specific thrombospondin motif instead of a transmembrane domain [27–29].

Growing evidence indicates that ADAM proteases are expressed in an inactive form. It has been proven that the activity of ADAMs and ADAMTS is regulated via endogenous inhibitors called tissue inhibitors of metalloproteinases (TIMPs) as well as proprotein convertases. In addition, they might also be controlled by protein kinase C activators,

G-protein coupled receptor agonists or Ca2+ ionophores. Various ADAMs are usually kept in an inactive state because of the interaction of a cysteine residue at the propeptide domain with zinc in the metalloproteinase module. Therefore, ADAMs and MMPs are activated by the cysteine switch mechanism that disrupts the cysteine–zinc interaction to expose the catalytic site. It has been observed that levels of these proteins are regulated at the transcriptional level. However, current knowledge concerning the role of physiological inhibitors of ADAMs is still limited. It has been proven that only TIMP3 inhibits the crystal structure of the protease domain of human ADAM17, while ADAM10 might be inhibited by TIMP1 and 3, and by hydroxamates [35]. TIMP3 may be an inhibitor of various ADAMs as well as ADAMTS members [27–29]. Increasing numbers of reports have demonstrated that GI cancer cells might be transformed by aberrant and uncontrolled mechanisms that may produce alternative splicing. It was found that the *APC* gene, aberrant splice skipping of exon 4, as well as *Ron* gen, skipping of exon 11 are involved in colon cancer progression. An alternative 5′ splice site in BCL-X, involved in apoptosis, is overexpressed in hepatocellular carcinoma, similar to the *CDH17* gene (exclusion of exon 13) that regulates incidence of tumour recurrence. In addition, the *TACC1* gene has splicing variants associated with GC. These findings suggest the expression of aberrant and abnormal splice variants in GI cancer development [36–39].

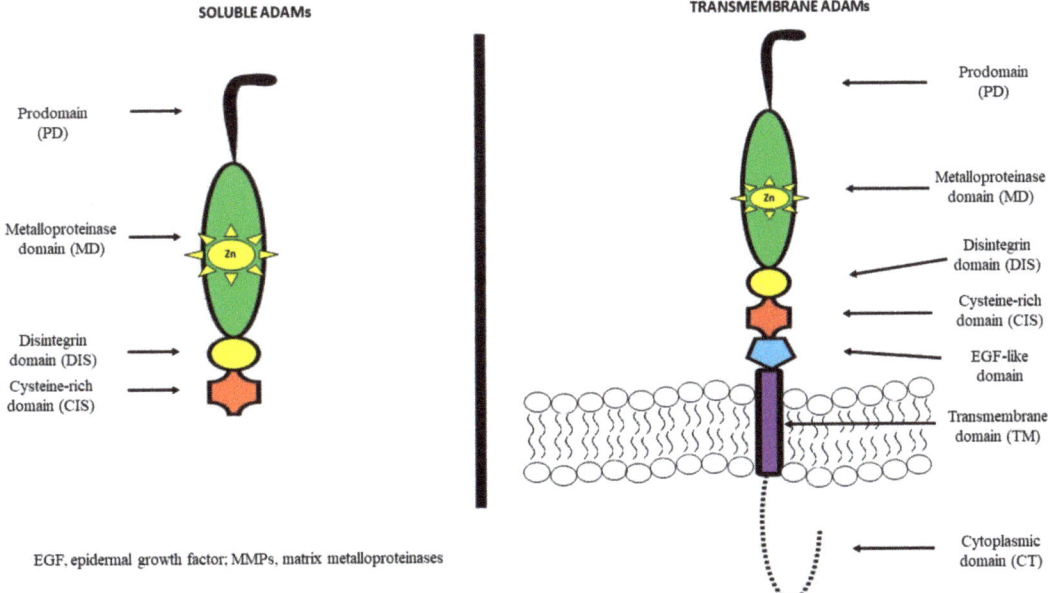

Figure 1. Structure of ADAMs of transmembrane and soluble ADAMs [30–32].

ADAMs, similarly to MMPs, possess various physiological functions and the ability to regulate many processes such as cell migration, proliferation, angiogenesis, apoptosis, wound healing, tissue repair and survival. By way of illustration, ADAM1 and 2 are able to modulate cell adhesion or sperm–egg fusion. In addition, ADAM12 plays a role in myoblast fusion, while ADAM9, 10 and 17 regulate ectodomain shedding of cell-surface proteins [27–29]. However, these molecules might also be involved in some pathological conditions such as cardiovascular and malignant diseases, including GI cancers [40–43].

3. A Disintegrin and Metalloproteinase (ADAM)—Their Role in Tumour Development

A growing body of evidence suggests that cancer growth is not only driven by tumour cell-intrinsic mechanisms, but might be dependent on paracrine signals, such as growth factors or cytokines, produced by the tumour microenvironment (TME). These molecules are synthesized as trans-membrane proteins and must be released by limited proteolysis defined as ectodomain shedding. It has been proven that ADAMs are major mediators of ectodomain shedding and thus are able to initiate paracrine signal transduction [25]. Changes in the activation process of paracrine signal transduction is a crucial step in the development of GI malignancies. Therefore, ADAM proteases play an important role in inflammation as well as pathogenesis of several tumours because of their ability to interact with a variety of substrates [25].

The multiple functional roles of ADAMs prove their involvement in a variety of normal and pathophysiological conditions, including cancer progression [32,41,42,44]. Characteristics of selected ADAMs [32] and their significance in tumour biology are presented in Table 1.

Table 1. Characteristics of selected ADAMs [32].

ADAMs	Other Name	Involvement in Cancer Biology	Inhibitors
ADAM8	MS2 (CD156)	Promotion of migration	-
ADAM9	MDC9, MCMP, Meltrin-γ	Promotion of cell adhesion and invasion, binding to integrins ($\alpha 6\beta 4$ and $\alpha 2\beta 1$)	-
ADAM10	MDAM, Kuzbanian	Type I membrane glycoprotein L1 shedding, promotion of cell growth and migration	TIMP1 TIMP3
ADAM12	Meltrin-α, MCMP, MLTN, MLTNA	HB-EGF (heparin-binding epidermal growth factor) shedding, promotion of cell growth	TIMP3
ADAM15	Metargidin, MDC15, AD56, CR II-7	Promotion of cell growth	No data
ADAM17	TACE, cSVP	TGF-β (transforming growth factor) shedding, promotion of cell growth	TIMP2 TIMP3
ADAM19	Meltrin-β, FKSG34	No data	-
ADAM28	e-MDC II, MDC-Lm, MDC-Ls	IGFBP-3 (insulin-like growth factor binding protein-3) cleavage, promotion of cell growth	TIMP3 TIMP4
ADAMTS1	C3-C5, METH1, KIAA1346	HB-EGF (heparin-binding epidermal growth factor) and AR shedding, promotion of cell growth, survival and invasion	No data
ADAMTS4	KIAA0688, aggrecanase-1, ADMP-1	No data	TIMP3
ADAMTS5	ADAMTS11, aggrecanase-2, ADMP-2	Brevican cleavage, promotion of invasion	TIMP3

It has been reported that ADAM8 is involved in tumour cell migration and invasion, ADAM9 plays a role in tumorigenesis, invasion and metastasis through modulation of growth factor activity and integrin function, while overexpression of ADAM10 appears to promote the growth and proliferation of tumour cells. In addition, ADAM12 cleaves various ECM molecules including gelatin, type IV collagen and fibronectin, suggesting a potential role of this enzyme in ECM digestion in cancer invasion and metastasis. Thus, ADAM12 functions as a shedder, adhesion molecule and ECM-degrading proteinase and is involved in cancer progression. ADAM28 may play a key role in cancer cell proliferation and metastasis, whereas ADAM17 is a target of tumorigenesis, but the role of ADAM15 in cancer biology remains to be elucidated [32,44].

It has been established that ADAM12 and ADAM28 regulate the level of free IGF-1 by proteolysis of the IGFBP-3/IGF-1 protein complex [44]. In addition, ADAM17 protein is responsible for the activation of TNFα, initiating the signalling pathway associated with the EGF receptor for which it is a ligand, leading to tumour cell proliferation [45]. Adamalysines might be involved in the pathogenesis of gastric cancer via the EGFR signalling pathway and the TGF-α/Smad pathway [46]. In vitro assays indicate that ADAM8 overexpression promotes cell growth and increases migration and invasion abilities by decreasing the p-p38/p-extracellular regulated protein kinase (p-ERK) ratio. Several studies suggest that there are five most common pathways of ADAMs involvement in cancer biology. It has been reported that proADAM might be activated via furin or MMPs. As furin activates MMP activity, cancer cells have the potential to become metastatic. Another pathway leads to growth factors such as TGFα shedding, which may change signals on the cancer cell's surface. Soluble growth factors activate EGFR on cells, causing the enhanced cells proliferation via autocrine and paracrine manners. A third route involves the participation of ADAMs as adhesion molecules with integrins on cells, which may facilitate the digestion of the substrates of the ECM. Fourth, cell proliferation signals can be regulated indirectly by ADAMs via integrins; thus these molecules provide traction to migrating cells through the ECM using integrins. In addition, ADAMs are able to stimulate cancer development and metastasis via the interaction with other molecules, including cytokines and their receptors, that are also associated with cancer progression. ADAMs, similar to MMPs, are able to cleave ECM molecules. As a consequence, it allows neoplastic cells to adhere to new locations, which is responsible for, e.g., cancer metastasis [44]. All the pathways are presented in Figure 2.

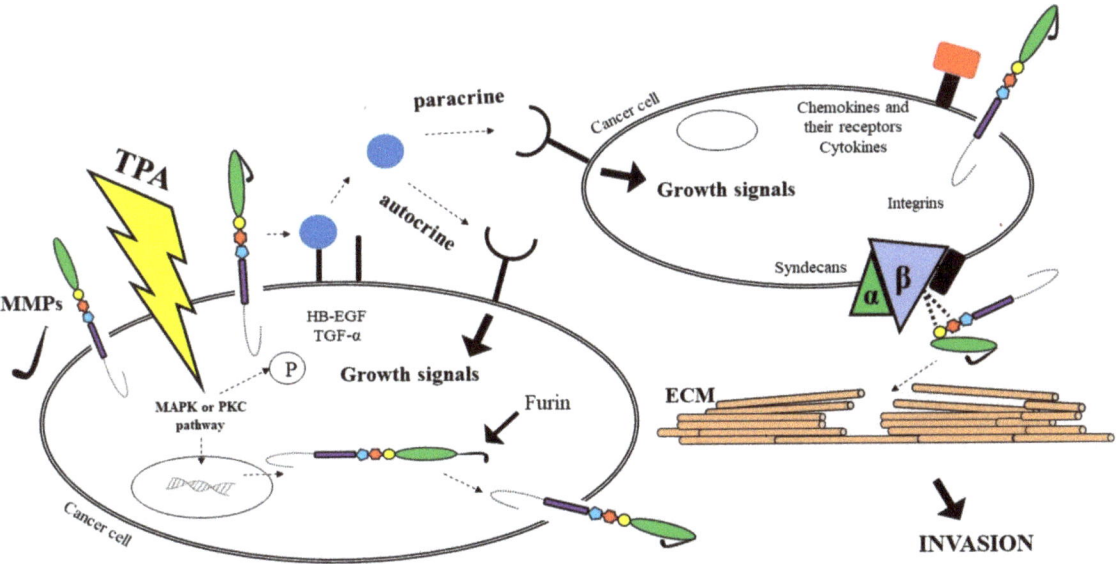

Figure 2. The significance of ADAMs in cancer biology [30–32].

Recent studies indicate the importance of the ADAM family in tumour formation, migration, proliferation and development [47,48]. There is increasing evidence that several ADAMs are differentially expressed in tumours. Some studies have confirmed the role of ADAMs in the biology of malignant cells, including breast [49,50], renal [51] and small cell lung [52] cancer as well as GI malignancies such as gastric [46–58], colorectal [59–62] and pancreatic [63–65] cancer and hepatocellular carcinoma [66–69].

4. A Disintegrin and Metalloproteinase (ADAMs)—Their Role in the Development and Prognosis of Gastrointestinal Cancers (GI)

Mounting evidence has associated an increased expression of individual ADAM family members with various types of cancer [46]. Among ADAM proteins, proteinase activities have been demonstrated for ADAM8, 9, 10, 12, 15, 17, 19, 28 and 33 [32]. Therefore, this review will focus of their significance in the pathogenesis of GI cancers. The significance of selected ADAMs in GI malignancies is presented in Table 2.

Table 2. The significance of selected ADAMs in GI malignancies.

ADAMs	GI Cancers	Results	References
ADAM8	GC	• overexpression in GC tissues compared with noncancerous tissues • correlation with tumour size (T factor), N (nodal involvement), vessel invasion and shorter survival	[54]
	CRC	• overexpression in CRC tissues compared with adjacent normal tissues • independent prognostic factor for patient survival	[60]
	PC	• overexpression in PC compared with normal pancreatic tissues • correlation with reduced patient survival	[64]
	LC	• overexpression in HCC tissues compared with normal liver tissues • correlation with higher concentrations of alpha-fetoprotein, tumour stage and size, histological differentiation, tumour recurrence and tumour metastasis • independent prognostic factor for patient survival	[68]
ADAM9	GC	• overexpression in GC compared with non-neoplastic foveolar epithelium	[46]
	PC	• overexpression in PC cell lines compared with normal epithelial cells • correlation with poor tumour differentiation and worse patient prognosis	[63,65,70]
Adam10	GC	• overexpression in GC lesions compared with adjacent non-cancerous tissues • correlation with TNM stage, size and location of tumour, depth of invasion, presence of lymph node and distant metastases • independent prognostic indicator of GC	[56]
	CRC	• elevated serum concentrations in CRC patients in comparison to healthy controls • correlation with clinical stage and histological grade of tumour • predictor of tumour progression	[61]
	HCC	• overexpression correlated with the presence of metastasis, grade, differentiation and size of tumour • correlation with reduced patient survival	[66,67,69]

Table 2. *Cont.*

ADAMs	GI Cancers	Results	References
ADAM12	GC	• upregulated expression in GC compared with non-neoplastic foveolar epithelium	[46]
	CRC	• serum levels were higher in the sera of CRC patients in comparison to healthy subjects • highest concentrations found in advanced stage of CRC	[43,61]
ADAM15	GC	• upregulated in GC compared with non-neoplastic foveolar epithelium • implicated in malignant growth of GC cells	[46]
	CRC	• reduced expression of ADAM15 in cancer cells • correlation with histologically poorly differentiated malignancies	[62]
	PC	• overexpression in PC cells compared with normal pancreatic epithelial cells	[63]
ADAM17	GC	• overexpression promoted migration of GC cells and tumour growth • overexpression was associated with advanced TNM stage and presence of lymph node metastasis • a significant biomarker for poor prognosis in GC	[71,72]
	CRC	• decreased serum levels in CRC patients in comparison to healthy controls	[43,59,61]
ADAM28	GC	• overexpression in GC cells regulated cell proliferation, migration and apoptosis	[58]
	CRC	• elevated serum levels in CRC patients in comparison to healthy subjects • correlation with clinical TNM stage, presence of distant metastases (M factor) and histopathological grading (G factor)	[61]

5. A Disintegrin and Metalloproteinase 8 (ADAM8)

Several studies have demonstrated that adamalysines are highly expressed in gastric cancer and play an important role in gastric cancer proliferation and invasion [46,55,56]. A disintegrin and metalloprotease 8 (ADAM8) is a member of the ADAM family which is involved in tumour development by enhancing cellular abilities of invasion and migration [60,64,73], stimulating angiogenesis [73,74] and inhibiting cancer cell apoptosis [75]. In GI malignancies, overexpression of this protease has been reported in pancreatic [64], gastric, colorectal and hepatocellular carcinomas [68].

ADAM8 plays an important role in GC proliferation and invasion [54]. A study by Huang et al. evaluated the clinical significance of ADAM8 in GC and explored its biological effects on GC. Using quantitative reverse transcription-polymerase chain reaction (q-RT-PCR), Western blotting and immunohistochemical (IHC) staining analysis, the authors revealed that ADAM8 mRNA expression was significantly upregulated in GC tissues compared with noncancerous tissues. Positive ADAM8 expression was more frequent in GC tissues in comparison to normal tissues and correlated with tumour size (T factor), N (nodal involvement), vessel invasion as well as shorter GC patient overall survival [54].

In addition, ADAM8 overexpression promoted cell growth and increased their migration and invasion abilities. The authors concluded that ADAM8 is able to promote proliferation and invasion of GC cells, and its expression is positively correlated with poor survival. Therefore, this glycoprotein might be a promising target in GC therapy [54].

Yang et al. assessed the expression of ADAM8 in CRC using q-RT-PCR Western blot and IHC staining analysis [60]. Expression of mRNA and protein levels of ADAM8 were significantly elevated in CRC tissues in comparison to adjacent normal tissues, which may suggest its importance in CRC carcinogenesis [47]. In addition, knockdown of ADAM8 in two CRC cell lines stimulated apoptosis and reduction of cellular growth and proliferation [60]. There was no significant association between ADAM8 expression and the clinicopathological characteristics of the tumour, which was confirmed using the IHC method [60]. Moreover, survival analysis indicated that CRC patients with ADAM8-positive tumours had worse 5-year overall survival and 5-year disease free survival in comparison with patients with ADAM8-negative tumours. Additionally, multivariate analysis revealed that ADAM8 expression was an independent prognostic factor for the survival of CRC patients [60]. The authors concluded that ADAM8 is overexpressed in CRC and may promote tumour growth as well as serve as an independent biomarker for the survival of CRC patients [60].

A study by Valkovskaya et al. [64] demonstrated that ADAM8 mRNA was significantly overexpressed in PC compared to normal pancreatic tissues, while elevated ADAM8 mRNA and protein expression levels correlated with reduced survival among PC patients. In addition, silencing of ADAM8 expression did not have a significant impact on PC cell growth but was able to suppress the invasiveness of this malignancy. The authors concluded that ADAM8 is overexpressed in PC tissue and may promote cancer cell invasiveness as well as correlate with reduced PC survival [64].

It has been reported that ADAM8 expression is markedly elevated in hepatocellular carcinoma (HCC) tissues in comparison to normal liver tissues. In addition, enhanced expression of this protein is positively correlated with elevated concentrations of the classical tumour marker for HCC—alpha-fetoprotein (AFP), tumour stage and size, histological differentiation, tumour recurrence and tumour metastasis [65]. Moreover, significantly shorter overall survival rates are observed among HCC patients with elevated ADAM8 expression in comparison to patients with low expression of this glycoprotein. Furthermore, multivariate analysis suggests that ADAM8 expression might be an independent prognostic factor for the survival of patients with HCC [65].

6. A Disintegrin and Metalloproteinase 9 (ADAM9)

ADAM metalloproteinase domain-containing protein (ADAM9) has been reported to be overexpressed in several GI cancers. Using immunohistochemistry and q-RT-PCR, it was demonstrated that this molecule was significantly upregulated in GC compared to non-neoplastic foveolar epithelium [46]. The administration of anti-ADAM9 antibodies inhibited the development of this malignancy, while ADAM9 promoted malignant growth of GC cells. The authors suggest that ADAM9 influences tumour cells via two possible ways—interaction with adhesion molecules, or the proteolytic 'shedding' of signalling molecules, which leads to the activation of their receptors, including the EGF receptor and its ligands [46]. These investigations indicate that modulation of the tumour–host interface may contribute to the pathogenesis, development and progression of GC [46].

It has also been reported that ADAM9 is overexpressed in PC and its cell lines, which has been proven using gene expression profiling by microarray. Moreover, based on the IHC method, the authors report that ADAM9 expression is associated with poor tumour differentiation and a worse prognosis of PC patients [65,70]. In addition, a study by Yamada et al. [63] revealed that PC cells expressed significantly higher levels of ADAM9 in comparison to normal pancreatic epithelial cells, which may suggest that this protein plays a role in the progression of PC and may present promising target for the diagnosis of this malignancy and treatment of patients [63].

7. A Disintegrin and Metalloproteinase 10 (ADAM10)

The metalloproteinase domain-containing protein 10 (ADAM10) has been implicated in the development and progression of several GI malignancies, including GC, HCC and CRC [56].

Protein levels of ADAM10 were upregulated in GC tissues compared with adjacent non-cancerous tissues, which was assessed using the IHC method. In addition, positive ADAM10 expression correlated with TNM stage, size and location of the tumour, depth of invasion as well as lymph node and distant metastases. The 5-year survival rate for patients with stage I, II and III GC with high expression of ADAM10 was significantly lower than for patients with low immunoreactivity of this protein. In addition, multivariate analysis determined that upregulation of ADAM10 was an independent prognostic indicator of GC [56]. The authors concluded that the expression of this protein is significantly associated with the presence of lymph node and distant metastases and poor prognosis and proved that ADAM10 could be a predictor of tumour progression and prognosis [56].

A study by Walkiewicz et al. [61] evaluated the concentrations of serum ADAM10 in CRC patients using the ELISA method. The authors revealed that serum ADAM10 levels were significantly higher in CRC patients in comparison to healthy controls and correlated with the clinical stage of CRC. In addition, there was a relationship between ADAM10 concentrations and the histological grade of the tumour, as serum ADAM10 levels were elevated in G1 tumours when compared to G3 malignancies. In conclusion, this protein might be a predictor of tumour progression [61].

Some clinical investigations have reported ADAM10 overexpression in HCC, which correlated with the presence of metastasis, grade, differentiation and size of the tumour. Moreover, the authors indicated that ADAM10 protein expression was significantly associated with reduced patient survival and may serve as a useful molecular marker for HCC [69]. Elevated ADAM10 expression has also been found in HCC cells, which correlated with the increased capacity of HCC cells for proliferation, invasion and migration, suggesting that this protein plays an important role in HCC progression [66,67].

8. A Disintegrin and Metalloproteinase 12 (ADAM12)

ADAM12 is a proteolytic glycoprotein that is located almost exclusively in tumour cells [61]. Moreover, tumour-associated stroma may also stimulate the expression of this protein in tumour cells via the synthesis of tumour growth factor β1 (TGF β1) that promotes carcinogenesis [76]. Some clinical investigations have revealed that ADAM12 overexpression may lead to increased tumour size and metastasis. Two isoforms of this glycoprotein have been discovered. However, only the secreted form of ADAM12 may enhance the ability of tumour cells to migrate and invade as well as stimulate local and distant metastasis in vivo. Moreover, it has been indicated that the stimulatory effect of ADAM12 on the migration and invasion of tumour cells is probably dependent on its proteolytic activity, and thus ADAM12 may represent a potential therapeutic target [30,36]. Using IHC and q-RT-PCR, the transcription and expression pattern of ADAM12 in GC cells and the corresponding non-tumour tissue as well as in GC cell lines were examined. Furthermore, immunoreactivity of this glycoprotein was significantly upregulated in GC compared to non-neoplastic foveolar epithelium [46]. Moreover, ADAM-specific antibodies enhanced the proliferation of GC cell lines. The authors concluded that this protein is implicated in the malignant growth of GC cells due to the interaction with adhesion molecules, the proteolytic 'shedding' of signalling molecules and the activation of their receptors, including the epithelial growth factor (EGF) receptor and its ligands [46].

Serum ADAM12 levels in patients with CRC have also been evaluated using the immunoenzyme method [43,61]. Concentrations of this glycoprotein were higher in the sera of CRC patients in comparison to healthy controls, while the highest concentrations were found in advanced stages of CRC, which may suggest the significance of ADAM12 in the pathogenesis of this malignancy [43,61].

9. A Disintegrin and Metalloproteinase 15 (ADAM15)

ADAM15 as a membrane protein with an adhesion domain is able to bind to a5b1 integrin via a unique arginine–glycine–aspartic acid (RGD) motif domain.

ADAM15 was found to be significantly upregulated in GC compared to non-neoplastic foveolar epithelium, with the expression being higher in intestinal neoplasms than in diffuse-type tumours, which was assessed using IHC and q-RT-PCR analyses [46]. The authors also demonstrated that the anti-ADAM15 antibodies inhibited GC cell growth, while the protein was also implicated in the malignant growth of GC cells, similarly to ADAM12, via the interaction with proteolytic 'shedding' of signalling molecules or adhesion molecules [46].

It has been shown that 63% of CRC cells demonstrate reduced expression of ADAM15 in cancer cells, which has been evaluated at the mRNA level. Moreover, downregulation of this molecule is associated with histologically poorly differentiated malignancies. Toquet et al. [62] assessed ADAM15 expression in colon carcinomas using both IHC and mRNA quantitative methods [49]. The authors observed decreased expression of ADAM15 in CRC associated with a loss of differentiation in a subset of colon carcinomas, which indicates that the role of ADAM15 in cancer progression is tissue-specific [62].

Some clinical investigations have revealed that the mRNA expression of ADAM15 is significantly higher in PC cells than in normal pancreatic epithelial cells, which may indicate the involvement of ADAM15 in the development of this malignancy [63].

10. A Disintegrin and Metalloproteinase 17 (ADAM17)

A disintegrin and metalloproteinase 17 (ADAM17) is also known as tumour necrosis factor-alpha (TNFα) converting enzyme (TACE). A growing body of evidence has revealed that this protein is associated with inflammation and cancer [53,77–79]. In addition, the significance of ADAM17 in cancer development is based on its direct effect on the release of TNFα [43,45]. Therefore, the relationship between ADAM17 levels and GI malignancies has been described in several studies [71,72,80–82].

The overexpression of ADAM17 may enhance the migratory ability of GC cells and tumour growth [72,80]. The authors demonstrated that ADAM17 overexpression was associated with an advanced TNM stage and presence of lymph node metastasis, while there was no significant correlation between ADAM17 expression and tumour differentiation [71,72,80–82]. In addition, elevated ADAM17 levels correlated with reduced overall survival rates, and thus ADAM17 was found to be a significant biomarker for poor prognosis in GC [71,72,80–82] and shown to play an important role in the development and progression of this malignancy [81]. Similar results were presented in a study by Ni et al. who evaluated the prognostic significance of ADAM17 and its association with the clinicopathological characteristics of GC [53]. The meta-analysis revealed that lower ADAM17 levels were correlated with longer overall survival rates in GC, while ADAM17 overexpression was associated with an advanced TNM stage and the presence of lymph node metastasis. The authors concluded that ADAM17 is a significant prognostic factor for GC [53].

It has been reported that ADAM17 may enhance the malignant potential of CRC cells via increasing their motility and the expression of proangiogenic factors, promoting tumour progression and metastasis [43,61]. A study by Walkiewicz et al., based on the ELISA method, revealed a statistically significant relationship between serum levels of ADAM17 and the clinical stage of CRC. The concentrations of this protein were lower in the sera of CRC patients in comparison to the control group [43,61]. Moreover, elevated serum concentrations of ADAM17 were found in obese CRC patients, which may explain the relationship between a Western diet and the activation of malignant processes [43,61]. Other investigations have confirmed the crucial role of ADAM17 in the pathogenesis of CRC and revealed that the use of a specific anti-ADAM17 antibody may inhibit the growth of CRC cell lines [43,59,61].

11. A Disintegrin and Metalloproteinase 28 (ADAM28)

Disintegrin and metalloproteinase 28 (ADAM28) is also associated with the growth and metastasis of various GI malignancies. ADAM28 protease supports cancer cell proliferation, survival and migration as well as metastatic progression [83]. A study by Yin et al. [58], which used, i.a., Western blot, q-PCR, wound healing assay and flow cytometry, demonstrated ADAM28 overexpression in GC cells, which correlated with shorter overall survival in comparison to those with low ADAM28 expression [58]. In addition, the authors revealed that ADAM28 from the endothelium and GC may cleave von Willebrand Factor (WF) to eliminate vWF-induced apoptosis of GC cells and promote a pro-metastasis effect [58]. These findings indicate that ADAM28 is able to regulate GC cell proliferation, migration and apoptosis.

The significance of ADAM28 in CRC pathogenesis has also been studied. Serum levels of ADAM28 were shown to be significantly higher in CRC patients than in healthy controls. Moreover, there was a relationship between serum levels of ADAM28 and clinical TNM stage as well as the presence of distant metastases (M factor). ADAM28 concentrations were highest in patients with stage IV CRC and presence of distant metastasis. In addition, there was a significant relationship between serum ADAM28 levels and histopathological grading (G factor). Serum concentrations of this molecule were higher in G3 patients in comparison to G1 and G2 subjects [61]. The authors indicated the potential usefulness of this molecule in the pathogenesis of CRC.

12. Conclusions

GI cancers are among the five most common malignancies in both men and women worldwide. Therefore, there is an urgent need for more research on early biomarkers of these malignancies. Pro-tumour functions have been mostly related to proteolytic enzymes from the metalloproteinase family including A disintegrin and metalloproteinases (ADAMs). Some clinical investigations suggest the potential role of these proteins in the pathogenesis of GI cancers. In this paper, we reviewed the involvement of selected ADAMs in GI cancer development and progression. The present paper demonstrates that of all ADAMs, ADAM8 is able to promote progression of CRC, PC, GC and HCC cells and may serve as a prognostic factor. ADAM9 contributes to the pathogenesis of GC and PC and poor PC patient prognosis. ADAM10 is significantly associated with the presence of lymph node and distant metastases in GC and histological grading in CRC patients. In addition, elevated ADAM10 levels correlate with a worse prognosis of GC and HCC patients. ADAM12 and ADAM15 are implicated in the malignant growth of GC, CRC and CRC. ADAM17 is associated with an advanced TNM stage and the presence of lymph node metastasis and is a significant biomarker for poor prognosis in GC. It might also play a role in the pathogenesis of CRC. ADAM28 levels correlate with the TNM stage, the presence of distant metastasis and the histological grading of CRC and may produce a pro-metastasis effect on GC.

In conclusion, our review paper confirms that selected ADAMs, particularly those with proteolytic properties, play an important role in the development of GI tumours and patient prognosis. However, given the non-specific nature of adamalysines, further research needs to be performed before selected ADAMs can be established as biomarkers for GI malignancies.

Author Contributions: M.Ł.-Z., S.P. and B.M. put forward the idea of the study. M.Ł.-Z. coordinated project funding. All authors have read and agreed to the published version of the manuscript.

Funding: This research was funded by the Medical University of Bialystok, Poland, grant number SUB/1/DN/22/004/2207, SUB/1/DN/22/003/1198. The APC was funded by Medical University of Bialystok, Poland, grant number SUB/1/DN/22/004/2207, SUB/1/DN/22/003/1198.

Acknowledgments: The presented project was supported by the Medical University of Bialystok, Poland. B.M. received consultation and/or lecture honoraria from Abbott, Wiener, Roche, Cormay and Biameditek; M.Ł.-Z. received consultation and/or lecture honoraria from Roche.

Conflicts of Interest: The authors declare no conflict of interest.

References

1. Cancer Facts & Figures 2018. Atlanta: American Cancer Society. 2018. Available online: https://www.cancer.org/content/dam/cancer-org/research/cancer-facts-and-statistics/annual-cancer-facts-and-figures/2018/cancer-facts-and-figures-2018.pdf (accessed on 26 April 2022).
2. Dizdar, Ö.; Kılıçkap, S. *Global Epidemiology of Gastrointestinal Cancers*; Yalcin, S., Philip, P.A., Eds.; Springer International Publishing: Cham, Switzerland, 2019; pp. 1–12.
3. Available online: https://www.cancer.org/content/dam/cancer-org/research/cancer-facts-and-statistics/annual-cancer-facts-and-figures/2019/cancer-facts-and-figures-2019.pdf (accessed on 26 April 2022).
4. Siegel, R.L.; Miller, K.D.; Fuchs, H.E.; Jemal, A. Cancer statistics, 2022. *CA Cancer J. Clin.* **2022**, *72*, 7–33. [CrossRef] [PubMed]
5. Flanagan, L.; Schmid, J.; Ebert, M.; Soucek, P.; Kunicka, T.; Liska, V.; Bruha, J.; Neary, P.; Dezeeuw, J.; Tommasino, M.; et al. Fusobacterium nucleatum associates with stages of colorectal neoplasia development, colorectal cancer and disease outcome. *Eur. J. Clin. Microbiol. Infect. Dis.* **2014**, *33*, 1381–1390. [CrossRef] [PubMed]
6. Mima, K.; Nishihara, R.; Qian, Z.R.; Cao, Y.; Sukawa, Y.; Nowak, J.A.; Yang, J.; Dou, R.; Masugi, Y.; Song, M.; et al. Fusobacterium nucleatum in colorectal carcinoma tissue and patient prognosis. *Gut* **2016**, *65*, 1973–1980. [CrossRef] [PubMed]
7. Abed, J.; Maalouf, N.; Manson, A.L.; Earl, A.M.; Parhi, L.; Emgård, J.E.M.; Klutstein, M.; Tayeb, S.; Almogy, G.; Atlan, K.A.; et al. Colon Cancer-Associated Fusobacterium nucleatum May Originate From the Oral Cavity and Reach Colon Tumors via the Circulatory System. *Front. Cell. Infect. Microbiol.* **2020**, *10*, 400. [CrossRef]
8. Yoshimura, T.; Tomita, T.; Dixon, M.F.; Axon, A.T.R.; Robinson, P.A.; Crabtree, J.E. ADAMs (a disintegrin and metalloproteinase) messenger RNA expression in Helicobacter pylori-infected, normal, and neoplastic gastric mucosa. *J. Infect. Dis.* **2002**, *185*, 332–340. [CrossRef]
9. D'Elia, L.; Galletti, F.; Strazzullo, P. Dietary salt intake and risk of gastric cancer. *Cancer Treat. Res.* **2014**, *159*, 83–95.
10. Yavuzsen, T.; Kazaz, N.; Tanriverdi, Ö.; Akman, T.; Davis, M.P. *Symptom Management in Gastrointestinal Cancers*; Yalcin, S., Philip, P.A., Eds.; Springer International Publishing: Cham, Switzerland, 2019; pp. 669–685.
11. Hui, D.; Shamieh, O.; Paiva, C.E.; Perex-Cruz, P.E.; Kwon, J.H.; Muckaden, M.A.; Park, M.; Yennu, S.; Kang, J.K.; Bruera, E. Minimal clinically important differences in the Edmonton Symptom Assessment Scale in cancer patients: A prospective, multicenter study. *Cancer* **2015**, *121*, 3027–3035. [CrossRef]
12. Karaosmanoglu, A.D.; Onur, M.R.; Arellano, R.S. *Imaging in Gastrointestinal Cancers*; Yalcin, S., Philip, P.A., Eds.; Springer International Publishing: Cham, Switzerland, 2019; pp. 445–464.
13. McCawley, L.J.; Matrisian, L.M. Matrix metalloproteinases: Multifunctional contributors to tumor progression. *Mol. Med. Today* **2000**, *6*, 149–156. [CrossRef]
14. Łukaszewicz-Zając, M.; Gryko, M.; Pączek, S.; Szmitkowski, M.; Kędra, B.; Mroczko, B. Matrix metalloproteinase 2 (MMP-2) and its tissue inhibitor 2 (TIMP-2) in pancreatic cancer (PC). *Oncotarget* **2019**, *10*, 395–403. [CrossRef]
15. Mroczko, B.; Kozłowski, M.; Groblewska, M.; Łukaszewicz, M.; Nikliński, J.; Jelski, W.; Laudański, J.; Chyczewski, L.; Szmitkowski, M. The diagnostic value of the measurement of matrix metalloproteinase 9 (MMP-9), squamous cell cancer antigen (SCC) and carcinoembryonic antigen (CEA) in the sera of esophageal cancer patients. *Clin. Chim. Acta* **2008**, *389*, 61–66. [CrossRef]
16. Mroczko, B.; Łukaszewicz-Zając, M.; Wereszczyńska-Siemiątkowska, U.; Groblewska, M.; Gryko, M.; Kędra, B.; Jurkowska, G.; Szmitkowski, M. Clinical significance of the measurements of serum matrix metalloproteinase-9 and its inhibitor (tissue inhibitor of metalloproteinase-1) in patients with pancreatic cancer. Metalloproteinase-9 as an independent prognostic factor. *Pancreas* **2009**, *38*, 613–618. [CrossRef] [PubMed]
17. Mroczko, B.; Łukaszewicz-Zając, M.; Guzińska-Ustymowicz, K.; Gryko, M.; Czyżewska, J.; Kemona, A.; Kędra, B.; Szmitkowski, M. Expression of matrix metalloproteinase-9 in the neoplastic and interstitial inflammatory infiltrate cells in gastric cancer. *Folia Histochem. Cytobiol.* **2009**, *47*, 491–496. [CrossRef] [PubMed]
18. Mroczko, B.; Groblewska, M.; Łukaszewicz-Zając, M.; Bandurski, R.; Kędra, B.; Szmitkowski, M. Pre-treatment serum and plasma levels of matrix metalloproteinase 9 (MMP-9) and tissue inhibitor of matrix metalloproteinases 1 (TIMP-1) in gastric cancer patients. *Clin. Chem. Lab. Med.* **2009**, *47*, 1133–1139. [CrossRef] [PubMed]
19. Mroczko, B.; Łukaszewicz-Zając, M.; Gryko, M.; Kędra, B.; Szmitkowski, M. Clinical significance of serum levels of matrix metalloproteinase 2 (MMP-2) and its tissue inhibitor (TIMP-2) in gastric cancer. *Folia Histochem. Cytobiol.* **2011**, *49*, 125–131. [CrossRef] [PubMed]
20. Melton, S.D.; Genta, R.M.; Souza, R.F. Biomarkers and Molecular Diagnostic Tests in Gastrointestinal Tract and Pancreatic Neoplasms. *Nat. Rev. Gastroenterol. Hepatol.* **2010**, *7*, 620–628. [CrossRef] [PubMed]
21. Łukaszewicz-Zając, M.; Mroczko, B. Circulating Biomarkers of Colorectal Cancer (CRC)—Their Utility in Diagnosis and Prognosis. *J. Clin. Med.* **2021**, *10*, 2391. [CrossRef]

22. Łukaszewicz-Zając, M.; Mroczko, B.; Gryko, M.; Kędra, B.; Szmitkowski, M. Comparison between clinical significance of serum proinflammatory proteins (IL-6 and CRP) and classic tumor markers (CEA and CA 19-9) in gastric cancer. *Clin. Exp. Med.* **2011**, *11*, 89–96. [CrossRef]
23. Pawluczuk, E.; Łukaszewicz-Zając, M.; Gryko, M.; Kulczyńska-Przybik, A.; Mroczko, B. Serum CXCL8 and Its Specific Receptor (CXCR2) in Gastric Cancer. *Cancers* **2021**, *13*, 5186. [CrossRef]
24. Valacca, C.; Tassone, E.; Mignatti, P. TIMP-2 Interaction with MT1-MMP Activates the AKT Pathway and Protects Tumor Cells from Apoptosis. *PLoS ONE* **2015**, *10*, e0136797. [CrossRef]
25. Schumacher, N.; Rose-John, S.; Schmidt-Arras, D. ADAM-Mediated Signalling Pathways in Gastrointestinal Cancer Formation. *Int. J. Mol. Sci.* **2020**, *21*, 5133. [CrossRef]
26. Edwards, D.R.; Handsley, M.M.; Pennington, C.J. The ADAM metalloproteinases. *Mol. Asp. Med.* **2008**, *29*, 258–289. [CrossRef] [PubMed]
27. Mentlein, R.; Hattermann, K.; Held-Feindt, J. Lost in disruption: Role of proteases in glioma invasion and progression. *Biochim. Biophys. Acta* **2012**, *1825*, 178–185. [CrossRef] [PubMed]
28. Englund, A.T.; Geffner, M.E.; Nagel, R.A.; Lippe, B.M.; Braunstein, G.D. Pediatric germ cell and human chorionic gonadotropin producing tumors. Clinical and laboratory features. *Am. J. Dis. Child.* **1991**, *145*, 1294–1297. [CrossRef]
29. Uhm, J.H.; Dooley, N.P.; Villemure, J.G.; Yong, V.W. Glioma invasion in vitro: Regulation by matrix metalloprotease-2 and protein kinase C. *Clin. Exp. Metastasis* **1996**, *14*, 421–433. [CrossRef] [PubMed]
30. Haoyuan, M.A.; Yanshu, L.I. Structure, regulatory factors and cancer-related physiological effects of ADAM9. *Cell Adhes. Migr.* **2020**, *14*, 165–181. [CrossRef] [PubMed]
31. Giebeler, N.; Zigrino, P. A Disintegrin and Metalloprotease (ADAM): Historical Overview of Their Functions. *Toxins* **2016**, *8*, 122. [CrossRef]
32. Mochizuki, S.; Okada, Y. ADAMs in cancer cell proliferation and progression. *Cancer Sci.* **2007**, *98*, 621–628. [CrossRef]
33. Lorenzen, I.; Lokau, J.; Düsterhöft, S.; Trad, A.; Garbers, C.; Scheller, J.; Rose-John, S.; Grötzinger, J. The membrane-proximal domain of A Disintegrin and Metalloprotease 17 (ADAM17) is responsible for recognition of the interleukin-6 receptor and interleukin-1 receptor II. *FEBS Lett.* **2012**, *586*, 1093–1100. [CrossRef]
34. Düsterhöft, S.; Michalek, M.; Kordowski, F.; Oldefest, M.; Sommer, A.; Röseler, J.; Reiss, K.; Grötzinger, J.; Lorenzen, I. Extracellular Juxtamembrane Segment of ADAM17 Interacts with Membranes and Is Essential for Its Shedding Activity. *Biochemistry (Moscow)* **2015**, *54*, 5791–5800. [CrossRef]
35. Schlondorff, J.; Blobel, C.P. Metalloprotease-disintegrins: Modular proteins capable of promoting cell–cell interactions and triggering signals by protein-ectodomain shedding. *J. Cell Sci.* **1999**, *112*, 3603–3617. [CrossRef]
36. Ghigna, C.; Giordano, S.; Shen, H.; Benvenuto, F.; Castiglioni, F.; Comoglio, P.M.; Green, M.R.; Riva, G.; Biamonti, S. Cell motility is controlled by SF2/ASF through alternative splicing of the Ron protooncogene. *Mol. Cell* **2005**, *20*, 881–890. [CrossRef] [PubMed]
37. Takehara, T.; Liu, X.; Fujimoto, J.; Friedman, S.L.; Takahashi, H. Expression and role of Bcl-xL in human hepatocellular carcinomas. *Hepatology* **2001**, *34*, 55–61. [CrossRef] [PubMed]
38. Line, A.; Slucka, Z.; Stengrevics, A.; Li, G.; Rees, R.C. Altered splicing pattern of TACC1 mRNA in gastric cancer. *Cancer Genet. Cytogenet.* **2002**, *139*, 78–83. [CrossRef]
39. Kim, Y.-J.; Kim, H.-S. Alternative Splicing and Its Impact as a Cancer Diagnostic Marker. *Genom. Inform.* **2012**, *10*, 74–80. [CrossRef] [PubMed]
40. Chute, M.; Jana, S.; Kassiri, Z. Disintegrin and metalloproteinases (ADAMs and ADAM-TSs), the emerging family of proteases in heart physiology and pathology. *Curr. Opin. Physiol.* **2018**, *1*, 34–45. [CrossRef]
41. Duffy, M.J.; Mullooly, M.; O'Donovan, N.; Sukor, S.; Crown, J.; Pierce, A.; McGowan, P.M. The ADAMs family of proteases: New biomarkers and therapeutic targets for cancer? *Clin. Proteom.* **2011**, *8*, 9. [CrossRef] [PubMed]
42. Duffy, M.J.; McKiernan, E.; O'Donovan, N.; McGowan, P.M. Role of ADAMs in cancer formation and progression. *Clin. Cancer Res.* **2009**, *15*, 1140–1144. [CrossRef]
43. Walkiewicz, K.; Koziel, P.; Bednarczyk, M.; Błażelonis, A.; Mazurek, U.; Muc-Wierzgoń, M. Expression of Migration-Related Genes in Human Colorectal Cancer and Activity of a Disintegrin and Metalloproteinase 17. *Biomed. Res. Int.* **2016**, *2016*, 8208904. [CrossRef]
44. Mochizuki, S.; Shimoda, M.; Shiomi, T.; Fujii, Y.; Okada, Y. ADAM28 is activated by MMP-7 (matrilysin-1) and cleaves insulin-like growth factor binding protein-3. *Biochem. Biophys. Res. Commun.* **2004**, *315*, 79–84. [CrossRef]
45. Gao, M.Q.; Kim, B.G.; Kang, S.; Choi, Y.P.; Yoon, J.H.; Cho, N.H. Human breast cancer-associated fibroblasts enhance cancer cell proliferation through increased TGF-α cleavage by ADAM17. *Cancer Lett.* **2013**, *336*, 240–246. [CrossRef]
46. Carl-McGrath, S.; Lendeckel, U.; Ebert, M.; Roessner, A.; Röcken, C. The disintegrin-metalloproteinases ADAM9, ADAM12, and ADAM15 are upregulated in gastric cancer. *Int. J. Oncol.* **2005**, *26*, 17–24. [CrossRef] [PubMed]
47. Wagstaff, L.; Kelwick, R.; Decock, J.; Edwards, D.R. The roles of ADAMTS metalloproteinases in tumorigenesis and metastasis. *Front. Biosci.* **2011**, *16*, 1861–1872. [CrossRef] [PubMed]
48. Herat, L.; Rudnicka, C.; Okada, Y.; Mochizuki, S.; Schlaich, M.; Matthews, V. The Metalloproteinase ADAM28 Promotes Metabolic Dysfunction in Mice. *Int. J. Mol. Sci.* **2017**, *18*, 884. [CrossRef] [PubMed]
49. Roy, R.; Moses, M.A. ADAM12 induces estrogen-independence in breast cancer cells. *Breast Cancer Res. Treat.* **2012**, *131*, 731–741. [CrossRef]

50. Roy, R.; Rodig, S.; Bielenberg, D.; Zurakowski, D.; Moses, M.A. ADAM12 transmembrane and secreted isoforms promote breast tumor growth: A distinct role for ADAM12-S protein in tumor metastasis. *J. Biol. Chem.* **2011**, *286*, 20758–20768. [CrossRef]
51. Fritzsche, F.R.; Wassermann, K.; Jung, M.; Tölle, A.; Kristiansen, I.; Lein, M.; Johannsen, M.; Dietel, M.; Jung, K.; Kristiansen, G. ADAM9 is highly expressed in renal cell cancer and is associated with tumour progression. *BMC Cancer* **2008**, *26*, 179. [CrossRef]
52. Shao, S.; Li, Z.; Gao, W.; Yu, G.; Liu, D.; Pan, F. ADAM-12 as a diagnostic marker for the proliferation, migration and invasion in patients with small cell lung cancer. *PLoS ONE* **2014**, *9*, e85936. [CrossRef]
53. Ni, P.; Yu, M.; Zhang, R.; He, M.; Wang, H.; Chen, S.; Duan, G. Prognostic Significance of ADAM17 for Gastric Cancer Survival: A Meta-Analysis. *Medicina* **2020**, *56*, 322. [CrossRef]
54. Huang, J.; Bai, Y.; Huo, L.; Xiao, J.; Fan, X.; Yang, Z.; Chen, H.; Yang, Z. Upregulation of a disintegrin and metalloprotease 8 is associated with progression and prognosis of patients with gastric cancer. *Transl. Res.* **2015**, *166*, 602–613. [CrossRef]
55. Kim, J.M.; Jeung, H.C.; Rha, S.Y.; Yu, E.J.; Kim, T.S.; Shin, Y.K.; Zhang, X.; Park, K.H.; Park, S.W.; Chung, H.C.; et al. The effect of disintegrin-metalloproteinase ADAM9 in gastric cancer progression. *Mol. Cancer Ther.* **2014**, *13*, 3074–3085. [CrossRef]
56. Wang, Y.Y.; Ye, Z.Y.; Li, L.; Zhao, Z.S.; Shao, Q.S.; Tao, H.Q. ADAM 10 is associated with gastric cancer progression and prognosis of patients. *J. Surg. Oncol.* **2011**, *103*, 116–123. [CrossRef] [PubMed]
57. Xu, M.; Zhou, H.; Zhang, C.; He, J.; Wei, H.; Zhou, M.; Lu, Y.; Sun, Y.; Ding, J.W.; Zeng, J.; et al. ADAM17 promotes epithelial-mesenchymal transition via TGF-β/Smad pathway in gastric carcinoma cells. *Int. J. Oncol.* **2016**, *49*, 2520–2528. [CrossRef] [PubMed]
58. Yin, Q.; Gu, J.; Qi, Y.; Lu, Y.; Yang, L.; Liu, J.; Liang, X. ADAM28 from both endothelium and gastric cancer cleaves von Willebrand Factor to eliminate von Willebrand Factor-induced apoptosis of gastric cancer cells. *Eur. J. Pharmacol.* **2021**, *898*, 173994. [CrossRef] [PubMed]
59. Dosch, J.; Ziemke, E.; Wan, S.; Luker, K.; Welling, T.; Hardiman, K.; Fearon, E.; Thomas, S.; Flynn, M.; Rios-Doria, J.; et al. Targeting ADAM17 inhibits human colorectal adenocarcinoma progression and tumor-initiating cell frequency. *Oncotarget* **2017**, *8*, 65090–65099. [CrossRef] [PubMed]
60. Yang, Z.; Bai, Y.; Huo, L.; Chen, H.; Huang, J.; Li, J.; Fan, X.; Yang, Z.; Wang, L.; Wang, J. Expression of A disintegrin and metalloprotease 8 is associated with cell growth and poor survival in colorectal cancer. *BMC Cancer* **2014**, *14*, 568. [CrossRef]
61. Walkiewicz, K.; Strzelczyk, J.; Waniczek, D.; Biernacki, K.; Muc-Wierzgoń, M.; Copija, A.; Nowakowska-Zajdel, E. Adamalysines as Biomarkers and a Potential Target of Therapy in Colorectal Cancer Patients: Preliminary Results. *Dis. Markers* **2019**, *2019*, 5035234. [CrossRef]
62. Toquet, C.; Colson, A.; Jarry, A.; Bezieau, S.; Volteau, C.; Boisseau, P.; Merlin, D.; Laboisse, C.L.; Mosnier, J.F. ADAM15 to α5β1 integrin switch in colon carcinoma cells: A late event in cancer progression associated with tumor dedifferentiation and poor prognosis. *Int. J. Cancer* **2012**, *130*, 278–287. [CrossRef]
63. Yamada, D.; Ohuchida, K.; Mizumoto, K.; Ohhashi, S.; Yu, J.; Egami, T.; Fujita, H.; Nagai, E.; Tanaka, M. Increased expression of ADAM 9 and ADAM 15 mRNA in pancreatic cancer. *Anticancer Res.* **2007**, *27*, 793–799.
64. Valkovskaya, N.; Kayed, H.; Felix, K.; Hartmann, D.; Giese, N.A.; Osinsky, S.P.; Friess, H.; Kleeff, J. ADAM8 expression is associated with increased invasiveness and reduced patient survival in pancreatic cancer. *J. Cell Mol. Med.* **2007**, *11*, 1162–1174. [CrossRef]
65. Alldinger, I.; Dittert, D.; Peiper, M.; Fusco, A.; Chiappetta, G.; Staub, E.; Lohr, M.; Jesnowski, R.; Baretton, G.; Ockert, D.; et al. Gene expression analysis of pancreatic cell lines reveals genes overexpressed in pancreatic cancer. *Pancreatology* **2005**, *5*, 370–379. [CrossRef]
66. Yuan, S.; Lei, S.; Wu, S. ADAM10 is overexpressed in human hepatocellular carcinoma and contributes to the proliferation, invasion and migration of HepG2 cells. *Oncol. Rep.* **2013**, *30*, 1715–1722. [CrossRef] [PubMed]
67. Shiu, J.S.; Hsieh, M.J.; Chiou, H.L.; Wang, H.L.; Yeh, C.B.; Yang, S.F.; Chou, Y.E. Impact of ADAM10 gene polymorphisms on hepatocellular carcinoma development and clinical characteristics. *Int. J. Med. Sci.* **2018**, *15*, 1334–1340. [CrossRef] [PubMed]
68. Zhang, Y.; Tan, Y.F.; Jiang, C.; Zhang, K.; Zha, T.Z.; Zhang, M. High ADAM8 expression is associated with poor prognosis in patients with hepatocellular carcinoma. *Pathol. Oncol. Res.* **2013**, *19*, 79–88. [CrossRef] [PubMed]
69. Zhang, W.; Liu, S.; Liu, K.; Wang, Y.; Ji, B.; Zhang, X.; Liu, Y. A disintegrin and metalloprotease (ADAM)10 is highly expressed in hepatocellular carcinoma and is associated with tumor progression. *J. Int. Med. Res.* **2014**, *42*, 611–618. [CrossRef]
70. Grutzmann, R.; Luttges, J.; Sipos, B.; Ammerpohl, O.; Dobrowolski, F.; Alldinger, I.; Kersting, S.; Ockert, D.; Koch, R.; Kalthoff, H.; et al. ADAM9 expression in pancreatic cancer is associated with tumour type and is a prognostic factor in ductal adenocarcinoma. *Br. J. Cancer* **2004**, *90*, 1053–1058. [CrossRef]
71. Fang, W.; Qian, J.; Wu, Q.; Chen, Y.; Yu, G. ADAM-17 expression is enhanced by FoxM1 and is a poor prognostic sign in gastric carcinoma. *J. Surg. Res.* **2017**, *220*, 223–233. [CrossRef]
72. Sun, J.; Jiang, J.; Lu, K.; Chen, Q.; Tao, D.; Chen, Z. Therapeutic potential of ADAM17 modulation in gastric cancer through regulation of the EGFR and TNF-alpha signalling pathways. *Mol. Cell. Biochem.* **2017**, *426*, 17–26. [CrossRef]
73. Romagnoli, M.; Mineva, N.D.; Polmear, M.; Conrad, C.; Srinivasan, S.; Loussouarn, D.; Barillé-Nion, S.; Georgakoudi, I.; Dagg, A.; McDermott, E.W.; et al. ADAM8 expression in invasive breast cancer promotes tumor dissemination and metastasis. *EMBO Mol. Med.* **2014**, *6*, 278–294. [CrossRef]

74. Guaiquil, V.H.; Swendeman, S.; Zhou, W.; Guaiquil, P.; Weskamp, G.; Bartsch, J.W.; Blobel, C.P. ADAM8 is a negative regulator of retinal neovascularization and of the growth of heterotopically injected tumor cells in mice. *J. Mol. Med.* **2010**, *88*, 497–505. [CrossRef]
75. Zhang, W.; Wan, M.; Ma, L.; Liu, X.; He, J. Protective effects of ADAM8 against cisplatin-mediated apoptosis in non-small-cell lung cancer. *Cell Biol. Int.* **2013**, *37*, 47–53. [CrossRef]
76. Fröhlich, C.; Nehammer, C.; Albrechtsen, R.; Kronqvist, P.; Kveiborg, M.; Sehara-Fujisawa, A.; Mercurio, A.M.; Wewer, U.M. ADAM12 produced by tumor cells rather than stromal cells accelerates breast tumor progression. *Mol. Cancer Res.* **2011**, *9*, 1449–1461. [CrossRef] [PubMed]
77. Rossello, A.; Nuti, E.; Ferrini, S.; Fabbi, M. Targeting ADAM17 Sheddase Activity in Cancer. *Curr. Drug Targets* **2016**, *17*, 1908–1927. [CrossRef] [PubMed]
78. Lisi, S.; D'Amore, M.; Sisto, M. ADAM17 at the interface between inflammation and autoimmunity. *Immunol. Lett.* **2014**, *162*, 159–169. [CrossRef] [PubMed]
79. Moss, M.L.; Minond, D. Recent Advances in ADAM17 Research: A Promising Target for Cancer and Inflammation. *Mediat. Inflamm.* **2017**, *2017*, 9673537. [CrossRef]
80. Li, W.; Wang, D.; Sun, X.; Zhang, Y.; Wang, L.; Suo, J. ADAM17 promotes lymph node metastasis in gastric cancer via activation of the Notch and Wnt signaling pathways. *Int. J. Mol. Med.* **2019**, *43*, 914–926. [CrossRef]
81. Zhang, T.C.; Zhu, W.G.; Huang, M.D.; Fan, R.H.; Chen, X.F. Prognostic value of ADAM17 in human gastric cancer. *Med. Oncol.* **2012**, *29*, 2684–2690. [CrossRef]
82. Shou, Z.X.; Jin, X.; Zhao, Z.S. Upregulated expression of ADAM17 is a prognostic marker for patients with gastric cancer. *Ann. Surg.* **2012**, *256*, 1014–1022. [CrossRef]
83. Hubeau, C.; Rocks, N.; Cataldo, D. ADAM28: Another ambivalent protease in cancer. *Cancer Lett.* **2020**, *494*, 18–26. [CrossRef]

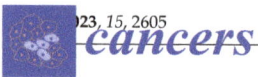

Article

Preoperative CA125 Significantly Improves Risk Stratification in High-Grade Endometrial Cancer

Marike S. Lombaers [1,2,*], Karlijn M. C. Cornel [1,3], Nicole C. M. Visser [4], Johan Bulten [5], Heidi V. N. Küsters-Vandevelde [6], Frédéric Amant [7,8], Dorry Boll [9], Peter Bronsert [10], Eva Colas [11], Peggy M. A. J. Geomini [12], Antonio Gil-Moreno [11,13], Dennis van Hamont [14], Jutta Huvila [15], Camilla Krakstad [16,17], Arjan A. Kraayenbrink [18], Martin Koskas [19], Gemma Mancebo [20], Xavier Matías-Guiu [21], Huy Ngo [22], Brenda M. Pijlman [23], Maria Caroline Vos [24], Vit Weinberger [25], Marc P. L. M. Snijders [26], Sebastiaan W. van Koeverden [27], ENITEC-Consortium [†], Ingfrid S. Haldorsen [16,28], Casper Reijnen [29] and Johanna M. A. Pijnenborg [1,2,*]

1. Department of Obstetrics and Gynaecology, Radboud University Medical Center, 6525 GA Nijmegen, The Netherlands
2. Radboud Institute of Health Sciences, 6525 GA Nijmegen, The Netherlands
3. Department of Obstetrics and Gynecology, Division Gynecologic Oncology, University of Toronto, Toronto, ON M5G 1E2, Canada
4. Department of Pathology, Eurofins PAMM, 5623 EJ Eindhoven, The Netherlands
5. Department of Pathology, Radboud University Medical Center, 6525 GA Nijmegen, The Netherlands
6. Department of Pathology, Canisius-Wilhelmina Hospital, 6532 SZ Nijmegen, The Netherlands
7. Department of Oncology, KU Leuven, 3000 Leuven, Belgium
8. Center for Gynecologic Oncology Amsterdam, Netherlands Cancer Institute and Amsterdam University Medical Center, 1066 CX Amsterdam, The Netherlands
9. Department of Gynecology, Catharina Hospital, 5623 EJ Eindhoven, The Netherlands
10. Institute of Pathology, University Medical Center, 79104 Freiburg, Germany
11. Biomedical Research Group in Gynecology, Vall Hebron Institute of Research, Universitat Autònoma de Barcelona, Centro de Investigación Biomédica en Red Cáncer, 08193 Barcelona, Spain
12. Department of Obstetrics and Gynaecology, Maxima Medical Centre, 5631 BM Veldhoven, The Netherlands
13. Department of Gynecology, Vall Hebron University Hospital, Centro de Investigación Biomédica en Red Cáncer, 08035 Barcelona, Spain
14. Department of Obstetrics and Gynaecology, Amphia Hospital, Breda, 4818 CK Breda, The Netherlands
15. Department of Pathology, University of Turku, 20500 Turku, Finland
16. Department of Obstetrics and Gynaecology, Haukeland University Hospital, 5021 Bergen, Norway
17. Centre for Cancer Biomarkers, Department of Clinical Science, University of Bergen, 5020 Bergen, Norway
18. Department of Obstetrics and Gynaecology, Rijnstate Hospital, 6815 AD Arnhem, The Netherlands
19. Department of Obstetrics and Gynaecology, Bichat-Claude Bernard Hospital, 75018 Paris, France
20. Department of Obstetrics and Gynaecology, Hospital del Mar, Parc de Salut Mar, 08003 Barcelona, Spain
21. Department of Pathology and Molecular Genetics and Research Laboratory, Hospital Universitari Arnau de Vilanova, University of Lleida, IRBLleida, Centro de Investigación Biomédica en Red Cáncer, 25003 Lleida, Spain
22. Department of Obstetrics and Gynaecology, Elkerliek Hospital, 5751 CB Helmond, The Netherlands
23. Department of Obstetrics and Gynaecology, Jeroen Bosch Hospital, 5223 GZ 's-Hertogenbosch, The Netherlands
24. Department of Obstetrics and Gynaecology, Elisabeth-TweeSteden Hospital, 5000 LC Tilburg, The Netherlands
25. Department of Gynecology and Obstetrics, University Hospital Brno, Faculty of Medicine, Masaryk University, 601 77 Brno, Czech Republic
26. Department of Obstetrics and Gynaecology, Canisius-Wilhelmina Hospital, 6532 SZ Nijmegen, The Netherlands
27. Department of Radiology and Nuclear Medicine, Radboud University Medical Center, 6525 GA Nijmegen, The Netherlands
28. Mohn Medical Imaging and Visualization Centre, Department of Radiology, Haukeland University Hospital, 5021 Bergen, Norway
29. Department of Radiation Oncology, Radboud University Medical Center, 6525 GA Nijmegen, The Netherlands
* Correspondence: marike.lombaers@radboudumc.nl (M.S.L.); hanny.ma.pijnenborg@radboudumc.nl (J.M.A.P.)
† All members of the ENITEC Consortium are included as authors on this work.

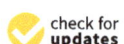

Citation: Lombaers, M.S.; Cornel, K.M.C.; Visser, N.C.M.; Bulten, J.; Küsters-Vandevelde, H.V.N.; Amant, F.; Boll, D.; Bronsert, P.; Colas, E.; Geomini, P.M.A.J.; et al. Preoperative CA125 Significantly Improves Risk Stratification in High-Grade Endometrial Cancer. *Cancers* 2023, 15, 2605. https://doi.org/10.3390/cancers15092605

Academic Editors: Daniel L. Pouliquen and Cristina Núñez González

Received: 28 February 2023
Revised: 3 April 2023
Accepted: 22 April 2023
Published: 4 May 2023

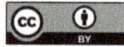

Copyright: © 2023 by the authors. Licensee MDPI, Basel, Switzerland. This article is an open access article distributed under the terms and conditions of the Creative Commons Attribution (CC BY) license (https://creativecommons.org/licenses/by/4.0/).

Simple Summary: Patients with high-grade uterine cancer (UC) have a risk of around 20% of the cancer spreading to the lymph nodes, while this is only around 10% in patients with low-grade uterine cancer. CA125 is a marker that can be detected in blood and is associated with increased tumor spread. Studies on CA125 and its association with tumor spread within low-grade UC exist but are limited for high-grade UC. The primary aim of this retrospective study was to assess whether elevated CA125 is predictive for UC spread and survival. Secondarily, we studied the additional value of preoperative imaging by CT scan in relation to CA125 specifically in high-grade UC. We observed that elevated CA125 was related to advanced stage and LNM in high-grade UC and a worse prognosis. If CA125 was normal, the additional value of CT to predict lymph node spread was limited.

Abstract: Patients with high-grade endometrial carcinoma (EC) have an increased risk of tumor spread and lymph node metastasis (LNM). Preoperative imaging and CA125 can be used in work-up. As data on cancer antigen 125 (CA125) in high-grade EC are limited, we aimed to study primarily the predictive value of CA125, and secondarily the contributive value of computed tomography (CT) for advanced stage and LNM. Patients with high-grade EC (n = 333) and available preoperative CA125 were included retrospectively. The association of CA125 and CT findings with LNM was analyzed by logistic regression. Elevated CA125 ((>35 U/mL), (35.2% (68/193)) was significantly associated with stage III-IV disease (60.3% (41/68)) compared with normal CA125 (20.8% (26/125), [$p < 0.001$]), and with reduced disease-specific—(DSS) ($p < 0.001$) and overall survival (OS) ($p < 0.001$). The overall accuracy of predicting LNM by CT resulted in an area under the curve (AUC) of 0.623 ($p < 0.001$) independent of CA125. Stratification by CA125 resulted in an AUC of 0.484 (normal), and 0.660 (elevated). In multivariate analysis elevated CA125, non-endometrioid histology, pathological deep myometrial invasion $\geq$50%, and cervical involvement were significant predictors of LNM, whereas suspected LNM on CT was not. This shows that elevated CA125 is a relevant independent predictor of advanced stage and outcome specifically in high-grade EC.

Keywords: endometrial cancer; advanced stage; outcome; high-grade; CA125

1. Introduction

Endometrial carcinoma (EC) is the most common gynecological malignancy in industrialized countries. Primarily, distinction on outcome is based on tumor grade, with favorable outcomes in low-grade tumors and poor outcomes in high-grade tumors. In high-grade EC, i.e., grade 3 endometrioid and non-endometrioid histology, there is an increased risk of advanced stage and lymph node metastasis (LNM) [1]. As the risk of LNM in grade 3 EC varies between 15–44% depending on the histological subtype and myometrial invasion (MI), determination of lymph node status by lymphadenectomy or sentinel node (SN) biopsy is recommended in patients without clinical suspicion of advanced stage EC [2–5]. In the preoperative work-up abdominal computed tomography (CT), pelvic magnetic resonance imaging (MRI), and 18FDG positron emission tomography (PET)-CT can be considered to detect extra-uterine tumor spread or distant metastases, as this may impact the surgical approach [2,3,6,7]. After primary surgico-pathological staging, information about tumor stage, histopathological subtype, tumor grade, presence of deep myometrial invasion $\geq$50% (DMI), cervical stromal invasion (CI), lymphovascular space invasion (LVSI), or LNM guides adjuvant radiotherapy and/or chemotherapy [2,3]. The recently introduced molecular classification may increasingly guide adjuvant therapy, yet for high-grade EC surgical staging is still recommended according to the ESGO-ESTRO-ESP guideline [2]. In a systematic review and meta-analysis, it was shown that elevated cancer antigen 125 (CA125) serum level is associated with increased risk of LNM both in low-grade and high-grade ECs [8]. In addition, CA125 has been incorporated in several predictive models that have shown an improved risk classification for advanced stage and LNM in

EC and remains an independent prediction compared to molecular classification [9–14]. Furthermore, imaging findings indicating extra-uterine spread and/or distant spread predict advanced stage and poor prognosis [6,8]. However, preoperative CT and MRI have limited sensitivity for the identification of LNM [6,8,13,15,16]. So far, preoperative CA125 has not been selectively studied in patients with high-grade EC in relation to imaging findings. Therefore, our primary aim is to determine the predictive value of CA125 in relation to LNM and advanced stage in high-grade EC. Our secondary aim is to determine the predictive value of CA125 combined with preoperative imaging in relation to LNM and advanced stage in high-grade EC.

2. Materials and Methods

2.1. Patient Cohort

A retrospective multicenter study was performed including patients with preoperative high-grade EC with all histological subtypes, diagnosed by endometrial sampling by pipelle, dilatation and curettage, or hysteroscopic biopsy. Patients were retrieved from three well-documented study cohorts [13,17–19]. Patients who underwent surgical staging but with either preoperative or postoperative grade 3 tumors, remained included for analysis. Patients without available preoperative CA125 were excluded. In all study cohorts, histopathological analysis was performed by gynecological pathologists. Approval for the original studies was obtained by the Review Board Radboud University Medical Center Nijmegen, the Netherlands (institutional study protocol 2015-2101) and by the medical ethical committee of the Elisabeth-Tweesteden Hospital Tilburg, the Netherlands (protocol 1129).

2.2. Data Collection

Collected data consisted of patient characteristics (age, body mass index [BMI], comorbidity), preoperative CA125, modality and results of preoperative imaging as reported in the routine radiology report, type of surgical procedure, pathological lymph node status, histology type, and stage of disease. Lymphadenopathy on imaging was defined as lymph nodes with short axis diameter $\geq$10 mm and with or without suspected distant spread on imaging [20]. Scans were read and reported by radiologists at the hospital where the patient was treated. When imaging findings reported in the radiology report were 'inconclusive' for lymph node status, they were excluded from analysis. Surgical lymph node staging was defined as pelvic and/or para-aortic lymph node sampling, with or without omental sampling, peritoneal biopsies, or both. Both preoperative and postoperative histopathological data on tumor histology and grade were documented. Patients who underwent staging with distant metastases but without LNM were excluded. Due to a limited number of performed MRIs (n = 14), myometrial invasion (MI) and cervical stromal invasion (CI) were documented from the postoperative pathology report only. When CI findings did not specify whether there was stromal or only endocervical invasion, they were excluded from analysis. The presence of LNM, LVSI and the final FIGO stage were documented from the final postoperative pathology report after surgical staging. Adjuvant treatment was classified into: none, radiotherapy including external beam radiation (EBRT) with or without vaginal brachytherapy (VBT), VBT only, chemotherapy, and combined chemoradiotherapy. Follow-up data including disease-specific- and overall survival were collected for an average of 32 months after diagnosis.

2.3. Statistical Analysis

Clinicopathological differences between the three cohorts and subgroups were compared using Pearson's chi-square test or Fisher's exact test for categorical data. The Mann–Whitney U test was used for continuous data. It has been shown that different cut-off values for CA125 serum levels (25 U/mL and 35 U/mL) had comparable diagnostic accuracy for the prediction of LNM [8]. We used the cut-off value of 35 U/mL as dichotomous variable for 'normal' ($\leq$35 U/mL) and 'elevated' (>35 U/mL) CA125, according the widely used cut-off value in hospital laboratories [11,21,22]. Kaplan–Meier curves were created for 5-year disease-specific survival (DSS) and overall survival (OS) for all patients within the cohort with available data on recurrence and death. Patients with progression of disease were excluded from DSS analysis. A log rank (Mantel–Cox) test was run to compare DSS and OS in groups with and without elevated CA125. For the analysis on LNM and advanced International Federation of Gynecology and Obstetrics (FIGO) stage, defined as FIGO stage III and IV, all patients who underwent surgical staging were included. A p value less than 0.05 was considered significant. Sensitivity, specificity, positive predictive value (PPV), negative predictive value (NPV), and Clopper–Pearson exact confidence intervals for CA125 and CT imaging versus LNM were calculated. Receiver operating characteristics (ROC) were made to calculate the area under the curve (AUC). Age, BMI, non-EC histology, MI, and CI were identified from earlier studies as additional predictive variables for LNM and included in univariable analysis for LNM [1,8,13,23]. Significant predictive variables from univariate logistic regression analysis ($p < 0.02$) were included in a multivariate logistical regression analysis. Statistical Package for the Social Sciences (SPSS) version 25 (SPSS IBM, New York, NY, USA) software was used for data management and to perform the statistical analyses.

In accordance with the journal's guidelines, we will provide our data for independent analysis by a selected team by the Editorial Team for the purposes of additional data analysis or for the reproducibility of this study in other centers if such is requested.

3. Results

3.1. Study Cohort

A total of 333 patients with preoperative CA125 serum level and high-grade EC were included. An overview of the inclusion of patients is shown in Figure S1. The baseline characteristics in relation to CA125 serum level are shown in Table 1, specified for patients with (n = 193) and without (n = 140) surgical lymph node (LN) staging. The median age was 66 and 72 years, respectively, and median BMI 26.8 kg/m^2 versus 28.2 kg/m^2, respectively. The differences in age and BMI were not statistically significant. Of all patients, 2.4% (8/333) did not undergo surgery. Overall, 44.1% (147/334) of the patients had an elevated CA125 serum level. Patients without surgical LN staging had elevated CA125 serum levels in 56.4% (79/140) of patients and presented with FIGO IV in 30.0% (42/140), whereas patients with surgical staging presented with elevated CA125 in 35.2% (68/193) and FIGO IV in 9.8% (19/193). Preoperative imaging was performed in 68.2% (n = 227) of the patients; abdominal/chest CT in 64.3% (214/333) and pelvic MRI in 4.2% (14/333). In one patient, both CT and MRI were performed. According to the radiology report, LNM were suspected in 16.3% (37/227) of patients and extra-uterine or distant spread in 8.8% (20/228). Both LNM and extra-uterine or distant spread were reported in 1.8% (4/227) of the patients. Patients with preoperative imaging underwent surgical LN staging in 67.8% (154/227) compared to 34.0% (14/40) in patients without preoperative imaging ($p < 0.001$). Excluded patients (n = 185) due to lack of CA125 did not differ with respect to baseline characteristics from the included patients.

Table 1. Baseline characteristics of patients with preoperative high-grade EC and surgical staging versus no staging, in association with CA125 level.

		Total (n = 193)	Surgical LN Staging (n = 193)			Total (n = 140)	No Surgical LN Staging (n = 140)		
			CA125 <35 U/mL (n = 125)	CA125 >35 U/mL (n = 68)	p Value		CA125 <35 U/mL (n = 61)	CA125 >35 U/mL (n = 79)	p Value
Age (years)		66 (35–83)	66 (35–83)	66 (44–82)	0.477	72 (48–93)	74 (48–91)	71 (51–93)	0.234
BMI (kg/m^2)		26.8 (17.6–56.0)	26.8 (17.6–56.0)	28.2 (18.0–42.6)	0.750	28.2 (16.4–49.5)	27.9 (19.5–47.8)	29.1 (16.4–49.5)	0.486
Imaging modality	CT	145 (86.3)	94 (84.7)	51 (89.5)	0.393	69 (69.7)	30 (55.6)	39 (86.7)	<0.001
	MRI	10 (12.0)	8 (15.4)	2 (8.0)	0.485	4 (16.0)	3 (18.8)	1 (11.1)	1

Table 1. Cont.

		Total (n = 193)	Surgical LN Staging (n = 193)			Total (n = 140)	No Surgical LN Staging (n = 140)		
			CA125 <35 U/mL (n = 125)	CA125 >35 U/mL (n = 68)	p Value		CA125 <35 U/mL (n = 61)	CA125 >35 U/mL (n = 79)	p Value
CT results	No extra-uterine disease	101 (69.7)	77 (81.9)	24 (47.1)	<0.001	43 (62.3)	22 (73.3)	21 (53.8)	0.052
	Suspected LNM with or without suspected distant metastasis	28 (19.3)	9 (9.6)	19 (37.3)		11 (15.9)	6 (20.0)	5 (12.8)	
	Suspected distant metastasis without suspected LNM	5 (3.4)	2 (2.1)	3 (5.9)		14 (20.3)	2 (6.7)	12 (30.8)	
	Inconclusive	11 (7.6)	6 (6.4)	5 (9.8)		1 (1.4)	0 (0.0)	1 (2.6)	
FIGO stage [a]	IA	69 (35.8)	59 (47.2)	10 (14.7)	<0.001	32 (22.5)	25 (41.0)	7 (8.9)	<0.001
	IB	40 (20.7)	30 (24.0)	10 (14.7)		36 (25.7)	22 (36.1)	14 (17.7)	
	II	17 (8.8)	10 (8.0)	7 (10.3)		10 (7.1)	5 (8.2)	5 (6.3)	
	IIIA	7 (3.6)	5 (4.0)	2 (2.9)		12 (8.6)	3 (4.9)	9 (11.4)	
	IIIB	1 (0.5)	1 (0.8)	0 (0.0)		5 (3.6)	1 (1.6)	4 (5.1)	
	IIIC1-2	40 (20.7)	17 (13.6)	23 (33.8)		3 (2.1)	0 (0.0)	3 (3.8)	
	IVA	1 (0.5)	1 (0.8)	0 (0.0)		7 (5.0)	1 (1.6)	6 (7.6)	
	IVB	18 (9.3)	2 (1.6)	16 (23.5)		37 (25.0)	4 (6.6)	31 (39.2)	
Tumor grade [a]	1	3 (1.6)	0 (0.0)	3 (4.4)	0.020	6 (4.3)	5 (8.3)	1 (1.3)	0.040
	2	12 (6.2)	10 (8.0)	2 (2.9)		4 (2.9)	3 (5.0)	1 (1.3)	
	3	178 (92.2)	115 (92.0)	63 (92.6)		129 (92.8)	52 (86.7)	77 (97.5)	

		Total (n = 193)	CA125 <35 U/mL (n = 125)	CA125 >35 U/mL (n = 68)	p value	Total (n = 140)	CA125 <35 U/mL (n = 61)	CA125 >35 U/mL (n = 79)	p value
Histology [a]	Endometrioid	80 (41.5)	54 (43.2)	26 (38.2)	0.480	56 (40.0)	38 (62.3)	18 (22.8)	<0.001
	Serous	89 (46.1)	53 (42.4)	36 (52.9)		74 (52.9)	19 (31.1)	55 (69.6)	
	Clear cell	9 (4.7)	7 (5.6)	2 (2.9)		1 (0.7)	1 (1.6)	0 (0.0)	
	Other	15 (7.8)	11 (8.8)	4 (5.9)		9 (6.4)	3 (4.9)	6 (7.6)	
MI [a]	<50%	94 (48.7)	70 (56.0)	24 (35.3)	0.006	55 (41.7)	30 (50.0)	25 (34.7)	0.076
	=/>50%	99 (51.3)	55 (44.0)	44 (64.7)		77 (58.3)	30 (50.0)	47 (65.3)	
CI [a]	No	143 (74.1)	102 (83.6)	41 (62.1)	<0.001	94 (71.8)	47 (78.3)	47 (66.2)	0.124
	Yes	45 (23.3)	20 (16.4)	25 (37.9)		37 (28.2)	13 (21.7)	24 (33.8)	
LVSI [a]	No	110 (57.0)	91 (72.8)	19 (27.9)	<0.001	70 (52.6)	39 (65.0)	31 (42.5)	0.010
	Yes	83 (43.0)	34 (27.2)	49 (72.1)		63 (47.4)	21 (35.0)	42 (57.5)	
LNM [b]	No (N0)	136 (70.5)	107 (85.6)	29 (42.6)	<0.001	-	-	-	-
	Yes (N1)	57 (29.5)	18 (14.4)	39 (57.4)		-	-	-	
Adjuvant therapy	Radiotherapy	82 (42.5)	60 (48.0)	22 (32.4)	0.006	59 (42.1)	36 (59.0)	23 (29.1)	<0.001
	Chemotherapy	60 (31.1)	28 (22.4)	32 (47.1)		32 (22.9)	4 (6.6)	28 (35.4)	
	Radio- and chemo-therapy	10 (5.2)	7 (5.6)	3 (4.4)		5 (3.6)	2 (3.3)	3 (3.8)	
	No adjuvant therapy	41 (21.2)	30 (24.0)	11 (16.2)		44 (31.4)	19 (31.1)	25 (31.6)	
Radio-therapy	VBT	36 (39.1)	24 (35.8)	12 (48.0)	0.287	23 (35.9)	15 (39.5)	8 (30.8)	0.476
	EBRT ± VBT	56 (60.9)	43 (64.2)	13 (52.0)		41 (64.1)	23 (60.5)	18 (69.2)	
Follow up (months)		39.0 (0–193)	47.5 (0–193)	33.8 (0–123)	0.003	21.0 (0–132)	36.0 (0–132)	9.0 (0–83)	<0.001
Recurrence	No	120 (62.5)	92 (74.2)	28 (41.2)	<0.001	64 (46.0)	41 (68.3)	23 (29.1)	<0.001
	Yes	53 (27.6)	27 (21.8)	26 (38.2)		40 (28.8)	17 (28.3)	23 (29.1)	
	Progression	19 (9.9)	5 (4.0)	14 (20.6)		35 (25.2)	2 (3.3)	33 (41.8)	
Death	No	125 (65.4)	94 (75.8)	31 (46.3)	<0.001	68 (49.6)	43 (70.5)	25 (32.9)	<0.001
	Yes, caused by EC	54 (28.3)	23 (18.5)	31 (46.3)		56 (40.9)	12 (19.7)	44 (57.9)	
	Yes, not caused by EC	6 (3.1)	5 (4.0)	1 (1.5)		8 (5.8)	4 (6.6)	4 (5.3)	
	Yes, unknown cause	6 (3.1)	2 (1.6)	4 (6.0)		5 (3.6)	2 (3.3)	3 (3.9)	

Values are presented as median (range) or number (%), [a] = based on postoperative pathology, [b] = based on surgical staging, LN = lymph node, CA125 = cancer antigen 125, BMI = body mass index, CT = computed tomography, MRI = magnetic resonance imaging, LNM = lymph node metastasis, FIGO = International Federation of Gynecology and Obstetrics, MI = myometrial invasion, CI = cervical stromal invasion, LVSI = lymphovascular space invasion, VBT = vaginal brachytherapy, EBRT = External Beam Radiation Therapy, EC = endometrial cancer. Missing values are not shown or used in analysis for this table.

3.2. CA125 in Relation to Extra-Uterine Disease and LNM

Surgically staged patients with elevated CA125 were significantly more often diagnosed with FIGO stage III-IV (60.3% [41/68]) compared to patients with normal CA125 (20.8% [26/125], $p < 0.001$). In addition, in patients with elevated CA125 the prevalence was significantly higher for DMI, CI and LVSI (Table 1). In surgically staged patients (n = 194), LNM were present in 29.4% (57/194), respectively in 56.5% (39/69) of the patients with elevated CA125 and in 14.4% (18/125) of patients with normal CA125 ($p < 0.001$). The specificity, sensitivity, NPV, PPV, and AUC of CA125 > 35 U/mL for predicting LNM are summarized in Table 2. The AUC for CA125 in relation to pathological confirmed LNM was 0.721, and 0.675 for FIGO III/IV.

Table 2. Performance of preoperative CA125 serum level and preoperative CT alone and combined versus LNM in patients who underwent surgical LN staging.

			Total (n)	Sensitivity % [95% CI] (n)	Specificity % [95% CI] (n)	PPV % [95% CI] (n)	NPV % [95% CI] (n)	ROC AUC (95% CI)	p Value
LNM	CA125 [a]		193	68.4 [54.8–80.1] (39/57)	78.7 [70.8–85.2] (107/136)	57.4 [44.8–69.2] (39/68)	85.6 [78.2–91.2] (107/125)	0.721 (0.619–0.824)	<0.001
	CT [b]		129	40.5 [24.8–7.9] (15/37)	85.9 [77.1–92.3] (79/92)	53.6 [33.9–72.5] (15/28)	78.2 [68.9–85.8] (79/101)	0.623 (0.520–0.744)	<0.001
	CA125 <35 U/mL	CT [b]	86	7.7 [0.0–36.0] (1/13)	89.0 [79.5–95.2] (65/73)	11.1 [0.0–48.3] (1/9)	84.4 [74.4–91.7] (65/77)	0.484 (0.316–0.652)	1.000
	CA125 >35 U/mL	CT [b]	43	58.3 [36.6–77.9] (14/24)	73.7 [48.8–90.9] (14/19)	73.7 [48.8–90.9] (14/19)	58.3 [36.6–77.9] (14/24)	0.660 (0.495–0.826)	0.036

[a] = cut-off for positive test of 35 U/mL, [b] = cut-off for positive test is suspected LNM on CT for predicting LNM. CA125: cancer antigen 125, LNM: lymph node metastases, CT: computed tomography, PPV: positive predictive value, NPV: negative predictive value, ROC: receiver operating characteristic, AUC: area under the curve, CI: confidence interval.

3.3. Imaging in Relation to Extra-Uterine Disease and LNM

For the imaging analysis, only patients who underwent preoperative imaging by CT with conclusive results (n = 134) were included, as the number of patients who underwent MRI was limited (n = 10). Patients with suspected extra-uterine disease on CT (33/134), either LNM (n = 27), distant spread (n = 5), or both LNM and distant spread (n = 1) had significantly more often FIGO stage III-IV (54.5% [18/33] vs. 23.8% [24/101], $p < 0.002$). In patients with suspected extra-uterine disease on CT, the prevalence of DMI, CI, and LVSI was comparable. In patients with preoperative CT with suspected LNM (n = 28), 53.6% (15/28) had histologically confirmed LNM compared to 21.8% (22/101) in patients with no signs of LNM on CT ($p < 0.001$). The AUC for suspected LNM on CT in relation to confirmed LNM was 0.623 (Table 2) and 0.633 for FIGO III/IV.

3.4. CA125 and CT Results in Relation to LNM

Combined preoperative CA125 and CT results in relation to LNM are shown in Figure 1 and illustrate the relevance of CA125 in accordance with the summarized data in Table 2. Within patients with elevated CA125, CT scan with suspicion of LNM resulted in an AUC of 0.660, while with normal CA125, the AUC was 0.484. For advanced FIGO stage, similar results were observed, as the AUC for CT within patients with elevated CA125 was 0.633, while it was 0.545 in patients with normal CA125. In univariate logistic regression analysis, non-endometrioid (NEEC) histology, suspected LNM on preoperative imaging, elevated CA125, DMI and CI (from hysterectomy specimen) were significant predictive variables for LNM (Table 3). In multivariate logistic regression analysis, NEEC histology, elevated CA125 serum level, DMI, and CI remained significantly associated with LNM, whereas suspected LNM on preoperative CT was not significant.

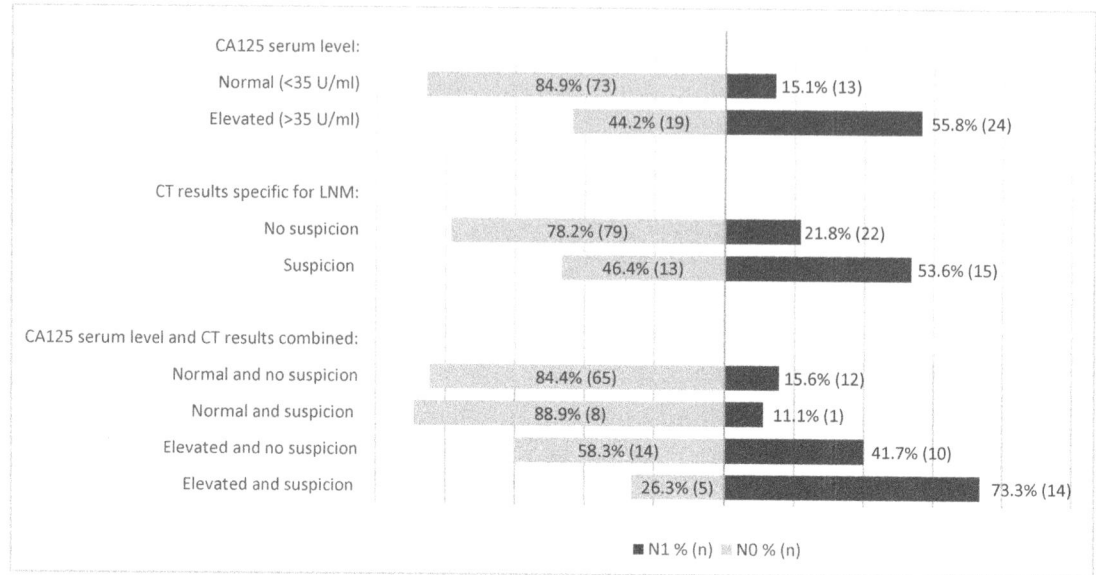

Figure 1. Study population proportion of LNM in relation to CA125 levels and LNM on imaging. N0: no LNM, N1: presence of LNM. CA125 = cancer antigen 125, LNM = lymph node metastases.

Table 3. Logistic regression analysis of clinicopathological variables in relation to LNM.

	Univariate Analysis			Multivariate Analysis		
	p Value	Adjusted OR	95% CI	p Value	Adjusted OR	95% CI
Age > 65 years *	0.964	0.99	0.53–1.83	-	-	-
BMI >30 kg/m^2 *	0.790	0.91	0.46–1.81	-	-	-
NEEC histology	<0.001	3.75	1.82–7.70	0.028	3.72	1.16–11.95
CA125 > 35 U/mL	<0.001	7.99	4.00–15.99	0.003	6.25	1.85–21.09
CT with suspected LNM	0.002	4.14	1.72–9.99	0.427	1.680	0.48–6.05
Deep myometrial involvement	<0.001	3.45	1.76 6.74	0.007	4.88	1.54–15.46
Cervical stromal involvement	0.009	4.21	1.42–12.50	0.018	7.87	1.42–43.78

OR: odds ratio, CI: confidence interval for adjusted OR, BMI: body mass index, NEEC: non-endometrioid endometrial carcinoma, CT: computed tomography. * = not included for multivariate analysis as $p > 0.02$.

3.5. CA125 in Relation to Outcome

Of all 333 patients, 331 patients had available recurrence data with a mean of 19 months until recurrence. The disease-specific survival (DSS) for patients with normal and elevated CA125 is shown in Figure 2a and was significantly different ($p < 0.001$). Endometrial cancer-related mortality data were available for 320 patients. The overall survival (OS) for patients with normal and elevated CA125 is shown in Figure 2b and was significantly different ($p < 0.001$). Both the DSS and OS remained significantly different for normal and elevated CA125 within the surgically staged patients (n = 193).

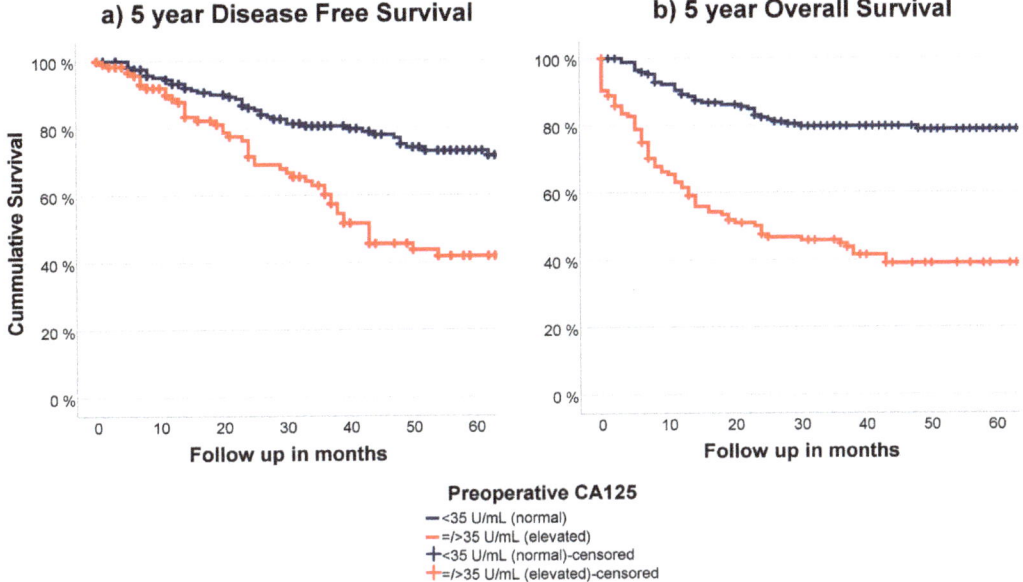

Figure 2. (a) 5 year DFS in relation to preoperative CA125 (b) 5 year OS in relation to preoperative CA125.

4. Discussion

4.1. Summary of Main Results

In the current study we have demonstrated that preoperative CA125 is a statistically significant predictor for advanced stage and LNM in high-grade EC. In addition, it was shown that suspected LNM on preoperative CT was a significant predictor for histologically confirmed LNM in high-grade EC but had no additional predictive value when preoperative CA125 was normal. We also demonstrated that DSS and OS are significantly worse for patients with elevated CA125. To our knowledge this is so far the largest study evaluating CA125 as prognostic biomarker specifically in patients with high-grade EC. The overall prevalence of 29.5% LNM is in line with previous studies [1,24,25]. With normal CA125, the negative predictive value for LNM was 85.6%.

Within patients with normal serum CA125 levels, preoperative CT with suspected LNM was not significant for predicting risk of LNM, and results were similar for CT and predicting advanced FIGO stage, supporting the limited additional benefit of preoperative CT imaging for staging in these patients. In the current study cohort, within patients with normal CA125, distant metastases including pulmonary metastases were present in 1.5% (2/135).

4.2. Results in the Context of Published Literature

The prognostic value of CA125 for advanced FIGO stage has been repeatedly shown in EC [22,26]. In a meta-analysis by Reijnen et al., both CA125 and imaging results were shown to predict the risk of LNM [8]. Within subgroup analysis of high-grade patients, preoperative CA125 resulted in an AUC of 0.745 compared to 0.638 for preoperative CT scan, both in line with our findings. Two other studies reported on the use of CA125 as predictor for LNM in high-grade EC and showed a significant association of CA125 with FIGO stage. However, only patients with either serous EC (n = 26) or clear cell EC (n = 61) histology were included without incorporation of other clinicopathological risk factors [27,28]. The low sensitivity of detection of LNM by CT is in line with previous studies and is likely attributed to the fact that the lymph nodes should be enlarged to be suspicious for metastatic on CT [20]. Although 18-FDG PET-CT scan is more sensitive than

CT scan, microscopic metastasis still might be easily missed by any imaging method and require histological evaluation of the lymph nodes [29]. Multiple studies have reported on the different imaging modalities for detecting LNM in EC patients [6,20]. Both 18-FDG PET-CT and conventional CT are mostly used in clinical practice to evaluate LNM and distant metastases, with PET-CT being superior with a pooled sensitivity of 72% [29]. Our observed sensitivity of 40.5% to detect LNM on CT is in line with the aforementioned publications. The lack of association between LNM and preoperative imaging in the multivariate analysis is most likely attributed to the low sensitivity of CT. The importance of DMI and CI as independent predictors of LNM in our multivariate analysis is in line with previous studies [1,8,23]. A recent study of Fasmer et al. demonstrated how selective use of 18-FDG PET-CT scan in patients with increased risk of extended EC, based on MRI (i.e., LNM, DMI, or CI) could be incorporated. Unfortunately, CA125 was not available in this study cohort, which might be interesting to add in future refined diagnostic work-up strategies [7]. Interestingly, elevated CA125 was significantly associated with the presence of LVSI, and thus could serve as a surrogate biomarker given its association with LNM in the multivariate analysis.

While CA125 is a very sensitive marker that can be used in postmenopausal women in the diagnostic work-up for endometrial cancer, it might be less suitable in premenopausal women. This is due to the fact that elevated CA125 is seen in several benign and physiological processes such as menstrual periods, endometriosis, and pregnancy [30,31]. For patients with a wish of fertility preservation, evidence-based oncofertility counseling is an important part of the preoperative work-up [32]. So far, it is not clear whether preoperative CA125 in these young women can equally contribute to the risk stratification of endometrial cancer.

The use of MRI or expert ultrasound to determine myometrial invasion has been recommended by the recent ESGO-ESTRO-ESP guideline, but so far not yet incorporated in the SGO guideline [3,10,13,24,25,33]. Selective use of preoperative MRI, specifically in patients with high-grade and elevated CA125, could aid in improving a cost-effective surgical approach in a preoperative setting. The reported sensitivity of MRI for assessment of CI is up to 59% with a specificity up to 91% [20,34].

While this study has shown that CA125 has a good predictive value for LNM and advanced stage, its discriminatory value is not enough to forgo surgical staging based solely on CA125 with or without CT. The results do however confirm that CA125 is a valuable marker that could be used in prediction models, such as the ENDORISK model which incorporates CA125, imaging and other factors [13].

Since the introduction of molecular classification in EC, prognostication has significantly improved by allocating patients to four molecular subgroups [14,35]. These subgroups may guide tailored adjuvant therapy, but as demonstrated by Jamieson et al. could also assist in the primary risk estimation of LNM. Interestingly, it was demonstrated that in addition to the molecular subgroup, CA125 remained relevant in the multivariate analysis, which underlines the relevance of our findings even within molecular classification. In the future, other molecular and genetic markers such as non-coding RNA (ncRNA) might further stratify tumor characterization and therapeutic targeting [36,37]. Further research will be needed to assess CA125 in relation to these markers but may enable the possibility to base the need of surgical staging and/or adjuvant treatment solely on these variables.

4.3. Strengths and Weaknesses

Inherent to the retrospective character of our study there are limitations that need to be addressed. Overall, 41.9% (n = 140) of patients with high-grade EC were not surgically staged and thus not included in the statistical analysis for LNM, which might have introduced selection bias. Yet, as 30% of patients without surgical staging were diagnosed with FIGO IV, omitting surgical staging is inherent to standard of care. Furthermore, selection bias might have been introduced due to using preoperative tumor grade, since this represents clinical practice where patients' treatment is based upon preoperative characteristics. However, occasionally this resulted in postoperative downgrading of EC after final pathological examination (n = 25). Based on the limited number, it is unlikely that this has significantly impacted our results. This discordance has been previously investigated in several studies who reported more extensive surgical treatment and an intermediate prognosis in patients who are 'over-graded' compared to correctly low-graded patients [28–30].

4.4. Implications for Practice and Future Research

The clinical applicability of incorporating CA125 in the diagnostic work-up of EC has been supported by several studies [3,14,25]. The well-established strong relation between LNM and histopathological DMI and CI, supports further research of the value of preoperative pelvic MRI, especially in patients with elevated CA125 serum levels. This might further improve identification of high-risk patients and individualized surgical approach even in the era of molecular profiling.

5. Conclusions

Preoperative CA125 is a relevant predictive marker for advanced stage and outcome in patients with high-grade EC. While CT was a valuable predictor of LNM and advanced stage in patients with elevated CA125, it was of limited additional value in patients with normal CA125. These results support that adding CA125 can improve preoperative risk stratification specifically for patients with high-grade EC.

Supplementary Materials: The following supporting information can be downloaded at: https://www.mdpi.com/article/10.3390/cancers15092605/s1, Figure S1: Inclusion of patients.

Author Contributions: Conceptualization, M.S.L., K.M.C.C., C.R. and J.M.A.P.; data curation: M.S.L. and C.R.; methodology: M.S.L., K.M.C.C. and J.M.A.P.; investigation: M.S.L.; formal analysis: M.S.L.; visualization: M.S.L. and K.M.C.C.; supervision: K.M.C.C. and J.M.A.P.; resources: C.R., J.M.A.P. and the ENITEC-Consortium; writing—original draft preparation: M.S.L., K.M.C.C. and J.M.A.P.; data acquisition: N.C.M.V., J.B., H.K, F.A., D.B., P.B., E.C., P.M.A.J.G., A.G.-M., D.v.H., J.H., C.K., A.A.K., M.K., G.M., X.M.-G., H.N., B.M.P., M.C.V., V.W., M.S.L., I.S.H. and the ENITEC-Consortium; data interpretation: S.W.v.K., I.S.H.; validation: K.M.C.C. and I.S.H.; writing—review and editing: M.S.L., K.M.C.C., N.C.M.V., J.B., H.V.N.K.-V., F.A., D.B., P.B., E.C., P.M.A.J.G., A.G.-M., D.v.H., J.H., C.K., A.A.K., M.K., G.M., X.M.-G., H.N., B.M.P., M.C.V., V.W., M.P.L.M.S., S.W.v.K., I.S.H., C.R. and J.M.A.P. All authors have read and agreed to the published version of the manuscript.

Funding: This research received no external funding.

Institutional Review Board Statement: The study was conducted in accordance with the Declaration of Helsinki, and approval for the original studies was obtained by the Review Board Radboud University Medical Center Nijmegen, The Netherlands (institutional study protocol 2015-2101) and by the medical ethical committee of the Elisabeth-Tweesteden Hospital Tilburg, The Netherlands (protocol 1129).

Informed Consent Statement: No written consent was obtained from patients in the original studies as data was used anonymously according to the "Code for Proper Use of Human Tissue". Included patients were informed about the use of tissue and data for scientific purpose in general. No drawbacks were made.

Data Availability Statement: The data presented in this study are available on request from the corresponding author. The data are not publicly available due to privacy and legal reasons.

Acknowledgments: We thank all participating patients for use of their data. We thank Steven Teerenstra, from the department of Health Evidence at the Radboud University Medical Center, for his statistical support.

Conflicts of Interest: The authors declare no conflict of interest.

References

1. Stålberg, K.; Kjølhede, P.; Bjurberg, M.; Borgfeldt, C.; Dahm-Kähler, P.; Falconer, H. Risk factors for lymph node metastases in women with endometrial cancer: A population-based, nation-wide register study-On behalf of the Swedish Gynecological Cancer Group. *Int. J. Cancer* 2017, *140*, 2693–2700. [CrossRef]
2. Colombo, N.; Creutzberg, C.; Amant, F.; Bosse, T.; González-Martín, A.; Ledermann, J.; Marth, C.; Nout, R.; Querleu, D.; Mirza, M.R.; et al. ESMO-ESGO-ESTRO Consensus Conference on Endometrial Cancer: Diagnosis, treatment and follow-up. *Ann. Oncol.* 2016, *27*, 16–41. [CrossRef]
3. Burke, W.M.; Orr, J.; Leitao, M.; Salom, E.; Gehrig, P.; Olawaiye, A.B. Endometrial cancer: A review and current management strategies: Part I. *Gynecol. Oncol.* 2014, *134*, 85–92. [CrossRef]
4. Holloway, R.W.; Abu-Rustum, N.R.; Backes, F.J.; Boggess, J.F.; Gotlieb, W.H.; Lowery, W.J.; Rossi, E.C.; Tanner, E.J.; Wolsky, R.J. Sentinel lymph node mapping and staging in endometrial cancer: A Society of Gynecologic Oncology literature review with consensus recommendations. *Gynecol. Oncol.* 2017, *146*, 405–415. [CrossRef] [PubMed]
5. Creasman, W.T.; Ali, S.; Mutch, D.G.; Zaino, R.J.; Powell, M.A.; Mannel, R.S.; Backes, F.J.; DiSilvestro, P.A.; Argenta, P.A.; Pearl, M.L.; et al. Surgical-pathological findings in type 1 and 2 endometrial cancer: An NRG Oncology/Gynecologic Oncology Group study on GOG-210 protocol. *Gynecol. Oncol.* 2017, *145*, 519–525. [CrossRef]
6. Haldorsen, I.S.; Salvesen, H.B. What Is the Best Preoperative Imaging for Endometrial Cancer? *Curr. Oncol. Rep.* 2016, *18*, 25. [CrossRef] [PubMed]
7. Fasmer, K.E.; Gulati, A.; Dybvik, J.A.; Wagner-Larsen, K.S.; Lura, N.; Salvesen, Ø. Preoperative pelvic MRI and 2-[(18)F]FDG PET/CT for lymph node staging and prognostication in endometrial cancer-time to revisit current imaging guidelines? *Eur. Radiol.* 2022, *33*, 221–232. [CrossRef]
8. Reijnen, C.; IntHout, J.; Massuger, L.F.; Strobbe, F.; Küsters-Vandevelde, H.V.; Haldorsen, I.S.; Snijders, M.P.; Pijnenborg, J.M. Diagnostic Accuracy of Clinical Biomarkers for Preoperative Prediction of Lymph Node Metastasis in Endometrial Carcinoma: A Systematic Review and Meta-Analysis. *Oncologist* 2019, *24*, e880–e890. [CrossRef]
9. Tuomi, T.; Pasanen, A.; Luomaranta, A.; Leminen, A.; Bützow, R.; Loukovaara, M. Risk-stratification of endometrial carcinomas revisited: A combined preoperative and intraoperative scoring system for a reliable prediction of an advanced disease. *Gynecol. Oncol.* 2015, *137*, 23–27. [CrossRef] [PubMed]
10. Kang, S.; Kang, W.D.; Chung, H.H.; Jeong, D.H.; Seo, S.-S.; Lee, J.-M.; Lee, J.-K.; Kim, J.-W.; Kim, S.-M.; Park, S.-Y.; et al. Preoperative identification of a low-risk group for lymph node metastasis in endometrial cancer: A Korean gynecologic oncology group study. *J. Clin. Oncol.* 2012, *30*, 1329–1334. [CrossRef]
11. Kang, S.; Nam, J.-H.; Bae, D.-S.; Kim, J.-W.; Kim, M.-H.; Chen, X.; No, J.-H.; Lee, J.-M.; Watari, H.; Kim, S.M.; et al. Preoperative assessment of lymph node metastasis in endometrial cancer: A Korean Gynecologic Oncology Group study. *Cancer* 2017, *123*, 263–272. [CrossRef]
12. Tsikouras, P.; Koukouli, Z.; Bothou, A.; Manav, B.; Iatrakis, G.; Zervoudis, S. Preoperative assessment in endometrial cancer. Is triage for lymphadenectomy possible? *J. Buon.* 2017, *22*, 34–43. [PubMed]
13. Reijnen, C.; Gogou, E.; Visser, N.C.M.; Engerud, H.; Ramjith, J.; Van Der Putten, L.J.M.; Van De Vijver, K.; Santacana, M.; Bronsert, P.; Bulten, J.; et al. Preoperative risk stratification in endometrial cancer (ENDORISK) by a Bayesian network model: A development and validation study. *PLoS Med.* 2020, *17*, e1003111. [CrossRef] [PubMed]
14. Jamieson, A.; Thompson, E.F.; Huvila, J.; Leung, S.; Lum, A.; Morin, C.; Ennour-Idrissi, K.; Sebastianelli, A.; Renaud, M.-C.; Gregoire, J.; et al. Endometrial carcinoma molecular subtype correlates with the presence of lymph node metastases. *Gynecol. Oncol.* 2022, *165*, 376–384. [CrossRef] [PubMed]
15. Anton, C.; e Silva, A.S.; Baracat, E.C.; Dogan, N.U.; Köhler, C.; Carvalho, J.P.; di Favero, G.M. A novel model to estimate lymph node metastasis in endometrial cancer patients. *Clinics* 2017, *72*, 30–35. [CrossRef]
16. Bogani, G.; Gostout, B.S.; Dowdy, S.C.; Multinu, F.; Casarin, J.; Cliby, W.A.; Frigerio, L.; Kim, B.; Weaver, A.L.; Glaser, G.E.; et al. Clinical Utility of Preoperative Computed Tomography in Patients With Endometrial Cancer. *Int. J. Gynecol. Cancer* 2017, *27*, 1685–1693. [CrossRef]
17. Steenbeek, M.P.; Bulten, J.; Snijders, M.P.; Lombaers, M.; Hendriks, J.; Brand, M.V.D.; Kraayenbrink, A.A.; Massuger, L.F.; Sweegers, S.; de Hullu, J.A.; et al. Fallopian tube abnormalities in uterine serous carcinoma. *Gynecol. Oncol.* 2020, *158*, 339–346. [CrossRef]
18. Visser, N.C.M.; Bulten, J.; Van Der Wurff, A.A.M.; Boss, E.A.; Bronkhorst, C.M.; Feijen, H.W.H.; Haartsen, J.E.; Van Herk, H.A.D.M.; De Kievit, I.M.; Klinkhamer, P.J.J.M.; et al. PIpelle Prospective ENDOmetrial carcinoma (PIPENDO) study, pre-operative recognition of high risk endometrial carcinoma: A multicentre prospective cohort study. *BMC Cancer* 2015, *15*, 487. [CrossRef]
19. Visser, N.C.; van der Wurff, A.A.; IntHout, J.; Reijnen, C.; Dabir, P.D.; Soltani, G.G.; Alcala, L.S.; Boll, D.; Bronkhorst, C.M.; Bult, P.; et al. Improving preoperative diagnosis in endometrial cancer using systematic morphological assessment and a small immunohistochemical panel. *Hum. Pathol.* 2021, *117*, 68–78. [CrossRef]
20. Faria, S.C.; Sagebiel, T.; Balachandran, A.; Devine, C.; Lal, C.; Bhosale, P.R. Imaging in endometrial carcinoma. *Indian J. Radiol. Imaging* 2015, *25*, 137–147. [CrossRef]
21. Lee, J.-Y.; Jung, D.-C.; Park, S.-H.; Lim, M.-C.; Seo, S.-S.; Park, S.-Y.; Kang, S. Preoperative prediction model of lymph node metastasis in endometrial cancer. *Int. J. Gynecol. Cancer* 2010, *20*, 1350–1355.

22. Reijnen, C.; Visser, N.C.; Kasius, J.C.; Boll, D.; Geomini, P.M.; Ngo, H.; van Hamont, D.; Pijlman, B.M.; Vos, M.C.; Bulten, J.; et al. Improved preoperative risk stratification with CA-125 in low-grade endometrial cancer: A multicenter prospective cohort study. *J. Gynecol. Oncol.* **2019**, *30*, e70. [CrossRef]
23. Solmaz, U.; Mat, E.; Dereli, M.; Turan, V.; Güngördük, K.; Hasdemir, P.S.; Tosun, G.; Dogan, A.; Ozdemir, A.; Adiyeke, M.; et al. Lymphovascular space invasion and cervical stromal invasion are independent risk factors for nodal metastasis in endometrioid endometrial cancer. *Aust. N. Z. J. Obstet. Gynaecol.* **2015**, *55*, 81–86. [CrossRef] [PubMed]
24. Concin, N.; Matias-Guiu, X.; Vergote, I.; Cibula, D.; Mirza, M.R.; Marnitz, S.; Ledermann, J.; Bosse, T.; Chargari, C.; Fagotti, A.; et al. ESGO/ESTRO/ESP guidelines for the management of patients with endometrial carcinoma. *Int. J. Gynecol. Cancer* **2021**, *31*, 12–39. [CrossRef] [PubMed]
25. Hamilton, C.A.; Pothuri, B.; Arend, R.C.; Backes, F.J.; Gehrig, P.A.; Soliman, P.T.; Thompson, J.S.; Urban, R.R.; Burke, W.M. Endometrial cancer: A society of gynecologic oncology evidence-based review and recommendations. *Gynecol. Oncol.* **2021**, *160*, 817–826. [CrossRef]
26. Sebastianelli, A.; Renaud, M.-C.; Grégoire, J.; Roy, M.; Plante, M. Preoperative CA 125 tumour marker in endometrial cancer: Correlation with advanced stage disease. *J. Obstet. Gynaecol. Can.* **2010**, *32*, 856–860. [CrossRef]
27. Schmidt, M.; Segev, Y.; Sadeh, R.; Suzan, E.; Feferkorn, I.; Kaldawy, A.; Kligun, G.; Lavie, O. Cancer Antigen 125 Levels are Significantly Associated With Prognostic Parameters in Uterine Papillary Serous Carcinoma. *Int. J. Gynecol. Cancer* **2018**, *28*, 1311–1317. [CrossRef]
28. Cetinkaya, N.; Selcuk, I.; Ozdal, B.; Meydanli, M.M.; Gungor, T. Diagnostic Impacts of Serum CA-125 Levels, Pap Smear Evaluation, and Endometrial Sampling in Women with Endometrial Clear Cell Carcinoma. *Oncol. Res. Treat* **2016**, *39*, 283–288. [CrossRef] [PubMed]
29. Bollineni, V.R.; Ytre-Hauge, S.; Bollineni-Balabay, O.; Salvesen, H.B.; Haldorsen, I.S. High Diagnostic Value of ^{18}F-FDG PET/CT in Endometrial Cancer: Systematic Review and Meta-Analysis of the Literature. *J. Nucl. Med.* **2016**, *57*, 879–885.
30. D'Ambrosio, V.; Brunelli, R.; Musacchio, L.; Del Negro, V.; Vena, F.; Boccuzzi, G.; Boccherini, C.; Di Donato, V.; Piccioni, M.G.; Panici, P.B.; et al. Adnexal masses in pregnancy: An updated review on diagnosis and treatment. *Tumori* **2021**, *107*, 12–16. [CrossRef]
31. Jacobs, I.; Bast, R.C., Jr. The CA 125 tumour-associated antigen: A review of the literature. *Hum. Reprod* **1989**, *4*, 1–12. [CrossRef]
32. Zaami, S.; Stark, M.; Signore, F.; Gullo, G.; Marinelli, E. Fertility preservation in female cancer sufferers: (only) a moral obligation? *Eur. J. Contracept. Reprod. Health Care* **2022**, *27*, 335–340. [CrossRef]
33. Zaami, S.; Stark, M.; Signore, F.; Gullo, G.; Marinelli, E. A systematic review of tests for lymph node status in primary endometrial cancer. *BMC Womens Health* **2008**, *8*, 8.
34. Haldorsen, I.S.; Berg, A.; Werner, H.M.; Magnussen, I.J.; Helland, H.; Salvesen, O.; Trovik, J.; Salvesen, H.B. Magnetic resonance imaging performs better than endocervical curettage for preoperative prediction of cervical stromal invasion in endometrial carcinomas. *Gynecol. Oncol.* **2012**, *126*, 413–418. [CrossRef] [PubMed]
35. Levine, D.A. Integrated genomic characterization of endometrial carcinoma. *Nature* **2013**, *497*, 67–73. [CrossRef]
36. Gulia, C.; Signore, F.; Gaffi, M.; Gigli, S.; Votino, R.; Nucciotti, R.; Bertacca, L.; Zaami, S.; Baffa, A.; Santini, E.; et al. Y RNA: An Overview of Their Role as Potential Biomarkers and Molecular Targets in Human Cancers. *Cancers* **2020**, *12*, 1238. [CrossRef]
37. Piergentili, R.; Zaami, S.; Cavaliere, A.; Signore, F.; Scambia, G.; Mattei, A.; Marinelli, E.; Gulia, C.; Perelli, F. Non-Coding RNAs as Prognostic Markers for Endometrial Cancer. *Int. J. Mol. Sci.* **2021**, *22*, 3151. [CrossRef] [PubMed]

Disclaimer/Publisher's Note: The statements, opinions and data contained in all publications are solely those of the individual author(s) and contributor(s) and not of MDPI and/or the editor(s). MDPI and/or the editor(s) disclaim responsibility for any injury to people or property resulting from any ideas, methods, instructions or products referred to in the content.

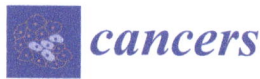 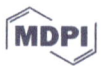

Article

The Atypical MAP Kinase MAPK15 Is Required for Lung Adenocarcinoma Metastasis via Its Interaction with NF-κB p50 Subunit and Transcriptional Regulation of Prostaglandin E2 Receptor EP3 Subtype

Fei-Yuan Yu [1], Qian Xu [2], Xiao-Yun Zhao [1], Hai-Ying Mo [1], Qiu-Hua Zhong [1], Li Luo [1], Andy T. Y. Lau [1,*] and Yan-Ming Xu [1,*]

[1] Laboratory of Cancer Biology and Epigenetics, Department of Cell Biology and Genetics, Shantou University Medical College, Shantou 515041, China
[2] Laboratory of Molecular Pathology, Department of Pathology, Shantou University Medical College, Shantou 515041, China
* Correspondence: andytylau@stu.edu.cn (A.T.Y.L.); amyymxu@stu.edu.cn (Y.-M.X.); Tel.: +86-754-8853-0052 (A.T.Y.L.); +86-754-8890-0437 (Y.-M.X.)

Simple Summary: Due to the lack of effective early diagnostic markers for lung cancer and the rich blood circulation in the lungs, it is very easy to cause lymph node metastasis and distant metastasis of lung cancer, making lung cancer as one of the top ten cancer types with the highest mortality rate in the world. This study found that MAPK15 is highly expressed in the tissues of patients with lung adenocarcinoma lymph node metastasis, and MAPK15 interacts with p50 to regulate the expression of EP3 at the transcriptional level, thereby promoting cancer cell migration. This suggests that MAPK15 plays a key role in the metastasis of lung cancer cells, and MAPK15 can be used as a molecular marker for the early diagnosis or prognosis assessment of lung cancer. Its molecular mechanism for regulating lung cancer metastasis can provide valuable information and insights on novel therapeutic options at molecular levels.

Abstract: Studying the relatively underexplored atypical MAP Kinase MAPK15 on cancer progression/patient outcomes and its potential transcriptional regulation of downstream genes would be highly valuable for the diagnosis, prognosis, and potential oncotherapy of malignant tumors such as lung adenocarcinoma (LUAD). Here, the expression of MAPK15 in LUAD was detected by immunohistochemistry and its correlation with clinical parameters such as lymph node metastasis and clinical stage was analyzed. The correlation between the prostaglandin E2 receptor EP3 subtype (EP3) and MAPK15 expression in LUAD tissues was examined, and the transcriptional regulation of EP3 and cell migration by MAPK15 in LUAD cell lines were studied using the luciferase reporter assay, immunoblot analysis, qRT-PCR, and transwell assay. We found that MAPK15 is highly expressed in LUAD with lymph node metastasis. In addition, EP3 is positively correlated with the expression of MAPK15 in LUAD tissues, and we confirmed that MAPK15 transcriptionally regulates the expression of EP3. Upon the knockdown of MAPK15, the expression of EP3 was down-regulated and the cell migration ability was decreased in vitro; similarly, the mesenteric metastasis ability of the MAPK15 knockdown cells was inhibited in in vivo animal experiments. Mechanistically, we demonstrate for the first time that MAPK15 interacts with NF-κB p50 and enters the nucleus, and NF-κB p50 binds to the EP3 promoter and transcriptionally regulates the expression of EP3. Taken together, we show that a novel atypical MAPK and NF-κB subunit interaction promotes LUAD cell migration through transcriptional regulation of EP3, and higher MAPK15 level is associated with lymph node metastasis in patients with LUAD.

Keywords: MAPK15; EP3; p50; LUAD; metastasis

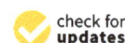

Citation: Yu, F.-Y.; Xu, Q.; Zhao, X.-Y.; Mo, H.-Y.; Zhong, Q.-H.; Luo, L.; Lau, A.T.Y.; Xu, Y.-M. The Atypical MAP Kinase MAPK15 Is Required for Lung Adenocarcinoma Metastasis via Its Interaction with NF-κB p50 Subunit and Transcriptional Regulation of Prostaglandin E2 Receptor EP3 Subtype. *Cancers* **2023**, *15*, 1398. https://doi.org/10.3390/cancers15051398

Academic Editors: Daniel L. Pouliquen and Cristina Núñez González

Received: 31 December 2022
Revised: 30 January 2023
Accepted: 30 January 2023
Published: 22 February 2023

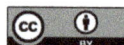

Copyright: © 2023 by the authors. Licensee MDPI, Basel, Switzerland. This article is an open access article distributed under the terms and conditions of the Creative Commons Attribution (CC BY) license (https://creativecommons.org/licenses/by/4.0/).

1. Introduction

The incidence of lung cancer is high among malignant tumors, which seriously affects human health. The mortality rate of lung cancer patients is high because lung cancer is usually in an advanced stage when diagnosed, with lymph node metastasis or even distant metastasis. Radiotherapy and chemotherapy have very limited therapeutic effects on advanced lung cancer. Targeted therapies, such as the use of targeted drugs EGFR tyrosine kinase inhibitors [1,2], can improve the survival of lung cancer patients to a certain extent, but they still face the problem of chemotherapy resistance, recurrence of targeted therapy, etc. Therefore, it is still not possible to effectively control the malignant development of lung cancer [2]. The study of molecular markers related to lung cancer metastasis and their corresponding molecular mechanisms still needs to be further explored.

The classical mitogen-activated protein kinases (MAPKs, e.g., ERK1/2, p38, and JNK/SAPK) play important roles in regulating gene expression, cell growth, proliferation, etc. Atypical MAPKs such as ERK3, ERK4, and NLK (nemo-like kinase) also play critical roles in many cellular responses [3,4]. MAPK15, alias extracellular signal-regulated kinase 7/8 (ERK7/8), is the most recently discovered atypical MAPK. Current research indicates that MAPK15 can promote the transformation of colon cancer by mediating the activation of the transcription factor c-Jun [5,6] or promoting the growth of gastric cancer cells [7]. MAPK15 has also been found to interact with autophagy-related proteins such as GABARAP and LC3 to control tumor development [8]. In addition, MAPK15 can be activated by carcinogenic factors such as RET/PTC3 [9] or involved in the regulation of telomerase activity [10] to participate in the development of tumors. Recently, our group has reported that MAPK15 can promote arsenic trioxide-induced apoptosis, as well as boosting the efficacy of combination therapy with cisplatin and TNF-α, in lung cancer cells [11,12]. At present, research about the function of MAPK15 is still limited, and its role in lung cancer metastasis remains unclear.

EP3 is one of the four G protein-coupled receptors of prostaglandin E2 (PGE2), which plays an important role in cell proliferation, differentiation, apoptosis, cardiovascular system regulation, and inflammation. It has been reported that tumor angiogenesis and tumor cell growth were significantly inhibited in a mouse lung cancer model with EP3 knocked out [13]. Yamaki et al. found that PGE2 promotes the growth of lung adenocarcinoma (LUAD) cell line A549 via the EP3 receptor-activated Src signaling pathway [14]. However, the molecular mechanism of EP3 in regulating lung cancer progression is still not fully clarified.

In this study, we detected the expression of MAPK15 in lung cancer tissues, and found that the expression of MAPK15 is positively correlated with lymph node metastasis in LUAD patients; remarkably, our results showed that the expression of EP3 was transcriptionally regulated by MAPK15, and the expression of EP3 was positively correlated with the expression of MAPK15 in LUAD tissues. Furthermore, we revealed the first time that MAPK15 promotes the expression of EP3 by interacting with p50, thereby enhancing the migration of lung cancer cells.

2. Materials and Methods

2.1. Immunohistochemistry

Lung cancer tissue microarray (BC041115c, US Biomax, Rockville, MD, USA) was purchased and all human tissues were collected according to HIPPA-approved protocols as described by US Biomax (https://www.biomax.us/FAQs, accessed on 14 June 2022). Immunohistochemistry was performed to detect the expression of MAPK15 and EP3. Briefly, tissue microarray was deparaffinized thrice in xylene (10 min for each) and rehydrated in gradient series ethanol (100%, 95%, 90%, 90%, 5 min for each), respectively. After being rinsed with water, tissue slides were incubated with 3% hydrogen peroxide for 40 min to block endogenous peroxidase. Tissue slides were then rinsed with PBS and immersed in 0.01 M citrate acid antigen retrieval solution and heated at 98 °C for 20 min using a water bath. After natural cooling, tissue slides were washed with PBS and incubated with 5%

BSA for 30 min. Tissue slides were then incubated with MAPK15 [15] or EP3 (Cat. 101760, Cayman Chemical, Ann Arbor, USA) antibody at 4 °C overnight. After being rinsed with PBS, tissue slides were incubated with secondary antibody for 45 min at RT. Subsequently, tissue slides were washed with PBS and reacted with 3,3′-diaminobenzidine (DAB, Zhongshan Golden Bridge Inc. Beijing, China) and counterstained with hematoxylin. Then, tissue slides were mounted with glycerogelatin and photographed with a light microscope.

Immunostaining of tissue microarray were scored according to immunoreactive score (IRS) [16,17]. Each tissue in the microarray was semiquantitatively scored for intensity (0, absent; 1, weak; 2, moderate; 3, strong) and extent of staining (percentage of the positive tumor cells: 0, ≤5%; 1, 6–25%; 2, 26–50%; 3, 51–75%; 4, >75%). Intensity and extent of each tissue were multiplied to give a composite score: 0–3, deemed as low expression, "−"; 4–12, deemed as high expression (4–6, "+"; 7–9, "++"; 10–12, "+++").

2.2. Cell Culture and Transfection

All cells were grown at 37 °C in a 5% CO_2 incubator. HEK293T, H1299, and A549 cells were purchased from ATCC Cell Bank of the Chinese Academy of Sciences (Shanghai, China) and maintained in MEM, RPMI-1640, or F12-K medium supplemented with 10% FBS and 1% PS, respectively. MAPK15 stable knockdown LUAD H1299 cells (H1299-shMAPK15) and control cells (H1299-shCtrl) were established previously [12]. For transfection, cells were mixed with siRNA/plasmids-polyethylenimine mixture and cultured for the indicated time point. Negative control siRNA (siN05815122147) and siRNA duplexes against EP3 were purchased from IGE Biotechnology LTD (Guangzhou, China) and listed in Supplementary Table S1.

2.3. RNA Extraction, cDNA Synthesis, and Real-Time PCR

RNA was extracted using RNAiso Plus (Takara, Dalian, China) from cells. Then, cDNA was synthesized using GoScript™ Reverse Transcription Mix (Promega, Madison, WI, USA) by following the manufacturer's instructions. Specific primers were used, and real-time PCR was performed using GoTaq qPCR Master Mix (Promega, Madison, WI, USA) on Applied Biosystems 7500 Real-Time PCR System. The $2^{\Delta\Delta CT}$ method was used to calculate the relative expression of target genes compared to internal control (β-Actin) as described previously [18]. Primers were synthesized by IGE Biotechnology LTD (Guangzhou, China) and listed in supplementary Table S1.

2.4. Immunoblot Analysis

Equivalent amounts of extracted protein were resolved by 10% SDS-PAGE and transferred onto polyvinylidene fluoride membranes. The membranes were blocked with 5% nonfat milk in PBS containing 0.05% Tween 20 followed by incubation with primary antibody overnight at 4 °C. After reacting with primary antibody, membranes were incubated with secondary antibody and proteins were visualized with ECL reagent using Tanon 5200 system (Tanon, Shanghai, China). The optical density of each protein band was quantified by Gel-Pro Analyzer 4 (Toyobo, Osaka, Japan) software. Original blots and blot quantification are shown in Figures S3–S5, S7 and S8.

2.5. Transwell Assay

Transwell assay was performed as described previously [16]. Briefly, 3.0×10^4 cells were seeded in the upper compartment of transwell inserts with 8 μm microporous membrane (cat no. 3422, Corning Inc., Corning, NY, USA). After being incubated for 24 h, unmigrated cells on the upper surface of the microporous membrane were wiped using a cotton swab. Cells on the lower surface of the microporous membrane were fixed with 4% PFA for 20 min and subsequently stained with 0.1% crystal violet for 15 min. The transwell chamber was rinsed with PBS to remove excess crystal violet, and images of migrated cells were captured using an Axiovert 40 CFL microscope (Carl Zeiss AG, Oberkochen,

Germany) with CCD camera (magnified 100×). Finally, the crystal violet in the migrated cells was dissolved with 33% acetic acid, and absorbance was measured at OD_{595}.

2.6. Immunofluorescence and Confocal Microscopy

Cells seeded on coverslip in 6-well plate were incubated for the indicated time point and fixed with 4% PFA for 15 min. After being rinsed with PBS, cells were permeabilized for 10 min with PBS containing 0.25% Triton X-100. Subsequently, cells were incubated with 5% BSA for 30 min to block unspecific binding of antibodies. Then, cells were incubated with primary antibody in a humidified chamber at 4 °C overnight. After decanting of primary antibody solution, cells were washed with PBS and incubated with secondary antibody for 1.5 h at room temperature in the dark. Coverslips were counterstained with 1 μg/mL Hoechst 33342 and mounted with mounting medium. Images were captured with Axiovert 40 CFL Microscope (Carl Zeiss AG, Germany) or Zeiss lsm 800 confocal microscope (Carl Zeiss AG, Germany).

2.7. In Vivo Peritoneal Metastasis Assay

In vivo peritoneal metastasis assay was performed as described previously [19]. Briefly, 5×10^6 MAPK15 stable knockdown H1299 or control cells in 200 μL of phosphate-buffered saline were injected intraperitoneally into BALB/c nude mice (Beijing Vital River Animal Technology Co., Ltd., Beijing, China, licensed by Charles River). After 7 weeks, the mice were sacrificed, and tumor nodules were quantified.

2.8. Co-Immunoprecipitation

HEK293T cells cultured in 10 cm dish were transfected with pcDNA4/Xpress-MAPK15 plasmids [15] and incubated for 24 h. Prior to immunoprecipitation, 1 μg of Xpress antibody or normal IgG was pre-adsorbed with 20 μL Protein A/G Sepharose slurry for 2 h at 4 °C with rotation. After transfection, cells were harvested and lysed with NP-40 lysis buffer using repetitive freeze-thawing method. An amount of 300 μg of lysates to be used for immunoprecipitation was precleared with 20 μL Protein A/G Sepharose at 4 °C for 1 h with rotation. The supernatant was then incubated with the Xpress antibody–Protein A/G Sepharose complexes overnight at 4 °C with rotation (anti-mouse IgG was used as negative control). In total, 10% of the supernatant was used as input. The Sepharose beads were collected by centrifugation and washed extensively in 500 μL of lysis buffer, and eluted in 20 μL of SDS sample buffer by heating to 98 °C for 5 min. After centrifugation at $10,000 \times g$, the supernatant was collected for immunoblot analysis.

2.9. Chromatin Immunoprecipitation Assay

Chromatin immunoprecipitation assay was performed using SimpleChIP® Enzymatic Chromatin IP Kit (Cell Signaling Technology, Danvers, MA, USA). Briefly, formaldehyde cross-linked H1299 cells were lysed, and chromatin was digested with micrococcal nuclease into DNA/protein fragments. Then, p50 antibody (Santa Cruz Biotechnology, Dallas, TX, USA) was added and the complex is captured by protein G magnetic beads. Seven p50 binding sites (site1–site7) in the EP3 promoter region (−2000 bp) were predicted by JASPAR databases and PCR was used to detect p50 binding.

2.10. Vector Construction and Luciferase Reporter Assay

Five repeats of p50 binding sequence (site5, sequence: GGGGCTTCCC) and 12 bp linker sequences with AflII and NsiI sites were synthesized by IGE Biotechnology LTD (Guangzhou, China) and ligated to a modified pJC6-GL3 plasmid [11] to construct luciferase reporter plasmid (5 × p50-Luc). Then, the 5 × p50-Luc plasmid was co-transfected with/without pCMV-p50 plasmid into equal amount of H1299 cells in 12-well plate. Afterward, cells were lysed for luciferase assay following manufacturer's instructions (dual-luciferase reporter assay system, Promega, Madison, WI, USA).

2.11. Statistical Analysis

Mean comparisons were performed using the GraphPad Prism 8 for unpaired t-test. Fisher's exact test was used to study the correlation between MAPK15 expression and clinical parameters. Spearman rank correlation analysis was used to compare the correlation between the expression of MAPK15 and EP3 in lung cancer tissues using SPSS 19 software. The above statistical analysis was two-tailed; $p < 0.05$ suggested that the difference was statistically significant.

3. Results

3.1. MAPK15 Is Correlated with Lymph Node Metastasis in LUAD Patients

To study the role of MAPK15 in lung cancer, we analyzed the relationship between MAPK15 and clinical–pathological parameters such as age, gender, depth of tumor invasion, lymph node metastasis, distant metastasis, tumor differentiation, clinical stage, etc. We found that there was a positive correlation between MAPK15 expression and lymph node metastasis ($p = 0.012$) as well as clinical stage ($p = 0.033$) (Supplementary Table S2). The expression of MAPK15 is higher in patients with lymph node metastasis (N1 + N2) as compared to patients without lymph node metastasis (N0) (Supplementary Table S2). Other clinical–pathological parameters such as age, gender, depth of tumor invasion, distant metastasis, and tumor differentiation were not significantly correlated with the expression of MAPK15 (Supplementary Table S2). Adenocarcinoma and squamous cell carcinoma are major types of non-small-cell lung cancer (NSCLC). As compared to squamous cell carcinoma, we revealed that the expression of MAPK15 is relatively higher in adenocarcinoma (Figure 1A, Supplementary Table S3) and is associated with lymph node metastasis ($p = 0.013$) (Table 1, Figure 1B).

3.2. Knockdown of MAPK15 Inhibits H1299 Cell Migration In Vitro and Metastasis In Vivo

The above results indicate that MAPK15 is expressed more highly in lymphatic metastatic LUAD. In MAPK15 stable knockdown LUAD H1299 cells (Figure 1C,D), cell migration was significantly inhibited (Figure 1E,F). The expression of Snail1 was decreased in MAPK15 knockdown cells (Figure 1G), which can down-regulate the expression of E-cadherin by post-translational modifications such as deacetylation and methylation during EMT [20]. Consequently, the expression of epithelial marker E-cadherin was increased, while mesenchymal marker integrin β1 is decreased after MAPK15 knockdown (Figure 1G). Then, we performed an in vivo peritoneal metastasis assay using H1299-shMAPK15 cells and found that loss of MAPK15 significantly reduces metastasis to mesentery in vivo (Figure 1H,I). The above results indicate that H1299 cells undergo mesenchymal–epithelial transition after MAPK15 knockdown, thereby decreasing migration and metastasis.

3.3. MAPK15 Regulates the Expression of Migration-Related Gene EP3

It has been reported that the expression of MMP2 was depressed in EP3 knock-out mice under hypoxic stress [21], which indicates a correlation between the expression of MMP2 and EP3. Our results showed that MMP2 was down-regulated in MAPK15 knockdown H1299 cells (Figure S1). To investigate whether EP3 is involved, we detect the expression of EP3 in H1299-shCtrl and H1299-shMAPK15 cells. We found that the mRNA and protein level of EP3 was significantly decreased in MAPK15-deficient cells (Figure 2A,B) and the protein level of EP3 was not affected by proteasome inhibitor MG132 (Figure 2B), suggesting that the decreased EP3 in H1299-shMAPK15 cells was transcriptionally regulated. Moreover, the migration of H1299 cells was inhibited (Figure 2F,G) after EP3 was knocked down (Figure 2C–E). The decreased EP3 in MAPK15 knockdown cells suggested that there might be a correlation between the expression patterns of these two molecules. Then, we detected the expression of EP3 in a serial section from the same tissue that we stained with MAPK15 antibody and found that the expression of EP3 is positively correlated with MAPK15 ($r = 0.589$, $p < 0.001$, Figure 2H and Table 2). Taken together, the above results show that MAPK15 affects cell migration through the regulation of EP3.

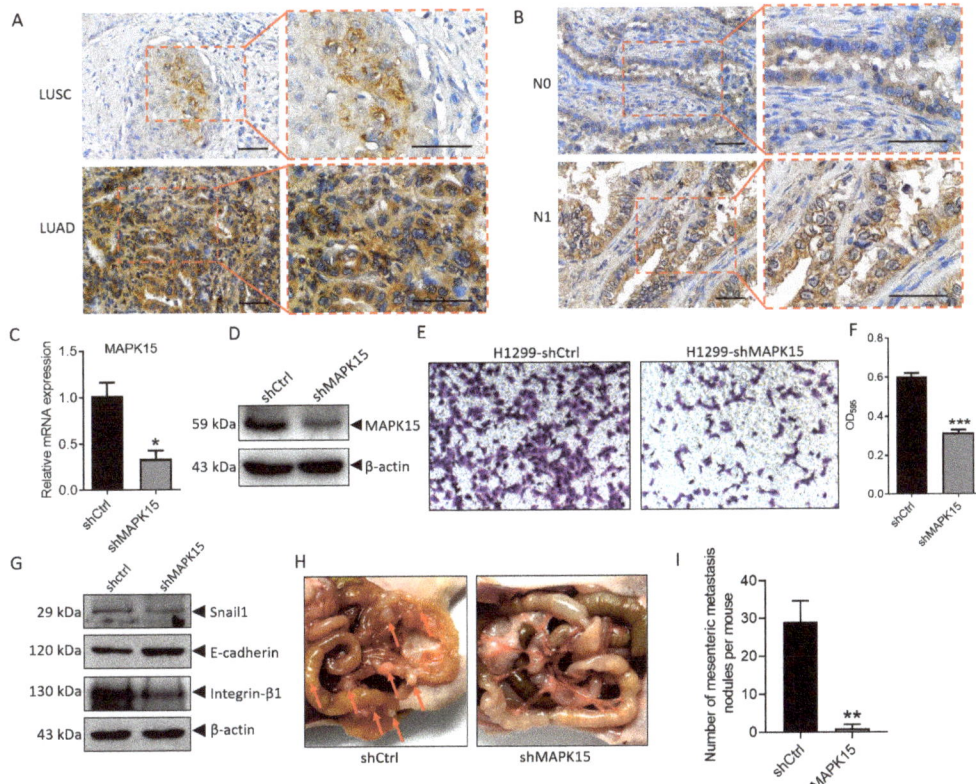

Figure 1. Knockdown of MAPK15 inhibits H1299 cell migration in vitro and in vivo. (**A**) MAPK15 staining in lung squamous cell lung carcinoma and adenocarcinoma tissues. (**B**) MAPK15 staining in LUAD tissues without lymph node involvement (N0) was compared with tissue with lymph node involvement (N1). Scale bar represents 60 μm. (**C,D**), real-time PCR and immunoblot analysis were used to detect the mRNA level (**C**) and protein level (**D**) of MAPK15 in H1299 cells. (**E,F**), transwell assay was used to detect the migration ability of H1299-shCtrl and H1299-shMAPK15 cells, migrated cells were stained with crystal violet (**E**) and absorbance of solubilized crystal violet was shown as bar chart graph (**F**). (**G**) The expression of Snail1/E-cadherin/Integrin-β1 was detected in H1299-shCtrl and H1299-shMAPK15 cells. (**H**) Metastatic nodules (red arrows) on intestinal mesentery of BALB/c nude mice. (**I**) Number of mesenteric metastasis nodules per mouse. * $p < 0.05$, ** $p < 0.01$, *** $p < 0.001$, Student's t-test.

Table 1. Correlation between MAPK15 expression and clinical parameters in patients with LUAD and LUSC.

Clinicopathological Parameters	Adenocarcinoma				Squamous Cell Carcinoma			
	MAPK15 Expression		Total	p Value	MAPK15 Expression		Total	p Value
	Low	High			Low	High		
Regional lymph nodes				0.013 *				0.486
N0	10	13	23		13	8	21	
N1	2	18	20		5	7	12	
N2	3	2	5		3	4	7	

Fisher's exact test. Statistically significant, * $p < 0.05$.

3.4. MAPK15 Interacts with NF-κB p50 Subunit and NF-κB p50 Transcriptionally Regulates EP3 Expression by Binding to EP3 Promoter

The molecular mechanism of how EP3 is transcriptionally regulated by MAPK15 is unknown. It has been reported that the expression of MAPK15, NF-κB1 (p50), and NF-κB2 (p52) were obviously decreased in ovarian cancer cell lines [22], which indicate there are correlations between MAPK15 and the NF-κB family. To investigate the relationship between MAPK15 and NF-κB family members, we transfected the pcDNA4/Xpress-MAPK15 plasmid into 293T cells and the immunoprecipitation assay revealed that MAPK15 interacts with p50 but not p65 and c-rel (Figure 3A). We also detected the localization of MAPK15 and p50 in H1299 cells by confocal microscopy and found that MAPK15 is distributed both in the cytoplasm and nucleus, and colocalizes with p50 (Figure 3B), indicating that there is an interaction between these two proteins in LUAD cells which might contribute to the expression of EP3. To study the relationship between MAPK15/p50 and EP3, we overexpressed MAPK15 (Figure 3C) and p50 (Figure 3D) in H1299 cells and found that the expression of EP3 was increased (Figure 3E), which indicates that MAPK15 and p50 positively regulate the transcription of EP3. The chromatin immunoprecipitation assay found that p50 binds to two p50 binding motifs in the EP3 promoter (Figure 3F, site2 and site5). Subsequently, we chose site 5 (Figure 3F) to construct the luciferase reporter plasmid and co-transfect with/without pCMV-p50 in H1299 cells for the luciferase reporter assay. Our results indicate that the luciferase activity is significantly increased in cells overexpressed with p50 (Figure 3G), which revealed that p50 can transcriptionally regulate EP3 by binding to the EP3 promoter.

3.5. TNF-α Promotes H1299 Cell Migration through Induction of MAPK15-NF-κB p50 Nuclear Localization and EP3 Expression

MAPK15 interacts with p50 intracellularly, indicating potential gene regulation and cellular phenotypic change. Beinke et al. reported that the p105 pathway can positively regulate gene transcription under TNF-α stimulation [23]. We hypothesize that TNF-α might promote the expression of EP3 through the p50 pathway, thereby contributing to cell migration. In TNF-α-treated H1299 cells, we found that TNF-α promoted EP3 expression in a dose- (Figure 4A) and time-dependent manner (Figure 4B). Furthermore, TNF-α promoted the migration of H1299 cells but had no significant effect on the migration of MAPK15 knockdown cells (Figure 4C,D). This result suggests that TNF-α promotes cell migration through MAPK15. In TNF-α-treated A549 cells, we found that TNF-α promotes nuclear localization of MAPK15 and p50 (Figure S2). In H1299 cells, we found that p50 is distributed in both cytoplasm and nucleus, whereas in MAPK15 knockdown cells, p50 is mainly located in the cytoplasm (Figure 4E), indicating that nuclear localization of p50 is dependent on MAPK15. At the same time, we treated H1299 cells with TNF-α and found that p50 is mainly located in the nucleus, whereas in MAPK15 knockdown cells, p50 is distributed in both the cytoplasm (white arrows) and the nucleus (Figure 4E). The above results indicate that TNF-α-induced nuclear translocation of p50 is dependent on MAPK15. In addition, we found that the expression of EP3 in TNF-α-treated H1299 cells was increased, while the expression changes of EP3 in MAPK15 knockdown H1299 cells were not significant (Figure 4F), and TNF-α could not promote H1299 cell migration while EP3 was knocked down (Figure 4G,H). Taken together, these results reveal that TNF-α promotes H1299 cell migration through induction of MAPK15-p50 nuclear localization and EP3 expression in cells with MAPK15 expression.

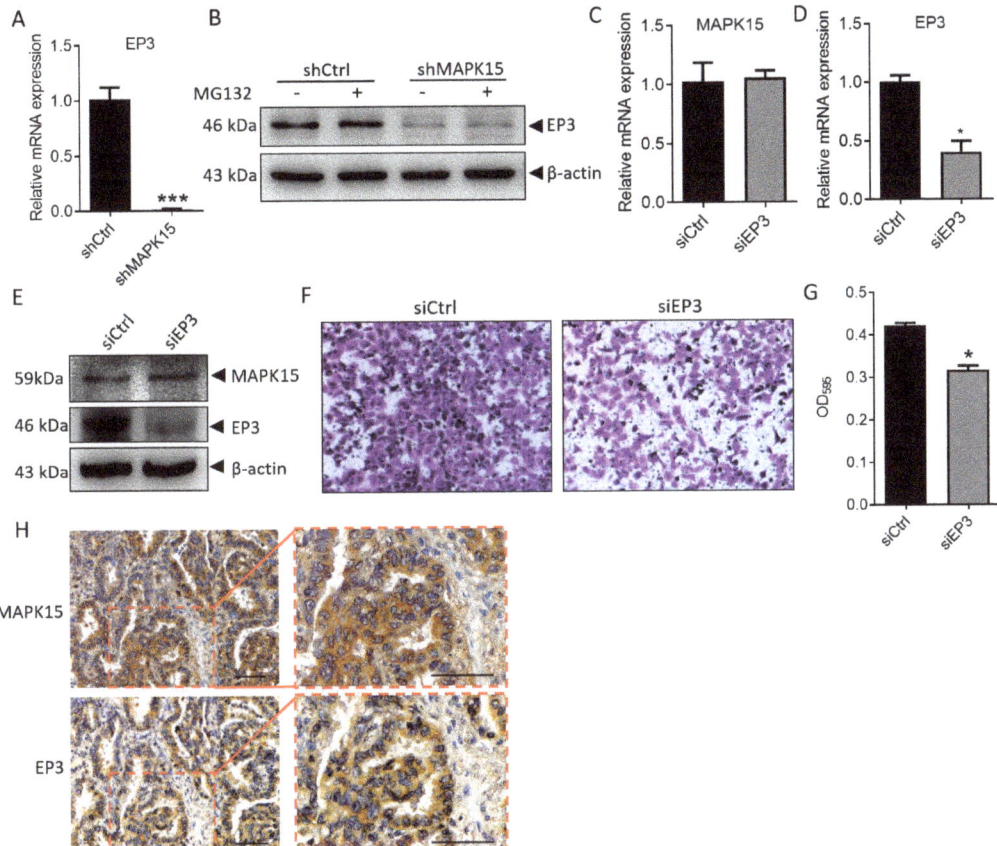

Figure 2. MAPK15 regulates the expression of migration-related gene EP3. (**A**) The expression of EP3 mRNA was detected in H1299-shctrl and H1299-shMAPK15 cells by real-time PCR. (**B**) H1299-shCtrl and H1299-shMAPK15 cells were treated with/without 10 μmol/L MG132 for 4 h, then the expression of EP3 was detected by immunoblot analysis. (**C–E**) An amount of 40 μmol/L of negative control siRNA and EP3 siRNA were transfected into H1299 cells, respectively, for 36 h and the expression of MAPK15/EP3 were detected. (**F,G**) H1299 cells transfected with negative control siRNA and EP3 siRNA for 36 h were seeded in transwell chamber for 24 h, then migrated cells were stained with crystal violet (**F**) and absorbance of solubilized crystal violet are shown as bar chart graph (**G**). (**H**) Serial section of the same LUAD tissue shows the similar expression pattern of MAPK15 and EP3. Scale bar represents 60 μm. * $p < 0.05$, *** $p < 0.001$, Student t test.

Table 2. Correlation between EP3 expression and MAPK15 in LUAD tissues.

		EP3				Total
		−	+	++	+++	
	−	10	5	0	0	15
MAPK15	+	3	12	1	0	16
	++	0	5	1	1	7
	+++	2	2	3	3	10
Total		15	24	5	4	48

Spearman correlation, r = 0.589, $p < 0.001$.

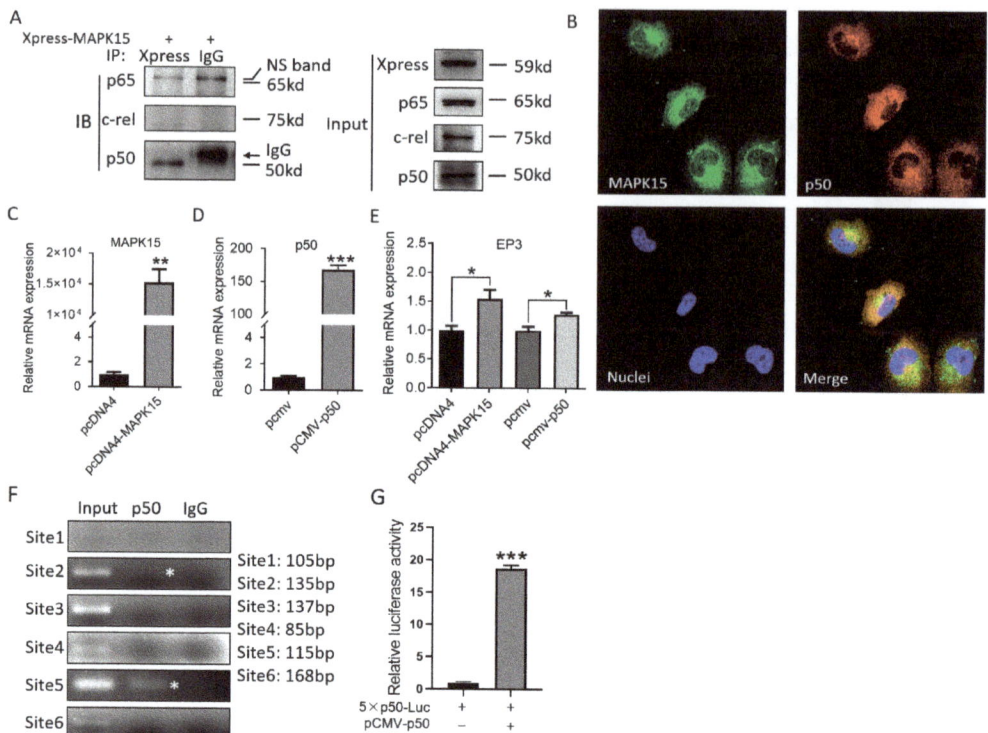

Figure 3. MAPK15 interacts with NF-κB p50 and p50 promotes EP3 expression by binding to EP3 promoter. (**A**) Immunoprecipitated proteins were resolved and the presence of MAPK15 and p50/c-rel/p65 were detected by anti-Xpress or anti-p50/c-rel/p65 antibodies. (**B**) The localization of MAPK15 and p50 in 4% paraformaldehyde-fixed H1299 cells were detected. (**C–E**) H1299 cells transfected with 2 μg pcDNA4, pcDNA4/Xpress-MAPK15, pCMV, and pCMV-p50 and the expression of MAPK15 (**C**)/p50 (**D**)/EP3 (**E**) was detected by real-time PCR. (**F**) Chromatin immunoprecipitation assay was used to detect the binding of p50 to EP3 promoter region; the asterisk indicates the immunoprecipitated EP3 promoter region. Original gels and gel quantification are shown in Figure S6. (**G**) In this study, 5 × p50-Luc plasmid was transfected with/without pCMV-p50 in H1299 cells and luciferase reporter assay was performed to detect the luciferase activity. * $p < 0.05$, ** $p < 0.01$, *** $p < 0.001$, Student's t-test.

3.6. JSH-23 Inhibits MAPK15-Induced EP3 Expression and Cell Migration

JSH-23 is an NF-κB inhibitor. When using JSH-23 to treat H1299 cells, we found that JSH-23 inhibited the expression of EP3 in a dose- (Figure 5A) and time-dependent manner (Figure 5B). Furthermore, JSH-23 inhibited the migration of H1299 cells but had no significant effect on the migration of knockdown MAPK15 cells (Figure 5C,D). This result suggests that JSH-23 inhibits cell migration through MAPK15. In addition, we found that the expression of EP3 in H1299 cells treated with JSH-23 was decreased, while the expression of EP3 in MAPK15 knockdown H1299 cells did not change significantly (Figure 5E), and JSH-23 could not inhibit H1299 cell migration when EP3 was knocked down (Figure 5F,G). The above results indicate that JSH-23 inhibits cell migration by inhibiting MAPK15-induced EP3 expression.

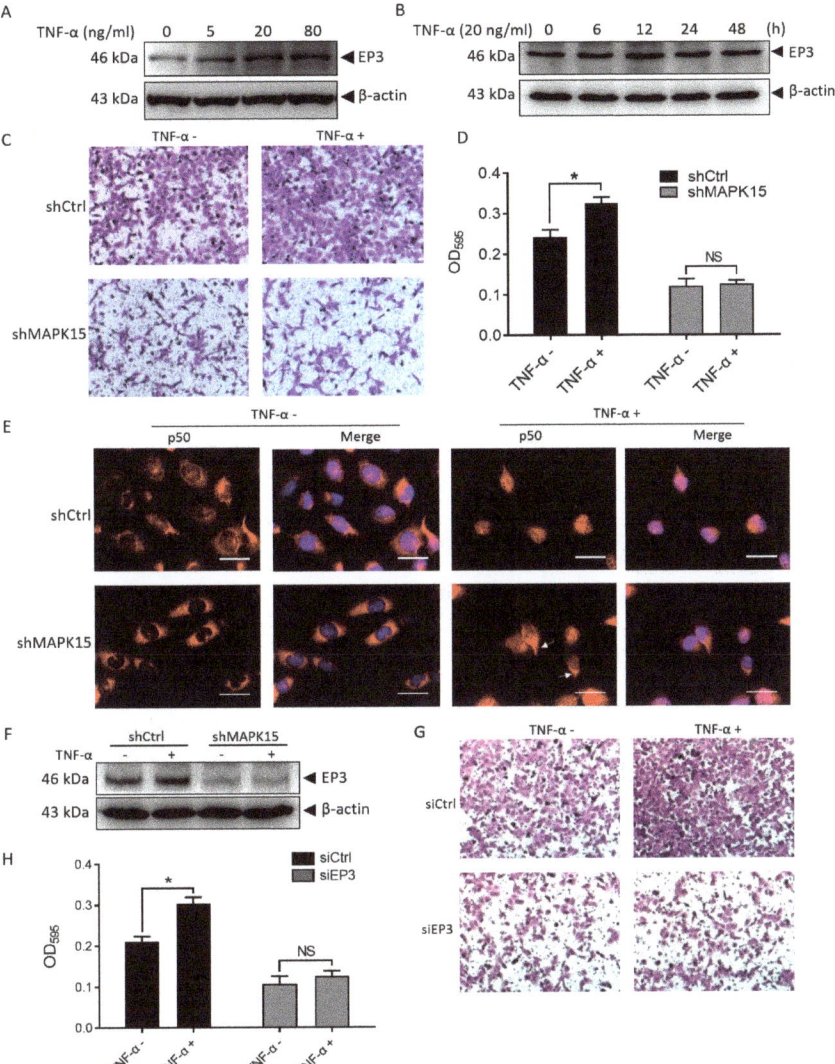

Figure 4. TNF-α promotes H1299 cell migration through induction of EP3 expression. (**A**) EP3 was detected in H1299 cells treated with different concentrations of TNF-α. (**B**) EP3 was detected in H1299 cells treated with 20 ng/mL TNF-α for different time points. (**C,D**) Transwell assay was used to detect migration effect of H1299-shCtrl and H1299-shMAPK15 cells with/without TNF-α treatment (20 ng/mL, 24 h), crystal violet in the migrated cells (**C**) was dissolved and absorbance was measured at OD_{595} (**D**). (**E**) H1299 cells cultured in serum-reduced medium (1% FBS) were stimulated with 20 ng/mL TNF-α for 1 h and p50 localization was detected in H1299 cells; scale bar represents 80 μm. (**F**) H1299-shCtrl and H1299-shMAPK15 cells cultured in serum-reduced medium (1% FBS) were treated with/without 20 ng/mL TNF-α for 12 h and the expression of EP3 was detected. (**G,H**) H1299 cells transfected with control siRNA or EP3 siRNA were resuspended in serum-reduced medium (1% FBS) and seeded to transwell chamber with/without 20 ng/mL TNF-α. Crystal violet in the migrated cells (**G**) was dissolved and absorbance was measured at OD_{595} (**H**). NS, non-significant; * $p < 0.05$, Student's *t*-test.

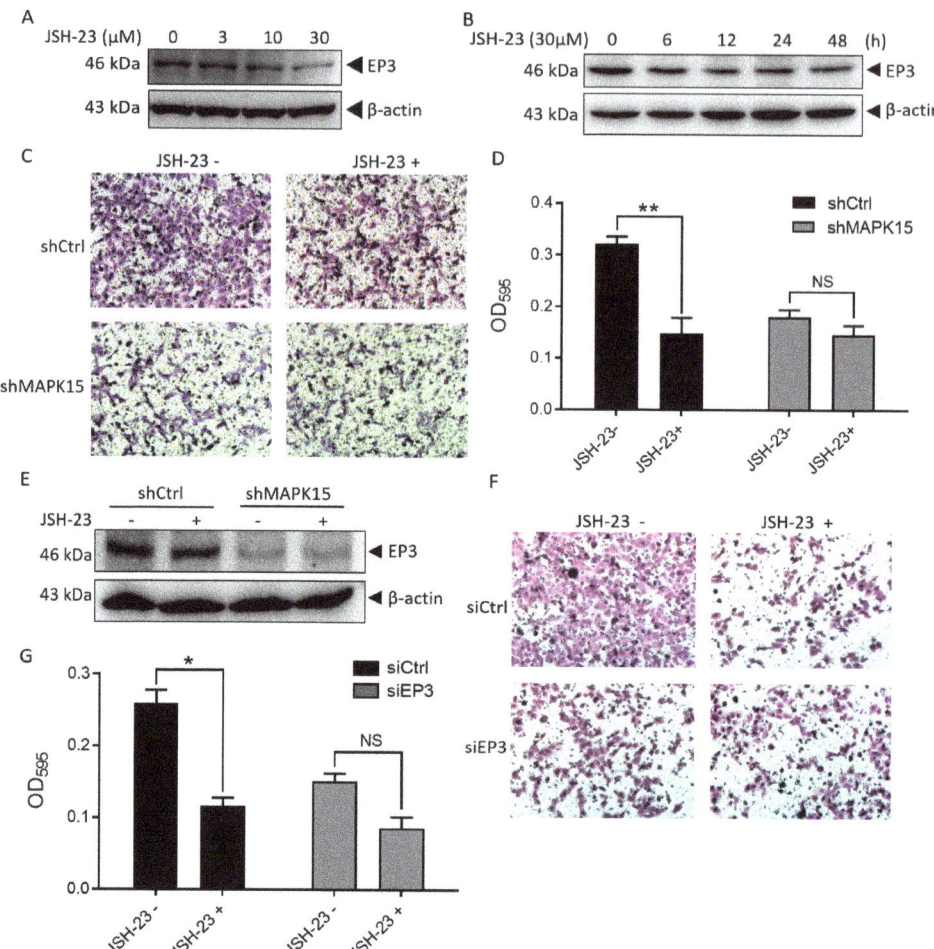

Figure 5. JSH-23 inhibits MAPK15-induced EP3 expression and cell migration. (**A,B**) H1299 cells were treated with/without different doses of JSH-23 for 12 h (**A**) or with 30 μM JSH-23 for different time points (**B**). The expression of EP3 was detected by immunoblot analysis. (**C,D**) H1299-shCtrl and H1299-shMAPK15 cells were resuspended in serum-reduced medium (1% FBS) and seeded to transwell chamber with/without 30 μM JSH-23, crystal violet in the migrated cells (**C**) was dissolved and absorbance was measured at OD_{595} (**D**). (**E**) H1299-shCtrl and H1299-shMAPK15 cells cultured in serum-reduced medium (1% FBS) were treated with/without 30 μM JSH-23 for 12 h and the expression of EP3 was detected. (**F,G**) H1299 cells transfected with control siRNA or EP3 siRNA were resuspended in serum-reduced medium (1% FBS) and seeded to transwell chamber with/without 30 μM JSH-23 for 24 h, crystal violet in the migrated cells (**F**) was dissolved and absorbance was measured at OD_{595} (**G**). NS, non-significant; * $p < 0.05$, ** $p < 0.01$, Student's *t*-test.

4. Discussion

Lung cancer is usually at an advanced stage with lymph node or distant metastasis when diagnosed, which leads to high mortality. Medical knowledge still lacks effective diagnostic molecular markers for metastatic lung cancer. In the present study, we revealed that MAPK15 is more highly expressed in the tissues of LUAD patients with lymph node metastasis (Figure 1B), and MAPK15 interacts with p50 to promote EP3 expression at the transcriptional level (Figure 6), thereby enhancing cancer cell migration and metastasis.

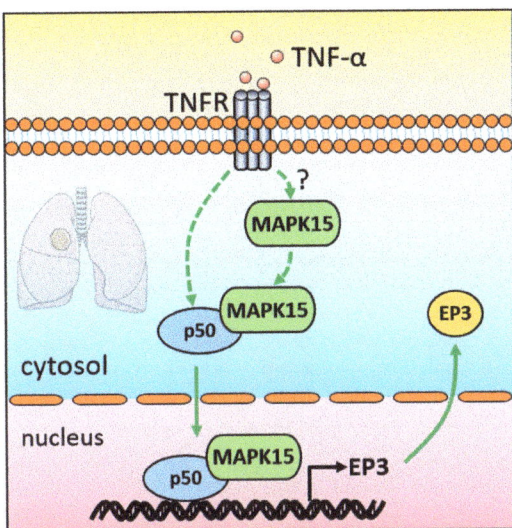

Figure 6. Schematic diagram of MAPK15 transcriptionally regulating EP3 by interacting with NF-κB p50 subunit and promoting LUAD metastasis. Question mark (?) indicates that how TNF-α affects MAPK15 in the cytosol is still unclear.

MAPK15 is a member of the ERK subfamily, which is involved in the regulation of cell growth and differentiation like other well-known ERKs. Previous research indicates that MAPK15 is involved in the transformation of colon cancer [6], promotes gastric cancer cell proliferation [7], and is associated with autophagy [8]. However, its clinical pathological role has, until now, not been examined in lung cancer. The correlation between MAPK15 and lymph node metastasis in LUAD described here suggests that MAPK15 plays an important role in lung cancer development, which may lead to poor clinical outcomes. Since we used a commercialized lung cancer tissue array in this study, there is a lack of relevant information on disease progression, so it is impossible to conduct a longitudinal assessment of the relationship between MAPK15 expression and patients' disease-free survival/overall survival, recurrence, metastasis, etc. However, with the in-depth study of MAPK15, we gradually realized its important role in LUAD. In future studies, multicenter, larger-sample-size studies should be conducted through longitudinal assessment of the patients' critical long-term clinical outcome to further clarify MAPK15 expression and the significance of clinical parameters. Due to the significant correlation between MAPK15 and the clinical features of the LUAD patients we observed, MAPK15 and its signaling pathway in LUAD may be a potential therapeutic target for metastatic LUAD. As a kinase, MAPK15 carries out different functions in various cancers, indicating the deregulation of key pathways. Studies have indicated a pivotal role of MAPK15 in mediating the effect of gene transcription. We have previously shown that MAPK15 promotes the transformation of colon cancer by mediating the activation of c-Jun [6]. Here, the identification of MAPK15 as an upstream regulator for EP3 unveiled a previously unknown mechanism for the MAPK15 or EP3 signaling pathway and their roles in the regulation of cell migration in LUAD.

The role of EP3 in tumor progression is still controversial. It has been reported that EP3 coupled with G proteins can effectively inhibit tumor growth. Shoji et al. found that EP3 can significantly inhibit the proliferation of tumor cells in advanced-stage colon cancer [24]. Sanchez et al. found that EP3 can promote the expression of p21 by reducing cAMP, thereby arresting the cell cycle in the S phase, and ultimately inhibiting the proliferation of 3T6 fibroblasts [25]. On the other hand, there are more and more studies showing that EP3 can promote the development of tumors. Finetti et al. found that EP3 is involved in regulating the formation of tumor blood vessels [26]. Amano et al. found that in an EP3-deficient mouse tumor model, tumor angiogenesis and tumor cell growth were effectively inhibited [13]. Yamaki et al. found that EP3 participates in the Src signaling pathway to promote the growth of LUAD A549 cells [14]. In this study, we reveal that knocking down EP3 can inhibit the migration of LUAD cells and that the expression of EP3 was positively regulated by MAPK15, which expands our understanding of EP3 and its regulation in lung cancer.

NF-κB is a type of transcription factor that plays an important role in the occurrence and development of tumors. The ERK family was linked to the NF-κB pathway [27,28]. As the most recently discovered MAPK family member, the relation between MAPK15 and NF-κB is mainly uncharacterized. Previous studies on the NF-κB protein family mainly focused on the activity of IκB or p65 in the p50/p65 complex to promote gene transcription. However, more and more studies have shown that p50 can bind to the promoter of the gene and activate gene transcription. The study of Hong et al. showed that overexpression of p50 in BAR-T cells significantly enhanced the activity of the DNMT1 gene promoter [29]. Karst et al. showed that overexpression of NF-κB p50 in melanoma cells MMRU can promote angiogenesis and up-regulate IL6 expression. They confirmed by Chip assay that p50 can bind to the promoter region of IL6 gene and activate its transcription [30]. Similarly, Southern et al. found that the BAG-1 protein can interact with the p50-p50 homodimer and bind to the promoter region of downstream genes to play a positive role in regulating gene transcription [31]. Beinke et al. reviewed that TNF-α/IL-1/LPS can activate the classic p50/p65 dimer NF-κB signaling pathway and the p100/RelB non-canonical signaling pathway, as well as the p105/p50 signaling pathway [23]. In this study, we found that MAPK15 interacts with p50 in LUAD cells, and the nuclear translocation of p50 may require the assistance of MAPK15. In addition, we also found that the mRNA expression level of EP3 increased when p50 was overexpressed in H1299 cells, indicating that p50 can regulate the expression of EP3 at the transcriptional level, and CHIP assay and luciferase reporter assay confirmed that p50 can bind to the promoter region of EP3 and promote the transcription of EP3. Our results revealed that MAPK15 interacts with p50 to promote the transcription of EP3, thereby affecting biological functions such as the migration of LUAD cells.

5. Conclusions

In conclusion, this study demonstrates the role of MAPK15 in the metastasis of LUAD. We revealed that MAPK15 promotes LUAD cell migration via p50 and EP3 signaling and is associated with lymph node metastasis in LUAD patients, which indicates that MAPK15 might be a potential prognostic biomarker for LUAD and a therapeutic target to inhibit metastasis in metastatic LUAD patients. The insights provided by this study could facilitate understanding the role of MAPK15 in lung cancer progression and its potential modulatory role in cancer metastasis.

Supplementary Materials: The following supporting information can be downloaded at: https://www.mdpi.com/article/10.3390/cancers15051398/s1, Table S1: Primer and siRNA used in this study; Table S2: Correlation between MAPK15 expression and clinicopathological parameters in patients with lung cancer; Table S3: Correlation between MAPK15 expression and tissue types; Figure S1: Matrix metalloproteinase-2 (MMP2) was significantly decreased in MAPK15 knockdown H1299 cells; Figure S2: Localization of MAPK15 and p50 in TNF-α treated A549 cells; Figure S3: Original blots and blot quantification of Figure 1; Figure S4: Original blots and blot quantification of Figure 2; Figure S5: Original blots and blot quantification of Figure 3; Figure S6: Original gels and gel quantification of Figure 3; Figure S7: Original blots and blot quantification of Figure 4; Figure S8: Original blots and blot quantification of Figure 5.

Author Contributions: F.-Y.Y.: conceptualization, methodology, validation, formal analysis, investigation, data curation, writing—original draft preparation, funding acquisition. Q.X.: validation, investigation, data curation. X.-Y.Z.: validation, investigation, data curation. H.-Y.M.: validation, investigation, data curation. Q.-H.Z.: validation, investigation, data curation. L.L.: validation, data curation. A.T.Y.L.: conceptualization, methodology, formal analysis, investigation, resources, writing—original draft preparation, writing—review and editing, supervision, project administration, funding acquisition. Y.-M.X.: conceptualization, methodology, formal analysis, investigation, resources, writing—original draft preparation, writing—review and editing, supervision, project administration, funding acquisition. All authors have read and agreed to the published version of the manuscript.

Funding: This work was supported by the grants from the National Natural Science Foundation of China (31271445, 31771582, and 31900468), the Guangdong Natural Science Foundation of China (2017A030313131 and 2019A1515011193), the "Thousand, Hundred, and Ten" Project of the Department of Education of Guangdong Province of China, the Basic and Applied Research Major Projects of Guangdong Province of China (2017KZDXM035 and 2018KZDXM036), the "Yang Fan" Project of Guangdong Province of China (Andy T. Y. Lau-2016 and Yan-Ming Xu-2015), and the Shantou Medical Health Science and Technology Plan (200624165260857).

Institutional Review Board Statement: The animal experiment in this study was approved by the Animal Ethics Committee of Shantou University Medical College (No. SUMC2021-042). The lung cancer tissue microarray was purchased from US Biomax Inc, Rockville, MD, USA.

Informed Consent Statement: Not applicable.

Data Availability Statement: The data presented in this study are available on request from the corresponding author.

Acknowledgments: We would like to thank members of the Lau And Xu laboratory for critical reading of this manuscript.

Conflicts of Interest: The authors declare no conflict of interest.

References

1. Singh, D.; Attri, B.K.; Gill, R.K.; Bariwal, J. Review on EGFR Inhibitors: Critical Updates. *Mini Rev. Med. Chem.* **2016**, *16*, 1134–1166. [CrossRef]
2. Melosky, B. Review of EGFR TKIs in Metastatic NSCLC, Including Ongoing Trials. *Front. Oncol.* **2014**, *4*, 244. [CrossRef]
3. Mao, L.; Zhou, Y.; Chen, L.; Hu, L.; Liu, S.; Zheng, W.; Zhao, J.; Guo, M.; Chen, C.; He, Z.; et al. Identification of atypical mitogen-activated protein kinase MAPK4 as a novel regulator in acute lung injury. *Cell Biosci.* **2020**, *10*, 121. [CrossRef]
4. De la Mota-Peynado, A.; Chernoff, J.; Beeser, A. Identification of the atypical MAPK Erk3 as a novel substrate for p21-activated kinase (Pak) activity. *J. Biol. Chem.* **2011**, *286*, 13603–13611. [CrossRef]
5. Lau, A.T.Y.; Xu, Y.M. Regulation of human mitogen-activated protein kinase 15 (extracellular signal-regulated kinase 7/8) and its functions: A recent update. *J. Cell. Physiol.* **2019**, *234*, 75–88. [CrossRef]
6. Xu, Y.M.; Zhu, F.; Cho, Y.Y.; Carper, A.; Peng, C.; Zheng, D.; Yao, K.; Lau, A.T.Y.; Zykova, T.A.; Kim, H.G.; et al. Extracellular signal-regulated kinase 8-mediated c-Jun phosphorylation increases tumorigenesis of human colon cancer. *Cancer Res.* **2010**, *70*, 3218–3227. [CrossRef]
7. Jin, D.H.; Lee, J.; Kim, K.M.; Kim, S.; Kim, D.H.; Park, J. Overexpression of MAPK15 in gastric cancer is associated with copy number gain and contributes to the stability of c-Jun. *Oncotarget* **2015**, *6*, 20190–20203. [CrossRef]
8. Colecchia, D.; Strambi, A.; Sanzone, S.; Iavarone, C.; Rossi, M.; Dall'Armi, C.; Piccioni, F.; Verrotti di Pianella, A.; Chiariello, M. MAPK15/ERK8 stimulates autophagy by interacting with LC3 and GABARAP proteins. *Autophagy* **2012**, *8*, 1724–1740. [CrossRef]
9. Iavarone, C.; Acunzo, M.; Carlomagno, F.; Catania, A.; Melillo, R.M.; Carlomagno, S.M.; Santoro, M.; Chiariello, M. Activation of the Erk8 mitogen-activated protein (MAP) kinase by RET/PTC3, a constitutively active form of the RET proto-oncogene. *J. Biol. Chem.* **2006**, *281*, 10567–10576. [CrossRef]
10. Cerone, M.A.; Burgess, D.J.; Naceur-Lombardelli, C.; Lord, C.J.; Ashworth, A. High-throughput RNAi screening reveals novel regulators of telomerase. *Cancer Res.* **2011**, *71*, 3328–3340. [CrossRef]
11. Wu, D.D.; Lau, A.T.Y.; Yu, F.Y.; Cai, N.L.; Dai, L.J.; Kim, M.O.; Jin, D.Y.; Xu, Y.M. Extracellular signal-regulated kinase 8-mediated NF-kappaB activation increases sensitivity of human lung cancer cells to arsenic trioxide. *Oncotarget* **2017**, *8*, 49144–49155. [CrossRef]
12. Wu, D.D.; Dai, L.J.; Tan, H.W.; Zhao, X.Y.; Wei, Q.Y.; Zhong, Q.H.; Ji, Y.C.; Yin, X.H.; Yu, F.Y.; Jin, D.Y.; et al. Transcriptional upregulation of MAPK15 by NF-κB signaling boosts the efficacy of combination therapy with cisplatin and TNF-α. *iScience* **2022**, *25*, 105459. [CrossRef]

13. Amano, H.; Hayashi, I.; Endo, H.; Kitasato, H.; Yamashina, S.; Maruyama, T.; Kobayashi, M.; Satoh, K.; Narita, M.; Sugimoto, Y.; et al. Host prostaglandin E(2)-EP3 signaling regulates tumor-associated angiogenesis and tumor growth. *J. Exp. Med.* **2003**, *197*, 221–232. [CrossRef]
14. Yamaki, T.; Endoh, K.; Miyahara, M.; Nagamine, I.; Thi Thu Huong, N.; Sakurai, H.; Pokorny, J.; Yano, T. Prostaglandin E2 activates Src signaling in lung adenocarcinoma cell via EP3. *Cancer Lett.* **2004**, *214*, 115–120. [CrossRef]
15. Cai, N.L.; Lau, A.T.Y.; Yu, F.Y.; Wu, D.D.; Dai, L.J.; Mo, H.Y.; Lin, C.M.; Xu, Y.M. Purification and characterization of a highly specific polyclonal antibody against human extracellular signal-regulated kinase 8 and its detection in lung cancer. *PLoS ONE* **2017**, *12*, e0184755. [CrossRef]
16. Yu, F.Y.; Xu, Q.; Wei, Q.Y.; Mo, H.Y.; Zhong, Q.H.; Zhao, X.Y.; Lau, A.T.Y.; Xu, Y.M. ACC2 is under-expressed in lung adenocarcinoma and predicts poor clinical outcomes. *J. Cancer Res. Clin. Oncol.* **2022**, *148*, 3145–3162. [CrossRef]
17. Li, M.; Tang, Y.; Zang, W.; Xuan, X.; Wang, N.; Ma, Y.; Wang, Y.; Dong, Z.; Zhao, G. Analysis of HAX-1 gene expression in esophageal squamous cell carcinoma. *Diagn. Pathol.* **2013**, *8*, 47. [CrossRef]
18. Livak, K.J.; Schmittgen, T.D. Analysis of relative gene expression data using real-time quantitative PCR and the 2(-Delta Delta C(T)) Method. *Methods* **2001**, *25*, 402–408. [CrossRef]
19. Li, A.; Morton, J.P.; Ma, Y.; Karim, S.A.; Zhou, Y.; Faller, W.J.; Woodham, E.F.; Morris, H.T.; Stevenson, R.P.; Juin, A.; et al. Fascin is regulated by slug, promotes progression of pancreatic cancer in mice, and is associated with patient outcomes. *Gastroenterology* **2014**, *146*, 1386–1396. [CrossRef]
20. Serrano-Gomez, S.J.; Maziveyi, M.; Alahari, S.K. Regulation of epithelial-mesenchymal transition through epigenetic and post-translational modifications. *Mol. Cancer* **2016**, *15*, 18. [CrossRef]
21. Lu, A.; Zuo, C.; He, Y.; Chen, G.; Piao, L.; Zhang, J.; Xiao, B.; Shen, Y.; Tang, J.; Kong, D.; et al. EP3 receptor deficiency attenuates pulmonary hypertension through suppression of Rho/TGF-beta1 signaling. *J. Clin. Investig.* **2015**, *125*, 1228–1242. [CrossRef] [PubMed]
22. Xiao, X.; Yang, G.; Bai, P.; Gui, S.; Nyuyen, T.M.; Mercado-Uribe, I.; Yang, M.; Zou, J.; Li, Q.; Xiao, J.; et al. Inhibition of nuclear factor-kappa B enhances the tumor growth of ovarian cancer cell line derived from a low-grade papillary serous carcinoma in p53-independent pathway. *BMC Cancer* **2016**, *16*, 582. [CrossRef] [PubMed]
23. Beinke, S.; Ley, S.C. Functions of NF-kappaB1 and NF-kappaB2 in immune cell biology. *Biochem. J.* **2004**, *382*, 393–409. [CrossRef] [PubMed]
24. Shoji, Y.; Takahashi, M.; Kitamura, T.; Watanabe, K.; Kawamori, T.; Maruyama, T.; Sugimoto, Y.; Negishi, M.; Narumiya, S.; Sugimura, T.; et al. Downregulation of prostaglandin E receptor subtype EP3 during colon cancer development. *Gut* **2004**, *53*, 1151–1158. [CrossRef]
25. Sanchez, T.; Moreno, J.J. GR 63799X, an EP3 receptor agonist, induced S phase arrest and 3T6 fibroblast growth inhibition. *Eur. J. Pharmacol.* **2006**, *529*, 16–23. [CrossRef]
26. Finetti, F.; Solito, R.; Morbidelli, L.; Giachetti, A.; Ziche, M.; Donnini, S. Prostaglandin E2 regulates angiogenesis via activation of fibroblast growth factor receptor-1. *J. Biol. Chem.* **2008**, *283*, 2139–2146. [CrossRef]
27. Hoesel, B.; Schmid, J.A. The complexity of NF-kappaB signaling in inflammation and cancer. *Mol. Cancer* **2013**, *12*, 86. [CrossRef] [PubMed]
28. Schulze-Osthoff, K.; Ferrari, D.; Riehemann, K.; Wesselborg, S. Regulation of NF-kappa B activation by MAP kinase cascades. *Immunobiology* **1997**, *198*, 35–49. [CrossRef]
29. Hong, J.; Li, D.; Wands, J.; Souza, R.; Cao, W. Role of NADPH oxidase NOX5-S, NF-kappaB, and DNMT1 in acid-induced p16 hypermethylation in Barrett's cells. *Am. J. Physiol. Cell Physiol.* **2013**, *305*, C1069–C1079. [CrossRef]
30. Karst, A.M.; Gao, K.; Nelson, C.C.; Li, G. Nuclear factor kappa B subunit p50 promotes melanoma angiogenesis by upregulating interleukin-6 expression. *Int. J. Cancer* **2009**, *124*, 494–501. [CrossRef]
31. Southern, S.L.; Collard, T.J.; Urban, B.C.; Skeen, V.R.; Smartt, H.J.; Hague, A.; Oakley, F.; Townsend, P.A.; Perkins, N.D.; Paraskeva, C.; et al. BAG-1 interacts with the p50-p50 homodimeric NF-kappaB complex: Implications for colorectal carcinogenesis. *Oncogene* **2012**, *31*, 2761–2772. [CrossRef]

Disclaimer/Publisher's Note: The statements, opinions and data contained in all publications are solely those of the individual author(s) and contributor(s) and not of MDPI and/or the editor(s). MDPI and/or the editor(s) disclaim responsibility for any injury to people or property resulting from any ideas, methods, instructions or products referred to in the content.

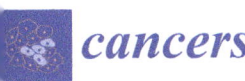

Article

IMP3 Expression as a Potential Tumour Marker in High-Risk Localisations of Cutaneous Squamous Cell Carcinoma: IMP3 in Metastatic cSCC

Maurice Klein [1,*], Merle Wefers [2], Christian Hallermann [3,4], Henrike J. Fischer [5], Frank Hölzle [1] and Kai Wermker [6]

1. Department of Oral, Maxillofacial and Facial Plastic Surgery, School of Medicine, University Hospital RWTH Aachen, Pauwelsstrasse 30, 52074 Aachen, Germany; fhoelzle@ukaachen.de
2. Orthodontics Meyer, Kurze Straße 6, 48151 Muenster, Germany; merle-wefers@gmx.de
3. Laboratory for Dermatopathology and Pathology Hamburg-Niendorf, Tibarg 7, 22459 Hamburg, Germany; c.hallermann@drrm.de
4. Department of Dermatology and Histopathology, Fachklinik Hornheide, Dorbaumstrasse 300, 48157 Muenster, Germany
5. Department of Immunology, School of Medicine, University Hospital RWTH Aachen, Pauwelsstraße 30, 52074 Aachen, Germany; hefischer@ukaachen.de
6. Department of Oral and Cranio-Maxillofacial Surgery, Klinikum Osnabrueck GmbH, Am Finkenhuegel 1, 49076 Osnabrueck, Germany; kai.wermker@klinikum-os.de
* Correspondence: mauklein@ukaachen.de; Tel.: +49-241-80-35-487; Fax: +49-241-80-82-430

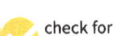

Citation: Klein, M.; Wefers, M.; Hallermann, C.; Fischer, H.J.; Hölzle, F.; Wermker, K. IMP3 Expression as a Potential Tumour Marker in High-Risk Localisations of Cutaneous Squamous Cell Carcinoma: IMP3 in Metastatic cSCC. *Cancers* 2023, *15*, 4087. https://doi.org/10.3390/cancers15164087

Academic Editors: Daniel L. Pouliquen and Cristina Núñez González

Received: 29 June 2023
Revised: 1 August 2023
Accepted: 5 August 2023
Published: 14 August 2023

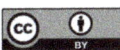

Copyright: © 2023 by the authors. Licensee MDPI, Basel, Switzerland. This article is an open access article distributed under the terms and conditions of the Creative Commons Attribution (CC BY) license (https://creativecommons.org/licenses/by/4.0/).

Simple Summary: High IMP3 expression is correlated with poorer prognosis in many tumour entities. To date, there have been no data on IMP3 expression and clinical outcome in high-risk localisations (lip, ear) of squamous cell carcinoma of the skin. These are almost twice as likely to metastasise compared to other sites. In this study, the tumour marker IMP3 showed clear correlations with aggressiveness features (lymph node metastases, local recurrences, and progression-free survival). The identification of these more-aggressive tumours could influence therapy and diagnostics (radicality of neck dissection, follow-up intervals, staging). The analysis method presented here is efficient and could be easily incorporated into a clinical workflow and used for prospective testing.

Abstract: Background: High IMP3 expression is correlated with a worse outcome. Until now, there have been no data about IMP3 expression and clinical outcome for high-risk localisation of squamous cell carcinoma of the skin (cSCC). Methods: One-hundred twenty-two patients with cSCC of the lip and ear were included, and IMP3 expression in the tumours was immunohistochemically assessed in different evaluation approaches. Subsequently, subgroups were analysed in a matched pair approach and correlated with clinical pathologic parameters. In the following, different IMP3 analysis methods were tested for clinical suitability. Results: We found a significant correlation between IMP3 expression and risk for lymph node metastasis, local relapse, and progression-free survival. Conclusions: On basis of our data, we suggest a prognostic benefit cutoff value for high (>50%) and low (<50%) IMP3 expression. Thus, IMP3 expression has a high scientific potential for further studies and could potentially be used as a prognostic marker in diagnostic and therapeutic decision-making.

Keywords: IMP3; lip cancer; squamous cell carcinoma; ear cancer; skin cancer; HNSCC

1. Introduction

Squamous cell carcinoma of the skin (cSCC) is the second-most-frequent skin cancer after basal cell carcinoma [1]. Risk localisations of cSCC include the ear and lip, which display an increased risk of lymph node metastases (LNMs) compared to other tumour localisations. Alam et al. showed that the localisations of cSCC at the external ear (ECSCC) and lip (LSCC) with recurrence and metastasis rates of 8–25% are more aggressive than other localisations [2]. Furthermore, the localisation in the lip area has an influence on the tumour aggressiveness, so that LSCC is more aggressive when oral mucosa is affected [3]. However, the lymph node metastasis status (N+ or N−) is one of the most-important prognostic factors in cSCC of the head and neck [2,4,5]. The distinction between N+ and N− patients is very important, as N+ patients have a worse prognosis and a lower 5-year survival rate. N− patient had a 5-year survival of 87–95%, and N+ had only survival rates of 25–50% [6]. Especially patients with high-risk localisations LSCC and ECSCC benefit from risk prediction. In addition to the prognostic assessment, the risk evaluation of LNMs and the indication for neck dissection are controversial topics among different disciplines [1].

In terms of individualised medicine, there is a particular need for research on predictive tumour markers. For example, a predictive model for LSCC has been created. A study by Wermker et al. showed that, with the help of tumour thickness and grading, a risk stratification and evaluation for LNMs could be made [6]. In contrast to the histopathomorphological risk constellations, immunohistochemical markers could also be helpful in the prognostic evaluation of high-risk localisations of cSCC.

The insulin-like growth factor 2 mRNA-binding protein 3 (IGF2BP3, also named IMP3) could be a tumour marker with such a potential. IMP3 is an RNA-binding oncofetal protein [7]. Different studies have shown that these proteins have important implications in cell function, polarisation, cell migration, morphology, cellular metabolism, proliferation, and differentiation [7–9]. Gong et al. presented that IMP3 expression supports tumour cell proliferation, tumour cell adhesion, and tumour cell invasion [10]. There is also evidence of a link between increased IMP3 expression and advanced tumour stage [11]. In a meta-analysis in 2017, Chen et al. showed that the level of IMP3 expression correlates significantly with a decreased overall survival (OS) in different tumour entities. The authors evaluated 53 studies covering numerous tumour entities including renal cancer, lung cancer, oral cancer, and gastrointestinal cancer. There were positive correlations of high IMP3 expression with worse overall survival, disease-specific survival, and metastasis-free survival. To summarise, a high IMP3 expression is associated with a worse prognosis [12].

In oral squamous cell carcinoma (oSCC), high IMP3 expression correlates with lymph node metastasis (N+) and decreased 5-year survival. If two patients had the same tumour stage, but different IMP3 expression levels, the patient with the higher IMP3 expression had a worse prognosis [13].

The aim of our study was to analyse if the marker IMP3 can be used in a clinical setting to assess the aggressiveness of high-risk localisations of cSCC. The aggressiveness was determined with the overall survival rate, disease-specific survival, occurrence of local relapses, and progression-free survival. The key question was if the IMP3 analysis methods (IMP3 Analysis Category I (<25%, 25–50%, 50–75%, >75%), IMP3 Analysis Category II (0%, 1–20%, 21–60%, >60%), IMP3 Analysis Category III (>50%; <50%)) were usable for risk prediction for N+ cases (correlated with worse prognosis). It seems that one of the IMP3 analysis categories (IMP3 Analysis Category II) is particularly suitable in terms of outcome prediction.

2. Materials and Methods
2.1. Ethics Statement

This study was approved by the local ethics committee (Ethical Committee of the Westphalian Wilhelms University Muenster, Approval No. 2013-063-f-S) and was conducted in accordance with the Guidelines for Good Clinical Practice and in compliance with the Declaration of Helsinki. All patients gave their written informed consent for participating in this study.

2.2. Patients

All included patients were > 18 years old and had a histologically proven cSCC of the lip (LSCC) or ear (ECSCC). Included localisations for LSCC were the upper lip and lower lip. The following localisations were defined for the ECSCC: helix, cavum conchae/anthelix/tragus, retroauricular/posterior side, or a combination with more than one of these regions. All patients were resected R0 in the primary tumour.

Each patient had a preoperative stay with a minimum diagnostic procedure of sonography of the head and neck, X-ray of the thorax, and abdominal sonography. All patients were presented in an interdisciplinary tumour board. After the therapy, all patients received a periodic recall. The exclusion criteria were: no written consent and condition according to neck dissection or different HNSCC than in the inclusion criteria. Further data included in the correlation analysis were: follow-up time, first diagnosis, tumour localisation, local recurrence, lymph node metastasis, distant metastasis, disease-specific death, and overall survival.

The electronic patient data were complete and had a follow-up of at least 24 months. The abuse of alcohol or tobacco was not part of the exclusion criteria.

All patients (n = 122) were divided into two main groups and subsequently into two subgroups. Allocation to the two main groups was based on the localisation: LSCC and ESCC. These were then further subdivided into cases of N+ or N−. In addition, subgroup division into LSCC and ECSCC and lymph node status was performed: LSCC N−, LSCC N+, ECSCC N−, ECSCC N+.

In addition, a subdivision was performed for nodal status with both cases: N+ (LSCC N+ and ECSCC N+) and N− (LSCC N− + ECSCC N−).

The matched pair approach was used, as it allows a certain homogeneity to be achieved. The following groups were compared: LSCC N− vs. LSCC N+ and ECSCC N− vs. ECSCC N+. Each patient from the respective group was contrasted with a patient from the other group and with clinically pathologically selected known risk factors with as few differences as possible.

Included parameters for matching were: age, gender, grading, T-stadium, primary tumour localisation, tumour infiltration depth, perineural growth, cartilage invasion (only for ECSCC), comorbidities, and immunosuppression (classification into none, weak, moderate, strong). Finally, IMP3 expression (different IMP3 expression ranges; see below) was correlated with clinical pathological data.

2.3. Immunohistochemistry Analysis of IMP3

The selection of suitable tumour samples was made on Haematoxylin-Eosin-stained slices. The tumour tissue (histologically proven LSCC and ECSCC) was fixed in 10% formaldehyde solution.

Incubation with a primary antibody against IMP3 (anti-IMP3 Clon 69.1, 1:50, Agilent/Dako (Glostrup, Denmark)) was performed in the Autostainer Plus (Dako REAL DETECTION SYSTEM K5005, Glostrup). The tissue slices were incubated with the secondary (Dako REAL Link Biotinylated secondary antibody (AB2), Glostrup) antibody (exposure time 15 min) and then with Dako Real Streptavidin Alkaline Phosphatase (AP) (Glostrup; exposure time 15 min). Afterwards the SCC tissue slices were exposed to chromogen (Dako RED Chromogen, Glostrup) for 8 min. Next, Haematoxylin (nucleus counterstain/eight-minute exposure time) was applied. Coverslip tape was used.

The cellular localisation of IMP3 staining was determined by the Olympus BX51 microscope (Hamburg, Germany).

Two investigators blinded to the patients' prognostic data analysed each slice with a first overview and then divided each slice into 5 high-power fields (HPFs) with a magnification of 400× after randomisation.

In every HPF, the investigator counted 5 × 10 tumour cells, totalling 50 cells per HPF and 250 cells in each slice. All tumour cells with a positive dark brown colour in the cytoplasm were counted as positive. Tonsil tissue was used as the positive control. The expression analysis was according to the literature [13,14]. In the event of discrepancies between the investigators, the case was reevaluated in a shared discussion.

The study focused on three different analysis categories. The aim was to find which expression range is most suitable for prognostic use. The expression was analysed in % ranges of expression: IMP3 Analysis Category I (<25%, 25–50%, 50–75%, >75%), IMP3 Analysis Category II (0%, 1–20%, 21–60%, >60%), IMP3 Analysis Category III (>50%; <50%). These three categories are presented in the Results Section.

2.4. Statistical Analysis

All statistical analyses were performed by using the Statistical Package for Social Sciences (SPSS) Version 22.0 for Windows® (SPSS Inc., Chicago, IL, USA).

Categorical variables were analysed using the chi-squared test and Fisher's exact test. For continuous variables, the Mann–Whitney U-test was used as a non-parametric test for abnormally distributed data, and an independent t-test was used to analyse normally distributed variables. Disease-specific survival (time from first diagnosis until tumour-dependent death; data on patients without tumour-dependent death were censored at the last follow-up time) and progression-free survival (time from first diagnosis until local recurrence or metastasising; data on patients without an event of progression were censored at the last follow-up time) were calculated using the Kaplan–Meier method, and group differences were analysed using the log-rank test.

3. Results

In the first part of the results, an overview of the patient cohort will be given, followed by the correlation of IMP3 expression with the nodal status groups in the second part. Finally, the evaluation methods of IMP3 expression (IMP3 Expression Categories I-III) are compared and correlated with clinical pathological outcome parameters.

3.1. Study Population

The patients' age range was 42.7–97 years (mean 75.8 years, median 75.7 years, standard deviation 10.1 years). The patients' subgroups were LSCC + ECSCC (n = 122, 100%, male n = 109, female n = 13). The subgroup data characteristics were: LSCC (n = 58, 47.5%, LSCC unilateral: n = 25; LSCC bilateral: n = 33) and ECSCC (n = 64, 52.5%).

The distribution of the classification of immunosuppression of the patients was as follows: none (n = 102), weak (n = 6), moderate (n = 13), strong (n = 1).

3.2. Clinical Pathology Data in the Study Cohort

Prognostic TNM data were collected: (all pT n = 122, 100%; pT1 n = 27, 22.5%; pT2 n = 31, 25.8%; pT3 n = 47, 37.5%; pT4 n = 17, 14.2%; all pN n = 120, 100%; pN0 n = 76, 63.3%; pN1 n = 26, 21.7%; pN 2a n = 14, 11.7%; pN 2b n = 3, 2.5%; pN 2c n = 1, 0.8%; all M n = 122, 100%; M0 n = 120, 98.4%; M1 n = 2, 1.6%). All patients showed an R0 status.

3.3. IMP3 Expression Distribution in the Study Cohort

As there were only marginal differences between the investigators, a shared decision was not necessary. The mean of IMP3 expression was 51.2%, and the median was 52.4% with a standard deviation of 19.5%. The range of IMP3 expression was between 0.0% and 88.4% IMP3 expression.

3.4. Higher IMP3 Expression Correlates with the Risk for Lymph Node Metastasis

The comparison between the N+ and N− groups showed that IMP3 expression in all cases with N+ had a mean of 61.4%, a median of 63.2%, and a standard deviation of 14.9.

Interestingly, IMP3 expression of all cases with N− showed a mean of 41.1%, a median of 45.6%, and a standard deviation of 18.4. Thus, a higher IMP 3 expression was correlated with pN+ in high-risk localisation of cSCC ($p < 0.001$). Figure 1 (left side) shows the correlation of the nodal status and IMP3 expression in the boxplot.

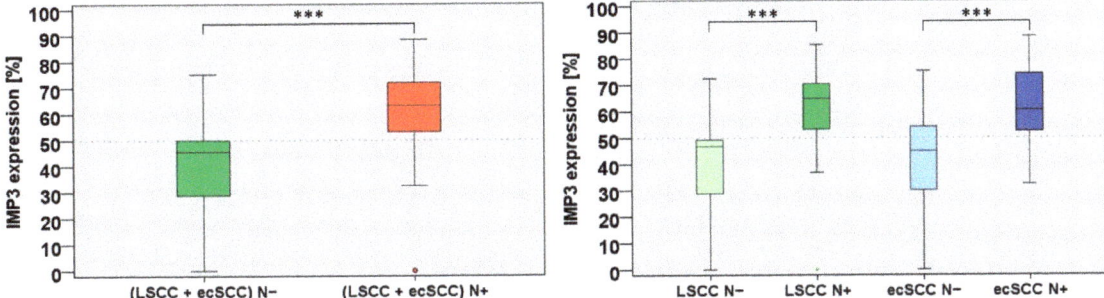

Figure 1. (**Left side**) IMP3 expression correlates positively with nodal status (N+/N−) in high-risk localisation of squamous cell carcinoma of the ear (ECSCC) and lip (LSCC) ($p < 0.001$). (**Right side**) The subgroups analysis of LSCC N+/N− and ECSCC N+/N− and IMP3 expression show each a significant correlation with nodal status ($p < 0.001$). *** $p < 0.001$.

In addition to the correlation of the total collective (including both LSCC and ECSCC) with N+, the analysis of the subgroups LSCC and ECSCC followed. Interestingly, both subgroups showed a higher expression of IMP3 in the N+ group. Figure 1 (right side) displays the risk for LNMs and the expression of IMP3 in the subgroups of LSCC N+/N− and ECSCC N+/N− and IMP3 expression.

LSCC N+ patients presented with a mean IMP3 expression of 60.3%, a range of 0.0–85.2%, and a standard deviation of 16.2. For LSCC N−, we found a mean of 40.3%, a range of 0.0–72.4%, and a standard deviation of 17.9. Interestingly, the difference of LSCC N+ vs. LSCC N− was significant in the Mann–Whitney U-test in the subgroup analysis ($p < 0.001$), proving that higher IMP3 expression is correlated with the risk for LNMs in LSCC. This was also revealed in the analysis of the ECSCC N+ subgroup. These patients presented with a mean IMP3 expression of 62.3%, a median of 60.4%, a range of 32.4–88.4%, and a standard deviation of 13.8, whereas the ECSCC N− subgroup showed a mean of 41.8%, a median of 45.0%, a range of 0.0–75.2%, and a standard deviation of 19.1. The difference of ECSCC N+ v. ECSCC N− was also significant ($p < 0.001$) in the Mann–Whitney U-test. Taken together, IMP3 could be a reliable marker for metastasis risk assessment as it consistently correlated with the LNM rates.

3.5. IMP3 Correlates with Disease Progression and Local Relapse

In addition to the prediction of N+ cases by the IMP3 expression rates, other prognostically significant outcome parameters were also analysed: A higher IMP3 expression significantly correlated with disease progression ($p < 0.001$) and local relapse ($p = 0.014$). However, IMP3 expression did not correlate with disease-specific death ($p = 0.090$) and distant metastasis ($p = 0.090$).

3.6. IMP3 Analysis Categories I–III

After proving the prognostic potential of IMP3 expression analysis for pN+, a simple clinically applicable semiquantitative IMP3 expression analysis needed to be established. For this purpose, we analysed the IMP3 expression using three different approaches (Analysis Categories I–III) to identify the most-reliable and -application-oriented method for the prognostic evaluation of IMP3 expression in LSCC and ECSCC. In addition, it should be investigated whether the correlation between increased IMP3 expression and the increased occurrence of LNMs also applies to IMP3 Analysis Categories I–III.

3.7. IMP3 Analysis Category I (<25%, 25–50%, 50–75%, >75% IMP3 Expression)

For the first screening of IMP3 expression ranges, a quarter-step classification (IMP3 Analysis Category I; <25%, 25–50%, 50–75%, >75% IMP3 expression) was performed.

In IMP3 Category I, the age at first diagnosis was as follows: <25% IMP3 expression: mean 76.1 years, median 73.6, 64.7–93.9 years; 25–50% IMP3 expression: mean 76.6 years, median 77.9 years, 42.7–94.8 years; 50–75% IMP3 expression: mean 74.9, median 75.2 years, 44.3–97.0 years; >75% IMP3 expression: mean 76.8 years, median 76.1 years, 65.2–91.7 years. The correlation was not significant in the Pearson chi-squared test ($p = 0.346$).

A distribution of IMP3 expression for the AJCC was also shown: <25% IMP3 expression: Stage I (n = 5), Stage II (n = 3), Stage III (n = 1), Stage IV (n = 3); 25–50% IMP3 expression: Stage I (n = 10), Stage II (n = 8), Stage III (n = 19), Stage IV (n = 9); 50–75% IMP3 expression: Stage I (n = 7), Stage II (n = 8), Stage III (n = 24), Stage IV (n = 14); >75% IMP3 expression: Stage I (n = 1), Stage II (n = 0), Stage III (n = 7), Stage IV (n = 3). The correlation failed to reach significance in the Pearson chi-squared test ($p = 0.179$).

In addition, IMP3 Analysis Category I is presented with the degree of differentiation (grading): <25% IMP3 expression: G1 (n = 4), G2 (n = 6), G 3 (n = 2); 25–50% IMP3 expression: G1 (n = 10), G2 (n = 27), G 3 (n = 9); 50–75% IMP3 expression: G1 (n = 11), G2 (n = 32), G 3 (n = 10); >75% IMP3 expression: G1 (n = 1), G2 (n = 8), G 3 (n = 3). The correlation was not significant in the Pearson chi-squared test ($p = 0.905$).

The distribution of the strength of immunosuppression could also be shown as dependent on the IMP3 expression: <25% IMP3 expression: none (n = 11), weak (n = 1), moderate (n = 0), strong (n = 0); 25–50% IMP3 expression: none (n = 38), weak (n = 4), moderate (n = 4), strong (n = 0); 50–75% IMP3 expression: none (n = 42), weak (n = 1), moderate (n = 9), strong n = 1); >75% IMP3 expression: no patient with immunosuppression. The correlation failed to reach significance in the Pearson chi-squared test ($p = 0.381$).

There were more cases in the N+ (LSCC N+ and ECSCC N+) group with an IMP3 expression range of 50–75% (63.9%) and an IMP3 expression range >75% (16.4%) as compared to the respective N− groups.

In line with this, the quartiles with lower IMP3 expression ranges showed fewer cases in the N+ (LSCC N+ and ECSCC N+) group (IMP3 expression range <25% (1.6%) and IMP3 expression range of 25–50% (18.0%)).

As expected, there were significantly more cases in the N− (LSCC N− + ECSCC N−) group with an IMP3 expression range <25% (18.0%) or IMP3 expression range of 25–50% (57.4%) and fewer cases for the high expression ranges (IMP3 expression range of 50–75% (23.0%) and IMP3 expression range >75% (1.6%)).

The cross-tabulation showed significance ($p < 0.001$) for IMP3 Analysis Category I with nodal status in the Pearson chi-squared test.

We then analysed this in further detail by comparing the individual subgroups (LSCC N−, LSCC N+, ECSCC N−, ECSCC N+) and found that, generally, the lower quartiles were more frequent in the N− subgroups, whereas in the N+ subgroups, the higher quartiles were prevalent: LSCC N−: IMP3 expression <25% (17.2%), IMP3 expression of 25–50% (65.5%), IMP3 expression of 50–75% (17.2%), IMP3 expression >75% (0%); LSCC N+: IMP3 expression <25% (3.4%), IMP3 expression of 25–50% (13.8%), IMP3 expression of 50–75% (75.9%), IMP3 expression >75% (6.9%); ECSCC N−: IMP3 expression <25% (18.8%), IMP3 expression of 25–50% (50.0%), IMP3 expression of 50–75% (28.1%), IMP3 expression >75% (3.1%); ECSCC N+: IMP3 expression <25% (0%), IMP3 expression of 25–50% (21.9%), IMP3 expression of 50–75% (53.1%), IMP3 expression >75% (25.0%).

After subgroup analysis, the correlations of IMP3 Analysis Category I with different clinical pathological outcome parameters were examined for all patients.

A significant correlation between IMP3 expression and N+ ($p < 0.001$) was demonstrated for IMP3 Analysis Category I.

There was no significant correlation ($p = 0.370$) of IMP3 Analysis Category I and disease-specific death in the Pearson chi-squared test. In contrast, there was a correlation in IMP3 Analysis Category I and disease progression ($p < 0.001$). In addition, trends could be shown for IMP3 Analysis Category I and distant metastasis ($p = 0.093$) and IMP3 Analysis Category I and local relapse ($p = 0.058$).

As we saw before that IMP3 expression correlates with disease-free progression, we also performed a Kaplan–Meyer analysis for progression-free survival for IMP3 Analysis Category I: Figure 2 shows that progression-free survival was reduced for an IMP3 expression range > 50%. The log-rank test (comparison with the <25% IMP3 expression range) showed a significant difference with the 50–75% IMP3 expression range ($p = 0.007$) and >75% IMP3 expression range ($p = 0.004$). For the 25–50% IMP expression range, no significant difference could be shown.

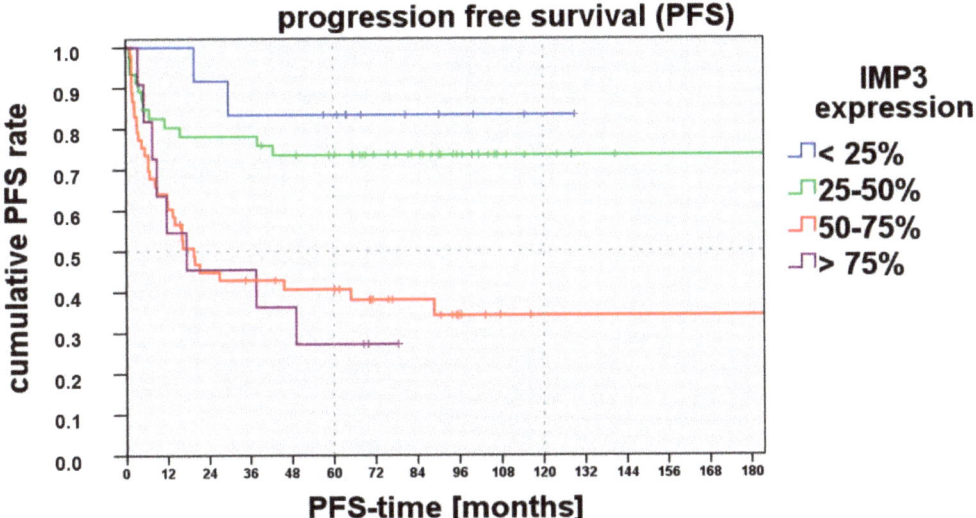

Figure 2. The progression-free survival was shortened depending on the IMP3 expression ranges (IMP3 Analysis Category I; <25%, 25–50%, 50–75%, >75%). A higher IMP3 expression of >50% was correlated with a less progression-free survival.

3.8. IMP3 Analysis Category II (0%, 1–20%, 21–60%, >60% IMP3 Expression)

After the analysis of the IMP3 Analysis Category I (<25%, 25–50%, 50–75%, >75% IMP3 expression), the IMP3 expression was subdivided into thirds (IMP3 Analysis Category II; 0%, 1–20%, 21–60%, >60% IMP3 expression).

In IMP3 Category II, the age at first diagnosis was as follows: 0% IMP3 expression: mean 69.5 years, median 71.6 years, 64.7–72.1 years; 1–20% IMP3 expression: mean 78.8 years, median 77.4 years, 69.5–93.9 years; 21–60% IMP3 expression: mean 75.8 years, median 76.5 years, 42.7–97.0 years; >60% IMP3 expression: mean 75.8 years, median 76.0 years, 44.3–97.0 years. The correlation was not significant in the Pearson chi-squared test ($p = 0.223$).

In addition, a distribution of IMP3 Analysis Category II could be shown for the AJCC: 0% IMP3 expression: Stage I (n = 2), Stage II (n = 1), Stage III (n = 0), Stage IV (n = 0); 1–20% IMP3 expression: Stage I (n = 2), Stage II (n = 2), Stage III (n = 1), Stage IV (n = 3); 21–60% IMP3 expression: Stage I (n = 13), Stage II (n = 15), Stage III (n = 29), Stage IV (n = 14); >60% IMP3 expression: Stage I (n = 6), Stage II (n = 1), Stage III (n = 21), Stage IV (n = 12). The correlation was significant in the Pearson chi-squared test ($p = 0.042$).

In addition, the IMP3 Analysis Category I is presented with the degree of differentiation (grading): 0% IMP3 expression: G1 (n = 2), G2 (n = 1), G 3 (n = 0); 1–20% IMP3 expression: G1 (n = 2), G2 (n = 4), G 3 (n = 2); 21–60% IMP3 expression: G1 (n = 16), G2 (n = 42), G 3 (n = 13); >60% IMP3 expression: G1 (n = 6), G2 (n = 26), G 3 (n = 8). The correlation was not significant in the Pearson chi-squared test ($p = 0.522$).

The distribution of the strength of immunosuppression could also be shown as a dependent on the IMP3 expression: 0% IMP3 expression: no immunosuppression (n = 3); 1–20% IMP3 expression: none (n = 7), weak (n = 1), moderate (n = 0), strong (n = 0); 21–60% IMP3 expression: none (n = 58), weak (n = 4), moderate (n = 8), strong (n = 1); >60% IMP3 expression: none (n = 34), weak (n = 1), moderate (n = 5), strong (n = 0). The correlation failed to reach significance in the Pearson chi-squared test (p = 0.922).

In the N+ group (LSCC N+ + ECSCC N+), most patients (54.1%) were in the >60% IMP3 expression range and 44.3% in the 21–60% IMP3 expression range. In the 0% IMP3 expression range, there were 1.6% of the cases, and in the 1–20% IMP3 expression range, no patients (0%).

The distribution in the N− group (LSCC N− + ECSCC N−) was different. Here, in the IMP3 expression range group 0%, 3.3% of the cases, in the IMP3 expression range 1–20%, 13.1% of the cases, in the IMP3 expression range 21–60%, 72.1% of the cases, and in the IMP3 expression range >60%, 11.5% of the cases fell.

IMP3 expression in the subgroups (LSCC N−, LSCC N+, ECSCC N−, ECSCC N+) was also examined:

LSCC N−: IMP3 expression range of 0%: 3.4%, IMP3 expression range of 1–20%: 10.3%, IMP3 expression range of 21–60%: 79.3%, IMP3 expression range >60%: 6.9%; LSCC N+: IMP3 expression range of 0%: 3.4%, IMP3 expression range of 1–20%: 0%, IMP3 expression range of 21–60%: 37.9%, IMP3 expression range >60%: 58.6%; ECSCC N−: IMP3 expression range of 0%: 3.1%, IMP3 expression range of 1–20%: 15.6%, IMP3 expression range of 21–60%: 65.6%, IMP3 expression range >60%: 15.6%, ECSCC N+: IMP3 expression range of 0%: 0%, IMP3 expression range of 1–20%: 0%, IMP3 expression range of 21–60%: 50.0%, IMP3 expression range >60%: 50.0%.

No correlation was found between IMP3 Analysis Category II and the risk of disease-related death and local relapse.

In contrast, the Pearson chi-squared test showed a positive correlation of IMP3 Analysis Category II with disease progression (p = 0.001), distant metastasis (p = 0.014), and LNM (p = 0.008).

3.9. IMP3 Analysis Category III (<50%, >50% IMP3 Expression)

A quick and clinically easy way to implement IMP3 analysis is the classification into the >50% and <50% IMP3 expression ranges (IMP3 Analysis Category III).

In IMP3 Category III, the age at first diagnosis was as follows: >50% IMP3 expression: mean 75.3 years, median 75.7 years, 44.3–97.0 years; <50% IMP3 expression: mean 76.5 years, median 76.1 years, 42.7–94.8 years. The correlation was not significant in the Pearson chi-squared test (p = 0.397).

A distribution of IMP3 expression for the AJCC was also shown: >50% IMP3 expression: Stage I (n = 8), Stage II (n = 9), Stage III (n = 33), Stage IV (n = 18); <50% IMP3 expression: Stage I (n = 15), Stage II (n = 10), Stage III (n = 18), Stage IV (n = 11). The correlation failed to reach significance in the Pearson chi-squared test (p = 0.80).

In addition, the IMP3 Analysis Category I is presented with the degree of differentiation (grading): >50% IMP3 expression: G1 (n = 12) G2 (n = 43) G 3 (n = 13); <50% IMP3 expression: G1 (n = 14) G2 (n = 30) G 3 (n = 10). The correlation was not significant in the Pearson chi-squared test (p = 0.530).

The distribution of the strength of immunosuppression could also be shown as dependent on the IMP3 expression: >50% IMP3 expression: none (n = 57), weak (n = 1) moderate (n = 9) strong (n = 1); <50% IMP3 expression: none (n = 45), weak (n = 5) moderate (n = 4) strong (n = 0). The correlation failed to reach significance in the Pearson chi-squared test (p = 0.141).

The >50% IMP3 expression range was positively correlated with the presence of LNMs at all sites (LSCC N+ + ECSCC N+): 83.6% of these cases showed an LNM and 27.9% no LNM. In contrast, 72.1% of patients in the <50% IMP 3 expression range group did not have an LNM (LSCC N− + ECSCC N−), and 16.4% had an LNM. Thus, a higher IMP3 expression of >50% was significantly ($p < 0.001$) correlated with the occurrence of an LNM.

We next analysed the localisation subgroups and also found significant correlations with IMP3 Expression Category III. In the LSCC group and IMP3 expression >50%, 82.8% of patients had an LNM and only 24.1% had no LNM. In the LSCC group and IMP3 expression <50%, 75.9% of patient cases showed no LNM and only 17.2% had LNM.

Comparable results were also found in the ECSCC group. In the ECSCC group and an IMP3 expression of >50%, 84.4% of patients had an LNM and 31.3% had no LNM. In line with this, in the ESCC group and an IMP3 expression of <50%, 68.8% of the patients had no LNM and 15.6% had an LNM. IMP3 Expression Category III (<50%, >50% IMP3 expression) was significantly correlated ($p < 0.001$) with the risk for LNMs in the subgroups.

Although we were able to show the significant correlation of >50% IMP3 expression and LNMs, we could unfortunately not demonstrate a significant correlation for IMP3 expression and distant metastasis in this category. Furthermore, there was a correlation between IMP3 Analysis Category III and disease progression ($p < 0.001$).

In addition, it was investigated whether IMP3 Analysis Category III correlated with the risk of local recurrence. There was a correlation ($p = 0.012$) for IMP3 Analysis Category III and local recurrence in the Pearson chi-squared test.

To examine whether the 50% expression cutoff was also able to predict the disease-specific survival, we analysed IMP3 Expression Category III with disease-related death. Higher IMP3 expression showed a tendency ($p = 0.092$) towards disease-related death in the IMP3 expression category in the log rank test (Mantel–Cox). A higher IMP3 expression of >50% showed a lower disease-specific survival (Figure 3).

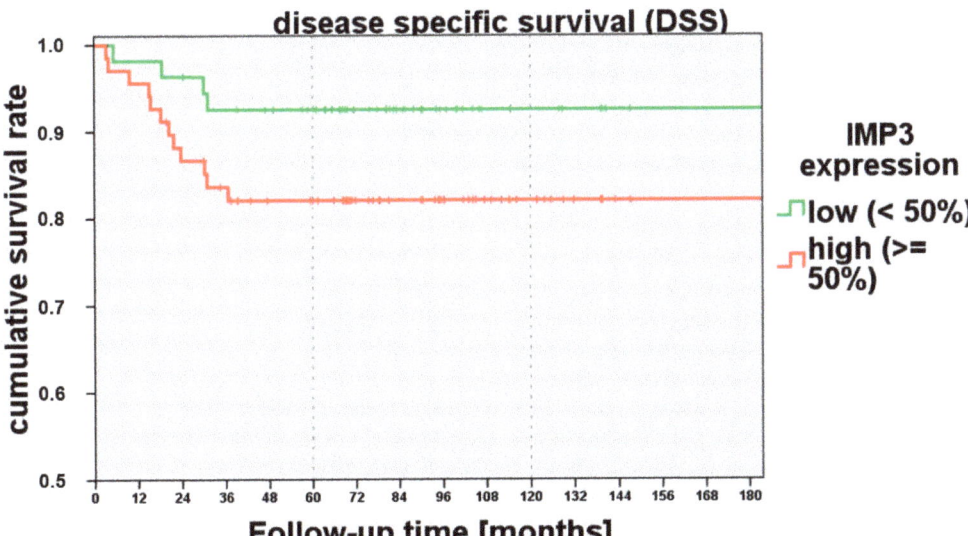

Figure 3. The disease-specific survival tended to be reduced ($p = 0.092$) from an IMP3 expression of >50% (IMP3 Analysis Category II).

Another important clinical outcome parameter is progression-free survival. A higher IMP3 expression >50% was correlated also with a shorter progression-free survival. The log rank test (Mantel–Cox) showed significant differences ($p < 0.001$). Figure 4 demonstrates the Kaplan–Meier curve for progression-free survival and IMP3 expression (IMP3 Analysis Category III (<50%, >50%)).

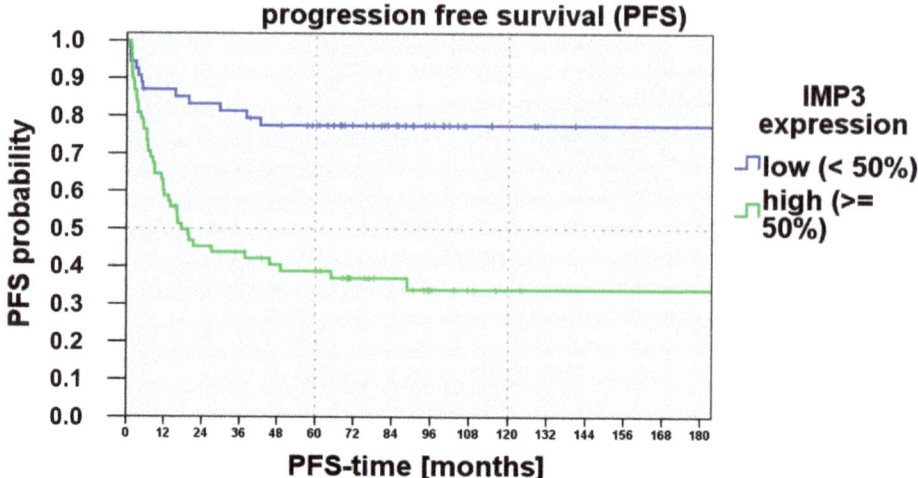

Figure 4. The IMP3 expression range >50%, <50% (IMP3 Analysis Category II) showed a significantly ($p < 0.001$) reduced progression-free survival with an IMP3 expression of >50%.

3.10. Concluding Remarks on the Results

The tumour marker IMP3 seems to be suitable for outcome prediction in LSCC and ECSCC. We observed a significant risk prediction potential for LNMs and, in particular, with IMP3 Analysis Category III (<50%, >50%). The evaluation was fast, efficient, and simple.

4. Discussion

4.1. Strengths and Weaknesses of the Study

The strength of the study is a high number of rare cases of cSCC of the ear and lip with lymph node metastasis. However, because of the distribution of the groups of N+ and N−, a selection bias is possible. Nevertheless, with the matched pair approach, it is possible to minimise the effects of known risk factors for bad prognosis and to work out the effect of the marker IMP3 in small cohorts. The matched pair approach nevertheless triggers a selection bias, which is why a multivariate analysis was deliberately omitted.

A weakness of retrospective analysis in general is that the data quality is lower than in a prospective approach, but for preclinical testing of IMP3, it is still more efficient than a prospective approach.

The classification of the expression ranges presented here can also be critically questioned. However, there is no standardised evaluation method for IMP3 in the literature, and different cutoff values have been published for when expression is considered positive [12]. It should be added that the evaluations also vary with regard to the semi-quantitative analysis.

Another strength of our study is that the IMP3 expression analysis was consistent between the two investigators, indicating that the analysis method seems to be reliable and independent of the examiner.

The origin of LSCC is often not detectable. It is possible that the origin is the oral mucosa, the white of the lip, or the red of the lip. This makes the exact onset of the disease and, thus, the precise classification into oSCC, cSCC, or LSCC difficult [15]. Unfortunately, this could have an impact on tumour aggressiveness. Oral SCCs are much more aggressive than SCCs of the skin [3]. The LSCC shows an intermediary status in aggressiveness. This is the reason why the LSCC is more and more seen as an independent tumour entity. In addition, the outer lip was found to be about 40-times more frequently affected by LSCC and other tumour entities than the inner lip [16]. Our study included upper lip and lower lip cancers because many studies did not show a prognostic difference between upper lip and lower lip cancers [1,17–19].

In the present study, the patient's phototype was not recorded. The phototype could also have an influence on the outcome in connection with IMP3 expression.

However, this is an academic discussion, and for the clinician, the assessment of aggressiveness is often, nonetheless, difficult. It might be reasonably assumed that lymph drainage is not the same in the comparison of the lip and ear. Likewise, the tumour biology is perhaps different. Nevertheless, we strongly believe that the strengths of our study outweigh the limitations.

4.2. Is IMP3 Expression Useful for the Clinical Outcome Prediction of High-Risk Localisation in cSCC?

In the literature, IMP3 is examined in many different tumour entities [20–22].

The RNA-binding protein IMP3 is known as a cancer-specific gene [10,12]. An increased IMP3 expression was observed in both malignant and benign neoplasm [7,12]. Furthermore, it is possible to differentiate between cSCC and keratoacanthoma with the marker IMP3 [23]. Chen et al. showed that an increased IMP3 expression is associated with a high recurrence and metastasising rates in many tumour entities [12]. This predisposes the protein IMP3 as a tumour marker for oncology decision-making. Many therapeutic decisions such as radiation or radio-chemotherapy are dependent on lymph node status. Liao et al. showed that IMP3 promotes the proliferation, cell growth, and robustness against ionising radiation [24]. Thus, one can speculate that IMP3 can be used to assess the response rate or indication for the radiotherapy of cSCC.

Another useful application of IMP3 could be the outcome prediction of cSCC during follow-up. In our study, we investigated this potential and aimed to identify the best assessment method. We found that a high IMP3 expression >50% showed a shortened progression-free survival into the seventh year. Especially in the first 24 months, the progression-free survival deteriorates strongly with an IMP3 expression >50%. After approximately 24–36 months, there is no or only marginal change in progression-free survival. Our data suggest that patients with an IMP3 expression >50% should be followed up more closely because of higher event risk. The marker IMP3 could thus be the basis for the decision of after-care duration of high-risk cSCC patients. However, this hypothesis must be controlled by bigger prospective cohorts.

In addition, we found a tendency (but a lack of significance) towards poorer disease-specific survival with increased IMP3 expression >50%. It seems sensible and exciting to investigate this connection in a larger collective.

It is known that IMP3 expression is different in the main tumour or satellite cells [13]. Future studies should also evaluate outcome differences when IMP3 expression is studied in the primarius tumours or in the LNMs.

Our study found no significant correlation between distant metastasis and IMP3 expression. However, this might be due to the small number of patients with distant metastasis. An increased risk for distant metastasis is permissible because of the correlation of lymph node metastasis and distant metastasis [25]. This fact must be controlled for IMP3 by bigger cohorts.

Taken together, the IMP3 expression is a promising candidate for risk assessment of high-risk cSCC in the clinic. Furthermore, it has a high scientific potential for further studies and could potentially be used as a prognostic marker in diagnostic and therapeutic decision-making.

4.3. Which Is the Best IMP3 Expression Category for Clinical IMP3 Outcome Prediction?

After confirming the beneficial outcome prediction of IMP3 in high-risk cSCC, the question of IMP3 expression range analysis (IMP3 analysis categories) should be discussed in terms of application areas and potential clinical use. Different clinical endpoints can be defined for outcome prediction. Lin et al. showed a correlation between increased

IMP3 expression and a decreased 5-year survival [13]. Our data showed that IMP3 Analysis Category III (<50%, >50%) could be used for follow-up assessment and prediction of progression-free survival. A shorter progression-free survival, especially in the first months, was correlated with IMP3 expression >50%. A new approach could be to adjust tumour follow-up care dependent on IMP3 expression. Since the risk of local relapse is increased with high IMP3 expression, this could support the call for IMP3-dependent closely monitored follow-up care.

In addition, the nodal status is important for the discussion of staging and therapy. The finding of significant differences in group and subgroup analysis made it necessary to find a suitable analysing system and cutoff value for the evaluation of potential clinical use for practitioners. The higher expression of IMP3 in the N+ group of LSCC and ECSCC requires the search for a cutoff value to use IMP3 as an LNM prediction marker. For this also, it seems that IMP3 Analysis Category III (>50%; <50%) is best suited. At an IMP3 expression >50%, the risk for LNMs increased. A similar correlation of IMP3 expression and the risk for LNMs was found in literature for oral cancer [13]. The few categories are advantageous for quick and cost-effective implementation for the clinician for prognostic prediction of LNMs. The discrimination of the expression level into just these two ranges is till sufficient for risk assessment and, then, is the easiest, yet still reliable method for clinical use.

4.4. IMP3 Expression Analysis Could Potentially Help in Decision-Making of Neck Dissection

There is wide knowledge about many tumour entities with a correlation between IMP3 and the risk for LNMs or DMs [12,13,26–28]. For oSCC and also for squamous cell carcinoma of the uterine cervix, a significant correlation between IMP3 and LNMs has been shown [13,26]. In contrast, in another tumour entity, prostate carcinoma, increased IMP3 expression of the primary tumour was shown in the presence of distant metastasis [28].

This correlation shows that IMP3 is unfortunately not specific to cSCC and can also be found in other tumour entities. Nevertheless, it also shows that IMP3 seems to play a role in many tumour entities with regard to metastasis.

Thus, we aimed to analyse if the IMP3 expression status is usable for LNM risk evaluation in high-risk localisations of cSCC. The LNM is an important clinical tool to estimate the prognosis. There is always a discussion about the extent of neck dissection in LSCC and ECSCC. The therapeutic consequence is often a neck dissection, but for the patient, it has a huge impact on the quality life. The decision of a neck dissection often depends on the orientation of a conservative or more-surgical medical discipline. IMP3 could help to support the decision for or against neck dissection in the high-risk localisations of cSCC.

The next question could be as follows: Should every patient with cSCC get an IMP3 expression status? Our opinion is that only the patients with high-risk localisation of the lip and ear benefit from this diagnostic tool because of the increased risk for LNMs. Without randomised, multi-centre, and controlled studies, there is no final statement for this biomarker. Nevertheless, there is a good cost–benefit for the reproducible immunohistochemical marker IMP3. More studies are needed to investigate this promising and exciting tumour marker in cSCC.

4.5. Outlook on IMP3 Vaccination/IMP3 Therapy

In advanced oesophageal cancer, IMP3 and other peptides (TTK, LY6K) have been used therapeutically as vaccines in phase II clinical trials. The authors postulate that an improvement in prognosis could be achieved [29]. Similarly, prognosis improvement by vaccination with IMP3 and other peptides (LY6K, CDCA1) has been used in advanced HNSCC in phase II clinical trials [30]. However, it remains to be seen whether these therapies will become established and whether they can find their way into the treatment of high-risk localisations of cSCC. Unfortunately, there is currently no therapy available that targets IMP3. However, due to the frequent occurrence of IMP3 expression, especially in aggressive tumours, the target structure appears to be interesting for system therapies. Interestingly, there is some evidence that IMP3 could be used to assess chemosensitivity in triple-negative breast cancers [31,32]. For example, Ohashi et al. showed that IMP3-positive tumours were significantly more likely to be non-responders to neoadjuvant chemotherapy [32]. It remains to be seen whether an influence of IMP3 on chemosensitivity can also be shown for cSCC.

5. Conclusion

In summary, the immunohistochemical marker IMP3 is suitable as a prognostic marker in high-risk localisation of cSCC. All three applied analysis categories showed significances in their correlation with the clinical outcome of the patients. A classification into <50% and >50% expression seems to be easily applicable, reproducible, and efficient and, thus, is the most-promising strategy to apply in the clinic. Furthermore, IMP3 assessment could help in the decision-making of radical neck dissection or could reduce non-indicated neck dissection in high-risk cSCC. Lastly, IMP3 expression can also be used to identify aggressive tumours early on and to adjust the patients' follow-up care.

Author Contributions: Conceptualisation, C.H. and K.W.; formal analysis, M.W. and C.H.; methodology, C.H. and K.W.; supervision, C.H., F.H. and K.W.; writing—original draft, M.K.; writing—review and editing, H.J.F. All authors have read and agreed to the published version of the manuscript.

Funding: This research received no external funding.

Institutional Review Board Statement: This study was approved by the local ethics committee (Ethical Committee of the Westphalian Wilhelms University Muenster, Approval No. 2013-063-f-S) and was conducted in accordance with the Guidelines for Good Clinical Practice and in compliance with the Declaration of Helsinki.

Informed Consent Statement: All patients gave their written informed consent for participating in this study.

Data Availability Statement: The research data can be requested after consultation with the corresponding author.

Acknowledgments: We thank the whole team of the Department of Histopathology of the Fachklinik Hornheide for the good cooperation.

Conflicts of Interest: The authors declare no conflict of interest.

Abbreviation

cSCC	cutaneous squamous cell carcinoma
ECSCC	ear cutaneous squamous cell carcinoma
IMP3	insulin-like growth factor 2 mRNA-binding protein 3
LSCC	lip squamous cell carcinoma
LNM	lymph node metastasis
N+	lymph node metastasis positive
N−	lymph node metastasis negative

References

1. Leiter, U.; Heppt, M.V.; Steeb, T.; Amaral, T.; Bauer, A.; Becker, J.C.; Breitbart, E.; Breuninger, H.; Diepgen, T.; Dirschka, T.; et al. S3 Guideline for Actinic Keratosis and Cutaneous Squamous Cell Carcinoma (CSCC)—Short Version, Part 2: Epidemiology, Surgical and Systemic Treatment of CSCC, Follow-up, Prevention and Occupational Disease. *J. Dtsch. Dermatol. Ges. J. Ger. Soc. Dermatol. JDDG* **2020**, *18*, 400–413. [CrossRef]
2. Alam, M.; Ratner, D. Cutaneous Squamous-Cell Carcinoma. *N. Engl. J. Med.* **2001**, *344*, 975–983. [CrossRef]
3. Bota, J.P.; Lyons, A.B.; Carroll, B.T. Squamous Cell Carcinoma of the Lip-A Review of Squamous Cell Carcinogenesis of the Mucosal and Cutaneous Junction. *Dermatol. Surg.* **2017**, *43*, 494–506. [CrossRef] [PubMed]
4. Breuninger, H.; Bootz, F.; Hauschild, A.; Kortmann, R.-D.; Wolff, K.; Stockfleth, E.; Szeimies, M.; Rompel, R.; Garbe, C. Short German Guidelines: Squamous Cell Carcinoma. *JDDG J. Dtsch. Dermatol. Ges.* **2008**, *6*, S5–S8. [CrossRef]

5. Schmults, C.D.; Karia, P.S.; Carter, J.B.; Han, J.; Qureshi, A.A. Factors Predictive of Recurrence and Death from Cutaneous Squamous Cell Carcinoma: A 10-Year, Single-Institution Cohort Study. *JAMA Dermatol.* **2013**, *149*, 541. [CrossRef]
6. Wermker, K.; Kluwig, J.; Schipmann, S.; Klein, M.; Schulze, H.J.; Hallermann, C. Prediction Score for Lymph Node Metastasis from Cutaneous Squamous Cell Carcinoma of the External Ear. *Eur. J. Surg. Oncol.* **2015**, *41*, 128–135. [CrossRef] [PubMed]
7. Bell, J.L.; Wächter, K.; Mühleck, B.; Pazaitis, N.; Köhn, M.; Lederer, M.; Hüttelmaier, S. Insulin-like Growth Factor 2 MRNA-Binding Proteins (IGF2BPs): Post-Transcriptional Drivers of Cancer Progression? *Cell. Mol. Life Sci. CMLS* **2013**, *70*, 2657–2675. [CrossRef] [PubMed]
8. Takizawa, K.; Yamamoto, H.; Taguchi, K.; Ohno, S.; Tokunaga, E.; Yamashita, N.; Kubo, M.; Nakamura, M.; Oda, Y. Insulin-like Growth Factor II Messenger RNA-Binding Protein-3 Is an Indicator of Malignant Phyllodes Tumor of the Breast. *Hum. Pathol.* **2016**, *55*, 30–38. [CrossRef]
9. Kanzaki, A.; Kudo, M.; Ansai, S.-I.; Peng, W.-X.; Ishino, K.; Yamamoto, T.; Wada, R.; Fujii, T.; Teduka, K.; Kawahara, K.; et al. Insulin-like Growth Factor 2 MRNA-Binding Protein-3 as a Marker for Distinguishing between Cutaneous Squamous Cell Carcinoma and Keratoacanthoma. *Int. J. Oncol.* **2016**, *48*, 1007–1015. [CrossRef]
10. Gong, Y.; Woda, B.A.; Jiang, Z. Oncofetal Protein IMP3, a New Cancer Biomarker. *Adv. Anat. Pathol.* **2014**, *21*, 191–200. [CrossRef]
11. Li, H.-G.; Han, J.-J.; Huang, Z.-Q.; Wang, L.; Chen, W.-L.; Shen, X.-M. IMP3 Is a Novel Biomarker to Predict Metastasis and Prognosis of Tongue Squamous Cell Carcinoma. *J. Craniofac. Surg.* **2011**, *22*, 2022–2025. [CrossRef]
12. Chen, L.; Xie, Y.; Li, X.; Gu, L.; Gao, Y.; Tang, L.; Chen, J.; Zhang, X. Prognostic Value of High IMP3 Expression in Solid Tumors: A Meta-Analysis. *OncoTargets Ther.* **2017**, *10*, 2849–2863. [CrossRef] [PubMed]
13. Lin, C.Y.; Chen, S.T.; Jeng, Y.M.; Yeh, C.C.; Chou, H.Y.; Deng, Y.T.; Chang, C.C.; Kuo, M.Y.P. Insulin-like Growth Factor II MRNA-Binding Protein 3 Expression Promotes Tumor Formation and Invasion and Predicts Poor Prognosis in Oral Squamous Cell Carcinoma. *J. Oral Pathol. Med.* **2011**, *40*, 699–705. [CrossRef] [PubMed]
14. Lu, D.; Yang, X.; Jiang, N.Y.; Woda, B.A.; Liu, Q.; Dresser, K.; Mercurio, A.M.; Rock, K.L.; Jiang, Z. IMP3, a New Biomarker to Predict Progression of Cervical Intraepithelial Neoplasia into Invasive Cancer. *Am. J. Surg. Pathol.* **2011**, *35*, 1638–1645. [CrossRef]
15. Klein, M.; Wermker, K.; Hallermann, C.; Pannier, F.; Hölzle, F.; Modabber, A. Immune Checkpoint Analysis in Lip Cancer. *J. Cranio-Maxillofac. Surg.* **2021**, *49*, 950–958. [CrossRef] [PubMed]
16. Czerninski, R.; Zini, A.; Sgan-Cohen, H.D. Lip Cancer: Incidence, Trends, Histology and Survival: 1970-2006. *Br. J. Dermatol.* **2010**, *162*, 1103–1109. [CrossRef]
17. Han, A.Y.; Kuan, E.C.; Mallen-St Clair, J.; Alonso, J.E.; Arshi, A.; St John, M.A. Epidemiology of Squamous Cell Carcinoma of the Lip in the United States: A Population-Based Cohort Analysis. *JAMA Otolaryngol. Neck Surg.* **2016**, *142*, 1216. [CrossRef]
18. Walton, E.; Cramer, J.D. Predictors of Occult Lymph Node Metastases in Lip Cancer. *Am. J. Otolaryngol.* **2020**, *41*, 102419. [CrossRef]
19. Wermker, K.; Belok, F.; Schipmann, S.; Klein, M.; Schulze, H.-J.; Hallermann, C. Prediction Model for Lymph Node Metastasis and Recommendations for Elective Neck Dissection in Lip Cancer. *J. Cranio-Maxillo-Fac. Surg.* **2015**, *43*, 545–552. [CrossRef]
20. Burdelski, C.; Jakani-Karimi, N.; Jacobsen, F.; Müller-Koop, C.; Minner, S.; Simon, R.; Sauter, G.; Steurer, S.; Clauditz, T.; Wilczak, W. IMP3 Overexpression Occurs in Various Important Cancer Types and Is Linked to Aggressive Tumor Features: A Tissue Microarray Study on 8,877 Human Cancers and Normal Tissues. *Oncol. Rep.* **2017**, *39*, 3–12. [CrossRef]
21. Maržić, D.; Marijić, B.; Braut, T.; Janik, S.; Avirović, M.; Hadžisejdić, I.; Tudor, F.; Radobuljac, K.; Čoklo, M.; Erovic, B.M. IMP3 Protein Overexpression Is Linked to Unfavorable Outcome in Laryngeal Squamous Cell Carcinoma. *Cancers* **2021**, *13*, 4306. [CrossRef]
22. Sjekloča, N.; Tomić, S.; Mrklić, I.; Vukmirović, F.; Vučković, L.; Lovasić, I.B.; Maras-Šimunić, M. Prognostic Value of IMP3 Immunohistochemical Expression in Triple Negative Breast Cancer. *Medicine* **2020**, *99*, e19091. [CrossRef] [PubMed]
23. Soddu, S.; Di Felice, E.; Cabras, S.; Castellanos, M.E.; Atzori, L.; Faa, G.; Pilloni, L. IMP-3 Expression in Keratoacanthomas and Squamous Cell Carcinomas of the Skin: An Immunohistochemical Study. *Eur. J. Histochem. EJH* **2013**, *57*, e6. [CrossRef] [PubMed]
24. Liao, B.; Hu, Y.; Brewer, G. RNA-Binding Protein Insulin-like Growth Factor MRNA-Binding Protein 3 (IMP-3) Promotes Cell Survival via Insulin-like Growth Factor II Signaling after Ionizing Radiation. *J. Biol. Chem.* **2011**, *286*, 31145–31152. [CrossRef]
25. Van Der Kamp, M.F.; Muntinghe, F.O.W.; Iepsma, R.S.; Plaat, B.E.C.; Van Der Laan, B.F.A.M.; Algassab, A.; Steenbakkers, R.J.H.M.; Witjes, M.J.H.; Van Dijk, B.A.C.; De Bock, G.H.; et al. Predictors for Distant Metastasis in Head and Neck Cancer, with Emphasis on Age. *Eur. Arch. Otorhinolaryngol.* **2021**, *278*, 181–190. [CrossRef] [PubMed]
26. Wei, Q.; Yan, J.; Fu, B.; Liu, J.; Zhong, L.; Yang, Q.; Zhao, T. IMP3 Expression Is Associated with Poor Survival in Cervical Squamous Cell Carcinoma. *Hum. Pathol.* **2014**, *45*, 2218–2224. [CrossRef] [PubMed]
27. Yan, J.; Wei, Q.; Jian, W.; Qiu, B.; Wen, J.; Liu, J.; Fu, B.; Zhou, X.; Zhao, T. IMP3 Predicts Invasion and Prognosis in Human Lung Adenocarcinoma. *Lung* **2016**, *194*, 137–146. [CrossRef] [PubMed]
28. Szarvas, T.; Tschirdewahn, S.; Niedworok, C.; Kramer, G.; Sevcenco, S.; Reis, H.; Shariat, S.F.; Rübben, H.; Vom Dorp, F. Prognostic Value of Tissue and Circulating Levels of IMP3 in Prostate Cancer: IMP3 in Prostate Cancer. *Int. J. Cancer* **2014**, *135*, 1596–1604. [CrossRef]
29. Kono, K.; Iinuma, H.; Akutsu, Y.; Tanaka, H.; Hayashi, N.; Uchikado, Y.; Noguchi, T.; Fujii, H.; Okinaka, K.; Fukushima, R.; et al. Multicenter, Phase II Clinical Trial of Cancer Vaccination for Advanced Esophageal Cancer with Three Peptides Derived from Novel Cancer-Testis Antigens. *J. Transl. Med.* **2012**, *10*, 141. [CrossRef]

30. Yoshitake, Y.; Fukuma, D.; Yuno, A.; Hirayama, M.; Nakayama, H.; Tanaka, T.; Nagata, M.; Takamune, Y.; Kawahara, K.; Nakagawa, Y.; et al. Phase II Clinical Trial of Multiple Peptide Vaccination for Advanced Head and Neck Cancer Patients Revealed Induction of Immune Responses and Improved OS. *Clin. Cancer Res.* **2015**, *21*, 312–321. [CrossRef]
31. Samanta, S.; Pursell, B.; Mercurio, A.M. IMP3 Protein Promotes Chemoresistance in Breast Cancer Cells by Regulating Breast Cancer Resistance Protein (ABCG2) Expression. *J. Biol. Chem.* **2013**, *288*, 12569–12573. [CrossRef] [PubMed]
32. Ohashi, R.; Sangen, M.; Namimatsu, S.; Yanagihara, K.; Yamashita, K.; Sakatani, T.; Takei, H.; Naito, Z. Prognostic Value of IMP3 Expression as a Determinant of Chemosensitivity in Triple-Negative Breast Cancer. *Pathol. Res. Pract.* **2017**, *213*, 1160–1165. [CrossRef] [PubMed]

Disclaimer/Publisher's Note: The statements, opinions and data contained in all publications are solely those of the individual author(s) and contributor(s) and not of MDPI and/or the editor(s). MDPI and/or the editor(s) disclaim responsibility for any injury to people or property resulting from any ideas, methods, instructions or products referred to in the content.

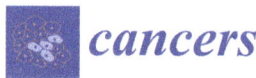

Article

Therapeutic Potential of BAY-117082, a Selective NLRP3 Inflammasome Inhibitor, on Metastatic Evolution in Human Oral Squamous Cell Carcinoma (OSCC)

Giovanna Casili [1,†], Sarah Adriana Scuderi [1,†], Marika Lanza [1], Alessia Filippone [1], Deborah Mannino [1], Raffaella Giuffrida [2], Cristina Colarossi [2], Marzia Mare [2], Anna Paola Capra [1], Federica De Gaetano [1], Marco Portelli [3], Angela Militi [1], Salvatore Cuzzocrea [1], Irene Paterniti [1,*] and Emanuela Esposito [1]

1. Department of Chemical, Biological, Pharmaceutical and Environmental Sciences, University of Messina, Viale Ferdinando Stagno D'Alcontres, 31, 98166 Messina, Italy; gcasili@unime.it (G.C.); sarahadriana.scuderi@unime.it (S.A.S.); mlanza@unime.it (M.L.); afilippone@unime.it (A.F.); deborah.mannino@unime.it (D.M.)
2. IOM Ricerca, Via Penninazzo 11, 95029 Viagrande Catania, Italy; cristina.colarossi@grupposamed.com (C.C.)
3. Department of Biomedical and Dental Science, Morphological and Functional Images, University of Messina, Via Consolare Valeria, 98125 Messina, Italy
* Correspondence: irene.paterniti@unime.it
† These authors contributed equally to this work.

Simple Summary: Each year, new cases of oral cancer occur and metastasis represents the primary determinant for survival. Thus, there is a need to improve the preoperative assessment of metastatic risk. Scientific evidence discovered that BAY 11-7082, a powerful inhibitor of the NLRP3 inflammasome, is able to modulate cell invasion and migration and counteract the apoptosis process. The purpose of this study was to evaluate the effect of BAY-117082 in an in vivo orthotopic model of OSCC and its role in the invasiveness and metastasis processes in neighbor organs such as lymph node, lung, and spleen tissues.

Abstract: Oral squamous cell carcinoma (OSCC) is a commonly occurring head and neck cancer and it is characterized by a high metastasis grade. The aim of this study was to evaluate for the first time the effect of BAY-117082, a selective NLRP3 inflammasome inhibitor, in an in vivo orthotopic model of OSCC and its role in the invasiveness and metastasis processes in neighbor organs such as lymph node, lung, and spleen tissues. Our results demonstrated that BAY-117082 treatment, at doses of 2.5 mg/kg and 5 mg/kg, was able to significantly reduce the presence of microscopic tumor islands and nuclear pleomorphism in tongue tissues and modulate the NLRP3 inflammasome pathway activation in tongue tissues, as well as in metastatic organs such as lung and spleen. Additionally, BAY-117082 treatment modulated the epithelial–mesenchymal transition (EMT) process in tongue tissue as well as in metastatic organs such as lymph node, lung, and spleen, also reducing the expression of matrix metalloproteinases (MMPs), particularly MMP2 and MMP9, markers of cell invasion and migration. In conclusion, the obtained data demonstrated that BAY-117082 at doses of 2.5 mg/kg and 5 mg/kg were able to reduce the tongue tumor area as well as the degree of metastasis in lymph node, lung, and spleen tissues through the NLRP3 inflammasome pathway inhibition.

Keywords: oral cancer; NLRP3; metastasis; lymph node; spleen; lung

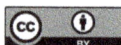

Citation: Casili, G.; Scuderi, S.A.; Lanza, M.; Filippone, A.; Mannino, D.; Giuffrida, R.; Colarossi, C.; Mare, M.; Capra, A.P.; De Gaetano, F.; et al. Therapeutic Potential of BAY-117082, a Selective NLRP3 Inflammasome Inhibitor, on Metastatic Evolution in Human Oral Squamous Cell Carcinoma (OSCC). *Cancers* **2023**, *15*, 2796. https://doi.org/10.3390/cancers15102796

Academic Editors: Daniel L. Pouliquen and Cristina Núñez González

Received: 17 April 2023
Revised: 11 May 2023
Accepted: 15 May 2023
Published: 17 May 2023

Copyright: © 2023 by the authors. Licensee MDPI, Basel, Switzerland. This article is an open access article distributed under the terms and conditions of the Creative Commons Attribution (CC BY) license (https://creativecommons.org/licenses/by/4.0/).

1. Introduction

Oral squamous cell carcinoma (OSCC) represents a common type of head and neck cancer; it is characterized by poor prognosis [1,2]. Radical resection represents the better strategy for patients with moderate to advanced oral cancer [3]. The multidisciplinary therapy of surgical resection, radiation, and chemotherapy in patients with an advanced stage resulted in 20% of patients being identified to have developed distant metastasis (DM) [4]; although the frequency of DM decreased, DM reduces a patient's quality of life and affects the clinical outcome. DM typically manifest itself in the lung (81.5%), followed by bone and liver (20%); only a few articles have reported a different localization of DM in the lymph nodes [5], spleen, kidney, and heart [6,7]. Despite the currently available therapeutic options for the treatment of oral cancer, the survival rate for patients with OSCC remains very low [8]. Oral cancer is characterized by a metastasis process which includes the detachment of cells from tumor tissue, and their invasion, proliferation, and evasion through the lymphatic or blood system [9]. Therefore, the identification of new therapeutic targets and new molecules capable of decreasing or preventing the progression of oral cancer represents a crucial purpose. In the field of cancer research, great interest has been dedicated to inflammasomes-mediated inflammation [10]. Inflammasomes are multi-protein complexes which consist of the nucleotide-binding and oligomerization domain (NOD)-like receptor (NLR), adapter protein apoptosis-associated speck-like protein-containing CARD (ASC), and caspase-1 [11]. The inflammasome complex can be activated by various stimuli which subsequently cleave pro-interleukine-1β (IL-1β) to its mature bioactive form via the activated caspase-1 [12]. The involvement of inflammasome in bladder cancer [13], gastric cancer [14], and leukemia [15] has been highlighted by several studies; however, the role of NLRP3 in DM due to OSCC has not been fully elucidated. Scientific evidence has shown that BAY 11-7082, a powerful inhibitor of the NLRP3 inflammasome [16], possesses various pharmacological abilities; it is also able to modulate the apoptosis process [17]. The purpose of this study was to evaluate the effect of BAY-117082, a selective NLRP3 inflammasome inhibitor, in an in vivo orthotopic model of OSCC and its role in the invasiveness and metastasis processes in neighbor organs such as lymph nodes, lung, and spleen tissues.

2. Materials and Methods

2.1. Animals

BALB/c nude male mice were obtained from Jackson Laboratory (Bar Harbor, Hancock, ME, USA) and fed with a typical regimen and water ad libitum under pathogen-free conditions with a cycle of 12 h light/12 h dark. Animal study was accepted by the University of Messina (n 368/2019-PR released on 14 May 2019) according to Italian regulations for the use of animals. This study was approved by the University of Messina review board for the care of animals. All animal experiments were carried out in agreement with Italian (DM 116192) and European Union regulations (2010/63/EU amended by Regulation 2019/1010).

2.2. Cell Line

The OSCC cell line CAL27 was acquired from ATCC (Manassas, VA, USA). CAL27 cells were grown in Dulbecco's modified Eagle's medium (Invitrogen, Waltham, MO, USA) supplemented with 10% fetal bovine serum (FBS) (Invitrogen) and 100 U/mL penicillin and 100 μg/mL streptomycin (Sigma-Aldrich, St. Louis, MO, USA) at 37 °C with 5% CO_2.

2.3. Experimental Design

The orthotopic model was performed as previously described [18,19]. Briefly, 1×10^6 CAL27 cells in 20 μL of phosphate-buffered saline (PBS) were injected into the lateral portion of the tongues of animals using a sterile 0.5 mL insulin syringe. Mice in the control group were injected with the vehicle only. Then, the animals were randomly divided into 4 groups to receive the vehicle or BAY-117082 at the doses of 2.5 and 5 mg/kg every 3 days according to [16,17] and as previously described in our study [16]. BAY-117082 was dissolved in PBS with 0.001% of DMSO. After 30 days, the mice were sacrificed, and the tongue, lung, lymph nodes, and spleen were excised and processed to perform several analyses.

Experimental Groups

Sham group (vehicle): mice only received vehicle (PBS).

OSCC group: intraperitoneal (ip) administration of PBS after OSCC model induction.

OSCC+ BAY-117082 2.5 mg/kg: mice received BAY-117082 2.5 mg/kg dissolved in PBS by intraperitoneal administration.

OSCC++ BAY-117082 5 mg/kg: mice received BAY-117082 5 mg/kg dissolved in PBS by intraperitoneal administration.

2.4. Hematoxylin and Eosin (H&E) Staining

The H&E assay was performed as shown previously [20]. Briefly, samples from tongue tumors and metastases from lung, spleen, and lymph node were deparaffinized with xylene and stained with H&E staining. The images are shown at 10× magnification (100 μm of the Bar scale) using an Axiovision Zeiss microscope (Milan, Italy). The degree of metastasis was quantified in the lymph node, lung, and spleen to evaluate the metastasis foci, as described previously [21].

2.5. Immunohistochemical Localization of N-cadherin, E-cadherin, MMP-2, MMP-9, and NLRP3

Immunohistochemistry was conducted as explained previously [22]. Sections from tongue tumors and metastases from lung, spleen, and lymph node were incubated overnight at room temperature with different primary antibodies: anti-N-cadherin (sc-393933, 1:100; Santa Cruz Biotechnology, Dallas, TX, USA), anti-E-cadherin (sc-8426, 1:100; Santa Cruz Biotechnology, Dallas, TX, USA), anti-MMP2 (sc-13595, 1:100; Santa Cruz Biotechnology, Dallas, TX, USA), anti-MMP9 (sc-393859, 1:100; Santa Cruz Biotechnology, Dallas, TX, USA), and anti-NLRP3 (sc-34411, 1:500; Santa Cruz Biotechnology, Dallas, TX, USA). Later, the pieces were cleaned with PBS and incubated for 1 h with the secondary antibody (Santa Cruz Biotechnology, CA, USA). This was performed using a negative control with no primary antibody. For the immunohistochemistry, magnifications of 20× (50 μm scale bar) are displayed.

2.6. Western Blot Analysis

Western blot analyses on samples from tongue, lung, and spleen metastases was performed as described previously [22]. The membranes were incubated with primary antibodies: anti-NLRP3 (sc-34411, 1:500; Santa Cruz Biotechnology, Dallas, TX, USA), anti-ASC (sc-22514, 1:500; Santa Cruz Biotechnology, Dallas, TX, USA), anti-IL-1β (sc-32294, 1:500; Santa Cruz Biotechnology, Dallas, TX, USA), anti-IL-18 (sc-80051, 1:500; Santa Cruz Biotechnology, Dallas, TX, USA), anti-N-cadherin (sc-393933, 1:100; Santa Cruz Biotechnology, Dallas, TX, USA), anti-E-cadherin (sc-8426, 1:100; Santa Cruz Biotechnology, Dallas, TX, USA), anti-MMP2 (sc-13595, 1:100; Santa Cruz Biotechnology, Dallas, TX, USA), anti-MMP9 (sc-393859, 1:100; Santa Cruz Biotechnology, Dallas, TX, USA), and anti-βactin for cytosolic fraction (1:500; Santa Cruz Biotechnology; Dallas, TX, USA. sc-8432). Signals were perceived with an enhanced chemiluminescence (ECL) detection system mixture according to the manufacturer's instructions (Thermo Fisher, Waltham, MA, USA).

2.7. Enzyme-Linked Immunosorbent Assay (ELISA) for NF-κB and IκBα

The levels of NF-κBp65 and IκBα in tongue samples were measured by an ELISA kit according to the manufacturer's instructions (NFκB-p65 ELISA Kit, Catalog No: E-EL-M0838; Elabscience; IκBα ELISA kit, Catalog No: MOES01330; AssayGenie). The homogenates were centrifuged for 5 min at $5000\times g$; then, the supernatants were collected and stored at $-20\,^\circ$C.

2.8. Materials

The reagents were obtained from Sigma-Aldrich (Milan, Italy). All stock solutions were made in PBS (Sigma-Aldrich, Milan, Italy).

2.9. Statistical Analysis

Data were analyzed with GraphPad Prism 7.04 software using one-way ANOVA analysis followed by a Bonferroni post hoc test for multiple comparisons. A *p*-value of less than 0.05 was considered significant. All values are indicated as a mean ± standard deviation (SD).

3. Results

3.1. BAY-117082 Treatment Reduced OSCC Growth

Histological analysis revealed that the OSCC group was characterized by the presence of microscopic tumor islands around the main tumor site, an archetypical feature of squamous cell carcinoma, irregular size, and nuclear pleomorphism compared to the sham group (Figure 1A,B). Nevertheless, BAY-117082 at doses of 2.5 mg/kg and 5 mg/kg significantly decreased the tumor area, restoring the tongue tissue architecture (Figure 1C,D). During the experiment, the OSCC group showed a significant reduction in body weight compared to the sham group; however, the BAY-117082 treatment at doses of 2.5 mg/kg and 5 mg/kg showed no significance (Figure 1E).

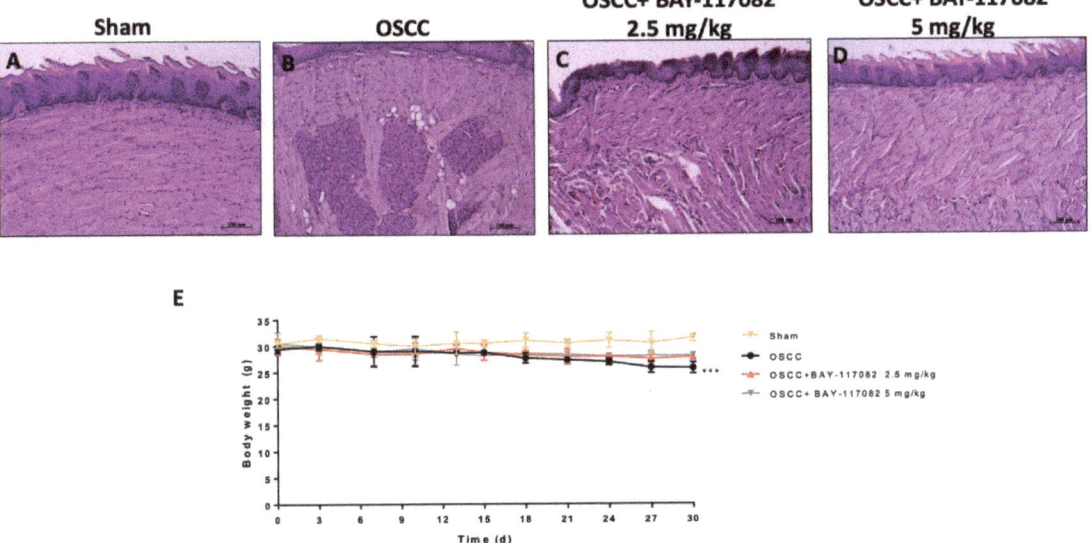

Figure 1. Effects of BAY-117082 treatment on tumor growth. The treatment with BAY-117082 2.5 mg/kg and 5 mg/kg significantly diminished the tumor mass (**C,D**) compared to the OSCC group (**B**). A significant decrease in animals' body weights was observed in the OSCC group compared to sham group; however, BAY-117082 at both doses did not show any significance (**E**). Sections were observed and photographed at 10× magnification. (**E**) *** $p < 0.01$ vs. sham group.

3.2. BAY-117082 Treatment Reduced NLRP3 Inflammasome Pathway Activation in OSCC

The NLRP3 inflammasome pathway overactivation could contribute to oral cancer progression [23]. Therefore, we decided to evaluate the effect of BAY-117082 on the NLRP3 and ASC expression by Western blot analysis, demonstrating that the expression of NLRP3 and ASC are very high in the OSCC group compared to the sham group; nevertheless, BAY-117082 at both doses significantly decreased their expression in a dose-dependent manner (Figure 2A,B). When activated, the NLRP3 inflammasome stimulates the release of pro-inflammatory cytokines IL-1β and IL-18, which promote the progression of cancer [16]. According to this, we found an increase in the IL-1β and IL-18 expressions in the OSCC group; however, the treatment with BAY-117082 at doses of 2.5 mg/kg and 5 mg/kg significantly decreased their expression in a dose-dependent manner (Figure 2C,D).

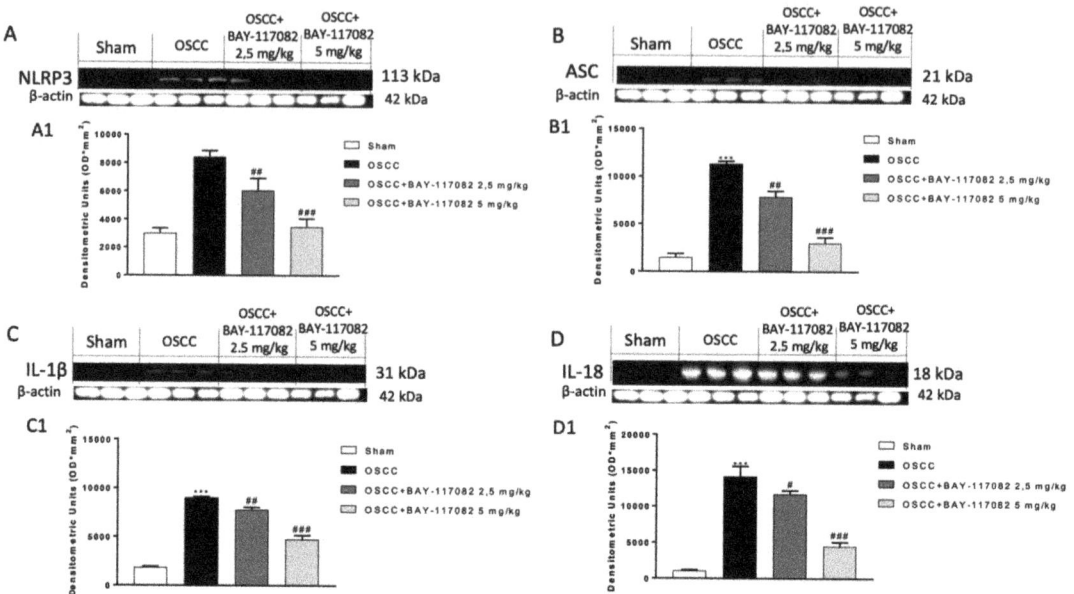

Figure 2. BAY-117082 reduced the NLRP3 inflammasome pathway activation in tongue samples. Western blot analysis showed that BAY-117082 2.5 mg/kg and 5 mg/kg decreased NLRP3, ASC, IL-1β, and IL-18 expression compared to the OSCC group. Data are representative of at least three independent experiments. (**A–C**) *** $p < 0.001$ vs. sham; ## $p < 0.01$ and ### $p < 0.001$ vs. OSCC; (**D**) *** $p < 0.001$ vs. control; # $p < 0.05$ and ### $p < 0.001$ vs. OSCC. The uncropped bolts are shown in Supplementary Materials.

3.3. BAY-117082 Treatment Modulated Epithelial–Mesenchymal Transition (EMT) and Matrix Metalloproteinases (MMPs) Expression in OSCC

Studies demonstrated that the epithelial–mesenchymal transition (EMT) plays a key role in the processes of oral cancer invasion and metastasis [24]. Thus, we decided to investigate the effect of BAY-117082 on N-cadherin and E-cadherin expression by immunohistochemical analysis, demonstrating that the OSCC group was characterized by an increase in N-cadherin and a decrease in E-cadherin expression compared to the sham groups (Figure 3A,B,F,G); however, the treatment with BAY-117082 at doses of 2.5 mg/kg and 5 mg/kg significantly reduced and increased the N-cadherin and the E-cadherin expressions, respectively, as shown in Figure 3C,D (see the % of the total tissue area score in Figure 3E) and Figure 3H,I (see the % of the total tissue area score in Figure 3J), respectively. Furthermore, we decided to evaluate the effect of BAY-117082 on the matrix metalloproteinase levels and particularly on MMP2 and MMP9, as markers of cell invasion and migration [25], showing that BAY-117082 at doses of 2.5 mg/kg and 5 mg/kg was able to significantly decrease their levels compared to the OSCC group, as shown in Figure 3K–N (see the % of the total tissue area score in Figure 3O); and in Figure 3P–S (see the % of the total tissue area score in Figure 3T).

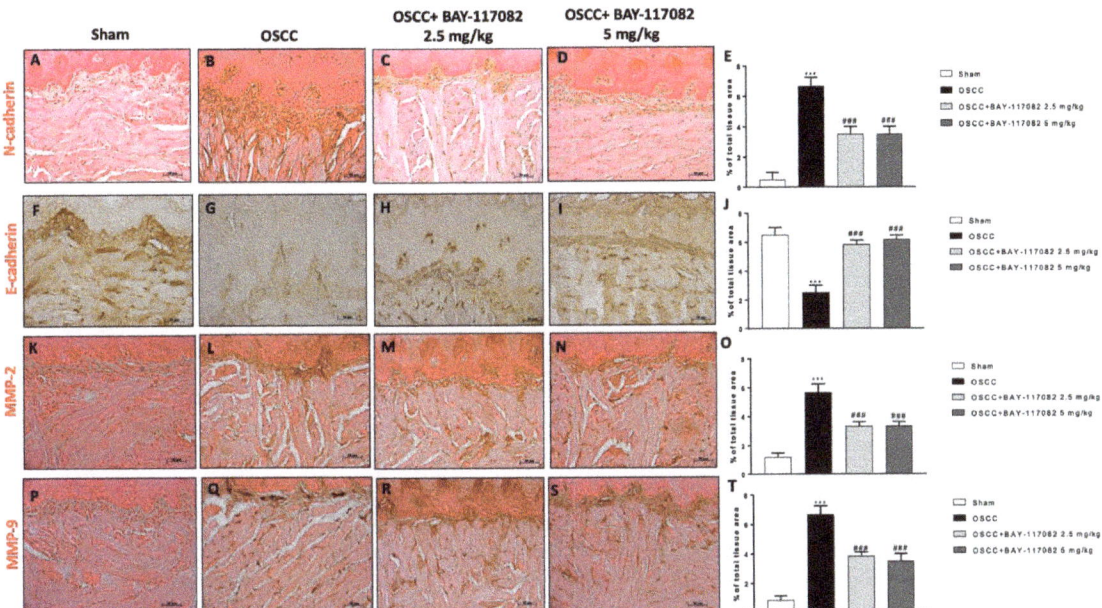

Figure 3. BAY-117082 treatment modulated the EMT process and MMP expression in tongue samples. Immunohistochemical analysis revealed that the treatment with BAY-117082 at doses of 2.5 and 5 mg/kg was able to reduce N-cadherin (**C,D,M,N,R,S**), MMP2, and MMP9 staining compared to the OSCC group (**B,L,Q**), increasing E-cadherin (H and I). Data are representative of at least three independent experiments. (**A–D**) *** $p < 0.001$ vs. sham; ### $p < 0.001$ vs. OSCC. (Scale bar: 50 µm).

3.4. BAY-117082 Treatment Reduced Metastasis Grade in OSCC Metastasis in Lymph Node, Lung, and Spleen

The metastasis process plays a pivotal role in oral cancer [26]. The most common site for OSCC metastasis is that of a cervical lymph node; however, tumor cells can move through lymphatic or blood vessels to distant metastatic sites such as the lung and the spleen [6]. Therefore, based on these considerations, we first decided to evaluate the ability of BAY-117082 to reduce the metastasis grade in the OSCC metastatic organs such as lymph nodes. Our results demonstrate that the OSCC group was characterized by the formation of an epidermoid cyst-like lesion lined by a layer of stratified squamous epithelium and nuclear pleomorphism compared to the sham group (Figure 4A,B,M); however, the treatment with BAY-117082 at doses of 2.5 mg/kg and 5 mg/kg was able to significantly decrease the lymphatic metastasis (Figure 4C,D,M). Additionally, we investigated whether BAY-117082 also reduced lung and spleen metastasis following OSCC induction. The histological analysis demonstrated that BAY-117082 at doses of 2.5 mg/kg and 5 mg/kg significantly reduced the diffuse tumor cell infiltration as well as the presence of multifocal cellular aggregates in lung tissues compared to the OSCC group (Figure 4E–H,N). Meanwhile, the histological analysis of spleen tissues showed that the tumor cells were spindled to polygonal with a poorly demarcated eosinophilic cytoplasm followed by the multinodular infiltration in the OSCC group compared to the sham group (Figure 4I,J); however, the treatment with BAY-117082 at both doses was able to significantly reduce the degree of metastasis (Figure 4K,L,O).

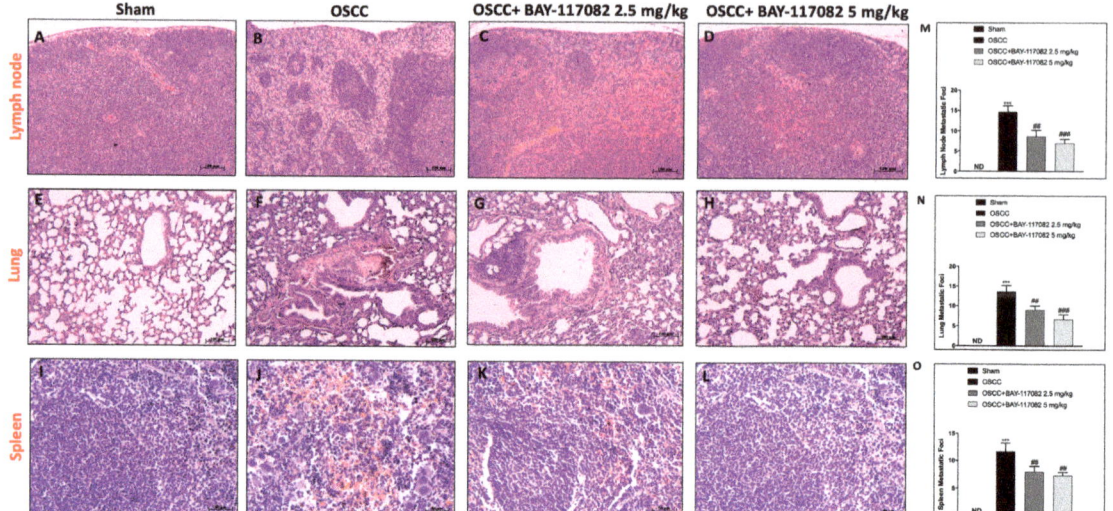

Figure 4. BAY-117082 treatment modulated the metastasis process in the lymph node, lung, and spleen. Histological analysis revealed that the treatment with BAY-117082 at doses of 2.5 and 5 mg/kg was able to reduce the degree of metastasis in the lymph node (**C,D,M**), lung (**G,H,N**), and spleen (**K,L,O**) in the C group compared to the OSCC group (**B,F,J**). (**A,E,I**) represents control groups in lymph node, lung and spleen. Data are representative of at least three independent experiments. ND, not designed. *** $p < 0.001$ vs. sham; ### $p < 0.001$ and vs. ## $p < 0.01$ OSCC.

3.5. BAY-117082 Treatment Reduced NLRP3 Inflammasome Pathway Activation in OSCC Metastasis in Lung and Spleen

Considering the great selectivity and inhibitor effect of BAY-117082 against the NLRP3 inflammasome [27], we also decided to evaluate its effect in OSCC metastatic organs namely the lung and spleen tissues. In this context, our results demonstrated that the OSCC groups were characterized by an increase in NLRP3, ASC, IL-1β, and IL-18 expressions in the lung as well as in spleen tissues compared to sham groups, respectively; however, the treatment with BAY-117082 at doses of 2.5 mg/kg and 5 mg/kg was able to significantly decrease the NLRP3, ASC, IL-1β, and IL-18 expressions in both OSCC metastatic organs (see the lung panel in Figure 5A–D and the spleen panel in Figure 5E–H).

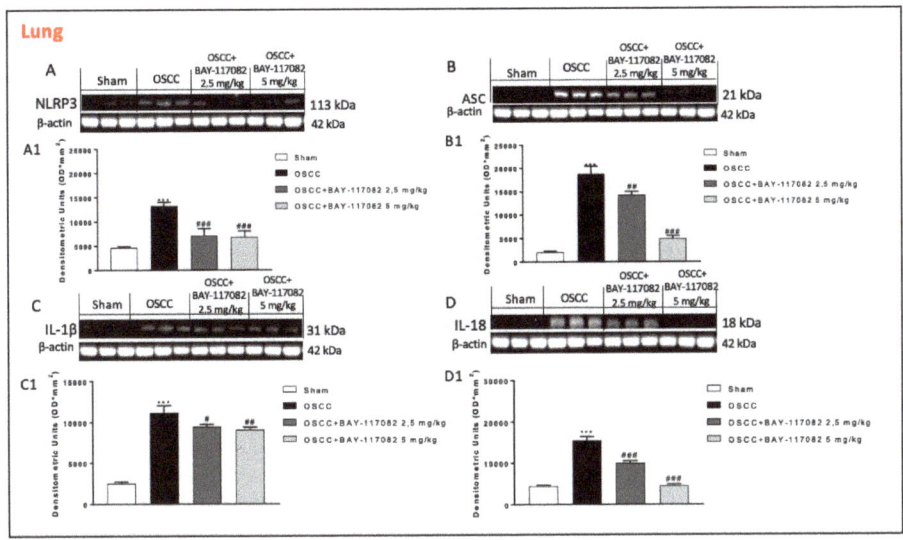

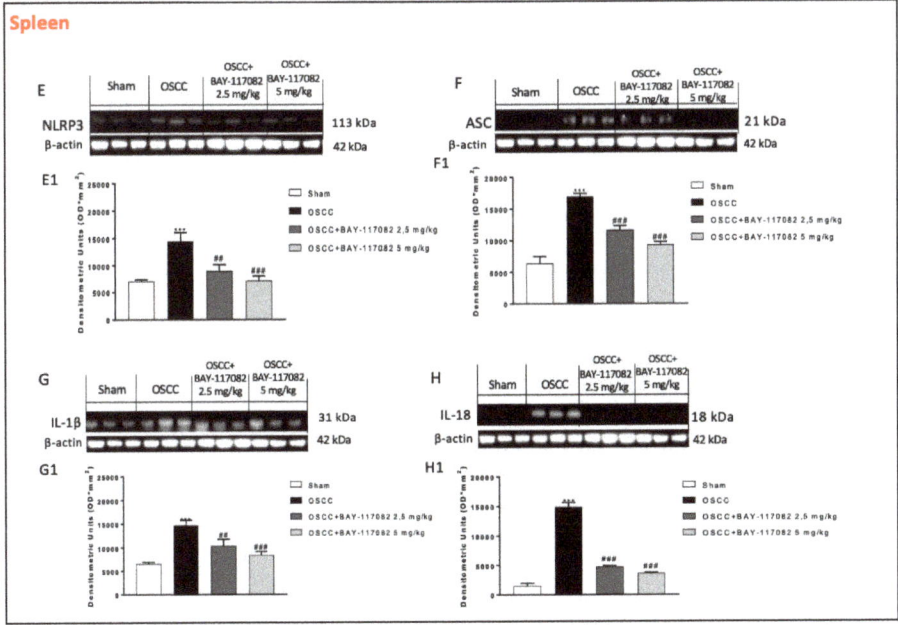

Figure 5. Effect of the BAY-117082 on the NLRP3 inflammasome pathway in lung and spleen samples. The blots revealed that the treatment with BAY-117082 at doses of 2.5 and 5 mg/kg was able to reduce the NLRP3, ASC, IL-1β, and IL-18 expressions compared to the OSCC group, in both the lung (**A–D**) and spleen (**E–H**). Data are representative of at least three independent experiments. (**A,D,F,H**) *** $p < 0.001$ vs. sham and ### $p < 0.001$ vs. OSCC; (**B,E,G**) *** $p < 0.001$ vs. sham; ## $p < 0.01$ and ### $p < 0.001$ vs. OSCC; and (**C**) *** $p < 0.001$ vs. sham; # $p < 0.05$ and ## $p < 0.01$ vs. OSCC.

3.6. BAY-117082 Treatment Modulated Epithelial–Mesenchymal Transition (EMT) and Matrix Metalloproteinases (MMPs) Expression in OSCC Metastatic Lymph Node, Lung, and Spleen

Considering the role of EMT in oral cancer progression [24], we also decided to evaluate the effect of BAY-117082 on E-cadherin and N-cadherin expression in the lymph node, lung, and spleen tissues following OSCC induction. Our data demonstrated that the OSCC group was characterized by a decrease in E-cadherin expression in all three OSCC metastatic organs (as shown in Figure 6A,B,F,G,K,L); however, the treatment with BAY-117082 at doses of 2.5 mg/kg and 5 mg/kg significantly restored the E-cadherin expression, as can be seen in the lymph node in Figure 6C,D (see the % of the total tissue area score in Figure 6E); in the lung in Figure 6H,I (see the % of the total tissue area score in Figure 6J; and in the spleen in Figure 6M,N (see the % of the total tissue area score Figure 6O). Moreover, the immunohistochemical analysis showed that the OSCC groups of the lymph node, lung, and spleen tissues were characterized by a significant increase in N-cadherin expression compared to the sham groups (Figure 7A,B,F,G,K,L, respectively); however, BAY-117082 at both doses reduced its expression in all three OSCC metastatic organs, as shown in Figure 7C,D for the lymph node (see the % of the total tissue area score in Figure 7E); in Figure 7H,I for the lung (see the % of the total tissue area score in Figure 7J); and in Figure 7M,N for the spleen (see the % of the total tissue area score Figure 7O).

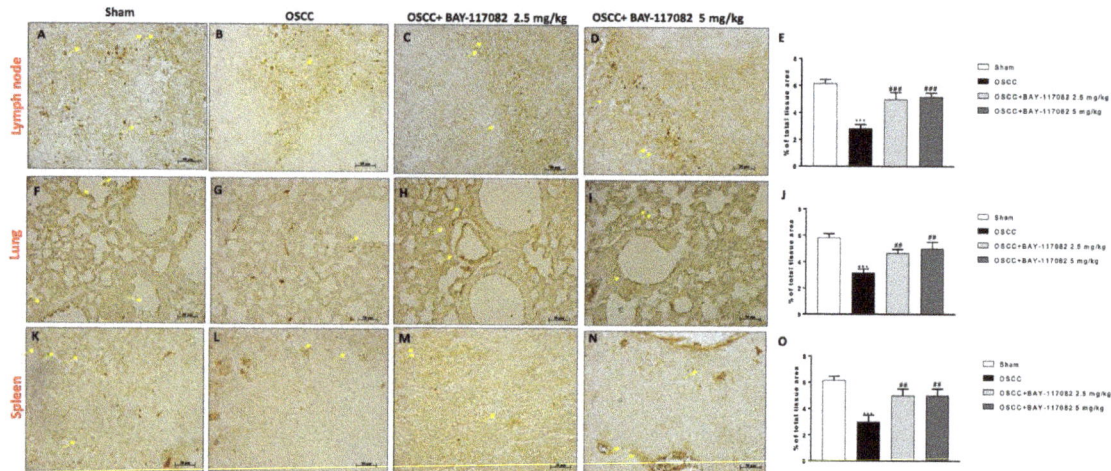

Figure 6. BAY-117082 treatment modulated the EMT pathway in the lymph node, lung, and spleen. Immunohistochemical analysis revealed that treatment with BAY-117082 at doses of 2.5 and 5 mg/kg was able to increase E-cadherin in the lymph node (**C,D**), lung (**H,I**), and spleen (**M,N**) compared to the OSCC group (**B,G,L**). Data are representative of at least three independent experiments. (**A–D**) *** $p < 0.001$ vs. sham; ## $p < 0.01$ and ### $p < 0.001$ vs. OSCC. (Scale bar: 50 µm).

Additionally, we investigated the MMP levels by immunohistochemical analysis, demonstrating that the OSCC groups were characterized by a significant increase in MMP2 and MPP9 levels in the lymph node, lung, and spleen tissues compared to the sham groups (as shown in Figure 8A,B,F,G,K,L and Figure 9A,B,F,G,K,L, respectively); however, the treatment with BAY-117082 at both doses was able to significantly reduce their levels in all three OSCC metastatic organs, as shown in Figure 8C,D (see the % of the total tissue area score in Figure 8E); in Figure 8H,I (see the % of the total tissue area score in Figure 8J); in Figure 8M,N (see the % of the total tissue area score in Figure 8O); in Figure 9C,D (see the % of the total tissue area score in Figure 9E); in Figure 9H,I (see the % of the total tissue area score in Figure 9J); and in Figure 9M,N (see the % of the total tissue area score in Figure 9O).

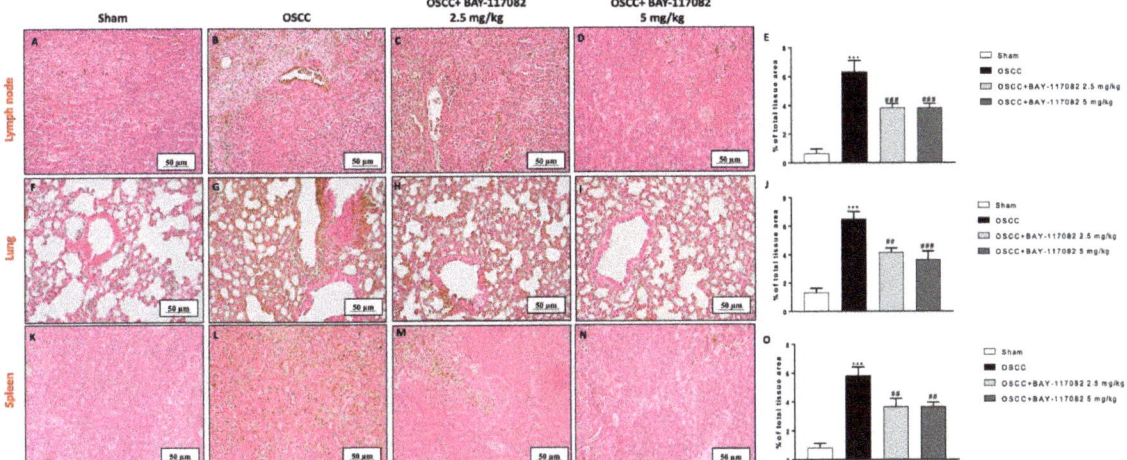

Figure 7. BAY-117082 treatment modulated the EMT pathway in the lymph node, lung, and spleen. Immunohistochemical analysis revealed that treatment with BAY-117082 at doses of 2.5 and 5 mg/kg was able to reduce N-cadherin in the lymph node (**C,D**), lung (**H,I**), and spleen (**M,N**) compared to the OSCC group (**B,G,L**). Data are representative of at least three independent experiments. (**A–D**) *** $p < 0.001$ vs. sham; ## $p < 0.01$ and ### $p < 0.001$ vs. OSCC.

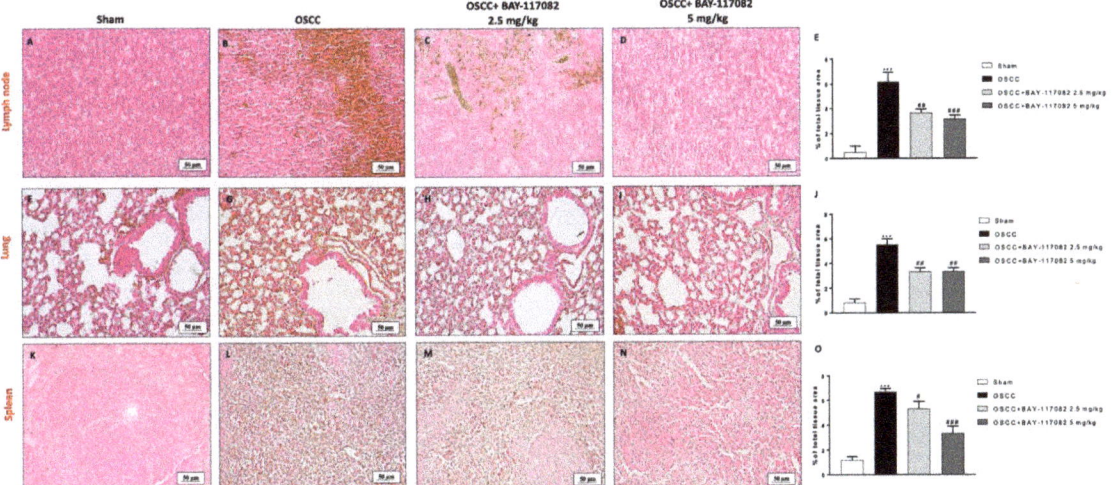

Figure 8. BAY-117082 treatment modulated MMP2 in the lymph node, lung, and spleen. Immunohistochemical analysis revealed that treatment with BAY-117082 at doses of 2.5 and 5 mg/kg was able to reduce MMP2 in the lymph node (**C,D**), lung (**H,I**), and spleen (**M,N**) compared to the OSCC group (**B,G,L**). Data are representative of at least three independent experiments. (**A–D**) *** $p < 0.001$ vs. sham; # $p < 0.05$, ## $p < 0.01$ and ### $p < 0.001$ vs. OSCC.

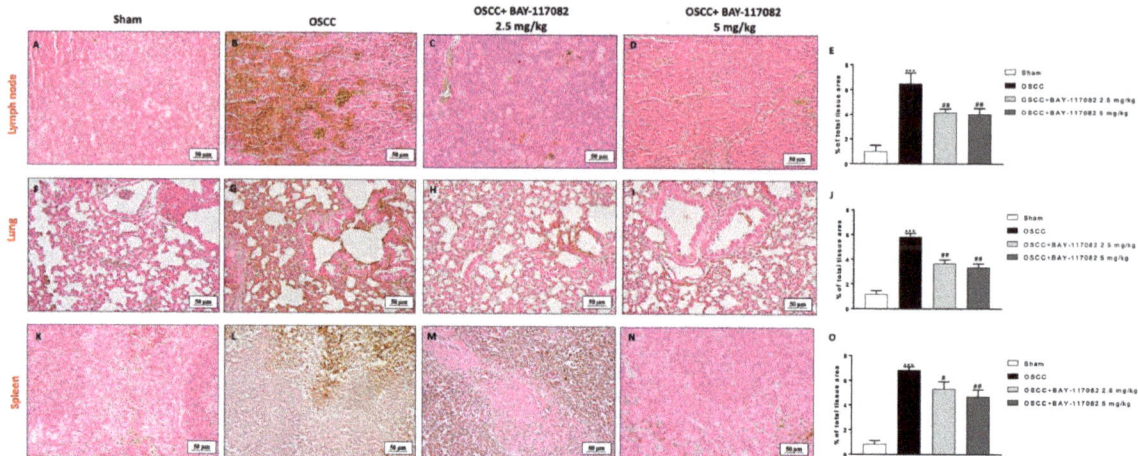

Figure 9. BAY-117082 treatment modulated MMP9 in the lymph node, lung, and spleen. Immunohistochemical analysis revealed that treatment with BAY-117082 at doses of 2.5 and 5 mg/kg was able to reduce MMP9 in the lymph node (**C–E**), lung (**H–J**), and spleen (**M–O**) compared to the OSCC group (**B,G,L**). Data are representative of at least three independent experiments. Control group (**A,F,K**) *** $p < 0.001$ vs. sham; # $p < 0.05$ and ## $p < 0.01$ vs. OSCC.

See Supplementary Files in Figures S1–S4.

4. Discussion

OSCC is a malignant neoplasm derived from the stratified squamous epithelium of the oral mucosa; OSCC has an incidence of 450,000 new cases per year [28]. Smoking and excessive alcohol consumption represent the main risk factors for OSCC development; however, human papillomavirus (HPV), dietary deficiencies, and genomic modifications are also involved [29]. OSCC can provoke regional as well as distant metastasis (DM) [6]; DM represents the major problem for oral cancer; it is associated with advanced stages of oral tumors [30]. Interestingly, nodal metastasis appears when cancer cells at the primary site pass through lymphatic channels and migrate to cervical lymph nodes [6]. Usually, oral carcinomas spread from the primary tumor site to an anatomically distant site; however, tumor cells extravasate from the vessels into the stroma of the metastatic site, colonizing neighboring organs and forming macroscopic metastasis. It is notable that the lung is the most common site for distant metastasis in cases of head and neck OSCC [31]. However, metastasis to other organs, such as the spleen and liver, can also occur [32]. The treatment for oral cancer includes surgical resection, followed by chemotherapy and radiotherapy; despite the advances in therapy against OSCC, no significant decrease in mortality or potential effects against DM have been revealed; furthermore, DM worsens the prognosis and reduces the chances of successful treatment [6]. Although the pathophysiology of oral cancer remains unclear, in vivo and in vitro studies have revealed the involvement of NLRP3 inflammasome activation in contributing to the initiation and progression of oral cancer [5,23]; NLRP3 also plays a role in activating the invasion and metastasis, which seems to be tissue- and context-dependent [33]. Interestingly, proteolytic enzymes such as MMPs are involved in the metastasis process and their augmented production could be linked with the invasive and metastatic phenotype in various tumors [34]. In the process of metastasis in oral cancer, numerous MMPs have played a key role; studies have suggested that tumor stromal cells produced MMPs to promote tumor invasion [35]. Recently, BAY-117082, as a strong inhibitor of NLRP3 inflammasome, showed significant anti-tumor effects, suggesting its possible use as a promising treatment for oral cancer [16]. Therefore, based on the key roles of the NLRP3 inflammasome, in this study, the DM-promoting property of NLRP3 was demonstrated for the first time, evaluating the beneficial effect of BAY-117082 on reducing metastasis in an in vivo orthotopic model of OSCC. In our previous study, we highlighted the protective effects of BAY-117082 treatment in oral cancer [16]; in this study, the histological analysis on OSCC tongue samples confirmed the capacity of BAY-117082 to significantly reduce the tumor area, restoring the tongue tissue architecture. Evidence demonstrated that the NLRP3 inflammasome controls the innate immunity response through ASC activation, which subsequently activates the inflammatory response [36] by cleaving the cytokines pro-IL-1β and pro-IL-18 into their biologically active forms [37]. It is particularly interesting that BAY-117082 is known to prevent the organization of the ASC pyroptosome and NLRP3 inflammasome function through the alkylation of the cysteine residues of the NLRP3 ATPase region [27]. In this study, a significant reduction in NLRP3, ASC, IL-1β, and IL-18 expression was shown in the tumor's samples from BAY-117082-treated mice compared to the OSCC group. The DM of oral cancer is a complex process involving the detachment of cells from the tumor tissue, the spread of cancer cells to tissues and organs beyond where the tumor originated, and the formation of secondary foci [38]; interestingly, OSCC can metastasize to the cervical lymph nodes and distant soft tissue metastases mostly occur in the lung [39]. Additionally, although DM incidence in the spleen is relatively low compared with that in other organs, cases have been recorded [40]. In this study, it was demonstrated for the first time that BAY-117082 treatment reduced DM in OSCC metastatic organs, namely the lymph node, lung, and spleen. The prodigious selectivity and inhibitor effect of BAY-117082 against the NLRP3 inflammasome was also demonstrated through the modulation of the NLRP3 pathway in OSCC metastatic organs, namely the lung and spleen tissues. The epithelial–mesenchymal transition (EMT) is a process in which epithelial cells change into mesenchymal cells, acquiring high mobility and an elevated migration grade, contributing to the progression of cancer [40]. In depth, it has been studied that, during EMT, epithelial cells undergo a suppression of genes responsible for the synthesis of components that form adherent junctions, such as E-cadherin, thereby causing the loss of cell adhesion and apical-basal polarity, followed by an increase in transcription factors associated with mesenchymal genes, such as N-cadherin, vimentin, fibronectin, and extracellular MMPs [41]. In this study, the treatment with BAY-117082 notably increased E-cadherin expression and significantly reduced the N-cadherin and MMP expression in the OSCC tumor samples; the same effects were also confirmed on the DM samples (for the lymph nodes, lung, and spleen), suggesting an innovative role of BAY-117082 as a modulator of the epithelial and mesenchymal transition process in oral cancer.

5. Conclusions

Therefore, BAY-117082 could represent an effective therapeutic strategy to reduce or counteract OSCC metastasis in lymph nodes, lung and spleen, thanks to its ability to modulate the NLRP3 inflammasome pathway and regulate the EMT process responsible for connecting the secondary metastatic tumors to the OSCC primary. Additional studies are necessary to better comprehend the role of these signaling pathways in metastases related to OSCC.

Supplementary Materials: The following supporting information can be downloaded at: https://www.mdpi.com/article/10.3390/cancers15102796/s1, Figure S1: Effect of BAY-117082 on NF-κB/IκBα pathway. ELISA kits revealed that BAY-117082 is able to significantly reduce NF-κB/IκBα pathway activation. (A) ** $p < 0.01$ vs. Sham; # $p < 0.05$ vs. OSCC; (B) ** $p < 0.01$ vs. Sham; # $p < 0.05$ vs. OSCC.; Figure S2. Effect of BAY-117082 on NLRP3 inflammasome. Immunoistochemical analysis demonstrated that BAY-117082 reduced cell-positive NLRP3 staining in tongue (C–E), lung (H–J), spleen (M–O) and lymph node tissue (R–T) compared to OSCC groups (B,G,L,Q). (E) *** $p < 0.001$ vs. Sham; ## $p < 0.01$ vs. OSCC. (J) *** $p < 0.001$ vs. Sham; ## $p < 0.01$ vs. OSCC (O) *** $p < 0.001$ vs. Sham; # $p < 0.05$ vs. OSCC; ## $p < 0.01$ vs. OSCC; (T) *** $p < 0.001$ vs. Sham;

$p < 0.01$ vs. OSCC. Figure S3. Effect of BAY-117082 on E-cadherin, N-cadherin, MMP2 and MMP9 expression in tongue and spleen samples. The blots reveal that treatment with BAY-117082 was able to restore E-cadherin and reduce N-cadherin, MMP2 and MMP9 expression compared to OSCC group, in tongue (A–D) as well as in spleen (E–H). Data are representative of at least three independent experiments. (A,G) *** $p < 0.001$ vs. Sham; ## $p < 0.01$ vs. OSCC; (B) ** $p < 0.01$ vs. Sham; ## $p < 0.01$ vs. OSCC; (C) ** $p < 0.01$ vs. Sham; ## $p < 0.01$ vs. OSCC; ### $p < 0.001$ vs. OSCC; (D) *** $p < 0.001$ vs. Sham; ### $p < 0.001$ vs. OSCC; (E) ** $p < 0.01$ vs. Sham; # $p < 0.05$ vs. OSCC; ## $p < 0.01$ vs. OSCC; (F) *** $p < 0.001$ vs. Sham; # $p < 0.05$ vs. OSCC; ## $p < 0.01$ vs. OSCC; (H) ** $p < 0.01$ vs. Sham; # $p < 0.05$ vs. OSCC. Figure S4. Effect of BAY-117082 on E-cadherin, N-cadherin, MMP2 and MMP9 expression in lung and lymph node samples. The blots reveal that treatment with BAY-117082 was able to restore E-cadherin and reduce N-cadherin, MMP2 and MMP9 expression compared to OSCC group, in lung (A–D) as well as in lymph node (E–H). Data are representative of at least three independent experiments. (A,G) ** $p < 0.01$ vs. Sham; # $p < 0.05$ vs. OSCC; ## $p < 0.01$ vs. OSCC; (B–D) *** $p < 0.001$ vs. Sham; ### $p < 0.001$ vs. OSCC; (E) ** $p < 0.01$ vs. Sham; # $p < 0.05$ vs. OSCC; ## $p < 0.01$ vs. OSCC; ## $p < 0.01$ vs. OSCC; (F) ** $p < 0.01$ vs. Sham; ## $p < 0.01$ vs. OSCC; ### $p < 0.001$ vs. OSCC; (H) *** $p < 0.001$ vs. Sham; # $p < 0.05$ vs. OSCC; ## $p < 0.01$ vs. OSCC.

Author Contributions: Conceptualization, G.C. and I.P.; methodology, S.A.S., D.M., A.F. and M.L.; software, A.P.C. and F.D.G. validation, R.G., C.C. and M.M.; formal analysis, G.C. investigation, G.C.; resources, E.E. and S.C.; data curation, G.C., M.P. and I.P.; writing—original draft preparation, G.C.; visualization, A.M.; supervision, I.P.; project administration, E.E.; funding acquisition, E.E. and S.C. All authors have read and agreed to the published version of the manuscript.

Funding: This research received no external funding.

Institutional Review Board Statement: Animal study was approved by the University of Messina (no 368/2019-PR released on 14 May 2019) in accordance with Italian regulations on the use of animals. This study was approved by the University of Messina review board for the care of animals.

Informed Consent Statement: Not applicable.

Data Availability Statement: The data can be shared up on request.

Conflicts of Interest: The authors declare no conflict of interest.

References

1. Nakagawa, T.; Ohta, K.; Naruse, T.; Sakuma, M.; Fukada, S.; Yamakado, N.; Akagi, M.; Sasaki, K.; Niwata, C.; Ono, S.; et al. Inhibition of angiogenesis and tumor progression of MK-0429, an integrin alphavbeta(3) antagonist, on oral squamous cell carcinoma. *J. Cancer Res. Clin. Oncol.* **2022**, *148*, 3281–3292. [CrossRef] [PubMed]
2. Chow, L.Q.M. Head and Neck Cancer. *N. Engl. J. Med.* **2020**, *382*, 60–72. [CrossRef] [PubMed]
3. Cramer, J.D.; Burtness, B.; Le, Q.T.; Ferris, R.L. The changing therapeutic landscape of head and neck cancer. *Nat. Rev. Clin. Oncol.* **2019**, *16*, 669–683. [CrossRef] [PubMed]
4. Takahashi, M.; Aoki, T.; Nakamura, N.; Carreras, J.; Kajiwara, H.; Kumaki, N.; Inomoto, C.; Ogura, G.; Kikuchi, T.; Kikuti, Y.Y.; et al. Clinicopathological analysis of 502 patients with oral squamous cell carcinoma with special interest to distant metastasis. *Tokai J. Exp. Clin. Med.* **2014**, *39*, 178–185.
5. Wang, H.; Luo, Q.; Feng, X.; Zhang, R.; Li, J.; Chen, F. NLRP3 promotes tumor growth and metastasis in human oral squamous cell carcinoma. *BMC Cancer* **2018**, *18*, 500. [CrossRef]
6. Bugshan, A.; Farooq, I. Oral squamous cell carcinoma: Metastasis, potentially associated malignant disorders, etiology and recent advancements in diagnosis. *F1000Research* **2020**, *9*, 229. [CrossRef]
7. Moriya, J.; Daimon, Y.; Itoh, Y.; Nakano, M.; Yamada, Z. Vegetative cardiac metastases of oral cavity cancer: An autopsy case report. *J. Cardiol.* **2004**, *44*, 33–38.
8. Rizvi, N.A.; Mazieres, J.; Planchard, D.; Stinchcombe, T.E.; Dy, G.K.; Antonia, S.J.; Horn, L.; Lena, H.; Minenza, E.; Mennecier, B.; et al. Activity and safety of nivolumab, an anti-PD-1 immune checkpoint inhibitor, for patients with advanced, refractory squamous non-small-cell lung cancer (CheckMate 063): A phase 2, single-arm trial. *Lancet Oncol.* **2015**, *16*, 257–265. [CrossRef]
9. Noguti, J.; De Moura, C.F.; De Jesus, G.P.; Da Silva, V.H.; Hossaka, T.A.; Oshima, C.T.; Ribeiro, D.A. Metastasis from oral cancer: An overview. *Cancer Genom.—Proteom.* **2012**, *9*, 329–335.
10. Schroder, K.; Tschopp, J. The inflammasomes. *Cell* **2010**, *140*, 821–832. [CrossRef]
11. Davis, B.K.; Wen, H.; Ting, J.P. The inflammasome NLRs in immunity, inflammation, and associated diseases. *Annu. Rev. Immunol.* **2011**, *29*, 707–735. [CrossRef] [PubMed]
12. Takeuchi, O.; Akira, S. Pattern recognition receptors and inflammation. *Cell* **2010**, *140*, 805–820. [CrossRef] [PubMed]

13. Poli, G.; Brancorsini, S.; Cochetti, G.; Barillaro, F.; Egidi, M.G.; Mearini, E. Expression of inflammasome-related genes in bladder cancer and their association with cytokeratin 20 messenger RNA. *Urol. Oncol. Semin. Orig. Investig.* **2015**, *33*, 505.e1–505.e7. [CrossRef]
14. Ng, G.Z.; Menheniott, T.R.; Every, A.L.; Stent, A.; Judd, L.M.; Chionh, Y.T.; Dhar, P.; Komen, J.C.; Giraud, A.S.; Wang, T.C.; et al. The MUC1 mucin protects against Helicobacter pylori pathogenesis in mice by regulation of the NLRP3 inflammasome. *Gut* **2016**, *65*, 1087–1099. [CrossRef] [PubMed]
15. Paugh, S.W.; Bonten, E.J.; Savic, D.; Ramsey, L.B.; Thierfelder, W.E.; Gurung, P.; Malireddi, R.K.; Actis, M.; Mayasundari, A.; Min, J.; et al. NALP3 inflammasome upregulation and CASP1 cleavage of the glucocorticoid receptor cause glucocorticoid resistance in leukemia cells. *Nat. Genet.* **2015**, *47*, 607–614. [CrossRef]
16. Scuderi, S.A.; Casili, G.; Basilotta, R.; Lanza, M.; Filippone, A.; Raciti, G.; Puliafito, I.; Colarossi, L.; Esposito, E.; Paterniti, I. NLRP3 Inflammasome Inhibitor BAY-117082 Reduces Oral Squamous Cell Carcinoma Progression. *Int. J. Mol. Sci.* **2021**, *22*, 11108. [CrossRef]
17. Chen, L.; Ruan, Y.; Wang, X.; Min, L.; Shen, Z.; Sun, Y.; Qin, X. BAY 11-7082, a nuclear factor-kappaB inhibitor, induces apoptosis and S phase arrest in gastric cancer cells. *J. Gastroenterol.* **2014**, *49*, 864–874. [CrossRef]
18. Yin, P.; Su, Y.; Chen, S.; Wen, J.; Gao, F.; Wu, Y.; Zhang, X. MMP-9 Knockdown Inhibits Oral Squamous Cell Carcinoma Lymph Node Metastasis in the Nude Mouse Tongue-Xenografted Model through the RhoC/Src Pathway. *Anal. Cell. Pathol.* **2021**, *2021*, 6683391. [CrossRef]
19. Eun, Y.G.; Yoon, Y.J.; Won, K.Y.; Lee, Y.C. Circulating Tumor DNA in Saliva in an Orthotopic Head and Neck Cancer Mouse Model. *Anticancer Res.* **2020**, *40*, 191–199. [CrossRef]
20. Casili, G.; Campolo, M.; Lanza, M.; Filippone, A.; Scuderi, S.; Messina, S.; Ardizzone, A.; Esposito, E.; Paterniti, I. Role of ABT888, a Novel Poly(ADP-Ribose) Polymerase (PARP) Inhibitor in Countering Autophagy and Apoptotic Processes Associated to Spinal Cord Injury. *Mol. Neurobiol.* **2020**, *57*, 4394–4407. [CrossRef]
21. Qi, C.L.; Wei, B.; Ye, J.; Yang, Y.; Li, B.; Zhang, Q.Q.; Li, J.C.; He, X.D.; Lan, T.; Wang, L.J. P-selectin-mediated platelet adhesion promotes the metastasis of murine melanoma cells. *PLoS ONE* **2014**, *9*, e91320. [CrossRef] [PubMed]
22. Scuderi, S.A.; Casili, G.; Lanza, M.; Filippone, A.; Paterniti, I.; Esposito, E.; Campolo, M. Modulation of NLRP3 Inflammasome Attenuated Inflammatory Response Associated to Diarrhea-Predominant Irritable Bowel Syndrome. *Biomedicines* **2020**, *8*, 519. [CrossRef]
23. Huang, C.F.; Chen, L.; Li, Y.C.; Wu, L.; Yu, G.T.; Zhang, W.F.; Sun, Z.J. NLRP3 inflammasome activation promotes inflammation-induced carcinogenesis in head and neck squamous cell carcinoma. *J. Exp. Clin. Cancer Res.* **2017**, *36*, 116. [CrossRef]
24. Krisanaprakornkit, S.; Iamaroon, A. Epithelial-mesenchymal transition in oral squamous cell carcinoma. *ISRN Oncol.* **2012**, *2012*, 681469. [CrossRef] [PubMed]
25. Imai, K. Matrix metalloproteinases and cancer cell invasion and metastasis. *Tanpakushitsu Kakusan Koso* **1997**, *42*, 1694–1700. [PubMed]
26. Cheng, Y.; Li, S.; Gao, L.; Zhi, K.; Ren, W. The Molecular Basis and Therapeutic Aspects of Cisplatin Resistance in Oral Squamous Cell Carcinoma. *Front. Oncol.* **2021**, *11*, 761379. [CrossRef]
27. Juliana, C.; Fernandes-Alnemri, T.; Wu, J.; Datta, P.; Solorzano, L.; Yu, J.W.; Meng, R.; Quong, A.A.; Latz, E.; Scott, C.P.; et al. Anti-inflammatory compounds parthenolide and Bay 11-7082 are direct inhibitors of the inflammasome. *J. Biol. Chem.* **2010**, *285*, 9792–9802. [CrossRef]
28. Johnson, N.W.; Jayasekara, P.; Amarasinghe, A.A. Squamous cell carcinoma and precursor lesions of the oral cavity: Epidemiology and aetiology. *Periodontology 2000* **2011**, *57*, 19–37. [CrossRef]
29. Marur, S.; D'Souza, G.; Westra, W.H.; Forastiere, A.A. HPV-associated head and neck cancer: A virus-related cancer epidemic. *Lancet Oncol.* **2010**, *11*, 781–789. [CrossRef]
30. Betka, J. Distant metastases from lip and oral cavity cancer. *Orl* **2001**, *63*, 217–221. [CrossRef]
31. Kotwall, C.; Sako, K.; Razack, M.S.; Rao, U.; Bakamjian, V.; Shedd, D.P. Metastatic patterns in squamous cell cancer of the head and neck. *Am. J. Surg.* **1987**, *154*, 439–442. [CrossRef]
32. Valastyan, S.; Weinberg, R.A. Tumor metastasis: Molecular insights and evolving paradigms. *Cell* **2011**, *147*, 275–292. [CrossRef] [PubMed]
33. Lin, T.Y.; Tsai, M.C.; Tu, W.; Yeh, H.C.; Wang, S.C.; Huang, S.P.; Li, C.Y. Role of the NLRP3 Inflammasome: Insights Into Cancer Hallmarks. *Front. Immunol.* **2020**, *11*, 610492. [CrossRef] [PubMed]
34. Mishev, G.; Deliverska, E.; Hlushchuk, R.; Velinov, N.; Aebersold, D.; Weinstein, F.; Djonov, V. Prognostic value of matrix metalloproteinases in oral squamous cell carcinoma. *Biotechnol. Biotechnol. Equip.* **2014**, *28*, 1138–1149. [CrossRef] [PubMed]
35. Thomas, G.T.; Lewis, M.P.; Speight, P.M. Matrix metalloproteinases and oral cancer. *Oral Oncol.* **1999**, *35*, 227–233. [CrossRef]
36. Kelley, N.; Jeltema, D.; Duan, Y.; He, Y. The NLRP3 Inflammasome: An Overview of Mechanisms of Activation and Regulation. *Int. J. Mol. Sci.* **2019**, *20*, 3328. [CrossRef] [PubMed]
37. Bauernfeind, F.G.; Horvath, G.; Stutz, A.; Alnemri, E.S.; MacDonald, K.; Speert, D.; Fernandes-Alnemri, T.; Wu, J.; Monks, B.G.; Fitzgerald, K.A.; et al. Cutting edge: NF-kappaB activating pattern recognition and cytokine receptors license NLRP3 inflammasome activation by regulating NLRP3 expression. *J. Immunol.* **2009**, *183*, 787–791. [CrossRef]
38. DeVita, V.T., Jr.; Young, R.C.; Canellos, G.P. Combination versus single agent chemotherapy: A review of the basis for selection of drug treatment of cancer. *Cancer* **1975**, *35*, 98–110. [CrossRef]

39. Irani, S. Distant metastasis from oral cancer: A review and molecular biologic aspects. *J. Int. Soc. Prev. Community Dent.* **2016**, *6*, 265–271. [CrossRef]
40. Gaponova, A.V.; Rodin, S.; Mazina, A.A.; Volchkov, P.V. Epithelial-Mesenchymal Transition: Role in Cancer Progression and the Perspectives of Antitumor Treatment. *Acta Nat.* **2020**, *12*, 4–23. [CrossRef]
41. Thiery, J.P.; Sleeman, J.P. Complex networks orchestrate epithelial-mesenchymal transitions. *Nat. Rev. Mol. Cell Biol.* **2006**, *7*, 131–142. [CrossRef] [PubMed]

Disclaimer/Publisher's Note: The statements, opinions and data contained in all publications are solely those of the individual author(s) and contributor(s) and not of MDPI and/or the editor(s). MDPI and/or the editor(s) disclaim responsibility for any injury to people or property resulting from any ideas, methods, instructions or products referred to in the content.

MDPI

St. Alban-Anlage 66

4052 Basel

Switzerland

www.mdpi.com

Cancers Editorial Office

E-mail: cancers@mdpi.com

www.mdpi.com/journal/cancers

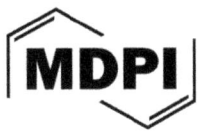

Disclaimer/Publisher's Note: The statements, opinions and data contained in all publications are solely those of the individual author(s) and contributor(s) and not of MDPI and/or the editor(s). MDPI and/or the editor(s) disclaim responsibility for any injury to people or property resulting from any ideas, methods, instructions or products referred to in the content.

www.ingramcontent.com/pod-product-compliance
Lightning Source LLC
LaVergne TN
LVHW070157100526
838202LV00015B/1961